OXFORD STUDIES IN BYZANTIUM

OXFORD STUDIES IN BYZANTIUM

Oxford Studies in Byzantium consists of scholarly monographs and editions on the history, literature, thought, and material culture of the Byzantine world.

Emperors and Usurpers in the Later Roman Empire
Civil War, Panegyric, and the Construction of Legitimacy
Adrastos Omissi

The *Universal History* of Step'anos Tarōnec'i
Introduction, Translation, and Commentary
Tim Greenwood

The Letters of Psellos
Cultural Networks and Historical Realities
Edited by Michael Jeffreys and Marc D. Lauxtermann

Holy Sites Encircled
The Early Byzantine Concentric Churches of Jerusalem
Vered Shalev-Hurvitz

Law, Power, and Imperial Ideology in the Iconoclast Era
c.680–850
M. T. G. Humphreys

Byzantium and the Turks in the Thirteenth Century
Dimitri Korobeinikov

Writing and Reading Byzantine Secular Poetry, 1025–1081
Floris Bernard

The Byzantine-Islamic Transition in Palestine
An Archaeological Approach
Gideon Avni

Shaping a Muslim State
The World of a Mid-Eighth-Century Egyptian Official
Petra M. Sijpesteijn

Niketas Choniates
A Historiographical Study
Alicia Simpson

Byzantines, Latins, and Turks in the Eastern Mediterranean World after 1150
Edited by Jonathan Harris, Catherine Holmes, and Eugenia Russell

Debating the Saints' Cults in the Age of Gregory the Great
Matthew Dal Santo

Innovation in Byzantine Medicine

The Writings of John Zacharias Aktouarios (c.1275–c.1330)

PETROS BOURAS-VALLIANATOS

OXFORD
UNIVERSITY PRESS

OXFORD
UNIVERSITY PRESS

Great Clarendon Street, Oxford, OX2 6DP,
United Kingdom

Oxford University Press is a department of the University of Oxford.
It furthers the University's objective of excellence in research, scholarship,
and education by publishing worldwide. Oxford is a registered trade mark of
Oxford University Press in the UK and in certain other countries

First Edition published in 2020
Impression: 1

Published in the United States of America by Oxford University Press
198 Madison Avenue, New York, NY 10016, United States of America

British Library Cataloguing in Publication Data
Data available

Library of Congress Control Number: 2020930014

ISBN 978–0–19–885068–7

DOI: 10.1093/oso/9780198850687.001.0001

Printed and bound by
CPI Group (UK) Ltd, Croydon, CR0 4YY

In memory of my grandfather
Ἄγγελος Βαλλιανᾶτος
1937–2008

Preface

This volume grew out of a King's College London PhD thesis on the same subject. It does, however, have one more chapter than my doctoral dissertation: Chapter 6, on John Zacharias Aktouarios' *On Psychic Pneuma*. There have also been several revisions of the text to make the book more concise and accessible. The research for this project started sometime in the summer of 2011. There are many people I wish to thank. I am most immensely grateful to my primary PhD supervisor, Dionysios Stathakopoulos, who first aroused my interest in Byzantine medicine in my undergraduate years. He has been a true teacher to me, demonstrating infinite generosity and patience with my various concerns over the last twelve years. I also wish to acknowledge a sincere debt to my secondary supervisor, Ludmilla Jordanova, who first initiated me into critical theory and read several drafts of my thesis, always providing thoughtful comments, which stimulated many ideas and prevented many mistakes.

I would also like to express my special thanks to Georgi Parpulov, whose continuous encouragement and support of my study of and research into numerous Greek manuscripts have been decisive. I am most grateful for his rare and unselfish friendship, transcending the strict boundaries of scholarship. Additionally, many thanks must go to my two PhD examiners, Peregrine Horden and Manfred Horstmanshoff, for their insightful suggestions during and after my examination. In particular, Peregrine's advice has been significant in opening up my research to a wider Mediterranean conceptual approach. Since then he has also been a very generous and devoted mentor, tirelessly committed to both my work and my professional development. Moreover, I have benefited significantly from the insightful comments of the anonymous reviewers at OUP, and from those scholars who have read sections of this book in various stages of its preparation: Sean Coughlin, Orly Lewis, Tassos Papacostas, Georgia Petridou, Alice Taylor, and Chiara Thumiger. I am grateful for bibliographical suggestions from their respective fields of expertise to Gerrit Bos, Fr Maximos Constas, Klaus-Dietrich Fischer, Erika Gielen, Florence Eliza Glaze, Monica Green, Fr Georgios Metallinos, Nikolai Serikoff, and Tess Tavormina. I am also indebted to all those Byzantinists and Historians of Medicine who encouraged me in crucial stages of my career to keep working on Byzantine medicine, and, in particular, Judith Herrin, the late Ruth Macrides, Maria Mavroudi, Julius Rocca, and Thomas Rütten. I would also like to thank Vassilios Kokkalis, my school science teacher, as well as my supervisors from my undergraduate days in London, particularly Hugh Bowden and Dominic Rathbone, and Marc Lauxtermann, my supervisor for my Master's at the University of Oxford. Special thanks should also go to Elizabeth Jeffreys, who encouraged me to submit this monograph to the Oxford Studies in Byzantium series and Charlotte Loveridge and Georgina Leighton from OUP for their constant kindness and professionalism.

I most grateful to the Alexander S. Onassis Public Benefit Foundation for the generous award it granted me to bring my doctoral thesis to its completion. I would also like to thank the Arts and Humanities Research Council, the A. G. Leventis Foundation, and Schilizzi Foundation, which awarded me further scholarships in the course of my graduate research. And I would not have been able to visit several libraries and archives abroad without the invaluable support of the Wellcome Trust (099354/Z/12/Z) and the Faculty of Arts and Humanities, King's College London.

A considerable period of my research was spent in Paris during an Erasmus Research studentship in the Université Paris–Sorbonne (Paris IV) and I am grateful to Béatrice Caseau for hosting me. I further benefited from a Junior Research Fellowship at the John W. Kluge Center of the Library of Congress, Washington DC, funded by the Arts and Humanities Research Council. The library itself was an ideal place for research and I am indebted to Mary Lou Reker, Special Assistant to the Director. While in Washington, I had the pleasure of visiting Dumbarton Oaks Research Library and using its collections at the kind invitation of Margaret Mullet, Director of Byzantine Studies. I am also grateful to Alain Touwaide for allowing me to access his rich microfilm collection at the Department of Botany in the Smithsonian. I am most grateful to the following libraries and institutions for allowing *in situ* access to manuscripts and for providing me with images and permission to reproduce them: Library of the Hellenic Parliament, National Library of Greece (both Athens); Library of Iviron Monastery (Mount Athos); Staatsbibliothek (Berlin); Bibliotheca Universitaria (Bologna); Bibliothèque royale de Belgique (Brussels); Gonville and Caius College Library, St John's College Library, Wren Library Trinity College (all Cambridge); Real Biblioteca del Monasterio (San Lorenzo de El Escorial); Biblioteca Medicea Laurenziana, Biblioteca Riccardiana (both Florence); University Library (Glasgow); Universiteitsbibliotheek (Leiden); Universitätsbibliothek (Leipzig); British Library, Wellcome Library, Woolff Gallery (all London); Biblioteca Nacional de España (Madrid); Biblioteca Ambrosiana (Milan); Bayerische Staatsbibliothek (Munich); Biblioteca nazionale (Naples); Bodleian Library (Oxford); Biblioteca centrale della Regione Siciliana (Palermo); Bibliothèque nationale de France (Paris); Biblioteca Angelica (Rome); Patriarchal Institute for Patristic Studies (Thessaloniki); Biblioteca nazionale universitaria (Turin); Biblioteca Apostolica (Vatican City); Biblioteca nazionale Marciana (Venice); Biblioteca capitolare, Biblioteca civica (both Verona); and Österreichische Nationalbibliothek (Vienna).

Finally, this thesis would not have been written without the love and support of my parents *Ἀγγελική* and *Ἀριστοτέλης*, my sisters *Βασιλική* and *Δέσποινα*, my brother *Γεράσιμος*, my aunt *Ἀργυρώ*, and my uncle *Γέρων Γεράσιμος Ἁγιοπαυλίτης*. The biggest thank you is reserved for my wife, Sophia Xenophontos, not only for helping unravel some of the abstruse language of John Zacharias Aktouarios in translation, but also for being the primary source of wise counsel and inspiration.

Petros Bouras-Vallianatos

Edinburgh
April 2019

Contents

List of Figures

List of Tables

Note to the Reader

All quotations from Greek and Latin have been translated into English by me, unless otherwise stated. Passages from John's works have not always been rendered word for word, since sometimes a more flexible translation can better convey the main ideas, especially given his dense prose. Where an implied word (or words) needs to be made explicit for reasons of clarity, it is supplied within angle brackets, e.g. 'The <patient> remained calm on the first day.' The original Greek text of the passages provided in English translation is always cited in the corresponding footnote. Greek terms or brief phrases are usually given in transliteration throughout the main text to facilitate the consultation of the book by those with very little or no knowledge of Greek. Transliteration of Greek and Arabic terms follows in most cases the Library of Congress system.

Proper names of ancient authors follow LSJ. The spelling of Byzantine names generally follows *The Oxford Dictionary of Byzantium* (*ODB*), e.g. 'Aetios of Amida' rather than 'Aetius of Amida'. The exact dates of ancient Greek, Latin, and Byzantine authors are rarely known and the dates given are only approximations following *Antike Medizin: ein Lexikon* (2005), *The Oxford Classical Dictionary* (*OCD*), and *ODB*. Primary sources are cited by the name of the author, followed by the title of the work, the numbering of the traditional division into books and/or sections where applicable, as well as a reference to the edition (volume in Roman numerals, page and line in Arabic numerals), e.g. Theophilos, *On Urines*, 7.1, ed. Ideler (1841) I.268.7–8. By convention, texts in the Hippocratic Corpus are referred to as being by [Hippocrates]. My references to John's edited works follow the division by Ideler (1841–2). John's *On the Activities and Affections of the Psychic Pneuma and the Corresponding Regimen* is abbreviated to *On Psychic Pneuma*. I prefer to place John's office (*aktouarios*) after his surname and to give it a capital letter (John Zacharias Aktouarios=JZA) in line with its most common use in secondary sources. For the unedited parts of John's *Medical Epitome* I always provide the reference to the early Latin printed edition by Mathys (1556). For secondary sources, I follow the Harvard author–date system, e.g. Biran (2015: 550–3).

Transcriptions of John's *Medical Epitome* are based on Vindobonensis med. gr. 17 (V) and occasionally important variant readings from Scorialensis Φ.III.12 (E) are also supplied (see also Appendix 5). Transcriptions from Greek retain the same spelling and punctuation as in the relevant codex, apart from the fact that I have supplied the iota subscript. Dates of manuscripts are from the most recent published catalogue in each case, unless a more accurate dating is given in a recent study, which is cited accordingly.

Lastly, I use the term 'clinical' throughout this book to denote the direct observation of a certain patient by a physician without implying a particular 'healing space', such as a clinic or hospital.

1

Introduction

In this book I examine the works of the late Byzantine practising physician and medical author John Zacharias Aktouarios (*c.*1275–*c.*1330), who lived and worked in Constantinople. It represents a substantial part of a project I have had in mind since my postgraduate studies, which involves placing the Byzantine medical tradition on equal terms alongside the Latin and Islamic medical traditions in the study of the medieval Mediterranean world. In this respect, it seeks to get away from prejudices that regard Byzantine medical literature as stagnant and not having made any significant contribution to the history of medicine, apart from the preservation and transmission of ancient Greek medical knowledge.[1] Furthermore, this book aims to motivate Byzantinists to make use of evidence from medical literature in the study and wider evaluation of Byzantine society and culture. I also hope this study inspires long overdue critical editions, commentaries, translations, and more comprehensive studies of Byzantine medical works.

John's works indisputably circulated in large numbers, which makes him a unique case, not only in Byzantine medical literature, but also in the entire literary production of the Byzantine world. Although his connections with other contemporary scholars and his basic biographical details have been delineated in the past, an evaluation of his medical corpus has not hitherto been attempted. Consequently, his reputation is based on the comments of earlier authorities, which have been being repeated uncritically since the nineteenth century. In this monograph, I would like to show that in John's writings it is clear that Byzantine medicine was remarkably open to foreign knowledge and had a significant degree of originality, in particular, in the fields of uroscopy, pharmacology, and human physiology.

My analysis of John's works is based on a close textual examination that aims to contextualize his contribution to the development of medical thought

[1] See, for example, Strohmaier (1998: 154, 169) [originally published in German (1996: 165, 181)], who states: 'medical thought in the Byzantine world had no truly new features' and 'the chief claim to credit of Byzantine science—which had developed even fewer ideas than Arabic science—was that it had preserved the original Galenic texts.' See also Nutton (1984: 2), who calls the early Byzantine medical authors 'refrigerators of antiquity'.

Innovation in Byzantine Medicine: The Writings of John Zacharias Aktouarios (c.1275–c.1330).
Petros Bouras-Vallianatos, Oxford University Press (2020). © Petros Bouras-Vallianatos.
DOI: 10.1093/oso/9780198850687.001.0001

and practice in Byzantium. Furthermore, by comparing John's contributions with examples from the Islamic and medieval Latin world, I place John's world of thought in a wider Mediterranean milieu and highlight the cultural exchanges between Byzantium and its neighbours. In this endeavour, I have used evidence from a wide variety of medical sources, including previously unedited material, and texts from other genres, such as epistolography and merchants' accounts, in order to see John's writings in the light of the contemporary social and cultural environment. In assessing John's corpus, I deal with each of his works in individual chapters. Each chapter and subsection follows a general-to-specific approach, providing background details to help the reader better understand the more specialized discussions on various sections of John's works.

This introduction (Chapter 1) aims to serve a dual role. Before embarking on the close examination of John's works, I wish first to situate John within his medical and social context. Secondly, this chapter gives an introductory account of John's biography and corpus. After Chapter 1, I examine John's original approach in *On Urines*, paying particular attention to his discussion of various urinary features and his introduction of a detailed graduated urine vial (Chapter 2). John's case histories discussing his interaction with patients, which are unique in Byzantine medical literature, are examined separately (Chapter 3). In contrast to *On Urines*, the *Medical Epitome* is mainly a compilation of earlier material and belongs to the genre of Byzantine 'encyclopedic' medical handbooks. Thus, the focus here is on John's sources, analysed through selected case studies. Ultimately, I argue that the work was primarily written for *philiatroi*, 'friends of medicine' or 'amateur physicians' (Chapter 4). John's pharmacology, which, as I shall show, attests a significant influence from Arabic pharmacological lore, is examined in Chapter 5. Since John's *Medical Epitome* is partly unedited, a study of all surviving manuscripts helps to reconstruct textual inconsistencies and make otherwise unedited material available to the reader (Appendix 5). Chapter 6 concentrates on John's original contributions to pneumatic physiology as presented in his *On Psychic Pneuma*. Lastly, Chapter 7 sums up John's achievements and outlines important aspects of the noteworthy reception of his works during the centuries following his death.

1. BYZANTINE MEDICAL LITERATURE

1.1 The ancient background

The single most influential premodern medical method for diagnosing and treating illness in the human body was the Hippocratic theory of the four humours, first outlined in the Hippocratic text *On the Nature of Man* composed in the late fifth century BC.[2] According to this theory, the body was made up of blood (*haima*), phlegm (*phlegma*), yellow bile (*cholē*), and black bile (*melaina cholē*). Later on, Galen (AD 129–216/17) aligned the four humours with the four elements.[3] Each humour was connected with a particular season and two of the four elementary qualities (hot or cold, and dry or moist). Blood was the dominant humour in spring and was marked by the hot and moist quality. Similarly, yellow bile was the main humour in summer and was hot and dry. Phlegm was cold and moist and associated with winter; finally, black bile, like autumn, was cold and dry. Galen refers to nine kinds of bodily mixtures, one 'good mixture' (*eukrasia*), in which all elementary qualities are in the same proportion and eight 'bad mixtures' (*dyskrasiai*), which were considered to be the result of an excess of one or two qualities and denoted a predisposition to certain kinds of disease.[4] Each human being had his or her own natural mixture (*krasis*). A physician was supposed to be able to counterbalance the qualities by prescribing a suitable diet or the administration of the appropriate drugs, to which particular qualities were assigned, or to remove the noxious humour using various techniques of bloodletting, thus restoring the patient's natural mixture.

By Galen's time there were three main 'schools' of medical thought and practice, i.e. the Dogmatists or Rationalists, who considered the search for the cause of disease an important part of their attempts to cure; the Empiricists, who gave a central role to the physician's past experience; and the Methodists, who applied a specific method or path in the process of healing.[5] Galen gave particular prominence to the Hippocratic concepts of health and disease, although his theories were often characterized by a considerable degree of eclecticism. He produced more works than any other author in antiquity, making a significant contribution to the understanding and establishing of numerous medical disciplines.[6] His medical ideas shaped ancient medicine and for well over a millennium Galenism, i.e. the medical system based on Galen's theories, would constitute the main dogma in rational medical approaches.[7] Hippocratic and

[2] For an introduction to the humoral theory, see Nutton (2013: 72–86). In particular, on the Hippocratic *On the Nature of Man*, see Craik (2015: 207–13).

[3] On the reception of the Hippocratic humoral theory by Galen, see Jouanna (2006).

[4] On Galen's theory on bodily mixtures, see van der Eijk (2015: 675–81).

[5] This categorization is based on Galen's *On Sects for Beginners*. On medical 'sects', see Caldwell (2018). On medicine in the Roman Empire, see Nutton, (2013: 160–221). More specifically on the various practitioners and their practices, see Jackson (1993).

[6] For an introduction to Galen's theory and practice, see Boudon-Millot (2007b); Nutton, (2013: 222–53); and Johnston (2018).

[7] On the rise of Galenism in the centuries following his death, see Temkin, (1973: 51–94). On Galen's reception, see the comprehensive edited volume by Bouras-Vallianatos and Zipser (2019).

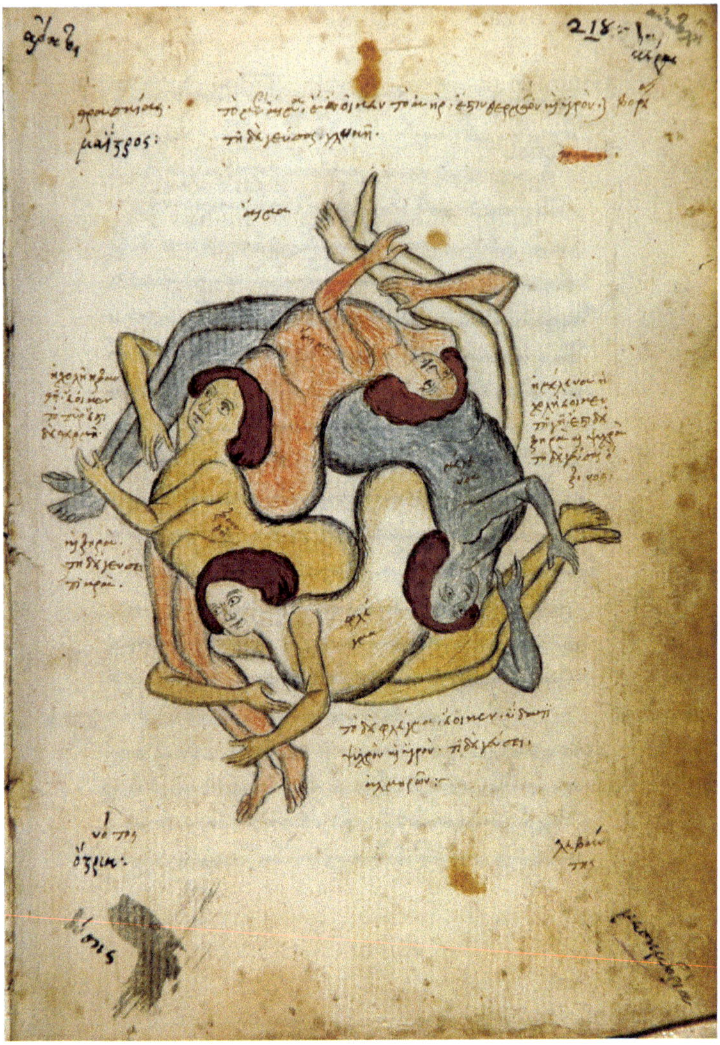

Figure 1.1. Personification of the four humours. Athous Iberiticus 218 (sixteenth century), f. 218r.

Galenic works were extensively copied and greatly influenced Byzantine authors and practitioners.[8]

[8] On the Hippocratic reception in Byzantium, see Mondrain (2014); and Ieraci Bio (2014). On the Galenic, see Bouras-Vallianatos (2019a) and (2019b). Galen was also widely appreciated by non-medical authors, who often cited Galenic passages or mentioned Galenic theories in their works throughout the Byzantine era. On this, see Stathakopoulos (2019).

1.2 The early Byzantine period (fourth–seventh centuries)

The medical literature of the early Byzantine period can be divided into two main categories, each corresponding to the basic purpose the texts were intended to serve.[9] First, this period saw the production of 'encyclopedic' medical handbooks intended to help their readers consult practical recommendations, mainly diagnostic and therapeutic, in the accessible format of a single volume.[10] Although these works consisted of quotations from earlier authors, recent studies have emphasized the important role of early Byzantine authors in the shaping of a medical tradition and rearranging otherwise chaotic material into a systematic and user-friendly form.[11]

Oribasios (AD *c.*325–after 395/6), friend and personal physician of the well-known pagan Emperor Julian (AD 361–3), was the first to produce a large-scale summary of primarily Galenic medical knowledge. His *Medical Collections* is a work originally consisting of seventy books, of which almost one third have survived. Alongside Galen, Oribasios also cites the Hippocratic corpus and Dioscorides (first century AD), as well as Antyllus (*c.* first half of the second century AD), Rufus of Ephesos (*fl.* AD 100), Soranus (second half of the first century/early second century AD), and Archigenes (second half of the first century–first half of the second century AD). An abridged version of the *Medical Collections* is the *Synopsis for Eustathios*, in nine books, composed for Oribasios' son; this is meant as a vade mecum used by travellers or for medical emergencies.[12] In another work, the *For Eunapios*, Oribasios was again heavily influenced by the *Medical Collections*, although in this case providing succinct medical advice to his friend Eunapios, a *philiatros*, is a central part of his agenda.

Oribasios' technique of using quotations from earlier authors was later followed by Aetios of Amida (*fl.* first half of the sixth century AD) in his vast work the *Tetrabiblos*, and Paul of Aegina (late sixth century–d. after AD 642) in his *Epitome*. Aetios seems to have been significantly less dependent on Galen than Oribasios was. Interestingly, Oribasios is often mentioned among Aetios' sources, alongside frequent references to Dioscorides, Hippocrates, Antyllus, Rufus, Soranus, Archigenes, Herodotus, Philumenus (second/third century AD),

[9] My discussion is not exhaustive and refers only to selected examples, which will be helpful in better understanding John's texts and context. The most detailed treatment of Byzantine medical literature is by Hunger (1978: II.287–320), although it is now outdated. See also Bouras-Vallianatos (2015c: 105–9) and (2016b), with a fresh overview of the Byzantine medical literature.

[10] For a critical overview, see Slaveva-Griffin (2018: 968–78). In my discussion, I focus on the Greek literary output. There are also examples in Latin by authors such as Theodore Priscianus (fourth/fifth century AD) and Marcellus (late fourth/early fifth century AD). See Formisano (2001: 63–92).

[11] See van der Eijk (2010).

[12] Oribasios, *Synopsis for Eustathios*, pr., ed. Raeder (1926) 5.7–13.

and many other minor authors,[13] including a certain Andrew the Count (*komēs*) and a woman author called Aspasia.[14] In the *Tetrabiblos*, there are also recipes attributed to Jewish prophets, Egyptian kings, and Christian apostles and bishops.[15] Unlike Oribasios and Aetios, Paul aimed to offer a condensed version of the most up-to-date medical knowledge for immediate consultation, which could be carried everywhere by physicians in the way lawyers carried legal synopses.[16] Perhaps book six, on surgery, was the single most influential part of Paul's work.[17] In it, Paul often quotes from various now-lost accounts on the subject by authors such as Antyllus and Leonides (*c.* first century AD).

Alexander of Tralles (AD *c.*525–*c.*605), on the other hand, as a result of his own extensive clinical experience, produced a medical handbook marked by his strong authorial presence and his persistent attempts to supplement pre-existing material with new elements.[18] His main work, the *Therapeutics*, is not a medical handbook *sensu stricto*; for example, Alexander excluded invasive surgery when used as a method of punishment rather than cure. Moreover, his independent attitude should be emphasized; he does not hesitate even to disagree with the 'most divine' (*theiotatos*) Galen.[19] His monographs *On Fevers* and *On Intestinal Worms* show his concern to provide up-to-date material on a variety of medical subjects. In close connection with these early Byzantine medical handbooks, we can also cite the *Hippiatrica*, a compilation of excerpts on horse medicine, which most probably dates to the fifth/sixth century AD.[20]

The fifth to the seventh centuries, in particular, was a period that was also marked by the production of texts of a clearly didactic nature, such as commentaries and summaries, which were connected with the teaching of medicine in the scholastic environment of Alexandria.[21] These texts were aimed at complementing the study of the Hippocratic and Galenic

[13] On Aetios' sources, see Bravos (1974).

[14] On Andrew and Aspasia, see Calà (2012b) and Flemming (2007: 270) respectively. See also Calà (2012a: 40–8).

[15] Martelli in Eijk et al. (2015: 203–4); and Calà (2016). In particular, on the Prophet Ezra and his association with the famous antidote bearing his name, see Martelli (2017).

[16] Paul of Aegina, *Epitome*, pr., ed. Heiberg (1921) I.2.8–16.

[17] Tabanelli (1964).

[18] See Bouras-Vallianatos (2014), who provides a fresh study of Alexander's clinical experience and pharmacology. Alexander thinks it immoral (*asebes*) not to provide all available methods of healing and thus includes a group of natural remedies, *physika*, reflecting contemporary popular healing practices. See Guardasole (2004b); and Bouras-Vallianatos (2016a).

[19] See Guardasole (2004a).

[20] See the detailed study on *Hippiatrica* and its various recensions by McCabe (2007).

[21] Recent excavations at the Kom el-Dikka in Alexandria have uncovered lecture halls dated to the sixth century, which might have served as auditoria for students of philosophy and medicine. See Majcherek (2008).

works that formed the Alexandrian curriculum.[22] Although only a small proportion of these texts, by authors such as Stephen and John of Alexandria, survives nowadays in the original Greek, others are accessible through Arabic translations.[23]

1.3 The middle and late Byzantine period (eighth–fifteenth centuries)

Similar medical handbooks were written over the next few centuries. Paul of Nicaea (before ninth/tenth century) composed his work in the form of an *erōtapokrisis* (questions and answers) in 137 short chapters.[24] Theophanes Chrysobalantes (*c.* tenth century), writing most probably for Constantine VII Porphyrogennetos (sole r. 945–59), penned his *Synopsis* summing up the findings of Greek and early Byzantine medical authors.[25] Leo the Physician (ninth[?] century), presumably writing for his pupil George,[26] produced the so-called *Synopsis of Medicine*, an epitome in often aphoristic form in seven books.[27] We can also place John Zacharias Aktouarios' *Medical Epitome*, which combines earlier Greek and Byzantine sources with recently introduced Arabic medical knowledge, in the same tradition.

The period was also marked by the writing of monographs on a variety of medical disciplines, based on the reworking of earlier material and supplemented according to the various authors' expertise. For example, in the field of diagnostics, Theophilos (seventh or ninth century) composed influential works on pulse, urine, and excrement.[28] Theophilos also composed the *On the Constitution of Man*, which takes its starting point from the teleological explanations of the human body as expounded by Galen in his *On the*

[22] For a description of the Alexandrian medical curriculum, see Iskandar (1976); and Roueché (1999). See also Pormann (2010). On the teaching of surgery, in particular, see Scarborough (2010).

[23] See Overwien (2018); and Garofalo (2019). There are also surviving commentaries in Latin, most probably produced by scholars based in sixth-century Ravenna; see Palmieri (2001).

[24] See the discussion on dating by Ieraci Bio (1996: 15–17). The earliest codex dates to the fourteenth century. I find a date after the eleventh century improbable, since the work lacks systematic references to oriental *materia medica* or the use of sugar in the preparation of liquid dosage forms, which became common from the late eleventh/early twelfth century onwards.

[25] In a large number of manuscripts, the work is dedicated to a certain Constantine Porphyrogennetos, most probably Constantine VII. See Sonderkamp's (1984) discussion of this. For a study of the various textual witnesses, see Sonderkamp (1987); and the recent study by Zipser (2017), who is working on a critical edition.

[26] Leo the Physician, *Synopsis of Medicine*, pr., ed. Ermerins (1840) 89.1–4.

[27] As Bliquez (1999) has convincingly argued, the information provided by the author is often insufficient to practise medicine without consulting other works on the topic, presumably the early Byzantine handbooks by Aetios of Amida or Paul of Aegina.

[28] For a recent summary of the *status quaestionis* on Theophilos' dating, see Grimm-Stadelmann (2008: 36–42). On his uroscopic treatise, see Chapter 2, Section 1.

Function of the Parts of the Body, and is supplemented with references to the Christian God, who created the human body with wisdom (*sophia*) and providence (*pronoia*).[29] More interesting in terms of the assembled material is the work on Christian anthropology, *On the Constitution of Man*, by Meletios (ninth[?] century).[30] Symeon Seth (*fl.* second half of the eleventh century) wrote his *Treatise on the Capacities of Foodstuffs* marking the introduction of Arabic medical knowledge to Byzantium.[31] Furthermore, he was the author of *Refutation of Galen*, a brief work, belonging to the genre of *antirrhēsis* (refutation), in which Symeon criticized a number of Galenic views on human physiology, which—given Galen's deified status in Byzantium—makes it unique in the entire Byzantine period.[32] The most extensive Byzantine work on pharmacology, the *Dynameron* by the so-called Nicholas Myrepsos was most probably compiled by the late thirteenth century.[33] The author under examination in this book, John Zacharias Aktouarios, composed long specialized works on uroscopy and human physiology in the early fourteenth century.

In addition to the aforementioned medical works, from at least the twelfth century onwards, a substantial number of collections of recipes, the so-called *iatrosophia*, were produced, often in the vernacular.[34] This is a somewhat neglected category of medical texts in which the main focus is on diagnosis and therapy. They are written in a simple way, so that they can be used in daily practice, and can fill an entire volume or just a couple of folia. As for their therapeutic recommendations, there is a strong emphasis on pharmacology, although they may include instructions on non-invasive surgical procedures, e.g. phlebotomy, and also popular elements, such as magic spells and biblical lore.

[29] See the recent study on the text by Grimm-Stadelmann (2008). [30] Gielen (2018).

[31] Symeon is best known as an astrologer and translator from Arabic into Greek. On Symeon Seth and his works, see Bouras-Vallianatos (2015a: 436–42). On the *Treatise on the Capacities of Foodstuffs*, see also Chapter 5, Section 1.

[32] See Bouras-Vallianatos (2015a: 442–57), who argues that Symeon Seth's criticism of Galen's theories is not based on practical experience or scientific observations, but is rather highly rhetorical, inspired by a close reading of the Galenic material. Symeon might have been inspired by cases of criticism in the Islamic world, such as, for example, Muḥammad ibn Zakarīyā᾽ al-Rāzī's (d. *c.*925) *Doubts About Galen* (*Kitāb al-Shukūk ʿalā Jālīnūs*). Temkin (1973: 118–19) was the first to relate Symeon to al-Rāzī. This suggestion was then contextualized in the framework of Symeon's *Refutation of Galen* by Bouras-Vallianatos (2015b: 447–8). It was also later proposed by Gutas et al. (2017: 96); and discussed with further evidence by Pietrobelli in Cronier et al. (2015: 91–3). Cf. Nutton (2007: 175). A brief response to Cronier et al. (2015: 72) might be necessary here. When I met Antoine Pietrobelli in Paris (19 February 2014), we found that we were both working independently on the same text. I deemed this likely to be particularly beneficial for the study of Byzantine medical texts, and welcomed the production of two individual studies, particularly as my work was already at an advanced stage.

[33] On the *Dynameron*, see Chapter 5, n. 17.

[34] See Temkin (1962: 113); Ieraci Bio (1982); Tselikas (1995); Touwaide (2007); Oberhelman (2015); and Zipser (2019). For some edited and unedited examples, see Chapter 5, n. 23.

Lastly, from the eleventh/twelfth century onwards, there is also growing circulation of Arabic and Persian works in Greek translation.[35] The most notable examples are the *Ephodia tou Apodēmountos* (Ar. *Zād al-Musāfir wa-Qūt al-Ḥāḍir/Provisions for the Traveller and Nourishment for the Sedentary/* Lat. *Viaticum*) of Ibn al-Jazzār (*fl.* tenth century),[36] a short text on smallpox and measles, *Peri Loimikēs* (Ar. *Kitāb fī al-Judarī wa-al-Ḥaṣbah/Treatise on Smallpox and Measles*), by Muḥammad ibn Zakarīyāʾ al-Rāzī (d. *c.*925),[37] and some antidotaries in Greek translation by George-Gregory Chioniades (*c.*1240/50–*c.*1320) and Constantine Melitiniotes (fourteenth century [?]).[38]

2. THE SETTING

2.1 Byzantium in the time of John

In April 1204 the armies of the Fourth Crusade conquered Constantinople and founded the short-lived Latin Empire of Constantinople (1204–61). The Byzantines managed to keep under their control some smaller regions, following the creation of the successor states of Epiros (mainly western Greece), Trebizond (the eponymous city on the south-eastern shore of the Black Sea and its hinterland), and Nicaea (chiefly western Asia Minor, including areas of Macedonia and Thrace from the late 1240s). At the same time, a number of Latin states emerged on the Greek mainland and in the Aegean islands, varying in extent and authority. The most notable and long-lasting example is certainly that of Venice, which managed to maintain its outposts until 1669 and 1797 in the case of Crete and the Ionian Islands respectively. The presence of Latins in the former territory of the Byzantine Empire gradually led to contact between East and West, which developed the exchange of ideas.[39]

[35] See Varella (1995); Touwaide (2002a); (2008a); (2011); (2016a); and Congourdeau (2012).

[36] On this translation, see Chapter 4, nn. 34–5, and Chapter 5, n. 13.

[37] Kousis (1909). The translator of this work is not known. Congourdeau (1996) suggested that the work might have been translated by Symeon Seth in the eleventh century, but there is not sufficient evidence to confirm this identification. See also n. 209, below.

[38] See Chapter 5, nn. 14–15. On Chioniades life and works, see Tihon (2008); on his contributions to astronomy, see n. 60, below.

[39] This contact also facilitated the circulation of Greek texts often previously unknown to Western scholars, and correspondingly of Latin texts that had been virtually unknown in the Byzantine East until then. On the Byzantine side, this led to many translations of Latin theological and secular texts; see nn. 56–7, below. We can also attest cases of Latin scholars travelling in the Byzantine East in order to consult manuscripts. The Flemish Dominican William of Moerbeke (*c.*1215–*c.*1286) translated into Latin a large number of Aristotle's and Proklos' works otherwise unknown in the West spending time in Nicaea and Thebes in 1260. On William of Moerbeke, see the edited volume by Brams and Vanhamel (1989); and the short article by Brams (2006), who sets William of Moerbeke in the context of contemporary Latin

Michael VIII Palaiologos, having meanwhile been proclaimed co-emperor of the Empire of Nicaea in 1259, managed to recapture Constantinople in 1261 without meeting any significant resistance and restored the Byzantine Empire.[40] The official ascent of the Palaiologan dynasty to the imperial throne of Byzantium, where it would remain until the Fall of Constantinople in 1453, went hand in hand with a steady decline in the Empire's territory. Asia Minor was gradually overrun by a number of post-Seljuk beyliks, in which the Ottoman Turks became the most powerful presence, ultimately conquering Byzantium itself. In addition to the Turks, Michael VIII was facing the danger of a new crusade, organized by Charles of Anjou (r. 1266–85) in order to recapture Constantinople. Among the measures immediately taken by Michael was accepting the Union of the Churches after sending his delegates to the Second Council of Lyons in 1274.[41] This caused a long internal ecclesiastical schism in Byzantium between Unionists and anti-Unionists.

Immediately after Michael VIII's death, his son and successor to the throne Andronikos II repudiated the Union and recalled from exile numerous anti-Unionists.[42] Meanwhile, bands of Turks had managed to reach Thrace, while Serbs and Bulgarians from the north were becoming an increasing threat. Andronikos' response was to increase the number of mercenaries, who—as in the case of the Catalan Company—sometimes proved extremely treacherous, and even subsequently established themselves in the territory of the Empire. Andronikos' last years were marked by internal and external instability. The problematic conditions on the frontiers were intensified by conflict between Andronikos II and his grandson Andronikos III (r. 1328–41), while the Hesychast religious controversy—an intense theological dispute starting in about 1337 between supporters and opponents of Gregory Palamas (*c.*1296–1359)—caused more troubles in an already turbulent environment.[43] In contrast to the territorial decline and political corruption of high imperial administrators, literary and artistic production flourished in this period.

translations of Greek philosophical works. Furthermore, the professor of medicine in Padua, Pietro d'Abano (*c.*1250–*c.*1315), sojourned in Constantinople at some time between 1270 and 1290 to investigate Greek medical manuscripts. See Thorndike (1923: 877); Paschetto (1984: 19–54); and Marangon (1984).

[40] On the history of the early Palaiologan period, see Nicol (1993: 39–167), although now outdated, and recently Stathakopoulos (2014: 150–65). See also the insightful historical overview by Laiou (2000). On Michael VIII's reign in particular, see Geanakoplos (1959).

[41] On the Union of Churches, see Papadakis (1997).

[42] For Andronikos II's reign, see Laiou (1972).

[43] On the civil war between the two Andronikoi, see Bosch (1965). In contrast to the Western Scholastic theology, Gregory Palamas put a new emphasis on prayer and meditation with the ultimate aim of divine revelation, something that was ridiculed by the southern Italian monk and philosopher Barlaam of Calabria (*c.*1290–1348), teacher of philosophy in Constantinople. The Palamists were ultimately victorious. For an overview, see Krausmüller (2006).

2.2 Early Palaiologan cultural revival (1261–1341)

The early Palaiologan period is marked by the prolific intellectual activity of an extremely large number of individuals and the wide variety of fields of expertise to which they often made original contributions.[44] Ihor Ševčenko has enumerated ninety-one Byzantine scholars who were active in the fourteenth century alone.[45] These intellectuals sometimes served in high imperial offices (e.g. Nikephoros Choumnos, Theodore Metochites).[46] Other scholars spent their lives as members of the clergy (e.g. George Pachymeres, Joseph Rhakendytes), or served in high ecclesiastical offices (e.g. George of Cyprus, who was Ecumenical Patriarch under the name of Gregory II between 1283 and 1289). Many of them have left surviving works—although they are usually only available in poor editions or are as yet unpublished—pointing to an active intellectual engagement with various subject areas, such as philosophy, rhetoric, and astronomy. I shall give a few representative examples of these literati which will offer interesting comparisons with John's career and writing activity, focusing on the early Palaiologan period, i.e. mainly from 1261 to 1341.

Already in the Empire of Nicaea (1204–61) we can see the first signs of this cultural movement. The temporary exile, combined with the strong anti-Latin sentiments of the period, created the need for an identity. Respect for the Greek past, including ancient Greek literature and the remains of Greek cities in Asia Minor, noticeably revived.[47] Emperor John III Vatatzes (r. 1222–54) proved a keen sponsor of education, founding libraries and supporting scholars such as Nikephoros Blemmydes (1197/8–*c*.1269), who wrote on a variety of subjects from theology to philosophy. Blemmydes is also well known as a teacher; among his students was the emperor and scholar Theodore II Laskaris (1254–8).[48] Later on, in Constantinople, both Michael VIII and

[44] In Byzantine studies, the term 'renaissance' has often been applied to the early Palaiologan cultural revival, as well as to the Macedonian and Komnenian revivals of classical knowledge in the ninth/tenth and the twelfth centuries respectively. On Byzantine 'renaissances', see the edited volume by Treadgold (1984); and *ODB*, s.v. renaissance. In particular on the Macedonian and Komnenian revival of knowledge, see the recent studies by Hanson (2010) and Kaldellis (2007: 225–316) respectively. On the early Palaiologan 'renaissance', see Runciman (1970) and Fryde (2000), although both now outdated; and Mergiali (1996: 43–112). See also the brief overview by Medvedev (1984). On the reception of classical authors in Palaiologan Byzantium, see Tinnefeld (1995). An up-to-date study looking at the activity of all Palaiologan scholars from various areas of expertise is still a *desideratum*.

[45] Ševčenko (1974).

[46] See Gaul (2016: 257–67), who discusses the role of *paideia* in group identity among top courtiers in Andronikos II's reign.

[47] On Hellenic identity in late Byzantium, see Kaldellis (2007: 317–88) and Page (2008: 94–242).

[48] On Nikephoros Blemmydes, see his unique *Partial Account* edited by Munitiz (1988). For a brief introduction to his works, see Gielen (2016: xv–xx). For his role in contemporary education, see Constantinides (1982: 5–27). On the scholarly activity of Theodore II Laskaris, see Angelov (2007: 204–52).

Andronikos II, as well as various patriarchs, were significant patrons of education and learning, restoring schools and funding teachers.[49]

Elementary education, the *enkyklios paideia*, consisted of the study of grammar, the *Iliad* and other poetry, logic, and rhetoric. Higher education involved the study of the so-called *quadrivium*, comprising arithmetic, music, geometry, and astronomy. The most notable schoolmasters and scholars of the late thirteenth century in Constantinople, such as George of Cyprus (*c.*1241–90), George Pachymeres (1242–*c.*1310), Maximos Planoudes (*c.*1255–*c.*1305), and Manuel Bryennios (*fl. c.*1300), composed their own *quadrivia* or commented on earlier versions thereof.[50] Scholars also had an active cultural life, connected to each other through exchanges of letters and also through gatherings, *theatra*, in which they could, for example, perform rhetorical set pieces or debate philosophy.[51]

Maximos Planoudes was certainly the leading figure in the early period, not only in the area of education, running his own school probably at the monastery of Chora before moving to the monastery of Akataleptos around 1300, but also in Palaiologan scholarship.[52] He edited a large number of ancient works of various genres, including historiography and mathematics, usually providing his own scholia.[53] Furthermore, he composed several orations and wrote grammars, paraphrases, and commentaries on the works of the poet Theocritus (*fl.* third century BC) and the rhetorician Hermogenes (*fl.* late second century AD) to facilitate the study of ancient Greek literature. He is also the author of a special treatise on Indian numbers,[54] which had been introduced to Byzantium some years earlier, and is credited with the revival of the study of geography by undertaking the enormous project of editing Ptolemy's *Geography*, including the creation of twenty-six revised regional maps.[55]

Among Planoudes' most remarkable achievements are undoubtedly his Greek translations of Latin texts on grammar, theology, and philosophy.[56] Other examples of translations from Latin into Greek include the work of

[49] During Andronikos II's reign higher education became more accessible than ever before. See Constantinides (1982: 90–110), who provides a detailed study of teachers of higher education in the late thirteenth and early fourteenth centuries.

[50] Constantinides (1982: 133–58). On early Palaiologan *Quadrivia*, see Cacouros (2006: 1–36).

[51] On *theatra*, see Medvedev (1993); Marciniak (2007); Toth (2007); Riehle (2011); and Gaul (2018).

[52] It is commonly believed that Planoudes' main residence was in the Chora before around 1300 when he moved to the monastery of Akataleptos; cf. Ševčenko (1975: 41–2); and Pérez Martin (1989). Constantinides (1982: 68–70) rejects the possibility that Planoudes ever spent time at the Chora.

[53] On Planoudes' editing skills, see Wilson (1996: 235–6).

[54] See Brown (2012).

[55] Chrysochoou (2014).

[56] Planoudes' translations include Augustine's *De Trinitate* (*On the Trinity*), ps.-Augustine's *De Duodecim Abusivis Saeculi* (*On the Twelve Abuses of the World*), Boethius' *De Consolatione Philosophiae* (*Consolation of Philosophy*), Cato's *Disticha*, Cicero's *Somnium Scipionis* (*Dream of Scipio*), Ovid's *Heroides* and *Metamorphoses*, and Macrobius' *Commentary on Cicero's Dream*

Demetrios Kydones (*c.*1324–*c.*1398), who translated many theological works, such as Thomas Aquinas' *Summa Theologica*.[57] We can also attest the introduction of a significant amount of scientific knowledge from the East in this period, manifested in the production of Greek translations of Arabic and Persian treatises in the fields of astronomy and medicine.[58] There was also considerable influence from this cultural milieu on the astronomical works of George-Gregory Chioniades and George Chrysokokkes (*fl.* 1335–50), a scholar from Trebizond.[59] Interestingly, Chioniades died in Trebizond, having first been appointed as a Christian bishop at the Ilkhanid capital Tabriz.[60]

Another notable scholar of the period is Theodore Metochites (1270–1332), who was also an active and influential statesman serving at the highest levels as *mesazōn* (personal adviser) and *megas logothetēs* (prime minister) in Andronikos II's reign.[61] Metochites wrote on a variety of subjects. His *Introduction to Astronomy* (*Stoicheiōsis Astronomikē*) consists of a three-part introduction to Ptolemaic astronomy, including an early proposal for the revision of the Julian calendar.[62] His other works include commentaries on Aristotle's works, contributing—together with the numerous paraphrases and commentaries by his contemporary George Pachymeres[63]—to a significant resurgence of Aristotelian philosophy; twenty long poems; the *Sententious Remarks* (*Sēmeioseis Gnōmikai*), a collection of 120 essays, often reflecting Metochites' personal experiences;[64] and eighteen orations, including his exhortation (*logos protreptikos*) on education, *Ēthikos*, and the *Presbeutikos*, which deals with an embassy to a foreign court.[65]

Metochites' influential role in the imperial administration allowed him to amass great wealth, which he then partly used to fund the renovation of the

of Scipio. For an overview of Planoudes' translation projects, see Schmitt (1968). See also the case study on the translation of Ovid's *Metamorphoses* by Fischer (2004).

[57] Glycofrydi-Leontsini (2003); Plested (2017: 543–7); and Kappes (unpublished). On Greek translations of Latin works in the Palaiologan period, see Nikitas (2001: 1043–51); Bianconi (2004: 554–68); and Kaldellis (2018: 41–55).

[58] On astronomy, see Tihon (2017: 191–2). On medicine, see Chapter 5, nn. 14–15. For a critical overview of the late Byzantine exchange of literature with Arabic writers, see Mavroudi (2004). For a survey of translations from Arabic into Greek, including those from before the thirteenth century, see Mavroudi (2002: 392–429); Gutas (2012: 252–4); and Kaldellis (2018: 25–40).

[59] For George Chrysokokkes' astronomical works, see Mercier (1984). On Chrysokokkes and medicine, see Lampsides (1938).

[60] On George-Gregory Chioniades' astronomical enterprises, see Pingree (1964); and Tihon (1987). See also n. 38, above.

[61] On Metochites' life and works, see Beck (1952); Ševčenko (1979); de Vries-van der Velden (1987); and Featherstone (2011).

[62] Paschos and Simelidis (2017: 1–6).

[63] Golitsis (2008).

[64] Hult (2002: xiv–xvi); see also Xenophontos (2018), who discusses Plutarch's reception by Metochites in light of his *Essay* 71.

[65] On *Ēthikos*, see the relevant study by Polemis (2002). For a fresh approach to *Presbeutikos* in the light of contemporary travel accounts, see Kaldellis (2013: 144–7).

Chora monastery between 1316–21, including the production of monumental mosaics and frescoes with sophisticated iconography and style,[66] and to acquire a large collection of manuscripts. This subsequently passed to his favourite student, the polymath Nikephoros Gregoras. In addition to his monumental *Roman History*, Gregoras (*c.*1293/4–*c.*1359/1360) wrote on grammar, theology, philosophy, mathematics, and astronomy.[67] He proposed a calendar reform for calculating the date of Easter to Andronikos II (almost two centuries before the Western calendar reform introduced by Pope Gregory XIII in 1582), although it was not ultimately adopted.[68] In his works Gregoras also demonstrates the appropriation of classical genres, as in his *Phlōrentios*, or *On Wisdom*, a contemporary dialogue in Platonic guise focusing on the theological controversy with Barlaam of Calabria.[69]

In addition to Constantinople, there were also notable scholars based in Thessaloniki, the second most important intellectual centre of the period.[70] Thomas Magistros (*c.*1280–after 1347/8) compiled a dictionary of Attic terms to help contemporary scholars make proper use of pure Attic Greek.[71] His scholia on Aeschylus' *Persians* provide links with the contemporary siege of the city by the Turks, thus showing his engagement with current politics. Another important intellectual active in the city is Demetrios Triklinios (*fl. c.*1300–25), scholiast and editor of Greek tragedies and comedies, including previously neglected ones such as Aeschylus' *Agamemnon* and *Eumenides*.[72]

3. STUDIES OF JOHN ZACHARIAS AKTOUARIOS AND HIS CORPUS

Charles du Cange, in his massive glossary of medieval Greek published in 1688, was the first to note John's dedications of his works to Joseph Rhakendytes

[66] On the Chora monastery, see Ousterhout (1987). On Palaiologan art patronage, see Kalopissi-Verti (2004).

[67] On the biography and literary production of Gregoras, see Beyer (1978); Wilson (1996: 266–8); and Manolova (2014: 10–26).

[68] His proposal for reforming the calculation of Easter may be found twice in his corpus, i.e. *Roman History*, 8.3, ed. Bekker (1829) I.364–73, and *Epistle* 20, ed. Bezdeki (1924) 330–6. Gregoras' reform was rejected by Barlaam of Calabria in his *Treatise on the Easter Computus*. See Tihon (2011: 393–407), who provides a commentary on Gregoras' proposal versus Barlaam's treatise.

[69] For Gregoras' theological views on the Hesychast controversy, see Beyer (1971). On *Phlōrentios*, see Manolova (2017).

[70] For an overview of literary activity in early Palaiologan Thessaloniki, see Tinnefeld (2003). See also Laiou (2003), who discusses the financial concerns of Thessalonikian intellectuals.

[71] On Magistros, see Gaul (2007) and (2011).

[72] Smith (1981/2); and Wilson (1996: 249–56).

(*c.*1260–*c.*1330) and Alexios Apokaukos (*c.*late 1280s–d. 1345).[73] Almost a century later, the English physician John Freind, in his *The History of Physick* published in 1724, made the first notable assessment of John's medical works.[74] Freind showed a particular interest in diagnosis and pharmacology. He concentrated on John's *Medical Epitome*, rightly pointing to Galen, Aetios of Amida, and Paul of Aegina as John's main sources.[75] Freind also emphasized John's numerous references to oriental *materia medica*, such as the various kinds of myrobalan.[76] It was not until the early nineteenth century that John's corpus attracted more interest from historians of medicine. In particular, the German physician and medical historian Justus Friedrich Karl Hecker made the first comprehensive study of John's works in his monumental *Geschichte der Heilkunde* published in 1829.[77] Hecker highlighted John's independent attitude in his *On Urines*, referring to various urinary characteristics treated by John in detail, such as his mention of the urine crown (*stephanē*).[78] On the other hand, he arbitrarily attributed the earliest mention of whipworm (*Trichocephalus dispar*) to John, although there is no explicit mention of it in John's *Medical Epitome*.[79] Overall, Hecker's analysis suffered from the fact that he based himself on the Latin editions of the works and from the trend among medical historians of his day for examining ancient and medieval medical works from a retrospective point of view, i.e. using modern terminology to refer to diseases and symptoms mentioned in ancient and medieval texts.[80] In 1887, the German ophthalmologist and historian Julius Hirschberg provided a German translation of John's section on ophthalmology, pointing out John's detailed description of various ophthalmic conditions.[81]

Although an edition of a large part of John's works in Greek was published in 1841–2 by the German philologist and naturalist Julius Ludwig Ideler,[82] all subsequent historians of medicine relied on Hecker's comments, making only general reference to the exceptional nature of John's contribution.[83] Their views were aptly illustrated by the Belgian-born American chemist and historian George Sarton who, in the first part of the third volume of his

[73] Charles du Cange (1688: I.46) s.v. *ΑΚΤΟΥΆΡΙΟΣ*. See also Fabricius (1724: 635–9).
[74] Freind (1744: 260–95). [75] Freind (1744: 261). [76] Freind (1744: 271–3).
[77] Hecker (1829: 335–58).
[78] Hecker (1829: 347–8). On the urine crown in John's work, see Chapter 2, n. 140.
[79] Hecker (1829: 349–50).
[80] On retrospective diagnosis, see Cunningham (1992); Leven (2004); and Mitchell (2011).
[81] Hirschberg (1887). [82] Ideler (1841–2).
[83] Meyer (1856: III.386–90); Haeser (1875: I.481–3); Bloch (1902: I.566–7); Neuburger (1911: II.133–7); Schelenz (1904: 193); Desnos (1914: I.191–7); Gossen (1916: 1799–800); Pournaropoulos (1942: 70–1); Diepgen (1949: I.168–9); Dampasis (1967: 947–61); Vogel (1967: 291); Sournia et al (1980: II.468–70); and Buchwald et al. (1982: 245). One must also note the three brief articles by Johann Stur who provided a German translation accompanied by brief comments, involving an analysis from a retrospective point of view of the sections on dermatology (1930), gynaecology (1931a), and sexual diseases (1931b) in John's *Medical Epitome*.

vast *Introduction to the History of Science* published in 1947, stated: 'The outstanding doctor of the age of the Palaiologoi was the court physician Joannes Actuarios. He closes the series of the great Byzantine physicians. His works were used considerably not only in the Christian East but also in the West, being read in Latin translation until the middle of the sixteenth century and even later.'[84]

Later on in the mid twentieth century, the great medical historian Oswei Temkin—attempting to revise our understanding of Byzantine medicine—underlined the lack of any serious study on John's work, stating bluntly: 'Yet I hesitate to include him in my discussion.'[85] The next noteworthy mention of John's works is found in Herbert Hunger's monumental history of Byzantine literature.[86] In his otherwise reliable handbook, Hunger misattributed John's active career to Andronikos III's reign. He expressed admiration for John's literary output and presented his *Medical Epitome* as his magnum opus—a view which continues to be held to this day. However, as will be shown in this book, if such a title must be awarded, it should go to *On Urines*. Hunger marginalized John's original contributions on uroscopy and made no reference to John's encounters with patients. It was not until the 1970s that particular attention was paid to *On Urines*. For example, Konstantin Dimitriadis offered the first brief critical overview of John's uroscopic theories.[87] Later on, Fridolf Kudlien argued that in his *On Urines* John attacked those doctors who relied solely on clinical experience (*peira*).[88] Nevertheless, John shows that both theoretical knowledge (*logos*) and the knowledge gained from *peira* are essential elements for a practising physician, and he does not consider one attribute more important than the other.[89]

In subsequent years, Stavros Kourousis' meticulous study of the collected letters of George Lakapenos—John's good friend and fellow scholar—provided important information about John's life and 'scholarly' networking in Constantinople.[90] He revealed details about John's studies in medicine and showed his clear connection with the circle of Maximos Planoudes' (*c.*1255–*c.*1305) students. In another study of letters relating to John's activity, he established John's approximate date of birth (1275) and confirmed the absence of any evidence about his life after 1328, thus connecting his *floruit* with the second half of the reign of Andronikos II (1282–1328).[91] Moreover, in the same study, Kourousis was the first to present brief summaries of John's

84 Sarton (1947: III.1.252).

85 Temkin (1962: 114).

86 Hunger (1978: II.312–13). It is also worth noting that in Krumbacher's (1897: 615) history of Byzantine literature John appears once again as practising in the reign of Emperor Andronikos III. The same mistake is also repeated by the otherwise meticulous German historian Klaus-Peter Matschke (2008: 370).

87 Dimitriadis (1971: 55–64).

88 Kudlien (1973).

89 I am in agreement with Hohlweg (1983: 314). See also Chapter 2, n. 55.

90 Kourousis (1978/9).

91 Kourousis (1980/2).

case histories. A few years later, he wrote a long monograph,[92] of which the greater part deals with his unconvincing argumentation, seeking to assign the authorship of three early Palaiologan texts in dialogic form (*Hermodotos*, *Mousoklēs*, and *Hermippos*) on philosophy and astronomy to John.[93] In his attempt to present the author of the anonymous texts as medically aware, Kourousis exaggerated the use of references with medical connotations in these dialogues and did not provide a critical assessment of his selection of supposed cross-referenced passages between these dialogues and John's medical corpus.[94] In his long study on the three dialogues, Armin Hohlweg advanced several counterproposals to Kourousis' argumentation, demonstrating that it was impossible to identify John as the author of the three dialogues. He argued instead in favour of the authorship by Nikephoros Gregoras.[95] Hohlweg's study was rejected by Kourousis, who reaffirmed his attribution of the dialogues to John in a new study some years later.[96] The evidence given by both scholars is inconclusive and I prefer to treat those three works as unattributed.

In Kourousis' monograph significant attention is given to John's work *On Psychic Pneuma*, which is also discussed by Hohlweg in a brief study.[97] Both Byzantine philologists presented John's work from a philosophical point of view, attempting to relate his theories to the writings of Neoplatonic philosophers and the Church Fathers, and thereby omitting John's medical contributions to human physiology. John and his corpus were the subject of an article written by Hohlweg in 1983, in which he announced his critical edition of the *Medical Epitome*, which was unfortunately never published.[98] Hohlweg rightly pointed out the innovative character of John's *On Urines* and provided a short description of its contents. He also gave a useful overview of the unedited part of the *Medical Epitome*. However, he made no particular attempt to investigate further and restricted himself to mentioning Hecker's comments uncritically. In conclusion, he considered John's *Medical Epitome* a specialized work written for contemporary physicians, contradicting the conclusion of the present volume, which shows that the work is primarily written for the non-expert.

[92] Kourousis (1984/8).

[93] *Hermodotos*, ed. Elter (1898) 5–38; *Mousokles*, ed. Elter (1898) 38–54; and *Hermippos*, ed. Kroll and Viereck (1895). It is important to note that the uniformity of the style in the three dialogues had already been pointed out in the early twentieth century by Kroll (1912: 854). A German translation of the three works was published by Schönberger and Schönberger (2010).

[94] Kourousis (1984/8: 258–88). Cf. Chapter 6, n. 104.

[95] Hohlweg (1995). See also Hohlweg (1996a), which reaffirms the authorship by Gregoras. Cf. Bianconi (2006: 70, n. 6).

[96] Kourousis (1997/9). See also Kourousis (1985/9).

[97] Kourousis (1984/8: 417–76); Hohlweg (1996b). A brief descriptive synopsis of John's work *On Psychic Pneuma* is also provided by Putscher (1973: 50–5, 110–11).

[98] Hohlweg (1983). The article reappeared in a slightly shorter version in English translation a year later (1984).

Timothy Miller's conclusions on John's activity in his monograph on Byzantine hospitals are often not substantiated by the available evidence in primary sources.[99] Although earlier studies by Kourousis and Hohlweg on John's basic biographical details had been available for at least a decade before the second revised edition of this work, Miller presented John as court physician in Andronikos III's reign. The erratic nature of Miller's statements is further illustrated in his description of the Mangana *xenōn* as a fully-functioning medicalized hospital and his identification of John as one of its physicians, without presenting any evidence for the restoration of this particular *xenōn* after 1261 or to support John's affiliation with it;[100] he consequently considered John's case histories an outcome of his *xenōn* experience.[101]

Scholars have generally given little attention to John's diagnostic methods. The only notable exception is Emilie Savage-Smith who, in her article on Byzantine ophthalmology, highlighted John's awareness of the differential diagnosis of eye affections.[102] Aristotelis Eftychiadis referred to some isolated examples of John's pharmacology in his book on Byzantine therapeutics, although his non-comparative approach limits the interpretive value of the study.[103] John's vast work on uroscopy was discussed from various perspectives in the collection of essays on the history of nephrology edited by the nephrologist Thanasis Diamandopoulos. This study often takes a retrospective analysis approach.[104] In Diamandopoulos' later study, co-written with Pavlos Goudas, the authors outlined for the first time some interesting data from John's work, including some inconclusive details on John's theory of the four digestions.[105] Moreover, in the doctoral thesis of Antonia Kakavelaki on the role of pneuma in the works of Greek and Byzantine authors from a philosophical point of view, there is a special section on John's *On Psychic Pneuma*, in which the author points to some additional philosophical sources not previously mentioned, such as John Philoponos' commentary *On Aristotle's on the Soul*.[106] Finally, mention must be made of a long doctoral thesis by Stavroula Georgiou, which provides the first-ever critical edition of the first book of *On Urines* accompanied by a French translation and commentary.[107]

[99] The first edition of Miller's book appeared in 1985; a revised edition was published in 1997.

[100] See also below, Section 4.1.1.

[101] Miller (1997: 158, 168, 185, 199). Miller's overall views on Byzantine *xenōnes* in this monograph have been strongly contested, initially by Nutton (1986) and then by Horden (2005). There is one case in which John refers to an *iatreion* as the place of his medical activity, but this term does not necessarily signify a *xenōn* or a place within it. See the discussion in Chapter 3, Section 2.3.

[102] Savage-Smith (1984: 184–5).

[103] Eftychiadis (1983).

[104] Diamandopoulos (2000).

[105] Diamandopoulos and Goudas (2009).

[106] Kakavelaki (2012: 341–83). This doctoral thesis was recently published in the form of a monograph: Kakavelaki (2018: 333–69).

[107] Georgiou (2013).

4. THE MAN

4.1 John's connections with contemporary intellectuals: evidence from Palaiologan epistolography

We can deduce various details of John's life and relationships with contemporary individuals from surviving letters addressed to him and one extant letter written by John.[108] The following letters (the particular letter(s) addressed to or concerning John is/are given in parenthesis) are of interest:[109] a) collection of letters by George Lakapenos and Andronikos Zarides (nos. 10, 18, and 20);[110] b) John's letter to Theodore Modenos;[111] c) a collection of letters by Michael Gabras (nos. 22, 52, 310, and 439);[112] d) a collection of letters by George Oinaiotes (nos. 43, 168, 171, and 174).[113]

The first collection consists of thirty-two letters and includes the correspondence of the Palaiologan intellectuals George Lakapenos (*fl.* *c.*1297–1310/11, d. before 1315) and Andronikos Zarides (*fl.* *c.*1300–15), both ex-students of Maximos Planoudes.[114] George Lakapenos is known as the author of

[108] For an exhaustive analysis of the surviving letters, see Kourousis (1980/2); reproduced in Kourousis (1984/8: 101–33).

[109] Kourousis (1980/2: 257–9) also believes that a letter in George-Gregory Chioniades' collection (*Epistle* 15, ed. Papadopoulos, 1927, 202.1–17), which has no addressee, is actually addressed to John. The letter does not offer any particular identificatory information, apart from revealing Chioniades' obvious desire to show his friendly feelings towards a certain physician by the name of John. I agree with Kourousis' (1980/2: 258, n. 1) suggestion that the reference to a physician in the letter is literal, not metaphorical. However, it is impossible to establish the identity of the addressee with any degree of certainty, although Chioniades and John might have known one another. On George-Gregory Chioniades, see nn. 38 and 60, above.

[110] The collection was first edited by Lindstam (1910) and included only the first ten letters. It was then re-edited, Lindstam (1924), containing all the letters and considering all the available manuscripts, of which there are almost 50. *Epistles* 10, 18, and 20, may be found in ed. Lindstam (1924) 80.4–82.25, 120.7–121, and 125.19–129.21. For a chronological table of the letters, see Kourousis (1984/8: 100).

[111] The letter was first edited by Treu (1899a) 39; and then re-edited by Kourousis (1984/8) 541. The title reads, Vindobonensis phil. gr. 219, f. 138r, l. 1: '*Ἰωάννου τοῦ τοῦ Ζαχαρίου: Θεοδώρῳ τῷ Μοδηνῷ*'. See also Kourousis (1984/8: 535–8).

[112] The collection edited by Fatouros (1973). In particular, *Epistles* 22, 52, 310, and 439 are found on II.48.1–49.39, II.87.1–88.21, II.493.1–494, and II.677.1–678.37. Six more letters by Gabras were recently edited by Stefec (2013), but without any references to John.

[113] The collection remains unedited, apart from a few isolated letters edited in individual studies. For example, see Ahrweiler (1996: 23–6) where letter no. 157 was edited by Fatouros. The letters survive in three manuscripts, Florentinus Laurentianus San Marco 356 (fourteenth century), Matritensis gr. 4796 (sixteenth century), and Monacensis gr. 198 (sixteenth century). The collection is anonymous and was first studied by Rein (1915); and then by Karlsson and Fatouros (1973), who also edited four letters. The identification of the author with George Oinaiotes is credited to Kourousis (1972: 99–121). For a recent study of a particular group of letters concerning Oinaiotes' interest in Plato, see Menchelli (2013). I am grateful to Diether Roderich Reinsch (Berlin) for providing me with access to the text of the forthcoming edition.

[114] Although there is no explicit reference indicating that both were students of Planoudes, this relationship convincingly deduced by Kourousis (1978/9: 301–6) on the basis of various

educational textbooks, including his epistles and associated *epimerismoi* (elementary word-by-word comments, grammar, syntax, and vocabulary, on texts intended for school use), works on grammar and syntax and an edition of a collection of Libanios' (fourth century AD) letters and scholia, thus suggesting his activity as a teacher in Constantinople.[115] Andronikos Zarides, the author of some surviving letters, was a low-level imperial administrator.[116]

Lakapenos sent *Epistle* 10 to John from Thessaloniki around autumn 1299.[117] He addresses him as 'Zacharias' (*tō Zacharia*), which is John's surname.[118] John wants to travel to Thessaloniki from Constantinople to meet his friend. Lakapenos urges his friend to stay in Constantinople and complete his studies in medicine. According to the letter, John was currently attending a daily *phrontistērion* but, since he had not finished his education, he would not be able to reach the appropriate level of knowledge on the 'secrets' of medicine (*orgiōn Hippokratous*) to acquire the *kērygmata*.[119] The word *phrontistērion* is associated with a place of education in Palaiologan sources,[120] and Lakapenos' reference to the term might be associated with some advanced tutorials on medicine by a contemporary schoolmaster, such as Planoudes. A later scholion in this letter provides another possibility associating the term with a *xenōn*,[121] a term which could denote one of Constantinople's hospitals.[122]

passages concerning education in the correspondence between George Lakapenos and George Zarides, brother of Andronikos Zarides, who was undoubtedly a student of Planoudes. This is confirmed in Planoudes' *Epistles* 39 and 42, ed. Leone (1991) 71.20–72.17 and 74.18–75.28 respectively, addressed to George Zarides. See also Constantinides (1982: 83–90).

[115] On Lakapenos' works, see Kourousis (1978/9: 295–6); and Constantinides (1982: 101). On the reception of Lakapenos' works, including their printed edition in the Renaissance West, see Constantinides (1982: 103).

[116] On Andronikos Zarides, see Kourousis (1978/9: 296, and *passim*).

[117] On the identification of the city with that of Thessaloniki, see Kourousis (1978/9: 307–9).

[118] See also the title of *Epistle* 22 by Michael Gabras, ed. Fatouros (1973) II.48: '*Τῷ Λακαπηνῷ κυρῷ Γεωργίῳ καὶ τῷ Ζαχαρίᾳ κυρῷ Ἰωάννῃ*', where the surname precedes the first name in the case of both John and his friend George Lakapenos. John's surname is well attested in Palaiologan Byzantium, see *PLP* 6481–97.

[119] George Lakapenos, *Epistle* 10, ed. Lindstam (1924) 82.5–25.

[120] See the discussion of this passage with associated references to primary sources in Kourousis (1980/2: 247–8); and Hohlweg (1983: 306–7) and (1989: 171–2). On the use of the term in the framework of a Palaiologan school, see Constantinides (1982: 68, 81, 138).

[121] Lindstam (1910: 21, *apparatus criticus*): '*ἐν τῷ φροντιστηρίῳ· ἐν τῷ ξενῶνι*'. Cf. Fuchs (1926: 61). It is worth emphasizing that there is no other surviving edited source in which the term is connected with a *xenōn*. See also n. 125, below.

[122] Only a few Constantinopolitan *xenōnes* are mentioned in the sources dating to after the recapture of the city by the Byzantines in 1261. See Thomas (1987: 244–67); Miller (1997: 192–9); and Stathakopoulos (2004). Perhaps, the most well-attested early-fourteenth-century *xenōn* is the so-called Kral *xenōn*, which was established by the Serbian King Stefan Uroš II Milutin (r. 1282–1321) in the Petra district of Constantinople. On this, see Birchler-Argyros (1988). We must also mention the unique case of the Lips *xenōn*, for which there is explicit mention in the late-thirteenth-century *Typikon* [ed. Delehaye (1921) 106–36] of the provision of a twelve-bed *xenōn* staffed by three doctors. Nevertheless, although there is no doubt about the restoration of the monastery by Theodora Palaiologina (d. 1303), which Talbot (2001: 336–8)

In fact, the foundation charter (*Typikon*) of the Pantokrator *xenōn* in Constantinople, which was established by John II Komnenos (r. 1118–43) in 1136, refers to the teaching of medicine in the framework of a medicalized hospital.[123] However, there are no other contemporary sources to confirm that such a school was actually functioning in the Pantokrator *xenōn*, which was in any case a short-lived institution.[124] Furthermore, there is no further evidence to support the idea that there was consistent provision of medical education in *xenōnes*.[125] The only exception is the case of John Argyropoulos (*c.*1393/4 or *c.*1415–87), who was giving lectures in medicine at the *Katholikon Mouseion* of the Kral *xenōn*, annexed to the monastery of St John the Baptist in Constantinople.[126] But there is a gap of almost three centuries between this and the descriptions of the Pantokrator *xenōn* in the *Typikon*. Consequently, it is not clear from Lakapenos' letter what kind of medical teaching John received and in what context, but it confirms some sort of medical teaching activity in Constantinople.

dates to sometime between 1294 and 1301, it is worth pointing out that there is no contemporary evidence confirming the actual functioning of the *xenōn*.

[123] The term 'medicalized' in this context was coined by Horden (2005) to describe an institution in which physicians were regularly present.

[124] The overall evidence suggests that the *xenōn* did not last long, not surviving beyond 1150, which was perhaps due to difficulties in sustaining such a large staff. See Kislinger (1987); and Horden (2005: 51–60). It is worth noting that Michael Italikos (d. before 1157), a prominent intellectual cleric of the mid twelfth century, taught physicians in different aspects of medical science such as anatomy and the pulse rate, as it is confirmed in his *Epistle* 5, ed. Gautier (1972) 97.19–28. He was ultimately elected a sort of professor of medicine [*didaskalos iatrōn*, in *Epistle* 33, ed. Gautier (1972) 209.1–3], after accepting an invitation from Irene Doukaina [*Epistle* 5, ed. Gautier (1972) 97.10–18], the widow of the Emperor Alexios I (1081–1118). However, there is not sufficient evidence to confirm the location and nature (e.g. whether private or public) of his teaching. One can also mention the inclusion of medicine, in the place of astronomy, among the subjects studied in the framework of the *quadrivium* in a school associated with the Church of Holy Apostles in Constantinople—otherwise unattested in other contemporary sources around 1200—according to Nicholas Mesarites' description of that church addressed to Patriarch John X Kamateros (1198–1206) [*Description of the Church of the Holy Apostles at Constantinople*, 42, ed. Downey (1957) 916–17]. On the 'idyllic' nature of this 'school', see Daskas (2016: 90 and n. 36) with references to previous studies.

[125] Miller (1997: 150) believes that the teaching of medicine, as described in the *Typikon* of the Pantokrator, must have applied to the majority of the later *xenōnes*. He also takes for granted the later manuscript scholion on Lakapenos' epistle (see n. 121, above) and states that 'John Zachariah was continuing to train in the healing art at a Constantinopolitan xenon' (1997: 158). I believe that the absence of any significant commentaries or extensive scholia on ancient medical works in the middle and late Byzantine period is another indication of the lack of consistent provision of medical education. In contrast to medicine, we can see extensive interpretive activity in the fields of philosophy and astronomy, both widely studied in Byzantium in the Komnenian and Palaiologan periods. See Bydén and Ierodiakonou (2018: Sections 1.1 and 1.3) and Tihon (2017: 197), respectively.

[126] John Argyropoulos' teaching was influenced by interpretations of Galenic theories by early Byzantine Alexandrian scholars and he also seems to have introduced into Byzantium interpretations by fourteenth- and fifteenth-century Italian scholars, perhaps due to his studies in Padua. See Mondrain (2000a) and (2003); Pietrobelli (2010); and Ieraci Bio (2010) and (2013).

As for the word *kērygmata*, it suggests a kind of medical licensing system, perhaps something similar to the *symbolon* mentioned by Patriarch Leo Stypes (1134–43) in the twelfth century.[127] In that case, the text states that those having received medical education and with long practical experience should be tested (*proexetasas*) before the supreme master of medical science (*iatrikēs proexarchōn*) like a 'Lydian rock' (*Lydia lithos*).[128] If the master found them not unsatisfactory (*ouk adokimon*), he endowed them with the symbols of approbation (*symbolon*). This could refer either to a licence or a specific object that could attest their medical proficiency. It is clear that both texts confirm the existence of a process for granting an educated physician the right to practise, but it is unclear whether it is regulated by the state or by a guild of physicians.[129]

To return to Lakapenos' *Epistle* 10, John had reported to Lakapenos in an earlier, no longer extant, letter that he lived in Constantinople with his mother, without referring to his father or a wife, but mentioning the financial difficulties he was currently facing.[130] More details about John's family are found in his sole surviving letter, addressed to a friend from Serres, Theodore Modenos. John wanted to visit his friend, who was ill,[131] but his father's lingering illness did not permit this.[132] Taking into consideration the absence of any reference to John's father in Lakapenos' letter, it would seem that John's letter to Theodore is likely to have preceded it and probably John's father had died at some point before 1299.[133] It is worth noting that John seems to have had friends in Serres, which—combined with the attestation of three, almost contemporary, people with the same surname as John in that city—could suggest it might have been John's place of origin.[134]

There are two more letters in Lakapenos' collection, which, although not addressed to John, refer to him indirectly. *Epistle* 18 was sent by Lakapenos to

[127] The text was edited by Rallis and Potlis (1855) V.76. See also Grumel (1949: 42–6).

[128] Lydian rock was used in ancient times to test the genuineness of gold. Consequently, the term was used metaphorically to indicate a thorough process for the identification of truth or precision. The metaphorical use of the term is attested as early as the *Hyporchemata*, fr. 1, ed. Irigoin (1993) 227, by the early-fifth-century BC lyric poet Bacchylides.

[129] On the regulation of medical practice in Komnenian and Palaiologan Byzantium, see Stathakopoulos (2013b: 227–31). On guilds of Byzantine physicians, cf. Maniatis (2001: 349–51). It is worth noting that in the same period in the West, the new medical schools in universities such as Bologna and Paris produced the first trained physicians. See Nutton (1995: 153–9).

[130] George Lakapenos, *Epistle* 10, ed. Lindstam (1924) 82.6–7, 12–18.

[131] JZA, *Epistle*, ed. Kourousis (1984/8) 541.1–10.

[132] JZA, *Epistle*, ed. Kourousis (1984/8) 541.11–12.

[133] Kourousis (1980/2: 243).

[134] We know of a priest in the Metropolis of Serres called Nicholas Zacharias in the last quarter of the thirteenth century, see Bénou (1998: 23, 28); another priest in Serres called Theodoulos Zacharias, Bénou (1998: 96); a local church official (*laosynaktēs*) and scribe Leo Zacharias (active between 1284 and 1313), *PLP* 6493 and Bénou (1998: 50, 95, 97); and one more official (*chartophylax*) of the Metropolis of Serres, John Zacharias (active between 1353 and 1378), *PLP* 6485, Bénou (1998: 277, 310).

Andronikos Zarides. Lakapenos is writing in connection with two books in which Zarides had shown an interest, one of which contains the Hippocratic *Aphorisms*. Zarides wanted to order a copy of it.[135] However, before giving various details about the delay in the preparation of the copy, Lakapenos passes on John's greetings to Zarides, calling John the chief (*koryphaion*) of their friends.[136] Thus, we can see that there is a friendly connection between John and Zarides, and also that Zarides had an interest in medical texts. In *Epistle* 20, sent by Lakapenos to Zarides between 1307 and 1309, John appears as the practising physician who had taken care of Lakapenos when he was ill.[137] Here Lakapenos calls John an 'able and mighty physician and philosopher' (*iatros tagathos krateros te philosophos*), stressing his all-round medical education and expertise, and presenting him in the Galenic fashion as 'physician cum philosopher'.[138] Kourousis proposes that John's friendship with Lakapenos and Zarides might suggest that John had also been a pupil of Planoudes,[139] but there is no conclusive evidence for this. Overall, we can deduce that John would probably have finished his studies and started practising medicine by around 1300 or shortly thereafter, and certainly before 1309. If John completed his advanced studies in medicine *c.*1300, he must have been born around 1275.[140]

The next groups of letters, which offers important details regarding John's connection with the imperial court, is that of the writer and official of the imperial chancery, Michael Gabras (*c.*1290–d. after 1350). The collection includes 462 letters in chronological order dating to between 1308 and 1327. In *Epistle* 22, which is addressed to both George Lakapenos and John, Michael pleads with them to intervene on his behalf and introduce him to the circle of intellectuals associated with Andronikos II.[141] He refers to some kind of meetings taking place in the evenings under the aegis of the emperor, probably alluding to a gathering of intellectuals. What Gabras says implies that both Lakapenos and John had good relations with the emperor.[142] Later on, Gabras sends John a letter (no. 52), including an oration, which he intends to perform in front of the emperor.[143] Gabras asks John to provide him with his comments, thus confirming their close acquaintance and John's contacts with the imperial court. In the next two letters (nos. 310 and 439), Gabras supplements

135 George Lakapenos, *Epistle* 18, ed. Lindstam (1924) 121.17–28.

136 George Lakapenos, *Epistle* 18, ed. Lindstam (1924) 121.14–17.

137 George Lakapenos, *Epistle* 20, ed. Lindstam (1924) 128.31–129.4.

138 As expressed in the Galenic treatise *The Best Doctor is also a Philosopher*, ed. Kühn (1821) I.53–63 = ed. Boudon-Millot (2007a) 283–92. Cf. Ieraci Bio (1991).

139 Kourousis (1980/2: 239).

140 Kourousis (1980/2: 244).

141 Michael Gabras, *Epistle* 22, ed. Fatouros (1973) II.48.3–9.

142 That George Lakapenos had access to the circle of intellectuals associated with Andronikos II is also implied in another letter sent to him by Andronikos Zarides between 1207 and 1209; see Andronikos Zarides, *Epistle* 24, ed. Lindstam (1924) 150.17–152.23.

143 Michael Gabras, *Epistle* 52, ed. Fatouros (1973) II.87.1–88.21.

John's title with the term *aktouarios*,[144] implying that John had at that point been appointed to this particular imperial office. In the second of these two letters, Gabras sends John a prayer, commenting on his admirable faith.[145] Given the chronological sequence of Gabras' letters, John must have been appointed *aktouarios* sometime between 1310 (*Epistle* 52) and 1323 (*Epistle* 310).[146] Lastly, it is notable that Gabras was once treated by a physician called Andronikos Zacharias.[147] Although the synonymy and the profession might suggest a relation of John's, we have no other information about Andronikos Zacharias from contemporary sources.

The last collection of letters is that of George Oinaiotes. Some of his unedited *Epistles* (nos. 43, 168, 171, and 174) are addressed to a certain *aktouarios* (*tō aktouariō*). Kourousis has convincingly shown that all four letters were addressed to the same person, who could not have been other than John, since the letters were sent between 1321 and 1327, a period when the office was held by him.[148] The letters contain details, which show that Oinaiotes was interested in the study of astronomy. According to *Epistle* 174, Oinaiotes received some sort of supervision from John in reading astronomical treatises.[149] Finally, in *Epistle* 43, Oinaiotes, having managed to attain a

[144] Michael Gabras, *Epistle* 310 and 439, ed. Fatouros (1973) II.493.1–2 and 677.1–2: '*τῷ ἀκτουαρίῳ κυρῷ Ἰωάννῃ τῷ Ζαχαρίᾳ*'.

[145] Michael Gabras, *Epistle* 439, ed. Fatouros (1973) II.677.1–678.37. John's piety can also be deduced from John's invariable invocation of God's blessing in starting or ending a particular section of his works using the words *Theou didontos* or *Theou eudokountos.* See, for example, JZA, *On Urines*, 3.18.8, ed. Ideler (1842) II.72.34–5; *Medical Epitome*, 1.57, ed. Ideler (1842) II.417.33–4; and *On Psychic Pneuma*, 1.20.13, ed. Ideler (1841) I.349.30–1. In one of his case histories John also appears to attend a religious feast and venerate the local saint, although the place and name are not specified, *On Urines*, 4.9.5, ed. Ideler (1842) II.92.10–13: '*ἀφικόμεθά ποτε περὶ Κυνὸς ἐπιτολὴν ἐντὸς τῆς πόλεως ἐπί τινα πανήγυριν προσκυνήσοντες μὲν τὸν ἐκεῖσε ἅγιον διαφερόντως τιμώμενον*'. In the unedited part of his *Medical Epitome*, John warns those who use poisonous drugs for human beings of the sin they are committing, which will, in turn, be the starting point for their eternal suffering, *Medical Epitome*, 5, Vindobonensis med. gr. 17, f. 161v, ll. 4–10: '*προαναφωνῶ δὲ πάντας τοὺς συντυγχάνοντας* (E: *ἐντυγχάνοντας*) *τῷ βιβλίῳ· καὶ μυουμένων τὰ τῆς τέχνης ὄργια, αὐτοὺς τὲ ἐπὶ σωτηρίᾳ τῶν ἀνθρώπων ταῦτα μανθάνειν μὴ παρασυρομένους ἐπὶ φθορὰν ἀνθρώπων…ἵνα μὴ ὁ Θεὸς δικάζων ὧ δέ τι* (E: *ὧδέ τε*) *τὴν ἁμαρτίαν σφῶν αὐτῶν θριαμβεύσῃ καὶ τὰς ἀξίας τίσαιεν ποινάς…αἰωνία καταδικάσας βασάνῳ·*'; ed. Mathys (1556) II.417.28–418.6. This also reminds the statement against the use of lethal drugs in the Hippocratic *Oath*. See also n. 203, below.

[146] Kourousis (1980/2: 252).

[147] *PLP* 6481; Michael Gabras, *Epistle* 445, ed. Fatouros (1973) II.682.1–684.56.

[148] Kourousis (1980/2: 260–9) suggests that the earlier letter is 168, then 171, 174, and the latest is 43. Furthermore, Kourousis argues that George Oinaiotes would probably have been John's nephew, based on his reference in *Epistle* 168 to: '*καὶ τῆς καθ' αἷμα πρὸς ἡμᾶς ἑταιρίας*'.

[149] There is also a mention of an astronomical manuscript, which John purportedly lent to George Oinaiotes, *Epistle* 174: '*δώσεις δὲ πῶς; εἰ τὴν τὰς τῶν σφαιρικῶν σωμάτων κινήσεις καὶ τῶν πλανωμένων καὶ ἀπλανῶν διευκρινοῦσαν βίβλον πέμψεις ἡμῖν, ὡς ἂν σημειωσάμενοι τὰ σελίδια καὶ ὡς ἐνὸν συνοπτικώτατα ἐγχαράξαντες πλαξὶ καρδίας πρότερον ἢ χάρτῃ ἔπειτα ἀποστείλωμεν. οὐδὲ γὰρ οὐδ' ἡμεῖς ἀγνοοῦμεν ὅπως ἀνάγκη τὴν καλλίστην βίβλον αἰεὶ συμπαρεῖναί σοι, δι' ἧς τὰ κατ' οὐρανὸν ἐποπτεύεις καὶ τοῖς ἄστρασι πλησιάζεις καὶ τὰ τ' ἐόντα τά τ' ἐσόμενα πρό τ' ἐόντα μανθάνεις, ἵνα καὶ προδιδάσκῃς ἀγνοοῦσι συλλήβδην περὶ τῶν πάντῃ χωριστῶν καὶ ἀιδίων καὶ ἀεὶ ἀμεταβλήτων*'.

considerable level of knowledge in astronomy, asks John to intercede on his behalf and introduce him to the circle of astronomers under Theodore Metochites, who at that point held the office of the *megas logothetēs*,[150] thus confirming John's eminent status among Palaiologan intellectuals.

4.1.1 The office of aktouarios

The office of *aktouarios* existed in early Byzantium, when it was related to the finances of the Empire.[151] From the twelfth century onwards there is consistent evidence of the association of this office with physicians. We first learn of an *aktouarios* who happened to be a physician in the Komnenian period, to be specific, in the monody of Michael Italikos on the physician and *aktouarios* Michael Pantechnes (d. *c.*1130).[152] Another notable physician and poet of the early twelfth century,[153] Nicholas Kalliklles, had also been an *aktouarios* at some point, as is confirmed by a reference in the *Ptōchoprodromika*.[154] Interestingly, Michael Pantechnes and Nicholas Kallikles were two of the three physicians attending the Emperor Alexios I Komnenos (r. 1081–1118) during his final illness. The episode is described by Anna Komnene in the *Alexiad*, where there is no use of the term *aktouarios* for any of the physicians, and thus we are unable to tell whether either of the two held the office at that particular time.[155] A further reference from the Empire of Nicaea associates

[150] George Oinaiotes, *Epistle* 43: '*ἐπεί σε καλῶς εἰδότα οἶδα δι' ὅσης ἐπιμελείας ὁ θειότατος καὶ ἅγιος ἡμῶν βασιλεὺς πεποίηται τὸ μὴ πολλοὺς χώραν λαμβάνειν τοῦ κορυφαίου τούτου μαθήματος. οὐ μὴν δ' ἀλλὰ καὶ τὰ μέγιστα τῷ μεγάλῳ λογοθέτῃ καὶ καθηγεμόνι ταύτης τῆς ὄντως ἀληθοῦς φιλοσοφίας—εἴπερ καὶ γνῶσις τῶν ὄντων ἡ φιλοσοφία κατονομάζεται—χαριζόμενος διατελεῖς, καὶ οὐδὲ τούτου χάριν δέδοικα*'. All the letters attest the profound interest of intellectuals in astronomy at that time, which is referred to as the 'chief subject'. The interpretation of this letter follows Kourousis (1980/2: 268–9).

[151] *ODB*, s.v. aktouarios; *LexLat*, s.v. *ἀκτουάριος*; and Zervan et al. (2019: 9–10). See also Karayannopulos (1958: 81, 102–3, 173, 201).

[152] Michael Italikos, *Monody on the aktouarios Pantechnes*, ed. Criscuolo (1972) 628–34 = ed. Gautier (1972) 110–15. For a commentary on the treatise, see Mavroudis (1993). There is also a monody dedicated to the brother of a certain *aktouarios* by the eleventh-century polymath Michael Psellos. Although the deceased brother of the *aktouarios* was a physician, it is not confirmed in the text whether the living brother who held the office of *aktouarios* was also a physician; see Michael Psellos, *Monody on the Brother of the aktouarios*, ed. Polemis (2014) 194–8. The name Theodore appears on two imperial documents dated to 1088 in association with the office of *aktouarios*, but there is no evidence to suggest his profession. See Vranousi (1980: 338, 345); and cf. Cheynet (2003: 94).

[153] On his poetry, see Romano (1979/80).

[154] *Ptōchoprodromika*, 4.605, ed. Eideneier (1991) 171. Eideneier has corrected the attested version of the manuscripts, i.e. *oktarios* to *aktarios*. *Oktarios* is a vernacular version of the term *aktouarios* which is also found in the titles of some manuscripts of John's works. See Chapter 3, n. 92 and Appendix 5, *passim*. The shorter version of *aktouarios*, i.e. *aktarios*, goes back to the first centuries AD. See the relevant evidence from Egyptian papyri in *LexLat*, s.v. *ἀκτουάριος*.

[155] Anna Komnene, *Alexiad*, 15.11.2–13, ed. Reinsch and Kambylis (2001) 494.29–499.7. The third one was a eunuch named Michael.

the office with a physician named Nicholas, who is presented as discussing the eclipse of the sun in 1239 with George Akropolites and the Empress Irene in the court of the Emperor John III Vatatzes.[156] The office survived in the Palaiologan period; an *aktouarios* and physician with the family name Kabasilas announced the imminent death of Michael VIII in 1282.[157] Interestingly, the office is not included in the fourteenth-century treatise on precedence by Pseudo-Kodinos, but it comes in forty-ninth place in the list of precedence in the appendix of the fourteenth-century *Hexabiblos* of jurist Constantine Harmenopoulos and occupies the same place in the contemporary versified list by the monk and theologian Matthew Blastares.[158]

So far the sources I have presented are silent on the responsibilities of the office and whether the *aktouarios* was also a permanent court physician, as has often been assumed by scholars.[159] Before drawing any conclusions about this, it is necessary to consider evidence from the group of so-called *xenōnika*, medical texts with a strong pharmacological focus, which are related to the Byzantine *xenōnes*.[160] More specifically, there are three more named physicians, who held the office and practised in Byzantine *xenōnes*, as is confirmed in surviving recipes bearing the name and title of the relevant author-physician. These are Abram the Saracen, *aktouarios* of the Mangana *xenōn* and *basilikos archiatros*, Stephen, *aktouarios* of the Mangana *xenōn*, and Michael, *aktouarios* of the Mauraganos *xenōn*.[161] In all cases, we can see that

[156] The *aktouarios* Nicholas is mentioned by George Akropolites, *Chronicle*, 39, ed. Heisenberg (1903) 63.12–16, and is traditionally identified with Nicholas Myrepsos, the author of the *Dynameron*. See Ieraci Bio (2017: 301–2); and cf. Hunger (1978: II.312). This identification has also recently been reproduced unquestioned in the dictionary of loanwords in the works of late Byzantine historians by Zervan et al. (2019: 10). However, this identification is not confirmed by any cross reference in the *Dynameron* where Myrepsos' identity remains unclear. Cf. the recent articles by Valiakos, in which he presents differing views on the identification of the author, although both articles were published in the same year. In the first article, Valiakos (2015a: 69) is convinced that Nicholas is to be identified with the physician at the Nicaean court, while in the second case (2015b: 241–2), he considers this identification to be uncertain.

[157] George Pachymeres, *Chronicle*, 6.35, ed. Failler and Laurent (1984) II.665.16–20. Kourousis (1980/2: 255) has also pointed out that Kabasilas owned a vineyard close to Thessaloniki and is mentioned in the source as having the rank of '*πανσεβάστου σεβαστοῦ*', ed. Giros, Kravari and Zivojinovic (1998) 165–6. On the *aktouarios* Kabasilas in the framework of thirteenth-century medical practice, see Stathakopoulos (2012: 145–6). The same appellation is also found in the title of John's works in some manuscripts (see Appendix 5, *passim*) and is included by Georgiou (2013: 398, 477–8) in the title of the first book of the critical edition of *On Urines*; see n. 186, below. It was also applied to other officials: see Ahrweiler (1966); Kontogiannopoulou (2012: 212–16); and Solomou (2016: 373–6).

[158] See Macrides, Munitiz, and Angelov (2013: 455–64), who, in their recent English translation and commentary of Pseudo-Kodinos' text, offer a very useful table containing the offices in all fourteenth-century *Lists of Court Precedence*.

[159] See, for example, Hunger (1978: II.312–13); and Miller (1997: 149).

[160] On these texts, see the recent monograph by Bennett (2017). See also Chapter 5, n. 130.

[161] Bennett (2003: 398): '*τοῦ Σαρακηνοῦ τοῦ Ἀβραμ· καὶ ἀκτουαρίου τῶν Μαγγάνων καὶ βασιλικοῦ ἀρχιϊάτρου·*'; Bennett (2003: 402): '*Στεφάνου ἰατροῦ καὶ ἀκτουαρίου τῶν Μαγγάνων*'; and Bennett (2003: 404, 405): '*συντεθέντος παρὰ Μιχαὴλ ἀκτουαρίου τοῦ Μαυραγάνου*', '*συντεθὲν*

the office is connected with a particular *xenōn*, while in the case of Abram the Saracen (most probably indicating an Arab physician), we can see that one *aktouarios* was also appointed imperial (*basilikos*) *archiatros*. Thus he was either associated with the court or he was employed in an imperial *xenōn* (*basilikos xenōn*).[162] As for the title of *archiatros*, it was used to signify a senior (head) physician in the early Byzantine period, but there is no evidence to attest the consistent existence of the post in later centuries.[163] Moreover, it is not connected with the office of *aktouarios* in any other source. David Bennett has convincingly shown that there is no evidence for the restoration of the Constantinopolitan Mangana *xenōn* after 1261 and the recipes concerned must be dated to between the mid tenth century (the assumed date of the foundation of the Mangana *xenōn*)[164] and 1204.[165] Thus, at some point, most probably between the eleventh and twelfth centuries, some physicians who held the office of *aktouarios* were practising in the Mangana *xenōn*, but there is no evidence that allows us to generalize about this affiliation with respect to *aktouarioi* active in the Palaiologan period like John, despite claims to this effect by Timothy Miller.[166] As for the reference to the Mauraganos *xenōn*, it remains an enigma, since we have no other evidence of a *xenōn* by this name.[167]

Overall, there is neither evidence that the *aktouarios* was an officially appointed court physician nor that the office was always associated with a position in a Constantinopolitan *xenōn*. In John's case, there is no significant

παρὰ τοῦ ὀκταρίου Μιχαὴλ τούτου Μαυραγάνου'. There are three more recipes ascribed to an *oktarios* of the Mauraganos *xenōn*, but without specifying his name; see Bennett (2003: 404–5). The Mangana recipes survive in the fourteenth-century Vaticanus gr. 299 and the Mauraganos ones in the fifteenth-century Parisinus gr. 2194. Finally, there is a recipe ascribed to a certain Kosmas *aktouarios* in the collection of *xenōnika* ascribed to Theophilos and surviving in the fourteenth-century manuscript Florentinus Laurentianus gr. plut. 75.19. The recipe has been edited by Kousis (1944a: 40). On this text, see Bennett (2017: 85–8).

162 Bennett (2017: 115).

163 On *archiatroi* in the Roman period with some evidence from early Byzantine Constantinople, see Nutton (1977: 210–12). Two epistles of Michael Choniates (*c.*1138–*c.*1222) are addressed to two *archiatroi*, George Kallistos and Nicholas Kalodoukes, 107, 131, ed. Lambros (1880) 201–3, 263–7. Later on, in the fifteenth century, Anthony Pyropoulos is also known as an *archiatros*. See Kousis (1946); and Appendix 5, V=Vindobonensis med. gr. 17.

164 Janin (1969: 560).

165 Bennett (2017: 110–18). It is worth noting that Michael VII restored the monastery of St George in the Mangana, but there is no evidence relating to the *xenōn*. See Janin (1969: 70–6); see also n. 125, above. Miller (1997: 185, 195, 205) believes that the Mangana *xenōn* was functioning in the fourteenth century solely on the basis of the dating of the surviving manuscript containing the recipes (Vaticanus gr. 299), without presenting any further evidence. This manuscript is a large medical miscellany and there is no evidence that the recipes are contemporaneous with the production of the codex. On this, see also the convincing argumentation by Bennett (2017: 112), based on evidence from other contents of the manuscript.

166 See n. 101, above.

167 Bennett (2017: 141) suggests that it might refer to the Maurianos *xenōn* founded by Emperor Romanos I Lakapenos (r. 919–44) in Constantinople.

surviving evidence to suggest either of these things.[168] It is certain, however, that John did hold this, most probably, honorific office, as is confirmed by contemporary letters and also its inclusion in the vast majority of the titles in surviving manuscripts of his works.[169] The award of this title implies some recognition of his medical services and expertise, might have been associated with a periodic income,[170] and shows Andronikos II's special respect for him.

4.2 John's literary output

4.2.1 Dating

John's earliest work is his monograph on uroscopy, *On Urines*. The chronology is confirmed by John in his *Medical Epitome* when, in writing about the diagnosis of urine, he refers to his long work on the subject where the reader would find a more detailed discussion.[171] The *Medical Epitome* was composed for the *parakoimōmenos* Alexios Apokaukos,[172] at some point after 1321, since Apokaukos was appointed to this office in the same year.[173] According to what John says in his proem to the first book of the *Medical Epitome*, his reason for writing it was so that it could be taken by Apokaukos on his diplomatic mission to the 'Hyperborean Scythians'.[174] By 'Hyperborean Scythians', John most probably referred to the Tatars of the Golden Horde.[175] We are not

[168] It is worth noting that there only two manuscripts, in which the title of John's *On Urines* includes the term *basilikos* [Venetus Marcianus V. 13 (coll. 1221), AD 1376, f. 25v: '*τοῦ σοφωτάτου καὶ λογιωτάτου βασιλικοῦ ἰατροῦ κυροῦ Ζαχαρίου τοῦ ἀκτουαρίου*'; and Parisinus gr. 2256, fifteenth century, f. 144v: '*τοῦ σοφωτάτου καὶ λογιωτάτου βασιλικοῦ ἰατροῦ, κυροῦ Ζαχαρίου, τοῦ ἀκτουαρίου*'], but this is not found in any title of his works in the numerous other surviving manuscripts and should most probably be considered a scribal addition. The term has rightly not been retained in the title of the critical edition of *On Urines* by Georgiou (2013: 398).

[169] See Appendix 5, *passim*.

[170] For example, Pseudo-Kodinos provides some information about sporadic payments linked to some high-ranking members of the court hierarchy. See Macrides, Munitiz, and Angelov (2013: 311–13). The rank of *aktouarios* is not found in Pseudo-Kodinos. On forms of payments connected with recipients of imperial offices in early Palaiologan Byzantium, see also Kyritses (1997: 165–84).

[171] JZA, *Medical Epitome*, 1.22, ed. Ideler (1842) II.383.31–3. Although John does not refer explicitly to the title of his work on uroscopy, he reports that the work consists of seven books: '*ἐν ἑπτὰ λόγοις βιβλίον*'.

[172] This is found in the dedication of the work, transmitted in a large number of the surviving manuscripts, and it either precedes or follows the main title of the work: '*τῷ παρακοιμωμένῳ τῷ Ἀποκαύκῳ*'. See Appendix 5, *passim*.

[173] *PLP* 1180. Apokaukos was in 1341 appointed *megas doux* by Andronikos III. Cf. Chapter 4, n. 31.

[174] JZA, *Medical Epitome*, 1.pr., ed. Ideler (1842) II.353.8–11. See also Chapter 4, Section 2.

[175] On the identification of the Scythians, see the long note by Kourousis (1984/8: 365–6, n.2), who provides copious references to primary and secondary sources. In particular, for references to Scythians by Palaiologan authors such as Pachymeres, Metochites, and Gregoras, see Kaldellis (2013: 156–66).

alerted to a particular embassy undertaken by Apokaukos by any contemporary source and thus we cannot be absolutely sure when John began to compose his *Medical Epitome*.[176] Apokaukos departed earlier than expected, as is confirmed in the last chapter of book one.[177] John started to work on his project again after Apokaukos' return, as we learn from the proem of book two.[178] Meanwhile, we are also informed that after the completion of book one, he wrote his treatise *On Psychic Pneuma* dedicated to Joseph Rhakendytes.[179] Joseph left Constantinople around 1326 and died around 1330.[180] Thus, not just the completion of the first book of the *Medical Epitome* but also John's work *On Psychic Pneuma* would most probably have been composed before 1326 and not later than 1330. At the end of the *Medical Epitome* there is mention of an Apokaukos going on another diplomatic mission, but John does not provide us with any further details.[181] Thus, we cannot date the completion of the *Medical Epitome* with certainty either. On the other hand, the potentially partly unfinished nature of John's work in the pharmacological section, as shown in Chapter 5,[182] could suggest that he died unexpectedly, around 1330.[183]

4.2.2 On Urines

The *On Urines* survives complete or in part in approximately forty manuscripts.[184] It was first published by Julius Ludwig Ideler,[185] who does not

[176] Kourousis (1984/8: 362–84) attempted to date Apokaukos' embassy by relating references in contemporary sources to the attested invasions of the Empire by the Mongols. He argues that the first book of the *Medical Epitome* and the treatise *On Psychic Pneuma* were written between January and March 1326. Although Kourousis provides an exhaustive study of all the available sources, his conclusions are debatable, since they are not based on a dated embassy attested in primary sources. Cf. Karpozilos (2008: 133), who dates the mission between 1323 and 1326.

[177] JZA, *Medical Epitome*, 1.57, ed. Ideler (1842) II.417.29–37. See also JZA, *On Psychic Pneuma*, 2.15.9, ed. Ideler (1841) I.380.4–14.

[178] JZA, *Medical Epitome*, 2.pr., ed. Ideler (1842) II.418.8–10, 419.10–15. See also JZA, *On Psychic Pneuma*, 2.15.10, ed. Ideler (1841) I.380.14–19.

[179] JZA, *Medical Epitome*, 2.pr., ed. Ideler (1842) II.418.21–5.

[180] On Joseph's departure from Constantinople, see Kourousis (1984/8: 363, n. 1). Regarding Joseph's death, see Treu (1899b: 33–4); and Sideras (1994: 55–6).

[181] JZA, *Medical Epitome*, 6, Vindobonensis med. gr. 17, f. 242v, ll. 18–20: '*σοὶ δὲ πρόκειται ἐπὶ πρεσβείαν αὖθις ἰέναι, ἔχεις μὲν ἀρκούντως ἐκ τῶν νῦν εἰρημένων ἐπὶ παντὸς ἀρρωστήματος διαγινώσκειν τε καὶ πράττειν τὰ δέοντα...*'; ed. Mathys (1556) II.563.13–17.

[182] Chapter 5, Section 4.2.

[183] See also Kourousis (1984/8: 390–5), who suggests that John might have left Constantinople around 1326 with Joseph Rhakendytes and spent the last years of his life in a monastery near Thessaloniki. It is worth noting that in the last chapter of *On Psychic Pneuma*, 2.17.27, ed. Ideler (1841) I.386.17–26, John expresses the hope that he may in the future be able to spend time with Joseph, which may help them to become closer and to manage collaboratively to understand better the intelligible cosmos (*noētos diakosmos*). On *noētos diakosmos*, see Chapter 6, n. 28.

[184] Diels (1906: II.109); Georgiou (2013: 175–307); *Pinakes: Textes et manuscrits grecs*, at http://pinakes.irht.cnrs.fr/notices/oeuvre/4315/ (accessed 29 September 2018); and Appendix 3.

[185] Ideler (1842) II.3–192. See Bühler (1990/3), who suggested some minor textual corrections to Ideler's text.

specify what manuscript(s) his edition is based on. The first book has been critically edited by Stavroula Georgiou,[186] who reproduces the long version of the title of the work, including a reference to John's office and all relevant appellations: 'Treatise on urines by the most wise and most erudite, most august, august *aktouarios*, *kyr* John Zacharias.'[187]

It is a specialized work on uroscopy for expert readers and is divided into seven books. The first serves as an introduction to the theoretical background to the method. The next six books concentrate on diagnosis (books two and three), aetiology (books four and five), and prognosis (books six and seven). John's approach is original both as regards its content and presentation. Several earlier theories on various urinary characteristics are revised and supplemented with the findings of the author himself, who is aware of wider medieval Mediterranean developments in the field. At some points, in presenting his theories, John expands his narration, first by using examples (*paradeigmata*) from his own engagement with the subject and secondly by embedding texts dealing with case histories (*historiai*) taken from his extensive clinical experience. This is the first time since Galen, almost twelve centuries earlier, that case histories have been seen in the Greek literature.

4.2.3 Medical Epitome

The *Medical Epitome* survives complete in twenty-six codices and there are thirteen more manuscripts that retain various fragments and excerpts.[188] It was partly published by Ideler (books one and two),[189] who—as in the case of *On Urines*—gives no details about the textual witness(es) that he used to establish the text. The remaining books (three to six) are unedited and are only available through a sixteenth-century Latin translation.[190] In citing passages from the unedited part, I use transcriptions from Vindobonensis med. gr. 17.[191] The work is usually mentioned in the literature by the Latin title, *Methodo Medendi* (*Method of Medicine*), given to it by its sixteenth-century translator.[192] I prefer to refer to it as the *Medical Epitome*, since this title corresponds to the title given in the majority of the manuscripts and fits better with its structure and contents.[193] It is dedicated to Alexios Apokaukos, who

[186] Georgiou (2013) 398–456.

[187] Georgiou (2013: 398): '*Τοῦ σοφωτάτου καὶ λογιωτάτου πανσεβάστου σεβαστοῦ τοῦ ἀκτουαρίου κυροῦ Ἰωάννου τοῦ Ζαχαρίου πραγματεία Περὶ Οὔρων*'.

[188] See Appendix 5. [189] Ideler (1842) II.353–463.

[190] Mathys (1554) 1–318 and (1556) II.153–563. There is also a partial edition of books five and six by Ruelle (1539). See Appendix 5, Section 2.3.

[191] See the relevant discussion in Appendix 5. [192] Mathys (1554).

[193] The usual title given in the manuscripts is: '*Βιβλίον ἰατρικόν, περιέχον πᾶσαν τέχνην ἐν ἐπιτόμῳ*' ('Medical book containing the entire art in an abridged version'). See Appendix 5, *passim*. As in the case of *On Urines*, there are some manuscripts which also include John's appellations.

took a lively interest in medicine. John refers consistently in his work to his friendship (*philia*) with Apokaukos,[194] which indicates a significant degree of intimacy between the two. Apokaukos is reported by the sources to be a tax collector of substance by 1321,[195] who has already managed to amass a great personal fortune. Thus, John's dedication can be also seen as a strategic plan to secure strong patronage.[196] A key player in the civil wars of the 1320s and 1340s, Apokaukos had managed to become the single most powerful individual, the de facto ruler of the Empire, shortly before his murder in 1345.[197]

As we will see in Chapter 4, the work is mainly written for the non-expert. It is divided into six books. The first two focus on diagnosis and the next two on various therapeutic methods. The last two books (five and six) concentrate solely on the composition of drugs, consisting of both traditional Greek and early Byzantine material, and newly introduced Arabic pharmacological lore. The work is mainly a compilation of earlier material and the author's presence is chiefly noticeable in the proem and epilogue of each book, where he presents his sources and outlines the structure of his work.

4.2.4 On the Activities and Affections of the Psychic Pneuma and the Corresponding Regimen

The *On Psychic Pneuma* survives in about thirty-five manuscripts dating to between the fourteenth and sixteenth centuries.[198] It was first printed in Greek in the sixteenth century.[199] Two further Greek editions were published in the late eighteenth century and early nineteenth century respectively.[200] It was written at the request of John's contemporary, the intellectual monk Joseph Rhakendytes, with the aim of helping the latter to keep his psychic pneuma in a purified state. In the text there is no evidence that John had been a student of

[194] See, for example, JZA, *Medical Epitome*, 1.pr. and 2.pr, ed. Ideler (1842) II.353.23–354.1 and 419.10.

[195] John Kantakouzenos, *History*, 3.14, ed. Schopen (1831) II.89.

[196] We are also aware of other prominent Byzantine *literati*, such as Theodore Hyrtakenos [*Epistle* 69, ed. Karpozilos and Fatouros (2017) 248–52], Michael Gabras [*Epistles* 197, 199, ed. Fatouros (1973) II.327.1–331.124, 331.1–332.12], and Nikephoros Gregoras [*Epistle* 119, ed. Leone (1982) 310–12], who sent congratulatory letters to Apokaukos, most probably, after his appointment as *parakoimōmenos*, in an attempt to secure his good will.

[197] Apokaukos was from a family of low social status in Bithynia and was educated in Constantinople (see Chapter 4, n. 29). On Apokaukos, see Stathakopoulos (forthcoming).

[198] Diels (1906: 108–9); and *Pinakes: Textes et manuscrits grecs*, at http://pinakes.irht.cnrs.fr/notices/oeuvre/3998/ (accessed 29 September 2018). See also Chapter 6, n. 21.

[199] Goupyl (1557).

[200] Fischer (1774) and Ideler (1841) I.312–86. The title of Ideler's edition reads: '*Περὶ Ἐνεργειῶν καὶ Παθῶν τοῦ Ψυχικοῦ Πνεύματος καὶ τῆς κατ' αὐτὸ Διαίτης*'. See also Chapter 6, n. 22. Hohlweg (1997) has proposed some textual emendations to Ideler's text. Furthermore, Kakavelaki (2016) proposed some useful new readings of corrupted passages in Ideler's edition, informed by her own consultation of manuscripts. In a personal communication, she confirmed that she is currently preparing a Modern Greek translation of John's *On Psychic Pneuma*.

Joseph Rhakendytes, as has previously been suggested.[201] The latter arrived in Constantinople around 1308[202] when John, as is confirmed in his correspondence with Lakapenos, was already a practising physician. John sometimes uses the term 'father' (*pateras*) when addressing Joseph, which should be seen in the light of Joseph's status as a member of the clergy and probably reflects a spiritual relationship.[203] In the text we are informed about meetings between John and Joseph in which they used to discuss philosophical matters. Joseph was also able to get involved in discussions about medicine with John and could perform venesection.[204]

The work is divided into two books as follows: theoretical aspects on the formation and roles of various kinds of pneumata (book one) and therapeutic agents (book two) with considerable attention given to diet. Throughout the treatise the psychic pneuma, which is dispersed through the body via the nerves and is responsible for sensory and motor activities, is the subject of significant attention. John introduces a new theory in which each of the four pneumata is correlated with two primary qualities (unnamed, 'gastric' pneuma: cold and moist; natural pneuma: warm and moist; vital pneuma: warm and dry; psychic pneuma: cold and dry). Any disturbance in the quality, for example, of the psychic pneuma may affect its flow and consequently it can be a cause of impairment. Ultimately, John made a direct connection between the quality of pneuma and someone's daily regimen, thus introducing a systematic classification of qualitative change in pneuma as an object of treatment.

4.2.5 John's other works

In the manuscript, Vindobonensis phil. gr. 219, which preserves John's only letter to Theodore Modenos, we find four short poems included immediately after the letter and ascribed to 'the same author' (*tou autou*).[205] They are iambic epigrams written in praise of certain icons.[206] The first epigram refers to the Annunciation, the next two to the Theotokos Brephokratousa

[201] Kousis (1933: 339, n. 3); and Pentogalos (1970: 10–11). Cf. Kourousis (1984/8: 353).

[202] Gielen (2016: lxxiii). See also Chapter 6, n. 3.

[203] JZA, *On Psychic Pneuma*, 1.pr.2, ed. Ideler (1841) I.313.1–2; and *Medical Epitome*, 2.pr, ed. Ideler (1842) II.418.19. A spiritual relationship between the two is implied in the following passages: JZA, *On Psychic Pneuma*, 1.pr.4, 1.20.14, and 2.17.25, ed. Ideler (1841) I.313.12–15, I.349.36–7, and I.386.16–17. John also twice asks Joseph to pray for him: JZA, *On Psychic Pneuma*, 1.20.14 and 1.17.25, ed. Ideler (1841) I.349.31–2 and I.386.10–13.

[204] On this and the meetings between John and Joseph, see Chapter 6, nn. 14 and 25.

[205] The part of the manuscript that contains the content in question (ff. 1r–176v) was written by John Anagnostes Apostolarios in 1337. See Hunger (1961: I.326–30), who provides a description of the codex and its contents; and Odorico (2017).

[206] On Palaiologan epigrams related to art, see Talbot (1999).

(Virgin Mary and Child), and the last one celebrates John the Baptist.[207] The latter epigram refers to brothers Andronikos and John Masgidas (*syngonōn Masgidadōn*) as the dedicators of the icon. They most probably belonged to the large family of the Masgigades attested in the area of Serres in the first half of the fourteenth century,[208] a place with which John was also connected. Unfortunately, there are no further details, which might permit us to identify the particular icons in question. Since the epigrams were copied together with John's letter, which was most probably written before 1299, it is probable that they were composed when he was young as a kind of school exercise.

In two more cases, we hear of other potential works by John through references in his *On Psychic Pneuma* and in the *Medical Epitome*.[209] In the first case, in the last chapter of book one of *On Psychic Pneuma*, John writes:

> This is not the right time to discuss whether character traits depend on the mixtures of the body; it is better to keep this idea for another instance. However, it is likely to talk specifically about the soul and the traits corresponding to it, and also about its activities and its association with the perceptible and intelligible order.[210]

[207] Epigram 1, 2, and 4 were edited by Treu (1899a) 39.21–40. These epigrams together with the fragmentary third one were (re-)edited by Kourousis (1984/8) 541–2. See also Kourousis' (1984/8: 145–7, 538–40) commentary, including his convincing discussion in favour of John's authorship of the epigrams.

[208] See Kourousis (1984/8: 146, n. 4); and Shukurov (2016: 197–200).

[209] These two cases were first pointed out by Kourousis (1984/8: 331–6). Furthermore, in the catalogue of manuscripts of the Greek libraries of Constantinople in the sixteenth century, which has survived in Vindobonensis hist. gr. 98, there is a reference to another potential work by John, actually a commentary on Aristotle's physiology. Papazoglou's (1983: 138) transcription of the title reads: '*Ἰωάννου Ὠκταρίου ἑρμηνεία εἰς τὴν φυσιολογίαν τοῦ Ἀριστοτέλους, τῶν τε ζώων πάντων*'. The relevant manuscript has not yet been identified. *Oktarios* is a vernacular version of *aktouarios*; on this see n. 151, above. Papazoglou suggests that the work might be identified with the one listed by Diels (1906: II.110) as having the title '*Περὶ ζῴων φθαρτικῶν*' and starting with the following phrase: '*ζῷα τοίνυν φθαρτικά ἐστι*'. However, this is not, in fact, a reference to a separate work by John, but is actually the title and the first sentence of the chapter on venomous animals at the end of the unedited book five of the *Medical Epitome*, Vindobonensis med. gr. 17, f. 161v, ll. 14–15: '*Περὶ ζῴων φθαρτικῶν: ζῷα τοίνυν φθαρτικὰ ἐστί…*'; ed. Mathys (1556) II.418.13–14: 'Itaque animalia lethalia sunt…'. Finally, John has sometimes been considered the translator into Greek of al-Rāzī's *Kitāb fī al-Judarī wa-al-Ḥaṣbah* [for a list of references, see Dimitradis (1971: 58); and Congourdeau (1996: 101, n. 10)], based on the title added by another hand ('*Περὶ λοιμικῆς τοῦ Ῥαζῆ: Ἑρμηνεία ἀκτουαρίου*', i.e. 'On Pestilential Disease by Rhazes: Explanation/Translation by Aktouarios') in the upper margin of Parisinus gr. 2228 (fourteenth/ fifteenth century), f. 39r. Taking into consideration John's role as a reviser of the Greek uroscopic treatise ascribed to Ibn Sīnā (see Section 4.2.6, below), we should not reject out of hand his potential involvement in a revised version of this treatise, too, especially in the absence of a critical edition and a detailed study of its textual transmission. The text survives in, at least, eleven manuscripts. A provisional list is available on *Pinakes: Textes et manuscrits grecs*, at https://pinakes.irht.cnrs.fr/notices/oeuvre/3526/ (accessed 29 September 2018).

[210] JZA, *On Psychic Pneuma*, 1.20.11, ed. Ideler (1841) I.349.13–18: '*Καὶ τὸ μὲν περὶ ἠθῶν μεταβαλλομένων ταῖς τοῦ σώματος κράσεσι λόγον, οὐ πάνυ τοι ὧδε προσήκοντα λέγεσθαι, ἐν ἄλλῃ σκέψει ἀποταμιεύεσθαι ἄμεινον. εἴη δ' ἄν ποτε ἰδίᾳ περὶ τε ψυχῆς καὶ τῶν κατ' αὐτὴν ἠθῶν φᾶναι, ἔτι δὲ ἐνεργειῶν καὶ κοινωνιῶν πρός τε τὸν αἰσθητὸν καὶ νοητόν διάκοσμον·*'.

Here John is clearly alluding to a subject that he would like to deal with in the future and which had been examined most famously in the past by Galen in his treatise *The Capacities of the Soul Depend on the Mixtures of the Body*.[211] However, we have no evidence that John eventually wrote about this topic.

In the second case, a passage from the unedited third book of his *Medical Epitome*, which deals with diet, gives further information about another potential work by John:

> The passions of the soul cannot be of any help to physicians because they do not follow any kind of <bodily> *dyskrasiai*. It is presumably better to adduce consolations in order to treat the soul that is swallowed by distress. For this reason I have tried to invent consolation every time I thought it appropriate, and it is possible to learn from there how to console those who happen to become distressed…you will learn all these things when you come across this book.[212]

It is evident from this that John had written a consolatory work (*paramythētikos logos*), intended to treat psychic distress. The work must have been written before his *Medical Epitome*, but it does not seem to have survived. This is not a medical treatise, but a psychotherapeutic work, something usually written by ancient philosophers in order to offer practical advice to combat distress.[213] The most illustrious example of a physician who is known to have written such a work is the 'physician-cum-philosopher' Galen with his *Avoiding Distress* (*Peri Alypias*).[214]

4.2.6 *John as a reviser of the Greek uroscopic treatise ascribed to Ibn Sīnā*

There is a short treatise in Greek on uroscopy ascribed to the Persian physician and polymath Ibn Sīnā (d. 1037). The text is found in many manuscripts in three textual forms. According to the title given in a group of textual

[211] Galen, *The Capacities of the Soul Depend on the Mixtures of the Body*, ed. Kühn (1822) IV.767–822 = ed. Bazou (2011).

[212] JZA, *Medical Epitome*, 3, Vindobonensis med. gr. 17, f. 62v, l. 21–63r l. 3: '*καὶ τὰ μὲν ψυχικὰ ταῦτα πάθη, οὐ ῥᾴδιον τοῖς ἰατροῖς βοηθεῖν· ἅτε μὴ ποιαῖς τισιν ἀκολουθήσαντα δυσκρασίαις· εἰ μή τισι μᾶλλον παραμυθοῦσι λόγοις οἵοίς τε οὖσι ψυχὴν καταποθεῖσαν λύπαις ἀνακαλέσασθαι· καί γε περὶ τούτου ἰδίᾳ ἡμῖν λόγος ἐξείργασται παραμυθίας ἐξευρίσκων ἐφ' ἑκάστῳ τῶν ἀτυχημάτων ὥς γ' ἐμοὶ δοκεῖ δεούσας, καὶ μαθεῖν ἐκεῖθεν ἔξεστιν οἷς τε παραμυθητέον τοὺς ἀτυχοῦντας λυπουμένους…κἄν που περὶ τύχης τῷ βιβλίῳ εἴσῃ περὶ τῶν εἰρημένων·*'; ed. Mathys (1556) II.176.19–26.

[213] Eratosthenes of Cyrene (third century BC), Diogenes of Babylon (second century BC), and Plutarch ('The catalogue of Lamprias', no. 172) were all said to have written a lost essay entitled *Peri Alypias*. Consolatory works written from a Christian perspective were also produced throughout the Byzantine era. See Hunger (1978: I.132–45); and Kourousis (1984/8: 332, n. 1).

[214] On Galen's theory of emotions, see Gill (2010: 243–329). More specifically, on psychotherapy in Galen's *Avoiding Distress*, see Xenophontos (2014). See also the volume by Singer (2014), which offers an English translation and commentary of Galen's psychological writings.

witnesses, John appears to be the reviser and editor of a version which has recently been critically edited by Mario Lamagna: 'Excellent treatise on urines by the most wise Alē among Indians, Avitzianos among Greeks, translated crudely into the Greek language by Christodoulos, most skilled in the medical art, and set out in Greek form and syntax by the *aktouarios*, *kyr* John Zacharias, most wise and most skilled in the medical art.'[215] Lamagna has discovered another, unedited, version of the text, which is only ascribed to the otherwise unknown physician mentioned above, one Christodoulos, without, this time, referring to his role as translator of the text.[216] In this form, which according to Lamagna seems to be the model for the later versions, the text is often characterized by improper use of Greek terms and incorrect syntax. Furthermore, the Greek translator/editor has added large sections of explanatory details on human physiology and some brief case histories situated in a Greek environment.[217] There is one more version, the briefest, which eliminates the sections on physiology and the case histories, although it is generally close to the Christodoulos version as regards the use of Greek terms.[218]

In my view, in the absence of the original text,[219] it is not certain that Christodoulos' version is a reworking of a translation from an oriental language into Greek, as has been suggested by Lamagna.[220] As I argue in Chapter 2, John was directly influenced by this treatise, since there are at least two uroscopic theories in this work, which are found in no other Byzantine work, apart from John's *On Urines*. The first of these involves the

[215] [Ibn Sīnā], *On Urines* (version edited by John Zacharias Aktouarios), ed. Lamagna (2017) 25.1–6: '*Τοῦ σοφωτάτου παρὰ μὲν Ἰνδοῖς Ἀλῆ, παρ' Ἕλλησι δὲ Ἀβιτζιάνου πραγματεία περὶ οὔρων ἀρίστη βαρβάρως εἰς τὴν Ἑλλάδα μετενεχθεῖσα γλῶτταν παρὰ τοῦ ἰατρικωτάτου Χριστοδούλου, εἰς ῥυθμὸν δὲ καὶ τάξιν Ἑλληνικὴν ἐκτεθεῖσα παρὰ τοῦ σοφωτάτου καὶ ἰατρικωτάτου Ἀκτουαρίου κυρίου Ἰωάννου τοῦ Ζαχαρίου*'. On the extensive manuscript transmission of the text and its various forms, see Lamagna (2011).

[216] See Lamagna (2016: 55). The text survives in two manuscripts. Parisinus Coislinianus 334 (fourteenth century), ff. 346r–335v, does not preserve the beginning of the text. Oxoniensis Bodleianus Thomae Roe 15 (fifteenth century), ff. 74r–83r, retains the following title: '*Περὶ οὔρων Χριστοδούλου ὡς ἐν συνόψει*' ('On urines by Christodoulos in the form of a synopsis').

[217] Lamagna (2017: 13).

[218] Lamagna (2017: 14). This was edited by Ideler (1842) II.286–302. The compiler of this version is unknown. For a comparison of this version with the one edited by John, see Lamagna (2003a).

[219] The uroscopic section in Ibn Sīnā's *Canon of Medicine* (*Kitāb al-Qānūn fī al-Ṭibb*), 1.2.3, (1593) I.68–74, has no content related to the treatise in question. This coincides with Lamagna's (2017: 11) conclusions. Cf. Lamagna (2017: 112, 114). There is only one known brief, unedited, and partly fragmentary, text on urines in Arabic by Ibn Sīnā, in Glasguensis Hunterianus 121 (AD 1339/40), which according to Lamagna (2011: 28) and (2017: 11) does not correspond to the text of the Greek translation.

[220] Lamagna (2017: 13): 'Già questa redazione attribuita a Cristodulo in realtà non è semplicemente una traduzione da una lingua orientale, ma piuttosto una rielaborazione di un testo arabo pensata per un pubblico di cultura greca…' ('In fact, this redaction attributed to Christodoulos is actually not simply a translation from an oriental language, but rather a reworking of an Arabic text conceived for an audience of Greek culture…').

particular importance given to a urinary characteristic called the ‘crown’ (*stephanē*) and the other is the notion of the relationship between certain areas in the uroscopic vial and parts of the human body.[221] Taking into consideration that the latter theory is first found in the works of Salernitan scholars of the twelfth century,[222] and that one of the versions of the name of Ibn Sīnā in Greek often appears in the title of some versions of the work in forms which suggest either a Latin or a vernacular Italian transliteration of his name into Greek,[223] it is tempting to suggest that the Byzantine version is the result of blending Arabic and Latin uroscopic lore through one or more stages of mediation.

Lamagna informs us that, compared to Christodoulos’ version, John’s version is indeed an improvement as regards the use of Greek vocabulary and syntax. Furthermore, the long sections on physiology in Christodoulos’ version are either summarized or omitted, and there are some additions, including further explanatory information, mainly derived from Theophilos’ *On Urines* and the

221 See Chapter 2, Section 2.7.

222 The earliest available text that provides details on this theory was written by Maurus of Salerno. On this, see Chapter 2, Section 2.7. Cf. Lamagna (2017: 119).

223 See the title of John’s version in n. 215, above. The title in the brief version provides a better transliteration of the Arabic version of Ibn Sīnā’s name, while when it refers to ‘*Ἀβιτζιανός*’, it specifies that this is what he is called by ‘Italians’. The title reads as follows, [Ibn Sīnā], *On Urines* (brief version), ed. Ideler (1842) II.286.1–6: ‘*Περὶ οὔρων πραγματεία ἀρίστη τοῦ σοφωτάτου παρὰ μὲν Ἰνδοῖς Ἄλλη Ἔμπνι τοῦ Σινᾶ ἤτοι Ἄλλη υἱοῦ τοῦ Σινᾶ, παρὰ δὲ Ἰταλοῖς Ἀβιτζιανοῦ*’ (‘Excellent treatise on urines by the most wise Allē Empni son of Sina, among Indians, or Allē son of Sina, <and> Avitzianos among Italians’). Ideler’s edition is not critical and does not provide sufficient information to identify the manuscript that his edition is based on. My examination of many manuscripts has shown that this is indeed a common version of the title of the brief version [see e.g. Parisinus gr. 2153 (fifteenth century), f. 170r; Parisinus gr. 2256 (fifteenth century), f. 529r; Parisinus gr. 2308 (fifteenth century), f. 1r; Londiniensis Harleianus 6295 (second half of the fifteenth century), f. 20v; Monacensis gr. 70 (c.AD 1550), f. 213r]. Furthermore, Scorialensis T.II.14 (fifteenth century), f. 186r, l. 2, (brief version) gives ‘*Ἀβιτζένα*’, and Venetus Marcianus gr. V. 8 (coll. 1334) (fourteenth century), f. 110r, l. 2 (version edited by John Zacharias Aktouarios) retains ‘*Ἀβετζιάνου*’; the latter has not been included by Lamagna (2017: 25) in his *apparatus criticus*. Lamagna (2017: 111) deals very briefly with this issue stating that ‘*Ἀβιτζιανος* è, infatti, una traslitterazione dell’arabo Abū ibn Sīnā…’ (‘*Ἀβιτζιανος* is, indeed, a transliteration of the Arabic Abū ibn Sīnā…’), although it is probably not as straightforward as he suggests. This is a complicated issue which cannot be fully investigated in the limited space of a footnote. It is clear that there is no stable version of Ibn Sīnā’s name in medieval Greek and it could also change also in line with the tastes and background of the scribe. For example, a sixteenth-century manuscript, Monacensis gr. 362, f. 215v, l. 22, of the brief version gives ‘*Ἀβικένα*’, which coincidentally is the version given by the fifteenth-century scholar Cardinal Bessarion in his philosophical work *Against the Slanderer of Plato* (e.g. 3.21.5 and 3.25.1, ed. Mohler, 1927, 352.27 and 400.30). The latter is the only other reference to Ibn Sīnā in the edited Byzantine literature. Linguistically, the Greek ‘*τζ*’ may be derived from the medieval Italian ‘z’. ‘Avizen(n)a’ is found in two thirteenth-century non-medical sources, actually notarial documents from Bologna [22 November 1268, ed. Zaccagnini (1927) 151] and Cividale [12 December 1291, ed. Scalon (1995) 149], which reflect vernacular oral versions of Ibn Sīnā’s name. I would like to thank Joël Chandelier (Paris) for these references. Lastly, it should be noted that I have not managed to locate any edited or unedited uroscopic treatise ascribed to Ibn Sīnā in Latin.

Hippocratic *Aphorisms* and the *Prognostic*.[224] Finally, it should be noted that there is not sufficient evidence to date John's own revision of Christodoulos' version precisely, but it must have been before the composition of his *On Urines*.[225]

4.3 John's use of language

Lastly, some remarks on John's use of language may be helpful in elucidating his intellectual background. Bearing in mind that all of John's works contain what is, for the most part, technical information, there is little room for any great degree of linguistic embellishment.[226] At times, however, we can glimpse an attempt to use syntactical structures or forms of words, which imitate classical Greek; this is usually more obvious in his proems and epilogues, which afford more opportunities for literary elaboration. Thus, there is occasional use of the verb *echō* accompanied by an infinitive to indicate capability,[227] use of the infinitive with the definite article as a noun,[228] and use of a singular verb with neuter plural as subject.[229] Furthermore, we can sometimes see use of the dual number,[230] use of the classical comparative form,[231] repeated use of krasis when *kai* comes before a preposition or adverb[232] and when the

[224] Lamagna (2017: 15–16). See also Lamagna's (2016) brief study, in which he provides some helpful examples of comparisons between the two versions.

[225] This is also in agreement with Kourousis (1984/8: 384).

[226] See, for example, Kourousis (1984/8: 142–5), who argues that John uses a simple Greek style. Kourousis goes a step further in suggesting that John follows Nikephoros Choumnos' advice on clarity concerning the use of language in contrast to Theodore Metochites, who preferred the use of elaborate Greek. On the supposed 'rivalry' between Choumnos and Metochites concerning language, see Ševčenko (1962: 51–67). More specifically, on Metochites' language, see Hinterberger (2001); and Polemis (2002: 155–9). For a brief introduction to the classicizing language of Palaiologan literature, see Browning (1978: 124–8); and Horrocks (2010: 268–71). On medieval Greek language in general, see Holton and Manolessou (2010).

[227] JZA, *Medical Epitome*, 1.pr, ed. Ideler (1842) II.353.14: '*ἔχῃς παραμυθεῖσθαι*'; and *On Psychic Pneuma*, 1.pr.1, ed. Ideler (1841) I.312.12–13: '*ἂν ἔχοις…εἰδέναι*'.

[228] JZA, *On Urines*, 2.pr.1, ed. Ideler (1842) II.31.24: '*τὸ μανθάνειν*'.

[229] JZA, *On Urines*, 1.21.5, ed. Ideler (1842) II.29.31–2: '*εἴτε τὰ χρώματα, εἴτ' ἀμφότερα ἀλλοιοῦται*'; and JZA, *On Urines*, 2.3.3, ed. Ideler (1842) II.34.12: '*τὰ οὖρα ψύχηται*'.

[230] JZA, *On Urines*, 2.5.8, ed. Ideler (1842) II.37.13–14: '*καὶ δὴ δυοῖν μὲν οὔσαιν ταῖν παθητικαῖν ποιητήταιν, δυοῖν δ' αὖ ταῖν δραστικαῖν τε καὶ ποιητικαῖν*'; *On Urines*, 4.13.1, ed. Ideler (1842) II.96.27–8: '*δυοῖν τοίνυν οὔσαιν ταῖν δραστικαῖν τε καὶ ποιητικαῖν ποιοτήταιν, δυοῖν δ' αὖ ταῖν παθητικαῖν*'; and *On Psychic Pneuma*, 1.11.5, ed. Ideler (1841) I.332.3: '*δυοῖν δυάδοιν τὸ τῆς ψυχῆς δοξαστικόν*'. On the use of the dual number in the Palaiologan period, see the brief case study by Perentidis (1980).

[231] JZA, *On Urines*, 1.20.5 and 2.3.4, ed. Ideler (1842) II.28.23 and II.34.20–1: '*πρωϊαίτερον*'; *On Urines*, 2.3.4, ed. Ideler (1842) II.34.19–20; *On Psychic Pneuma*, 1.12.4, ed. Ideler (1841) I.333.2; and *Medical Epitome*, 1.36, ed. Ideler (1842) II.393.21: '*σχολαίτερον*'.

[232] JZA, *On Psychic Pneuma*, 1.19.7, ed. Ideler (1841) I.347.7: '*κἀπί*'; and *Medical Epitome*, 2.5, ed. Ideler (1842) II.441.8: '*κἀνταῦθα*'.

preposition *pro* comes before a verb.[233] He also uses hyperbaton.[234] Finally, John's language shows some characteristics of contemporary Byzantine Greek. For instance, we can trace a flexibility in the use of moods in subordinate clauses, e.g. the use of *opotan* and *epeidan* with an optative (instead of subjunctive) as a response to a main verb in the present tense,[235] and use of the optative (instead of subjunctive) after *hina* as a response to a main verb in the present tense.[236] Moreover, we attest use of *ethelō* with the infinitive to indicate the future,[237] and of double negative.[238]

[233] JZA, *On Psychic Pneuma*, 2.3.11, ed. Ideler (1841) I.355.16: 'προὐθέμεθα'; *On Urines*, 6.4.3, ed. Ideler (1842) II.151.26: 'προὐξένησαν'; *On Psychic Pneuma*, 1.16.9, ed. Ideler (1841) I.343.8: 'προὐτρέπετο'; and *On Urines*, 6.13.18, ed. Ideler (1842) II.166.29–30: 'προὐχώρει'.

[234] JZA, *On Urines*, 7.pr.4, ed. Ideler (1842) II.171.29–172.1: 'τῆς ἐπὶ τοὺς κάμνοντας προγνώσεως'; and *Medical Epitome*, 2.pr, ed. Ideler (1842) II.418.8: 'τοῦ τῆς φιλίας καλοῦ'.

[235] JZA, *Medical Epitome*, 2.pr, ed. Ideler (1842) II.418.4–6: 'στέργουσί τε…ἐπειδάν…διαστήσειεν'.

[236] JZA, *On Urines*, 2.3.4, ed. Ideler (1842) II.34.21–5: 'προσήκει σκέπτεσθαι…ἵνα…μετατεθείη'.

[237] JZA, *On Psychic Pneuma*, 1.6.19, ed. Ideler (1841) I.324.23: 'προσέχειν τις ἐθέλει'. See *GMG*, p. 1868.

[238] JZA, *On Urines*, 7.3.5, ed. Ideler (1842) II.175.24: 'μὴ οὐχί'; and *On Urines*, 4.1.8, ed. Ideler (1842) II.80.26: 'μὴ οὐκ'.

2

On Urines

Byzantine Uroscopy between Tradition and Innovation

> Here begynneth the seynge of uryns, of all the colours that uryns be of: with medycynes annexed to euery uryne, and euery uryne his urynall . . . moche profytable for euery man to knowe.[1]

Modern techniques of urinalysis were only introduced at the end of eighteenth century. The isolation of uric acid from kidney stones by the pioneering Swedish chemist Carl Wilhelm Scheele (1742–86) and the analysis of diabetic urine by Matthew Dobson (1732–84) constituted the first steps towards the modern era of laboratory examinations by introducing chemical analysis.[2] In contrast to the highly developed modern microscopic techniques, ancient and medieval medical practitioners could only examine the urine sample macroscopically. Various features of the urine from colour to sediment were scrutinized by physicians in an attempt to diagnose and prognosticate the patient's clinical condition.

This chapter aims to contextualize John's *On Urines* by commenting on specific points of interest in light of the earlier and contemporary, Greek, Arabic, and Latin treatises on the subject. The first section deals with John's intended audience and how he constructs his authority based on his rich clinical experience. The notable division of John's work into individual diagnostic, aetiological, and prognostic sections will also be examined separately. The focus then shifts to a number of uroscopic theories such as on urine production, urine colour, and the urine vial, in order to get a better understanding of John's original contributions. It will also help us assess the extent to which he was influenced by the Greek uroscopic treatise ascribed to Ibn

[1] Title of an anonymous English epitome on uroscopy published for the first time in 1525, with at least ten subsequent printings in the sixteenth century.

[2] On the introduction of urinalysis, see Ramsey (2005).

Innovation in Byzantine Medicine: The Writings of John Zacharias Aktouarios (c.1275–c.1330). Petros Bouras-Vallianatos, Oxford University Press (2020). © Petros Bouras-Vallianatos.
DOI: 10.1093/oso/9780198850687.001.0001

Sīnā, especially on the notion of the analogies between parts of the human body and the areas marked in the urine vial. The chapter begins with a brief critical overview of the development of uroscopy since antiquity.

1. THE ART OF EXAMINING URINE

The examination of urine in the interpretation of a patient's clinical condition never occupied a central role in the ancient world.[3] Physicians showed a great interest in the examination of the pulse, which was studied in extreme detail. Medical authors such as Galen described several categories according to their various characteristics, and highly specialized, long treatises (e.g. *On Diagnosis by the Pulse*, *On Prognosis by the Pulse*, *On the Different Kinds of the Pulse*, *On the Causes of the Pulse*) were written on the subject.[4] The first references to uroscopy may be found in the Hippocratic corpus, in special sections devoted to the subject, mainly, in the *Aphorisms* and the *Prognostic* together with some scattered cases in the *Epidemics*.[5] In the Hippocratic texts various characteristics of urine such as the colour and the appearance of sediment (*hypostasis*) are considered. The presence of suspended (*enaiōrēma*) particles and 'clouds' (*nephelē*) is also noted, but no clear distinction is made between them. The best urine, which indicates a speedy recovery, is one which is smooth with white sediment (*leukē hypostasis*) for the entire period of the illness until the crisis according to the *Prognostic*,[6] while the focus may be either on diagnosis or prognosis. As regards nosology, several changes during fevers are first recorded in connection with urine—with a particular emphasis on crises.

Galen never wrote a single treatise on this topic. He described human digestion in terms of three phases. The first takes place in the stomach, producing faeces that pass through the pylorus into the duodenum and the intestines; from there the veins absorb the nutritious parts which are

[3] For the history of urology, including references to uroscopy, from ancient to medieval times, although most of them are now somewhat outdated, see Vieillard (1903); Desnos (1914: I.1–294); Neuburger (1937); and Wershub (1970). For an introduction to urine in the ancient world, see Muth (1968). On urine inspection in antiquity, see Stettler (1988).

[4] On Galenic sphygmology, see Harris (1973: 397–431).

[5] E.g. [Hippocrates], *Aphorisms*, 4.69–83 and 7.31–9, ed. Littré (1844) IV.526.7–532.8 = ed. Jones (1931) 152.18–156 and ed. Littré (1844) IV.584.8–588.7 = ed. Jones (1931) 198.10–200; *Epidemics*, e.g. 1.1.3, ed. Littré (1840) II.610.5–9 = ed. Jouanna (2016) 6.5–7; *Epidemics*, 3.1.2, 3.1.3, ed. Littré (1841) III.34.2–38.6, III.40.2–44.6 = ed. Jouanna (2016) 63.10–65.3, 65.9–68.12; *Epidemics*, 4.1.14, ed. Littré (1846) V.152.7–15; and *Epidemics*, 7.1.92, ed. Littré V.448.10–11 = ed. Jouanna (2000) 104.15–105.1. For a brief survey of Hippocratic uroscopy, see Marketos (1994).

[6] [Hippocrates], *Prognostic*, 12, ed. Littré (1840) II.138.15–142.15 = ed. Jouanna (2013) 32.5–37.2.

transferred through the portal vein into the liver, i.e. the place of the second digestion, in which a process of sanguification takes place producing blood. The blood is purified by the removal of the light waste-products that pass into the gall bladder and the heavy ones that pass into the spleen, where they turn into yellow and black bile respectively. Finally, through the vena cava the venous blood reaches the organs and parts of the body where the third digestion takes place, which is responsible for the creation of residues, such as sweat.[7] Meanwhile, at the end of the sanguification in the liver, a thin serous blood is also produced which must be eliminated; this is absorbed by the kidneys as a source of nutrition, where it is further purified, leading to the separation of the urine from the blood.[8] Colour gradually became the index of digestive power and thus an important element in the diagnosis of humoral excess. Galen identified various urinary characteristics as an outcome of partial digestion, while he describes the colour of healthy urine as yellowish (*hypoxanthon*) or reddish-yellow (*hypopyrron*).[9]

The most important step in moving uroscopy centre stage was made in the next few centuries.[10] Magnos (*c.*fourth/fifth century) was most probably the first author to write a treatise dealing solely with the examination of urine.[11]

[7] On Galen's theories about digestion and nutrition, see Cirenei (1961: 29–37); May (1968: 52–5); and Debru (2008: 273–5). The most detailed treatment of the subject is made in Galen's *On the Natural Capacities* and *On the Function of the Parts of the Body*, with scattered references throughout the works. In particular, on the numbering of the three digestions, see *On Good and Bad Humours*, 5, ed. Kühn (1823) VI.785–7 = ed. Helmreich (1923) 410–11. See also his discussion on the three kinds of nutriment in *On the Natural Capacities*, 3.13, ed. Kühn (1821) II.200.6–202.17 = ed. Helmreich (1893) III.246.10–248.7. A synoptic view of the ancient physicians who wrote on the subject is also given by the early Byzantine author Stephen, in his commentary on Hippocrates' *Prognostic*, 2.12, ed. Duffy (1983) 168.20–4.

[8] On the separation of urine from blood in the kidneys, see Siegel (1968: 126–32); and McVaugh (2012: 105–10).

[9] Galen, *On Crises*, 1.12, ed. Kühn (1825) IX.595.4–6 = ed. Alexanderson (1967) 97.18–22.

[10] For a study of Byzantine uroscopy, see Dimitriadis (1971); and Diamandopoulos (1997). Contributions by several authors and a selection of all original texts dealing with uroscopy in Byzantium are also available in the edited volume by Diamandopoulos (2000). On urology in Byzantium, see Malakates (1993).

[11] Bussemaker (1847) argues that chapters 1–28 and 30–6 of the treatise ascribed to Galen and edited by Kühn (1830) XIX.574–601 contain Magnos' work. There is also a synoptic version of this work edited by Ideler (1842) II.307–16. On the identification of Magnos, see Nutton in *DNP*, s.v. Magnus, [1] and [5]. See Touwaide (2002b), who provides a commentary on the treatise published by Kühn. Magnos also appears as the first authority on the subject after Hippocrates and Galen in the list of writers on urines in the proem of Theophilos' *On Urines*, ed. Ideler (1841) I.261.3–5. There is one more Pseudo-Galenic uroscopic treatise, edited by Moraux (1985), which has similarities with Magnos' version in Kühn, but it has clearly been elaborated in a late Byzantine milieu, as is attested by references to, for examples, sugar-based potions such as juleps. On sugar-based potions, see Chapter 5, Section 5.1. Furthermore, there is a uroscopic treatise attributed to Stephen, see Angeletti and Cavarra (1997); and Lamagna (2003b). The text was published by Bussemaker (1845). There are also some surviving scholia on Magnos' work by Stephen. See Lamagna (2010). Stephen is most probably to be identified with the early Byzantine (*c.*sixth/seventh century) author of Hippocratic and Galenic commentaries. For a recent summary of the *status quaestionis*, see Boudon-Millot (2016).

Undoubtedly the most influential Byzantine work was written by Theophilos (seventh or ninth century).[12] The treatise consists of twenty-six chapters written using division (*diairesis*), that is where the author divides and subdivides his work into individual sections, in this case concerning the various urinary characteristics, which are clearly connected with specific conditions of health and diseases.[13] The consistency (*systasis*) of the urinary liquid can be identified as thin (*leptē*), thick (*pacheia*) or symmetric (*symmetros*).[14] The colour spectrum has a total of twenty different shades, providing considerable detail in terms of variation as, for example, in the case of white. Apart from the crystal white (*leukon*), there are three more kinds: milk-white (*galaktōdes*), grey-white (*glaukon*), and greyish-white or grey (*charopon*).[15] Moreover, the various kinds of particles (*paryphistamena*) can be distinguished by colour, their place in the urine vial, shape, and consistency.[16] The work was translated into Latin, included in the earliest version of the *Articella* (the most popular medieval Latin medical textbook) and was widely circulated in the West.[17]

In Byzantium, interest in uroscopy never ceased, with several anonymous short treatises or synopses of early Byzantine works on the subject being compiled.[18] Among them, we can see a number of texts attributed to Syrian, Persian, and Arab physicians.[19] The most notable example is the treatise ascribed to Ibn Sīnā, one version of which was revised and edited by John.[20] This provides the first reference in Byzantine uroscopy to a potential 'crown' (*stephanē*),[21] which might be present in the urine and according to its colour and location in the urine vial may indicate various states of health.[22] Finally, mention should be made of the short treatise on uroscopy in the form of a

[12] The work is available in Ideler (1841) I.261–83. I would like to thank Piero Tassinari for allowing me to consult the text of his unpublished critical edition. See also Angeletti et al. (2009), who provides an English translation and commentary of Theophilos' text.

[13] Theophilos, *On Urines*, pr., ed. Ideler (1841) I.261.20–2. This method of division is known from antiquity; see Talamanca (1977: 3–189) and Mansfeld (1992: 326–31). On the Alexandrian method of division with additional examples in the later period, see Ieraci Bio (2003).

[14] Theophilos, *On Urines*, 4, ed. Ideler (1841) I.264.18–265.2.

[15] Theophilos, *On Urines*, 7.1, ed. Ideler (1841) I.268.7–8. On the colours *glaukon* and *charopon* in the ancient literature, see the special study by Maxwell-Stuart (1981: I.175–6, II.72–3), who provides a special section on Theophilos.

[16] Theophilos, *On Urines*, 11–21, ed. Ideler (1841) I.274.1–281.27.

[17] On the reception of Theophilos' treatise in the Latin West, see Angeletti and Gazzaniga (1999); and Wallis (2000a); and Moulinier-Brogi (2012: 49–57).

[18] See for example, ed. Ideler (1842) II.323–7.

[19] See, for example, ed. Ideler (1842) II.303–4, II.305–6. There are other treatises attributed to foreign physicians, as yet unedited; see Touwaide (2000) and (2004), who gives a list of manuscripts containing such works.

[20] On the various versions of the treatise, see the relevant discussion in Chapter 1, Section 4.2.6.

[21] It is literally translated as 'ring'; in the Latin literature it is attested as 'circulus' (see n. 31, below).

[22] [Ibn Sīnā], *On Urines* (brief version), 3, ed. Ideler (1842) II.287.9ff; and [Ibn Sīnā], *On Urines* (version edited by John Zacharias Aktouarios), 1, ed. Lamagna (2017) 25.7ff.

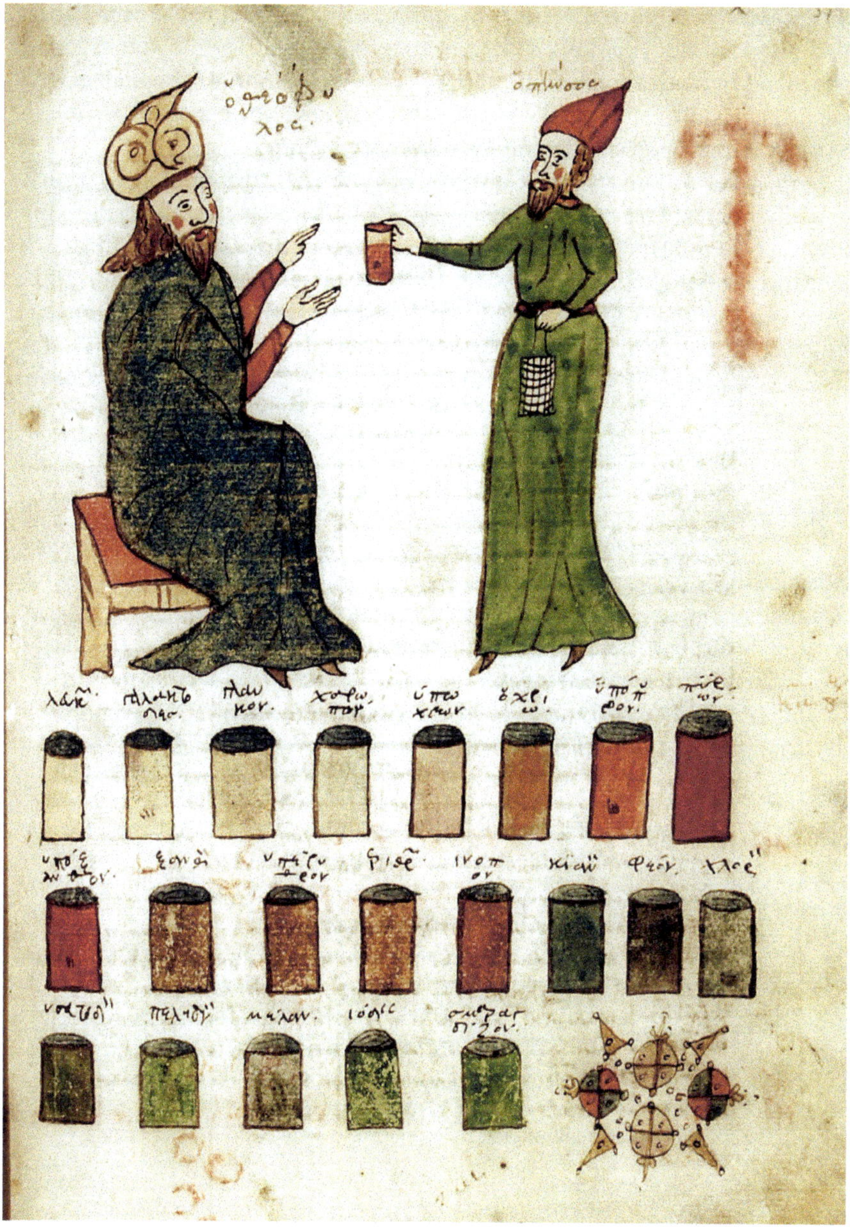

Figure 2.1. Theophilos examining a urine sample in the upper register and three rows of urine vials painted in various colours, as discussed in his treatise, in the bottom register. Bononiensis 3632 (mid fifteenth century), f. 51r.

liturgical canon attributed to Nikephoros Blemmydes.[23] Although the text offers nothing particularly new and seems to have been written for the non-expert, it shows late Byzantine interest in providing useful details in a memorable form and makes an interesting parallel with Gilles de Gorbeil's (*c.*1140–early thirteenth century) uroscopic poem, which will be discussed below.

Among the Arabic contributions to the subject,[24] the most popular one is certainly the *Book of Urine* (*Kitāb al-Bawl*) by the Jewish philosopher and physician from Egypt Isḥāq ibn Sulaymān al-Isrāʾīlī (d. *c.*932).[25] The treatise is divided into ten chapters in the Latin edition, and takes into consideration earlier Greek uroscopic lore, while it also includes a separate section on prognosis. A theory connecting four basic colours, including several variations thereof, with the four humours of the human body runs through the treatise, and seems to derive, directly or indirectly, from the now-lost work of the Nestorian Christian Job of Edessa, written in Syriac in the early ninth century.[26] More concise in terms of structure and organization is Ibn Sīnā's (d. 1037) uroscopic section in his long *Canon of Medicine* (*Kitāb al-Qānūn fī al-Ṭibb*).[27] This is divided into thirteen thematic parts, discussing several urinary characteristics, such as colour, consistency, odour, and sediment, and paying particular attention to age and gender. His emphasis on the need to collect urine in the early morning with the patient abstaining from sex on the night before, as well as his advice on examining urine out of direct sunlight, are noteworthy.

By the twelfth century urine vials had been established as the 'insignia' of physicians in the eyes of their contemporaries.[28] Uroscopy was studied in great

[23] Nikephoros Blemmydes, *Canon on Urines*, ed. Ideler (1842) II.318–22. See the discussion of the didactic and memorable nature of the treatise in Chapter 4, Section 1. For a commentary from a medical point of view, see Diamandopoulos (1995). A significant section on urines is also found in Michael Psellos' *Poem on Medicine*, 442–528, ed. Westerink (1992) 205–8. On this work, see Chapter 4, Section 1.

[24] On uroscopy in medieval Islamic medical tradition, see Massry et al. (1997: 239–40); Collins and Sussman (1999); Pormann and Savage-Smith (2007: 55); Massry (2009); and Visi (2015: 41–5).

[25] The text is available through a sixteenth-century Latin edition by Trot (1515: 156r–203r), reproduced by Fontana (1966: 143–239). An Italian translation by Fontana (1966: 25–139) based on the Latin version and accompanied by a commentary, is also available. The work was translated into Hebrew and Latin and was well received in both cultures. See Veit (2015) and Richler (2015). On the various versions of the text, see the preliminary comments by Visi (2015: 47–9).

[26] Visi (2015: 53–62).

[27] Ibn Sīnā, *Canon of Medicine* (*Kitāb al-Qānūn fī al-Ṭibb*), 1.2.3, (1593) I.68–74. The section does not discuss 'crowns', and its contents are not related to the Byzantine treatise on uroscopy ascribed to Ibn Sīnā. See also Chapter 1, n. 218. A shorter version of Ibn Sīnā's uroscopic theories, which does not, however, provide any further details, is also found in his *Poem on Medicine* (*Urjūzah fī al-Ṭibb*), 425–65, ed. Jahier and Noureddine (1956) 40–3. For an introduction and English translation, see Krueger (1963).

[28] For a detailed survey of uroscopic depictions in medieval visual culture, see Zglinicki (1982). McVaugh (1997) provides a study of the sociocultural context of the medieval Western 'bedside' examination, and Wallis (2000b) discusses the importance of pulse and urine examination in the medieval West. See also Moulinier-Brogi (2012: 166–90).

detail by Salernitan physicians and was taught at universities in the West.[29] Perhaps the most famous treatise on the subject in terms of content and structure was *On Urines*, composed by the French physician Gilles de Gorbeil, who studied at Salerno.[30] This is a Latin poem, 352 lines long, in an easily memorable form intended for contemporary students. He distinguishes twenty different colours in urine—mainly based on Theophilos. We also find a reference to the 'crown' (*circulus*), at the top of the urine vial, which is differentiated from the rest of the urine by its colour.[31] Uroscopy experienced a gradual decline in the later sixteenth century, losing its pre-eminent status by the seventeenth century, when learned physicians insisted on its limited diagnostic value.[32]

2. JOHN'S UROSCOPIC TREATISE

2.1 Audience and the construction of his authority

The work is 190 printed pages long, which makes it the longest medieval treatise produced on this topic. To give an indication, Theophilos' work is only 23 printed pages long, while Isḥāq al-Isrā'īlī's covers around 100 printed pages in its Latin version. In addition to the considerable length of John's work, it shows a good deal of originality, compared to his *Medical Epitome*, in which a substantial part of the content is a compilation of earlier material. Before we focus on John's theories, I will start by presenting his intentions regarding the writing of his work in order to give a better idea of his audience and his authority, as reflected in the text. Already in the proem John is attempting to communicate directly with his readers:

> A long time ago I wanted to engage myself with a work that would give honour and focused on theories which <, however,> do not produce pleasure in <the process of> reading; <so> I thought of doing something worthy of zeal. When I understood that I was engaged with other things which seemed vain, I decided to abstain completely from such an occupation, turn my attention to, and if possible write down, those accounts that would also serve others, once recorded.[33, 34]

[29] On Salernitan uroscopy, see Keil (1969); Oldoni (1994) and (2004); and Moulinier-Brogi (2012: 59–71). On Gilles de Corbeil, see Wallis (2005a).

[30] See Kliegel (1972), who provides the text, a German translation, and detailed commentary.

[31] Gilles de Corbeil, *On Urines*, 220–34, ed. Kliegel (1972) 44.

[32] Stolberg (2009: 167–212).

[33] Here I follow Georgiou's critical edition (2013) 401.7–8, which reads: '*τισιν ἑτέροις γραφέντα λυσιτελήσαιεν*' as compared to Ideler (1842) II.3.7–8: '*τίσιν ἄλλοις λυσιτελήσειεν*'.

[34] JZA, *On Urines*, 1.pr.1, ed. Ideler (1842) II.3.1–8: '*Πάλαι μὲν ἴσως φιλοτιμίας ἔργον τιθέμενος περὶ ἐκείνους μᾶλλον ἀναστρέφεσθαι τῶν λόγων, οἳ τὴν χάριν τῇ ἀναγνώσει συγκαταπαύουσι, διενοούμην τι πράττειν προθυμίας ἄξιον· ἐπεὶ δ' ἐμαυτὸν τοῖς ἄλλοις παιδευόμενον ἔγνων ἐπὶ κενῷ σπουδάζοντα, ἀφεκτέον τε εἶναι τοιαύτης λόγων σπουδῆς ἐνόμισα δεῖν, κἀκεῖνα μᾶλλον εἴ τις δύναμις γράφειν σπουδάζειν, ὅσα ἂν καὶ τίσιν ἄλλοις λυσιτελήσειεν.*'

John starts his work with a reference to *philotimia* (love of honour) revealing his yearning to achieve social prominence by writing scholarly works. The use of this term is common among authors of the Second Sophistic,[35] and it was revived in the works of the early Palaiologan authors.[36] It is in this environment, i.e. that of a highly educated elite, that John attempts to establish himself as a medical authority in the capital by contributing something novel to the most popular diagnostic method of his time. The last sentence of the passage cited above reveals one more classical *topos*, that is the idea of serving others through benevolent actions.[37] John also chooses to end his work in the same vein.[38] Although this could be seen as a highly rhetorical motif, whereby John tries to engage his readers by showing his eagerness to share his knowledge, it is also an indication of his awareness of the need to provide useful advice on diagnosing, prognosticating, and subsequently treating human disease effectively.

Later on, in the second chapter of the first book, John provides us with a brief background to the art of uroscopy:

> For I do not know the reason that wise men, who lived before us, showed little care about these things [i.e. uroscopic theories]. In fact, Hippocrates, the most wise, having said a little of this subject here and there, left the theory <on uroscopy> incomplete. On the other hand, the skilful Galen paid only a little attention to these things [i.e. uroscopic theories] . . . ; Magnos, Alexander, and in addition to them Theophilos and some others who have studied these <topics> appeared to pronounce more <theories> than the others. However, the subject <of uroscopy> was left incomplete even by them . . . ; they did not take into account the differences in or the causes or any other feature that appear necessary to a comprehensive treatment <of the subject of uroscopy>. Up to the present day, I have seen that the medical art has been exalted in a variety of treatises, and a great deal has been discovered by Hippocrates, Galen, and other men [i.e. medical authors] after them, but the subject of urine has been treated insufficiently and indeed this needs to be counterbalanced . . . [39]

[35] Whitmarsh (2005: 12, 38–9).

[36] See, for example, George Lakapenos, *Epistle* 32, ed. Lindstam (1924) 193.21; and Theodore Metochites, *Sententious Remarks*, 1.2, ed. Hult (2002) 24.1. See also the relevant discussion by Gaul (2011: 23–5).

[37] The notion is also prevalent in various Galenic treatises. For example in his *The Best Doctor is also a Philosopher*, 1, ed. Kühn (1821) I.57.8–9 = ed. Boudon-Millot (2007a) 288.5, he advances the social implications of medicine, asserting that its final end is to benefit mankind. In this respect, see Eichholz (1959: 70). For the relevant evidence from the Hippocratic corpus, see Horstmanshoff (1990: 194–6).

[38] Cf. JZA, *On Urines*, 7.18.14, ed. Ideler (1842) II.192.13–14: '*Τῷ δὲ πρὸς τὸ φιλάνθρωπον ἀφεωρακότι τῆς τέχνης* . . .' ('This work is meant to contribute to the benevolent <purpose> of the <medical> art . . .').

[39] JZA, *On Urines*, 1.2.1–3, ed. Ideler (1842) II.4.30–5.13: '*Ἐπεὶ γὰρ τοῖς πρὸ ἡμῶν περὶ τὰ τοιαῦτα σοφοῖς βραχύ τι περὶ τοῦδ' οὐκ οἶδα ὅπως ἐμέλησεν—ὁ μὲν γὰρ σοφώτατος Ἱπποκράτης ὀλίγα τινὰ περὶ τούτων εἰρηκὼς σποράδην, ἀτελῆ τὴν θεωρίαν παρῆκε, Γαληνῷ δὲ τῷ δεινῷ περὶ τὰ*

A similar account, which perhaps inspired John's, is also found at the beginning of Theophilos' treatise.[40] John does not hesitate to criticise Hippocrates[41] and Galen[42] for having dealt too briefly with the examination of urine. The sporadic presence of uroscopic advice in the Hippocratic corpus and the brief treatment by Galen have already been mentioned in the first part of this chapter. Although John acknowledges the considerable contribution of later medical authors such as Magnos, Alexander,[43] and Theophilos, he rightly identifies the lack of details, for example, on aetiology by those authors, which together with their brief, even aphoristic, treatment of prognosis never amount to a complete study of the topic. However, by referring to the earlier tradition and highlighting the gaps in uroscopy, John is also attempting to persuade his readers of his own profound knowledge and the firm theoretical underpinning he has given to the subject and to prepare them for what follows.

John's treatise was addressed to a specialized medical audience.[44] For example, its length makes it inaccessible to those lacking the necessary expertise. In fact, as we will see in the next section of this chapter, *On Urines* is a highly technical work and a reader has to read it step by step, since there

τοιαῦτα βραχύ τι καὶ αὐτῷ μελῆσαν.... Μάγνῳ δὲ καὶ Ἀλεξάνδρῳ καὶ πρὸς τούτοις ἔτι Θεοφίλῳ καί τισιν ἑτέροις περὶ τὰ τοιαῦτα ἐσπουδακόσι, πλέον τι τῶν ἄλλων εἰπεῖν δόξασι, καὶ αὐτοῖς ὁ λόγος ἀτελὴς διέμεινεν... καὶ μήτε διαφορὰς μήτε αἴτια, μήτε ἄλλ' ἄττα τὰ τῇ ἀρτιότητι δοκοῦντα προσήκειν ὑποθεμένοις. Ἔνθεν τοι ταῖς μὲν ἄλλαις ὁρῶν τὴν τέχνην σεμνυνομένην πραγματείαις, οὐκ ὀλίγα τοῦ θ' Ἱπποκράτους καὶ Γαληνοῦ καὶ τῶν μετ' αὐτοὺς ἐξευρηκότων ἀνδρῶν, τὴν δὲ περὶ οὔρων οἷον ὑποσκάζουσαν καί τινος εἰς τοῦτο συνάρσεως δεομένην...'

40 Theophilos, *On Urines*, pr., ed. Ideler (1841) I.261.1–262.9, refers to Galen, Hippocrates, and Magnos. A striking verbal similarity between the two authors is noted, for example, in reference to Hippocrates' sporadic treatment of the subject. Theophilos, *On Urines*, pr., ed. Ideler (1841) I.261.9–11: '*Ὁ μὲν γὰρ Ἱπποκράτης περὶ οὔρων ἐξηγησάμενος ἄλλοτε ἀλλαχοῦ ἐν ταῖς πραγματείαις αὐτοῦ κατασποράδην.*'

41 John refers three more times in his work to the wise (*sophos*) Hippocrates with positive comments about his contribution; cf. *On Urines*, 1.5.4, 1.6.5, 6.13.1, and 7.pr.1, ed. Ideler (1842) II.8.19–20, II.10.3–5, II.164.30–3, and II.171.14–15.

42 In the conclusion of his work, *On Urines*, 7.17.3, ed. Ideler (1842) II.190.20–34, John refers once more to the incomplete treatment of uroscopy by Galen. However, it is noteworthy that in all other mentions, John praises Galen and suggests his readers should consult particular works by him in order to increase their knowledge on certain medical topics in connection with uroscopy. This is particularly common in the last two books focusing on prognosis where, for example, in *On Urines*, 6.10.7, 7.2.7, 7.16.5, and 7.16.11, ed. Ideler (1842) II.158.22–3, II.174.36–175.4, II.187.20–4, II.188.8–10, John makes direct reference by name to Galen's *On Crises* and *On Critical Days*, calling him wise (*sophos*) or most wise (*sophōtatos*).

43 He is perhaps referring to an unedited text *On Pulse and Urine* ascribed to a certain Alexander the physician and found in one manuscript, Parisinus gr. 2316 (fifteenth century), ff. 207v–215r, dated to the fifteenth century. The title reads: '*Ἀλεξάνδρου ἰητροῦ, περὶ διαγνώσεως σφυγμῶν καὶ περὶ οὔρων, ἀφορισμοί*' ('Aphorisms on the diagnosis of the pulse and on urine by Alexander the physician').

44 An exception to John's concentration on a specialized audience can be found in his eleven case histories (in books two, three, four, six, seven), which—as I argue in Chapter 3—can also be seen as self-promotional material intended to impress even those without a medical background.

are many internal cross references, making it virtually impossible for the non-expert to navigate through it. This is in contrast, for example, to his *Medical Epitome* where each book and almost every chapter or recipe may be used separately and constitutes a brief, easily followed set of instructions on the diagnosis and therapy of various diseases for the non-specialist.[45]

That John was writing for a specialized readership is further confirmed by certain hints about physicians who were uneducated or not properly educated or indeed not even physicians (*apaideutos*) and whom John censures for their inability to examine urine properly.[46] Furthermore, John openly criticizes those having the 'audacity' (*authadeia*) to prognosticate without the proper theoretical background. He even refers to those attempting 'dream interpretation' (*oneiroskopiais*), perhaps indicating an element of competition between professional or educated physicians and those without a proper scientific background.[47] In fact, the vial's great popularity was, at times, exploited in medieval societies by malpractitioners or complete charlatans.[48]

John's authorial persona is constantly evident throughout the treatise. The first-person narrative either adopts a strong first-person pronoun in the singular (*egō/egōge/emoi/moi/eme*) or plural (*hēmeis*), sometimes followed by a second-person singular verb or pronoun (*sy*), which could be seen as an attempt to engage his readers more actively. To give an example, of the approximately fifty-five times that the first-person singular pronoun is used in his edited corpus, forty are in *On Urines*.[49] The first-person singular was used in the classical period by scientific and medical authors to draw the reader's attention to some innovative approach.[50] In John's case, it highlights the quality of his advice by providing his own assessment of the subject. The

[45] For the *Medical Epitome* and its audience, see the discussion in Chapter 4, Section 2.

[46] JZA, *On Urines*, 1.10.1, 1.10.10, and 3.pr.4, ed. Ideler (1842) II.16.22, II.17.27, II.53.24–5. In the first two cases, John uses the term to refer to those who mistakenly believe that the consistency of urine can vary according to changes in the external temperature. See the discussion in Section 2.4.

[47] JZA, *On Urines*, 5.pr.2–4, ed. Ideler (1842) II.145.12–24.

[48] We are aware, for example, of the case of Abū Bakr al-Rāzī (d. *c.*925), who was often critical of uroscopy, since it could be imitated by swindlers. On this in relation to charlatanism in medieval Islamic medicine, see Pormann (2005: 202–5). Another interesting case, almost five centuries later, which shows the interaction between professional physicians and uneducated practitioners with regard to the performance of uroscopy, is reported by Siraisi (1990: 32–3): 'Geralada Codines, a wisewoman active in the diocese of Barcelona in the late thirteenth and early fourteenth centuries... learned diagnosis by inspection of urines from a travelling *medicus* and for the next thirty years practiced this art along with conjuring away illnesses by charms.' Cf. Moulinier-Brogi (2012: 132–5).

[49] The vast majority of the remaining cases are found in the work on pneuma, which—as I show in Chapter 6—is also characterized by a large degree of originality with very little use of verbatim quotations from earlier sources compared to the *Medical Epitome*. See, for example, JZA, *On Psychic Pneuma*, 2.10.1, ed. Ideler (1841) I.373.2, on the use of *egō* in connection with a personal view of John on a certain dietary recommendation.

[50] See Lloyd (1987: 56–78); and von Staden (1994).

first-person plural could be seen as a further attempt to build a relationship with his reader through a spirit of 'communality'.[51]

In *On Urines*, we mainly see the use of the first-person singular or plural associated with a statement regarding a novel element of his theory or an important set of data as regards the understanding of the next chapter. For example, in referring to the definition of the 'crown' (*stephanē*), which is a urinary characteristic only recently introduced to Byzantine uroscopy,[52] he says: 'we call the outline that runs around the periphery of the surface of the urinary liquid a "crown"...'[53] In the same category, we can also include cross references to other parts of his work or allusions to what follows. For example: 'Now, we will give an account of all those things which provide a safe prognosis, since this part is missing from the books focusing on diagnosis.'[54]

Another feature of John's treatise are the brief references to or long accounts derived from his clinical experience (*peira*).[55] They emphasize the knowledge gained through John's contact with patients and contribute to his self-promotion as a skilful practising physician, which in turn adds validity to his account.[56] The most vivid examples of John's contact with patients are his illustrated case histories, of which there are eleven in total and which are discussed in detail in the next chapter of this book. In addition to his clinical accounts, we can see six cases of *paradeigmata* (examples), based on his observations and presented to the reader in connection with certain urinary characteristics.[57] For example, in the twenty-first chapter of the first book, which discusses the abnormal characteristics of various particles (*paryphistamena*) found in the urine, John states:

> In order to make the account clearer, we will make use of an example: if this kind of urine appears on the next two days, while that of the third day is different, and

[51] König (2011: 183–6) introduced the notion of 'communality' in connection with Galen and argued for a sort of didactic relationship between author and reader. On Galen's use of the first-person plural in his case histories, see Mattern (2008: 138–40).

[52] See nn. 21–2, above.

[53] JZA, *On Urines*, 1.18.6, ed. Ideler (1842) II.26.17–19: '*Στεφάνην τοίνυν ἡμεῖς φαμεν τὴν κατὰ τὸν κύκλον τῆς ἐπιφανείας τοῦ χύματος περιθέουσαν ἐσκιαγραφημένην γραμμήν...*'

[54] JZA, *On Urines*, 6.10.2, ed. Ideler (1842) II.157.31–3: '*Νῦν δ' ἐπιθῶμεν τῷ λόγῳ, ὅσον μὲν εἰς πρόγνωσιν ἀσφαλές, λέλειπται δ' ἐν τοῖς περὶ διαγνώσεως οὔρων λόγοις.*' Among the numerous cases, see also 4.9.2 and 6.15.1, ed. Ideler (1842) II.91.35 and II.168.26.

[55] JZA, *On Urines*, 1.12.1, ed. Ideler (1842) II.18.21–4. See also, JZA, *On Urines*, 2.14.1, 4.pr.2, 4.17.4, and 4.13.25, ed. Ideler (1842) II.46.4–8, II.79.9–11, II.105.11–12, and II.99.10–12, in which John refers to the importance of *peira* in conjunction with the theoretical training/knowledge (*logos*). In other cases, John's clinical experience could be expressed without explicit references to *peira*, as, for example, in *On Urines*, 4.8.3, ed. Ideler (1842) II.90.21–4, where he reports that he has seen (*eidon*) urine several times with yellow bile in patients who had had fever some time ago. See also John's references to *peira* in the pharmacological part of his *Medical Epitome* in Chapter 5, Section 3.

[56] For the use of the word *peira* and its connection with self-promotion strategies, see Bouras-Vallianatos (2014: 341–2), where I discuss the case of Alexander of Tralles.

[57] JZA, *On Urines*, 1.13.8, 1.20.8, 1.21.6, 4.19.7, 6.12.29, and 7.15.4, ed. Ideler (1842) II.20.35–6; II.28.32–5, II.29.27–30.1, II.107.17–18, II.163.37–164.3, and II.185.7–8.

> right after on the fourth and fifth day is similar to that of the first and second day . . . and this takes place over the following days with a certain periodicity, it results in the aforementioned abnormality <of the particles>.[58]

In another case, and in order to emphasize the instructional role of his *paradeigma* and at the same time enhance his attempts to keep his audience attentive, John includes the infinitive of the verb *manthanō* (= to learn): 'In order for you to clearly understand this account, it is possible to learn by the following example . . . '[59]

Finally, there is an example of a short anecdote from John's life in chapter eight of the first book, where he discusses the shade of various colours. By referring to *oinōpon* (literally the colour of wine), he states: 'For I remember having seen this kind of colour [i.e. *oinōpon*] in the market in the wine brought by traders . . . '[60] John gives a tangible example from everyday life by evoking a memory and thus providing a further clarification for his readers on a topic which could have caused problems of misidentification for contemporary physicians.[61] This is not part of a new theory on colours, but it could be seen as an 'addendum' to earlier accounts of this particular topic, and one emphatically marked by John's personal perspective.

2.2 Contents: from diagnosis to prognosis

Table 2.1 presents a synopsis of the contents of each book. The entire treatise and also each book follows a general rule of presentation, which is in effect a general-to-specific approach. We may theoretically divide the work into four parts—shown in the table as A, B, C, and D—corresponding to the main thematic areas. The first book starts with details on physiology connected with the production of urine; then come basic details on the nature of various urinary characteristics, including special mentions of the consistency

[58] JZA, *On Urines*, 1.21.6, ed. Ideler (1842) II.29.37–30.7: '*Ἵνα δὲ σαφέστερον προάγωμεν τὸν λόγον, ὧδ' ἐπὶ παραδείγματι τούτῳ χρησόμεθα· εἰ τοίνυν δυοῖν μὲν ἐφεξῆς ἡμεραῖν τὰ αὐτὰ δὴ οὖρα φαίνεται, τῇ τρίτῃ δ' αὖ ἑτεροῖα, καὶ αὖθις τῇ τετάρτῃ μὲν καὶ πέμπτῃ ὁποῖα καὶ τῇ πρώτῃ καὶ δευτέρᾳ . . . καὶ τοῦτο ἐπὶ πολλαῖς ἑξῆς ἡμερῶν γίνεται περιόδοις, τεταγμένη τις ἂν ὧδε ῥηθείη ἀνωμαλία.*'

[59] JZA, *On Urines*, 7.15.4, ed. Ideler (1842) II.185.7–8: '*Ἵνα δὲ σαφέστερον τὸν λόγον εἰδῇς, ἔστιν μαθεῖν ἐντεῦθεν ὡς ἐπὶ παραδείγματος . . .*' The use of the verb *manthanō* and its cognate *ekmanthanō* is common throughout John's *On Urines*. Among the numerous examples, see JZA, *On Urines*, 1.8.26, 2.1.7, 3.12.9, 5.18.6, 6.12.10, 6.13.25, and 7.11.2, ed. Ideler (1842) II.14.25, II.33.10, II.65.29, II.142.7, II.162.12, II.167.8, and II.180.2–3. See also Chapter 3, n. 28.

[60] JZA, *On Urines*, 1.8.20, ed. Ideler (1842) II.14.1–2: '*Μέμνημαι γὰρ καὶ ἔγωγε τοιοῦτον ἐν ἀγορᾷ πολλάκις ἑωρακὼς ἀπ' ἐμπόρων κομιζόμενον οἶνον . . .*' See also Chapter 3, n. 32.

[61] On the use of verbs related to memory, see Chapter 3, n. 29, in connection with John's case histories.

Table 2.1. Summary of contents of John's *On Urines*

Theoretical thematic division of the work	Reference to the edition	Contents of each Book
Part **A** Introduction	Book **1** [ed. Ideler (1842) II.3–31] **22** chapters	Introduction; production of urine (digestions); notes on other procedures of medical examination with a particular emphasis on pulse, colours, particles, urine vial, crowns, and bubbles.
Part **B** Diagnosis	Book **2** [ed. Ideler (1842) II.31–52] **19** chapters	Discussion of the appropriate urine vial; role of patient's mixture, age, exercise, and season; and diagnosis based on the colour of the urine.
	Book **3** [ed. Ideler (1842) II.53–78] **25** chapters	Diagnosis based on the urine consistency, particles, bubbles, and crowns; diagnosis of fevers based on the examination of urines; and diagnosis of other diseases based on the examination of urines.
Part **C** Aetiology	Book **4** [ed. Ideler (1842) II.79–111] **20** chapters	Cause of onset of indigestion; cause of the production of urine according to the colour and particles (shape, colour).
	Book **5** [ed. Ideler (1842) II.111–44] **20** chapters	Cause of the production of urine according to the particles (place in the vial), bubbles, and crowns; role of season, diet, exercise, and sleep in the production of urine; and cause of the production of urine related to fevers and other diseases.
Part **D** Prognosis	Book **6** [ed. Ideler (1842) II.145–71] **16** chapters	Role of pulse in prognosis; prognosis of various diseases and oncoming crises based on the examination of urine's colour, particles, bubbles, and crowns.
	Book **7** [ed. Ideler (1842) II.171–92] **18** chapters	Prognosis of fevers, heart, lung, liver, brain, stomach, splenic, kidney, intestinal, gynaecological diseases, and crises based on the examination of urine; prognosis of the duration of a disease; prognosis on whether a disease is likely to be fatal or not; and a brief synopsis of the entire treatise.

and colours of the urinary liquid, and various kinds of particles, bubbles, and crowns. A special section is also devoted to John's particular urine vial and the various areas within it. The next six books are divided into three groups of two books each focusing on diagnosis, aetiology, and prognosis respectively; special attention is also paid to the various characteristics denoting the type, periodicity, and duration of fevers. The importance of prognosis is not overlooked in favour of diagnosis and never before had such a significant part of a medical text of this type been devoted to aetiology. Thus, the significance of John's approach to uroscopy does not only lie in the equal amount of space devoted to each procedure, but also in the three-pronged approach to each urinary characteristic assessed.

Each book contains about twenty chapters. Each chapter varies in content and may be quite short (a few lines) or up to four–five printed pages long. As we can see in Table 2.1, there is a symmetry between the first book and the other three groups of books. For example, a certain urinary characteristic, discussed in an introductory fashion in the first book, is then treated separately as regards diagnosis in the second book, and then again in the fourth and sixth books in connection with the aetiology and prognosis respectively. John may take into consideration input coming from other techniques such as sphygmology or the examination of excrement and so on. I will return to this later, and, in particular, to the role of the pulse, but for now it is more appropriate to begin analysing how John thinks about these three procedures.

To this end, I have selected the chapters (see Table 2.2) concentrating on bubbles (*pompholyges*) for three reasons. They come from all four parts of the work and are neither too short nor too long. Furthermore, in contrast, for example, to the discussion of the various kinds of urine colours or particles, to which John devotes several chapters in each part of his work, here all the relevant details are included in a single chapter. And lastly, this is the first time in the history of uroscopy that such a detailed treatment of bubbles had been included.[62]

The first reference to bubbles appears in the first book, chapter eighteen, where John attempts to provide basic morphological characteristics, such as size and shape, on which a distinction could be based. Their place on the surface of the urine at the top of the vial is also important since it could be associated with a 'crown'; their particular place within a 'crown' and their number may also be crucial. Having provided all these details, John returns to the topic in the third book, chapter thirteen.

Table 2.2. Chapters in John's *On Urines* dealing with bubbles

Reference to the edition	Greek/English chapter title
Book 1, chapter 18 [ed. Ideler (1842) II.25.21–26.32]	*Περὶ διαφορᾶς πομφολύγων*/ On differences among bubbles
Book 3, chapter 13 [ed. Ideler (1842) II.66.1–67.30]	*Περὶ τῆς ἐκ τῶν κατὰ τὰ οὖρα πομφολύγων διαγνώσεως*/ On diagnosis based on the examination of bubbles
Book 5, chapter 3 [ed. Ideler (1842) II.114.31–116.23]	*Περὶ αἰτίας γεννήσεως τῶν ἐπιφαινομένων πομφολύγων*/ On the cause of the formation of displayed bubbles
Book 6, chapter 15 [ed. Ideler (1842) II.168.23–169.34]	*Περὶ τῆς ἐκ τῶν πομφολύγων προγνώσεως*/ On prognosis based on the examination of bubbles

62 See, for example, Theophilos, *On Urines*, 8, ed. Ideler (1841) I.270.6–8, who makes only one very brief mention of them.

The first paragraph of the chapter on diagnosis serves as a reminder of the various features which determine the differences between bubbles. Thus, John notices the significance of their shape, size, quantity, and location; in addition to these, a difference in colour is also suggested here. The main part deals with various kinds of bubbles related to various symptoms, such as pain and kidney affections. Twice in this chapter John informs his readers that they may find more details about the significance of bubbles in the relevant sections of his work, i.e. on the prognostication of disease through a specific kind of bubble and the cause of formation of a given kind of bubble.[63] On the one hand, John helps his reader to find the necessary data easily by using cross references. On the other hand, one cannot easily consult one of the later books (e.g. the seventh) without first having followed John's discussion in, for example, the first book, in which basic details are provided on their external appearance. This suggests a complementarity between the various parts and a thorough compositional redaction.

A similar pattern is followed in the subsequent books, which focus on aetiology and prognosis. John generally considers the identification of cause as something approaching the ability to provide a precise diagnosis, thus explicitly connecting the two procedures.[64] In the chapter on the aetiology of the formation of bubbles, this phenomenon is related to the production of pneuma as a result of indigestion, which in turn is responsible for the appearance of bubbles in urine. This is treated in considerable detail and related to the theory of digestion, which will be discussed below. Later on, John devotes one more chapter to bubbles, this time focusing on prognosis. A notable difference in terms of content can be seen in John's approach in this chapter. Here, there is greater emphasis on the connection between particular urinary characteristics and certain clinical conditions. For example, bubbles may be connected with fever, headache, and lung affections.

2.3 Urine versus pulse

From the very beginning of his treatise John was eager to highlight that none of the various diagnostic and prognostic examinations were absolutely accurate when used in isolation, and that it was important to consider a variety of clinical data in each case in dealing with a patient. He writes:

> If one chooses to make a precise diagnosis and prognosis of what happens in the affections, it is not fitting to take into consideration only the differences in urine... but <it is> also <necessary> to examine the pulse and to observe the

[63] JZA, *On Urines*, 3.13.12–13, ed. Ideler (1842) II.67.12–16.
[64] JZA, *On Urines*, 4.pr.3, ed. Ideler (1842) II.79.17–21.

> excrement, the rate of breathing, the position of the face, the way in which the entire body is lying down, and the production of speech[65] ...[66]

Thus the pulse is mainly useful for the indication of the warmth or coldness of the human body,[67] the excrement shows the degree of digestion in the stomach,[68] and urine the quality and quantity of the humours produced.[69] Speech shows the hegemonic activity (*hēgemonikē energeia*),[70] which is related to reasoning, memory, and imagination.[71] John maintains that neither the pulse nor excrement nor urine would by itself be a very precise indicator (*akribōs paragymnousi*[72] *ta pathē*) in revealing the various affections, but sometimes one of them could be more useful than another, depending on the particular case.[73] In an attempt to emphasize to his readers the need for an up-to-date comprehensive treatment of the subject of uroscopy, comparable to the already extensive treatment of sphygmology, he goes on to explain that, although the examination of urine is just as important as that of the pulse, uroscopy is a safer and easier technique (*asphalesteron te kai procheiroteron*[74]) to use.[75]

John supports his view by explaining that the accurate identification, for example, of the speed of each single movement of diastole and/or systole (*kinēseōn diastēmata*) or the frequency of a series of pulses (*parempiptontōn pyknotētas*) could often be problematic, since it involved the sense of touch.[76] He emphatically states that the physician should have an extremely sensitive hand (*euaisthēsias*[77] *cheiros*) and clear mind (*nou katharou*).[78] He seems to reflect a traditional concern connected with the examination of pulse, since the importance of the sense of touch and the associated training required is

[65] Here I follow Georgiou's critical edition (2013) 415.15–416.1, which reads: '*γλώττης προφοράν*' as compared to Ideler (1842) II.10.27: '*γλώττης προσφοράς*'.

[66] JZA, *On Urines*, 1.7.1–2, ed. Ideler (1842) II.10.20–7: '*Τῷ τοίνυν ἀκριβῶς διαγιγνώσκειν τε καὶ προγιγνώσκειν αἱρουμένῳ τῶν παθῶν τὰ συμβαίνοντα, οὐ μόνον οὔρων ἐπισκέπτεσθαι προσήκει διαφοράς ... ἀλλὰ καὶ σφυγμῶν αὐτῶν ἅπτεσθαι καὶ διαχωρήματα καθορᾶν καὶ κίνησιν ἀναπνοῆς, ἔτι δὲ θέσιν προσώπου, καὶ τοῦ παντὸς κατάκλισιν σώματος, καὶ αὐτῆς δὴ τῆς γλώττης προσφοράς ...*'

[67] JZA, *On Urines*, 1.7.2, ed. Ideler (1842) II.10.30–1.

[68] JZA, *On Urines*, 1.7.2, ed. Ideler (1842) II.10.32–3. On the importance of the examination of excrement, see also JZA, *On Urines*, 2.11.10, ed. Ideler (1842) II.44.7–10.

[69] JZA, *On Urines*, 1.7.2, ed. Ideler (1842) II.10.31–2.

[70] The agent of the hegemonic activity is the psychic pneuma. See John's special chapter in his *On Psychic Pneuma*, 1.18, ed. Ideler (1841) I.346.17–347.26, and Chapter 6, nn. 91–2.

[71] JZA, *On Urines*, 1.7.2, ed. Ideler (1842) II.10.33–4.

[72] Here I follow Georgiou (2013) 416.9. Ideler (1842) II.11.2 retains *paragymnōsi*.

[73] JZA, *On Urines*, 1.7.3, ed. Ideler (1842) II.11.1–5.

[74] Here I follow Georgiou (2013) 417.3. Ideler (1842) II.11.12 retains *procheiron*.

[75] JZA, *On Urines*, 1.7.5–6, 1.7.7, ed. Ideler (1842) II.11.11–17, II.11.27–8.

[76] JZA, *On Urines*, 1.7.6, ed. Ideler (1842) II.11.19–21.

[77] Here I follow Georgiou (2013) 417.8. Ideler (1842) II.11.18 retains *euaisthēseōs*.

[78] JZA, *On Urines*, 1.7.6, ed. Ideler (1842) II.11.17–18.

attested as far back as some ancient medical authors, such as Galen.[79] This said, there are some examples in John's treatise, where he is eager to show how sphygmology could be more beneficial or must be combined with uroscopy in practice.[80] This is also evident in his case histories, in which John also advertised his skills as a practising physician in pulse examination.[81]

2.4 Factors affecting urine

Throughout the text, John makes consistent attempts to include the influence of a person's daily regimen, such as diet, sleep, exercise, as well as age, mixture (*krasis*), and gender on various urinary features.[82] Although scattered references to seasonal, age, and gender factors could be seen in previous treatises, no such systematic recording of them in relation to urine is previously attested.[83]

Special chapters in the books on diagnosis and aetiology are devoted to the particularities of each factor, so that the physician might be informed before performing an examination and making his subsequent diagnosis. For example, the natural urine of men should be reddish-yellow (*hypopyrra*) or yellowish (*hypoxantha*) in colour with a regular consistency (*symmetrōs… systasin*) and sediment (*hypostasin*), although old men have thinner (*lepta*) and whiter (*leuka*) urine with smaller sediments (*brachyteras hypostaseis*); for children it is natural to have lots of sediment (*athroas hypostaseis*).[84] The urine of women is usually yellowish to white (*hypoxanthou pros to leukon*) in colour and of a somewhat thin consistency (*hypoleptoi… systaseis*).[85] Exercise and

[79] See, for example, Galen, *On the the Pulse for Beginners*, 1, ed. Kühn (1824) VIII.478.2–5. See also Lewis (2015: 202–10), who discusses the case of Marcellinus (second century AD[?]), who dealt specifically in his treatise, *On the Pulse*, with details of how to palpate the pulse.

[80] See, for example, JZA, *On Urines*, 3.25.1–2 and 6.1, ed. Ideler (1842) II.77.30–78.4 and II.146.11–147.12. John generally pays the same attention to the examination of the pulse as to that of urine in his *Medical Epitome*, 1.9–25 and 1.26–32, ed. Ideler (1842) II.362.32–375.10 and II.375.11–384.3; and *On Psychic Pneuma*, 1.13 and 1.15, ed. Ideler (1841) I.377.1–378.9 and I.379.1–380.4.

[81] For example, when referring to a pregnant patient, John uses special terminology in identifying her pulse. JZA, *On Urines*, 7.13.18, ed. Ideler (1842) II.182.7–8: '*Σφυγμοὶ δὲ οἱ πάνυ λεπτοὶ καὶ ἀνώμαλοι ἦσαν…*' ('<Her> pulse was very weak and irregular…'). See also, JZA, *On Urines*, 6.12.15, ed. Ideler (1842) II.162.26–8. For a detailed list of various diagnostic and prognostic techniques used in John's case histories, see Table 3.1.

[82] The first reference to regimen is in JZA, *On Urines*, 1.6.3, ed. Ideler (1842) II.9.23–6; further references in the diagnostic section, JZA, *On Urines*, 2.5, ed. Ideler (1842) II.36.17ff, and the part dealing with aetiology, JZA, *On Urines*, 5.7, ed. Ideler (1842) II.120.31ff.

[83] For example in Theophilos' treatise there is only one mention of old men, *On Urines*, 17, ed. Ideler (1841) I.279.36–7, and there is no reference to women.

[84] JZA, *On Urines*, 2.5.2, ed. Ideler (1842) II.36.24–31. On John's remarks on the performance of uroscopy in children, see the brief discussion by Hummel (1999: 245–6).

[85] JZA, *On Urines*, 2.5.5, ed. Ideler (1842) II.37.5–9.

season may also affect colour, while dietary habits and sleep are related to the digestion, which can cause a change in a great number of urinary features.[86] All these details clearly show the extraordinary effort John made to treat the examination of each patient's urine individually, something which is vividly attested in his case histories.

Finally, mention should be made of the impact of external temperature on the consistency of urine. John devotes a special chapter in the first book to refuting the idea that, if the consistency of the urine was thick, this could be the result of cooling due to the effect of the external temperature.[87] He does not specify at what time the examination should begin, but he clearly maintains that it is only some considerable time after collection that the various particles could be examined properly.[88] In fact, there was a debate among Byzantine authors as to whether the consistency of the urine is affected by the outside temperature. For example, Stephen, the author of an early Byzantine uroscopic treatise, suggests that urine becomes thickened due to external factors such as cold air, whereas it can be heated with hot water to make it thin.[89] John, however, maintains that urine could be thick (*pachytata*) in the summer or quite thin (*leptotata*) in the winter without the outside temperature changing its consistency.[90] In order to further persuade the reader, he suggests a simple test using two vials, one containing thick and the other thin urine, each exposed to the same low external temperature (*tō autō*... *aeri* [i.e. cold]). He ultimately reports that the consistency of the thin urine will remain the same (*leptēs menousēs*),[91] thus rejecting any effect of the external temperature.

2.5 Theory of digestion

A central aspect of uroscopy, as has already been noted in the section on the historical background, is the connection between digestion and the production of urine. John offers a much-needed systematization of the various phases of human digestion by providing a more detailed division and anatomical

[86] JZA, *On Urines*, 2.6–9, ed. Ideler (1842) II.38.8–41.8.

[87] JZA, *On Urines*, 1.10, ed. Ideler (1842) II.16.20–17.32. John believes that the consistency is mainly affected by the disposition (*diathesis*) of the body.

[88] JZA, *On Urines*, 2.3.3, ed. Ideler (1842) II.34.10–16. The only reference to a specific time after collection for the examination is given in the short, anonymous, uroscopic treatise preserved in the fifteenth-century Florentinus Laurentianus gr. plut. 75.8 [*On Diagnosis of Urines*, 1, ed. Lamagna (1999) 311.1], which suggests that the examination should take place within the first three hours after the sample has been collected.

[89] Stephen, *On Urines*, 6, ed. Bussemaker (1845) 428–9. For a discussion of this particular passage in Stephen's treatise, see Lamagna (2003b: 71–2).

[90] JZA, *On Urines*, 1.10.5, ed. Ideler (1842) II.17.3–6.

[91] JZA, *On Urines*, 1.10.8–10, ed. Ideler (1842) II.17.20–6.

Table 2.3. Digestion in Galen and John

Digestion	Place of each phase according to Galen	Place of each phase according to John's model in Book 1, *On Urines*
First	Stomach	Stomach
Second	Portal vein and liver	Portal vein and concave part of the liver
Third	Other organs and parts of the body	Convex part of the liver and successive veins
Fourth	n/a	Other organs and parts of the body

description than that of Galen.[92] He records four phrases in contrast to Galen's three (see Table 2.3).[93] Unlike Theophilos and Stephen, who do not number the various phases,[94] by assigning a particular number to each phase John is able to make quick and accurate reference to each of them and their products throughout his treatise. His account meets the needs for continuous development in the field of urine examination in the Middle Ages, especially as regards the scrutinizing of various particles (*paryphistamena*).

John starts by describing the traditional first phase, which takes place in the stomach and in which waste-products are excreted in the faeces.[95] However, he then proceeds to a more detailed treatment of the digestion that takes place in the liver, thus dividing the Galenic second phase into two further stages. John's second phase takes place in the portal vein (*stelechiaian phleba*) and the concave part of the liver (*ta koila tou hēpatos*) where the nutrients of the first phase are digested resulting in a 'diverse' group of humours (*heteroeideis chymoi*),[96] most probably referring to blood, yellow bile, black bile, and serous humour (*orrōdēs chymos*).[97] John's third phase happens in the convex part of the liver (*ta kyrta tou hēpatos*) and successive veins (*ephexēs phlebōdes genos*), where the products of the second phase are further digested.[98] From there, the thinnest (*leptoteron*) waste-product is attracted by the gall bladder, resulting in yellow bile, while the thickest (*pachyteron*) waste-product is absorbed by the

[92] John's approach has previously been noted by Diamandopoulos (2001), Diamandopoulos and Goudas (2009: 29–31), and Georgiou (2013: 516–17), but they did not put it in the context of previous theories.

[93] See also the influential medieval Latin treatise by Maurus of Salerno, *Rules on Urines* (*Regulae Urinarum*), ed. Renzi (1854), 5.24–5, in which the author refers to three phases taking place in the stomach, liver, and the other part of the body: 'prima in stomacho, secunda in epate, tertia in omnibus membris aliis'.

[94] Theophilos, *On Urines*, 1–2, ed. Ideler (1841) I.262.20–263.33. Another account is provided by Stephen, *On Urines*, 1–2, ed. Bussemaker (1845) 424–7.

[95] JZA, *On Urines*, 1.5.1, 4.1.6, and 4.1.13, ed. Ideler (1842) II.8.3–4, II.80.15–16, and II.81.10–12. On Galen's theory of digestion, see Section 1, above.

[96] JZA, *On Urines*, 1.5 and 4.1.6–7, ed. Ideler (1842) II.8.4–5, 10–11 and II.80.17–24.

[97] JZA, *On Urines*, 1.4.2–6, ed. Ideler (1842) II.7.1–27. Cf. JZA, *On Urines*, 4.1.13, ed. Ideler (1842) II.12–13.

[98] JZA, *On Urines*, 1.5.1, ed. Ideler (1842) II.8.5–7.

spleen, accumulating black bile.[99] Galen is somewhat unclear on the exact position of the biliary passages, although his account is in agreement with that of John on the nature of both the waste-products and their destination.[100] The same products are also recorded in Theophilos and Stephen, but in both authors the gall bladder is said to be attached to the concave part of the liver.[101]

Meanwhile, the blood and the serous humour enter the vena cava; the former reaches the heart and the other parts of the body, while the latter is transferred to the kidneys via the lambdoid part of the vena cava (*lambdoeidei*[102] *tēs koilēs phlebos*),[103] that is the branch connecting the vena cava with the kidneys. The lambdoid vein is not mentioned by any ancient nor any other Byzantine medical author.[104] It takes its name from its shape, which resembles the Greek letter lambda '*Λ*', and it most probably refers to the renal veins. The serous humour seems identical with the Galenic serous superfluity (*orrōdes perittōma*) that is moved from the liver to the kidneys for the production of urine.[105] John describes the urine as being filtrated in vessels inside the kidneys (*diylizontōn peri tous nephrous ta oura angeiōn*).[106] The third digestion that takes place in the convex part of the liver is responsible, according to John, for the production and subsequent appearance of various particles (*paryphistamena*) in the urine.[107] Consequently, the degree of digestion could be seen from

[99] JZA, *On Urines*, 1.4.2–3 and 4.1.8–10, ed. Ideler (1842) II.7.2–9 and II.80.25–81.1.

[100] Galen, *On the Function of the Parts of the Body*, 4.13, ed. Kühn (1822) III.301.5–302.1 = ed. Helmreich (1907) I.221.5–19. See also May (1968: 224, n. 52; and 227, n. 59).

[101] Theophilos, *On Urines*, 2, ed. Ideler (1841) I.263.2–5. Stephen, *On Urines*, 2, ed. Bussemaker (1845) 425.23–4.

[102] Here I follow Georgiou (2013) 409.6. Ideler (1842) II.7.19 retains *labdoeidei.*

[103] JZA, *On Urines*, 1.4–5, ed. Ideler (1842) II.7.9–22. See also, JZA, *On Urines*, 4.1.12, ed. Ideler (1842) II.81.1–5, referring to serous urine (*orrōdes ouron*).

[104] The same vein with the same role is also reported in John's *On Psychic Pneuma*, 1.6.16, ed. Ideler (1841) I.324.6–11 and *Medical Epitome*, 1.28, ed. Ideler (1842) II.378.7–11. Stephen, *On Urines*, 2, ed. Bussemaker (1845) 427.6–8, refers to the lambdoid shape (*labda gramma schēmatisthentes*) of the kidney passages (*poroi*), which absorb the serous superfluity. Theophilos' text in Ideler's (1841) I.263.18–19 edition has a lacuna, but Tassinari's unpublished edition based on fifteen surviving manuscripts is in line with Stephen's account: '*τῇ ῥάχει ἄνωθεν ἕως κάτω, κατ' αὐτὸ δὲ καὶ οἱ πόροι τοῦ νεφροῦ δεξιός τε καὶ ἀριστερὸς κατὰ τὸ* <u>*λάμβδα γράμμα σχηματισθέντες*</u> *ἐν τῇ θέσει αὐτῶν, ἕλκουσι δι' αὐτῶν ἀπὸ τῆς κοίλης φλεβὸς οἱ νεφροὶ καὶ εἰς οὔρου σύστασιν μεταβαλόντες.*' Galen and his Byzantine successors refer to the lambdoid suture (*lambdoeidēs rhaphē*) on the posterior aspect of the skull and the lambdoid or *hyioeides* bone. From among the many references to the lambdoid suture see, Galen, *On Bones for Beginners*, 1, ed. Kühn (1821) II.742.3–6 = ed. Garofalo (2005) 47.14–16, and Meletios, *On the Constitution of Man*, 1, ed. Cramer (1863) 53.7–9; for the lambdoid bone, see Galen, *On the Dissection of Muscles for Beginners*, ed. Kühn (1830) XVIIIb.957.1–959.2 = ed. Garofalo (2005) 140.1–141.20, and Oribasios, *Medical Collections*, 25.8, ed. Raeder (1931) II.1, 55.5–22.

[105] Galen, *On the Natural Capacities*, 1.16–17 and 2.2, ed. Kühn (1821) II.64–73 and II.79.5 = ed. Helmreich (1893) II.158.10–11. See also, Galen, *Causes of Symptoms*, 3.3, ed. Kühn (1824) VII.222.12–15.

[106] JZA, *On Urines*, 4.8.12, ed. Ideler (1842) II.91.21–3. See also, JZA, *On Urines*, 2.14.4, ed. Ideler (1842) II.46.16.–26.

[107] JZA, *On Urines*, 1.5.2 and 4.2.14, ed. Ideler (1842) II.8.11–12 and II.81.13–17. Among the various references to the production of the *paryphistamena* in the third digestion, see also JZA,

a number of urinary characteristics and played a decisive diagnostic and prognostic role. By distinguishing two different phases in the liver, John is able to establish where the particles in the urine are formed, unlike his predecessors who made vague connections between the formation of particles and the digestion, without indicating any particular location in which this might have occurred.[108] John's 'last' or 'fourth' digestion (*hystatēs de kai tetartēs*),[109] which corresponds to Galen's third, takes places in the organs and limbs (*peraiterō tou sōmatos*),[110] where the blood transfers the last remains of food (*to telos tēs trophēs*) through the vena cava. This is the phase in which all the body parts are nourished, while the by-products are excreted through the skin by perspiration (*adēlou diapnoēs*) resulting in sweat (*drosoeidōs exomoioutai*).[111]

2.6 Urine colours

The foremost and most commonly discussed feature in uroscopic treatises in medieval medical literature on the topic is the range of colours found in the examination of urine. John devotes a special chapter in the first book to dealing with the colours of urinary liquid (*chyma*).[112] There is one more chapter, focusing this time on the colours of various particles; however, he does not go into too much detail there and simply refers back to his detailed approach in the previous chapter.[113] Appendix 2 presents John's and Theophilos' sections on colour side by side. I selected Theophilos' text,[114] as it was for centuries the most popular account of uroscopy in Byzantium and the Latin West and makes a good comparison with John's chapter, allowing us to evaluate his extensive discussion of the topic and his additions. The underlined parts are those common to or nearly the same in both authors. Furthermore, Table 2.4 gives a list of the various colours in the two authors and in Gilles de Corbeil's account,[115] which is one of the longest treatments of this particular topic in medieval Western uroscopic treatises.

John identifies nine main colours (§3). These are: white, pale, fulvous, saffron-yellow, red, colour of red wine, blue, green, and black. After providing

On Urines, 1.11.1, 3.7.1, 4.2.1, and 5.6.2, ed. Ideler (1842) II.17.36–18.1, II.59.14–16, II.81.19–25, and II.119.14–17.

[108] See, for example, Theophilos, *On Urines*, 23, ed. Ideler (1841) I.283.1–3; and Stephen, *On Urines*, 24, ed. Bussemaker (1845) 560.5–12.

[109] JZA, *On Urines*, 1.5.2, ed. Ideler (1842) II.8.12.

[110] JZA, *On Urines*, 1.5.1–2, ed. Ideler (1842) II.8.7–9, 12–14.

[111] JZA, *On Urines*, 1.4.7, ed. Ideler (1842) II.7.27–32. See also, JZA, *On Urines*, 5.9.7, ed. Ideler (1842) II.127.14–17.

[112] JZA, *On Urines*, 1.8, ed. Ideler (1842) II.11.33–15.28.

[113] JZA, *On Urines*, 1.11, ed. Ideler (1842) II.17.33–18.19.

[114] Theophilos, *On Urines*, 6, ed. Ideler (1841) I.266.17–268.3.

[115] Gilles de Corbeil, *On Urines*, 19–207, ed. Kliegel (1972) 30–42.

Table 2.4. Urine colours in Theophilos, Gilles de Corbeil, and John

Theophilos	Gilles de Corbeil	John Zacharias Aktouarios	English translation[116]
Λευκόν (κρύσταλλος)	Albus	*Κρυσταλλοειδές*	White
Γαλακτῶδες	Lacteus	*Γαλακτῶδες*	Milk-white
Γλαυκόν	Glaucus	*Γλαυκόν*	Grey-white
Χαροπόν	Charopos	*Χαροπόν*	Grey
Ὕπωχρον	Subpallidus	*Ὕπωχρον*	Pale yellow
Ὠχρόν	Pallidus	*Ὠχρόν*	Yellow
Ὑπόπυρρον	Subrufus	*Ὑπόπυρρον*	Reddish-yellow
Πυρρόν	Rufus	*Πυρρόν*	Fulvous
—	Subcitrinus	—	Pale version of the colour of yellow apple
—	Citrinus	—	Colour of yellow apple
Ὑπόξανθον	—	*Ὑπόξανθον*	Yellowish
Ξανθόν	Rubeus	*Ξανθόν*	Saffron-yellow
Ὑπέρυθρον	Igneus	*Ὑπέρυθρον*	Reddish (red-purple)
Ἐρυθρόν	Rubicundus	*Ἐρυθρόν*	Red (blood-red)
Οἰνωπόν	Inopos	*Οἰνωπόν*	Colour of red wine (probably vivid red)
Κυανόν	Kyanos	*Κυανόν*	Blue or dark blue
Φαιόν	—	*Φαιόν*	Dark grey
Χλωρόν	Prasinus	*Χλωρόν*	Green
(Ἰῶδες		*(Κραμβίζον*	(Colour of green cabbage
Σμαραγδίζον		*Χλοάζον*	Bright green
Ἰσατῶδες)		*Ἰῶδες*	Greenish
		Σμαραγδίζον)	Emerald green Turquoise)
—	—	*Ἐλαιοφανές*	Between watery and oily
—	—	*Ἐλαιόχρουν*	Faintly oily
—	—	*Ἐλαιῶδες*	Oily
Πελιδνόν	Lividus	*Πελιδνόν*	Livid
Μελανόν	Niger	*Μελανόν*	Black

the names for the basic colours, he explains to his readers that there are other colours in between them (*emmesōn*) or close to them (*paramesōn*), thus indicating the existence of various shades in certain colours. For example, closely related tones are provided for pale, fulvous, saffron-yellow, and red: pale yellow, reddish-yellow, yellowish, and reddish. Interestingly, there are no colours to parallel de Corbeil's *citrinus* and *subcitrinus*.

Certainly the most important introduction to John's palette is the inclusion of three kinds of oily urine (§§27–9). Theophilos uses the same terms to name

[116] The English translation is mine and is based on a comparative study of the various supplementary details provided by all authors. Furthermore, I have considered Angeletti et al.'s (2009: 106–8) and Angeletti's and Cavarra's (1994: 286) studies on Theophilos, and Kliegel's (1972: 66–9) studies on Gilles de Corbeil, the tables by Willich (1670: 32–5), Vieillard (1903: 51), and Stolberg (2009: 48–50), and the relevant entries in LSJ.

oily urine; however, he does not include them among the colours, but as a characteristic of some urine in which a distinct film of oil appears, usually connected with various kinds of fevers.[117] John's choice is intentional since it is mentioned in between the green and livid colour, and he makes numerous references to this specific colour in various parts of his work, even devoting an entire chapter to it in the books on diagnosis and prognosis.[118]

The most notable elaboration, however, of John's account is the provision of a variety of supplementary details as part of his attempt to make things clearer and thus help his readers to differentiate properly between colours. As we can see in Appendix 2, this is also the main reason for John's account being considerably longer than Theophilos'. We have already mentioned his statement regarding the identification of the colour resembling red wine, which involves an authoritative first-person account (§20; see Section 2.1, above). A further interesting example relates to the identification of yellowish and saffron-yellow. Having specified yellowish (*hypoxanthon*) as the colour of the plant named *knikos* (blessed thistle), just like Theophilos, he goes a step further by providing a helpful tip to distinguish it from other candidates, in this case the *krokos* (saffron), which is similar to and may be confused with *knikos* (§14). In the next paragraph (§15), he continues with details on saffron-yellow (*xanthon*), which is related to the colour of Corycean *krokos*, in contrast to Theophilos, who simply mentions the 'genuine' *krokos* (*alēthinō krokō*). However, John thinks that the Corycean *krokos* might not be familiar to his readers (*tō xenō tou onomatos*).[119] Consequently, by using a strong first-person personal pronoun (*egō*), he provides further explanatory data for the identification of the colour, thus supplying his account with a reference to a *krokos* brought from Mt Athos (*apo tou Athō*), which was probably a variety of the plant that was more easily obtainable and more recognizable to his contemporaries.[120] Lastly, he clarifies that one must pay attention to the colour of this plant once it is dissolved in liquid (*xanthon*, saffron-yellow), and not to

[117] Theophilos, *On Urines*, 17, ed. Ideler (1841) I.278.34–280.2. See also Blemmydes' *Canon on Urines*, 8, ed. Ideler (1842) II.319.10 = ed. Kousis (1944a) 61.8, where he refers to '*τζίπαν ὡς ἐλαιώδη*'.

[118] JZA, *On Urines*, 2.18 and 6.8, ed. Ideler (1842) II.48.11–49.16 and II.156.15–157.3.

[119] The saffron from Corycus in Cilicia Trachea is considered be the best (*kratistos*) for medicinal use by, for example, Dioscorides, *De Materia Medica*, 1.26.1, ed. Wellmann (1907) I.29.9–13. Although the Corycean *krokos* is often mentioned by other ancient and early Byzantine authors, such as Galen, e.g. *On Antidotes*, 1.14, ed. Kühn (1827) XIV.68.5–7, and Aetios of Amida, *Tetrabiblos*, 2.196, ed. Oliveri (1935) I.224.24, it does not appear in any edited Palaiologan sources. The city of Corycus (mod. Kızkalesi in Mersin Province, Turkey) on the southern coast of Anatolia about 800 km from Constantinople was under Armenian rule (Armenian Kingdom of Cilicia) in the early fourteenth century.

[120] There is no reference to the *krokos* from Athos in any edited Byzantine text. Athos, the most important centre of Christian Orthodox monasticism from the tenth century onwards, was in constant contact with Constantinople. For an introduction to Athos, see *ODB*, s.v. Athos, Mount.

its natural colour which resembles red (*erythra*) or reddish (*hyperythra*) colours (§16). Further details are also provided by John in respect of red, blue, and black colours (§§ 17, 24, and 31).

2.7 The urine vial (*amis*)

Scholars mostly recognize John as an important figure in the history of uroscopy due to his graduated urine vial,[121] which became popular in the Renaissance West, after the translation of his treatise into Latin in 1519.[122] However, the practical application of John's complicated division of the urine vial and how John uses it in his discussion of urinary particles throughout the treatise has never been examined.

The important role that John ascribes to the best possible form of urine vial is shown by the fact that, unlike his predecessors,[123] he devoted a special chapter to its external appearance.[124] He considers fine, plain glass (*leukēs... kai leptēs hyelou*) the right material unlike vials made of greenish glass (*hypochlōrizousai*), since only the former allows easy observation of the various urinary colours and consistencies. As to the shape, there is an initial mention of a vial of irregular shape (*anōmalois amidesin*), which is elongated (*epimēkesi pany*) and has an extended base (*pythmena exechonta*); if it is large enough to contain plenty of urine, it may be useful. However, he thinks that the most appropriate vessel in which to examine urine is in the shape of a drinking cup or beaker (*ekpōma*), which suggests a cylindrical container with a flat bottom.[125]

The most significant part is found in the first book, where John discusses the division of the vial into particular areas.[126] The main difference between John and his predecessors lies not only in his extremely detailed discussion of the various features of particles found in urine, such as their colour, consistency,

[121] Vieillard (1903: 71–2); Desnos (1914: I.191–7); Neuburger (1937: 154); Dimitriadis (1971: 60–1); Diamandopoulos (1997: 226); and Moulinier-Brogi (2012: 148–66).

[122] See the discussion of John's reception in Chapter 7.

[123] There is no such chapter in any earlier Byzantine treatise on the topic. The appearance of the urine vial received some attention, although very brief, in Ibn Sīnā's *Canon of Medicine* (*Kitāb al-Qānūn fī al-Ṭibb*), 1.2.3, (1593) I.68, and Isḥāq al-Isrāʾīlī's *Book of Urine* (*Kitāb al-Bawl*), 2, ed. Trot (1515) 163r = repr. Fontana (1966) 152.

[124] JZA, *On Urines*, 2.1, ed. Ideler (1842) II.32.19–33.18.

[125] See Eustathios of Thessaloniki, *On the Capture of Thessaloniki*, ed. Kyriakidis (1961) 116.6–7, who in his account of the sack of Thessaloniki in 1185 mentions that the Normans used urine vials (*ourōn docheiois*) as beakers (*potēriois*) having been confused by their similar shape. Unfortunately, there are no surviving Byzantine urine vials. For a useful survey on glass containers in Byzantium, including references to medicinal uses, see Antonaras (2010), to whom I owe the reference to Eustathios.

[126] JZA, *On Urines*, 1.12–13, ed. Ideler (1842) II.19.21–2.22.

and shape, but also in his account of their place in the vial.[127] There are traditionally three kinds of particles identified in relation to their place in the vial: a) sediment (*hypostasis*) found on the bottom, b) the suspension (*enaiōrēma*) in the middle of the vial, and c) the cloud (*nephelē*) in the upper part. John, however, goes a step further by subdividing these three areas and introducing eleven sub-areas in the urine vial, each of them having the width of a finger (*daktylos*). Figure 2.2 shows my reconstruction based on John's text in association with evidence from all the surviving manuscripts of the work containing the diagram, which originates in John's treatise, as mentioned by him.[128]

Particles found in sub-areas 2 to 4 are considered sediments, the space between sub-areas 6 and 8 is connected with suspended particles, while clouds

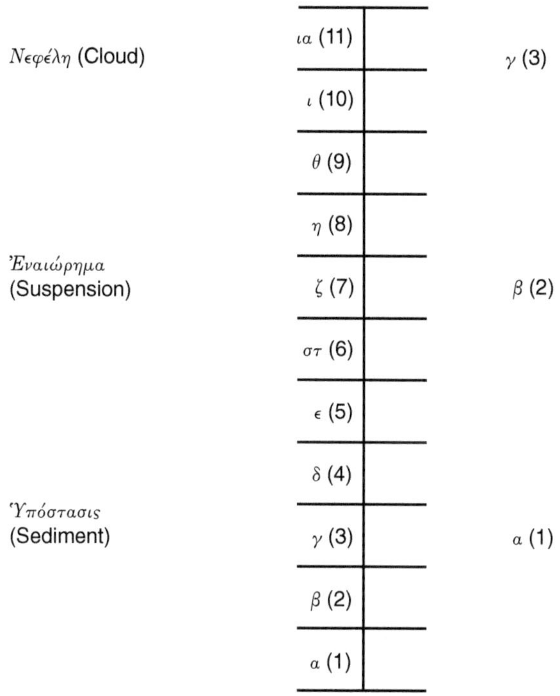

Figure 2.2. Diagram of John's urine vial. Reconstruction by Petros Bouras-Vallianatos.

[127] John devotes special chapters in each book of his treatise to particles. For example, in the second book, 2.1–12, ed. Ideler (1842) II.54.7–65.36, on diagnosis there are twelve chapters that discuss particles.

[128] This is a paratextual element to which John makes reference at the end of his chapter thirteen in the first book, *On Urines*, 1.13.13, ed. Ideler (1842) II.21.21: '*καὶ ἀπὸ τοῦ διαγράμματος γνοίη*'. For a list of the various versions of the diagram in surviving manuscripts with accompanying discussion, see Appendix 3.

may be located in either sub-areas 10, 11, or 1. Sub-areas 5 and 9 are theoretical spaces between the three kinds of particles. John clarifies further that the normal place for sediment and suspended particles is in the third and seventh sub-areas respectively. For both there are two additional places for those sediments and suspended parts settled down (*hyphizanousōn*) or elevated (*epairomenōn*): sub-areas 2 and 4, and 6 and 8 respectively. In the case of clouds, the symmetrical ones (*symmetrōn*) are found in sub-area 11, those which have settled are in sub-area 10, while those which are super-elevated are in sub-area 1 (*hyperērmenōs*).

John devotes three special chapters in the third, fifth, and sixth books to discussing diagnosis, aetiology, and prognosis based on identifying the location of particles.[129] In the chapter on diagnosis we can see what is clearly a new idea in Byzantine uroscopy. John relates the presence of particles in the various areas in the vial to parts of the human body,[130] although he never provides a detailed list of the parts of the body that correspond to specific areas in the urine vial as, for example, Maurus of Salerno does (see Table 2.5). This new theory has a special role in the field of prognosis. John gives more explicit references to these analogies in chapter thirteen of the sixth book, and they are further substantiated and highlighted by the inclusion of two case histories followed by concluding remarks on the outcome of the examination of urine. The introduction of case histories shows his eagerness to present the results of the new theory.[131] In the first case, he refers to particles found in the middle of the vial (*aiōroumena epi to meson chymatos*) connected with diseases of the hypochondrium (*hypochondriōn*),[132] while in the other case the appearance of clouds (*ōs nephelai*) is connected with diseases of head (*peri tēn kephalēn*).[133]

The analogies to the human body are known in Western uroscopy from as early as the twelfth century, when they are explicitly discussed in *Rules on Urines* (*Regulae Urinarum*), the uroscopic treatise by Maurus of Salerno (*c.*1130–1214), teacher of Gilles de Corbeil, and their popularity grew over the next few centuries.[134] Maurus refers to four areas, each of them connected with a particular part of the human body starting from the top, which could indicate diseases of the head and limbs. The second area is related to heart and

[129] JZA, *On Urines*, 3.12, 5.4, and 6.13, ed. Ideler (1842) II.64.20–65.36, II.116.24–118.27, and II.164.28–167.19.

[130] JZA, *On Urines*, 3.12.8, ed. Ideler (1842) II.65.21–6. See also JZA, *On Urines*, 5.4.1, ed. Ideler (1842) II.116.25–9.

[131] Case histories nos. 8 and 9; see Chapter 3, Table 3.1.

[132] JZA, *On Urines*, 6.13.16, ed. Ideler (1842) II.166.19–24. See also Chapter 3, n. 122.

[133] JZA, *On Urines*, 6.13.17, ed. Ideler (1842) II.166.24–7.

[134] Maurus of Salerno, *Rules on Urines* (*Regulae Urinarum*), ed. Renzi (1854) 41.10–16. On Maurus, see Wallis (2005b); and Moulinier-Brogi (2012: 144–8). For a discussion of the analogies to the human body in Maurus' text, see Oldoni (1994); and Moulinier-Brogi (2004: 268–9). On the reception of Maurus' uroscopy, see Moulinier-Brogi (2010).

Table 2.5. Statements on the analogy of the locations in the urine vial with parts of the human body in Maurus of Salerno, the Byzantine treatise ascribed to Ibn Sīnā, and John

---

Maurus of Salerno, *Rules on Urines* (*Regulae Urinarum*), ed. Renzi (1854) 41.14–16

Prima regio est cerebrum et membra animata. Secunda cor, et membra spiritualia. Tertia epar et membra nutritiva. Quarta renes, testiculi et cetera inferiora.[135]
The first region <of the urine vial> corresponds to the brain and moving parts. The second <region is related to the> heart and spiritual parts. The third <region is connected with the> liver and the nutritive parts. The fourth <region corresponds to the> kidneys, testicles, and other lower <parts>.

[Ibn Sīnā], *On Urines* (brief version), 20, ed. Ideler (1842) II.293.10–12

Εἰ ἡ ὑπόστασις εἰς μέρος ἵσταται τῆς ἀμίδος, δηλοῦται πάθος τοῦ μέρους τοῦ σώματος τῆς ἀμίδος ἐκείνου εἴτε ἄνω εἴτε κάτω.
The location in which the sediment occurs in the <urine> vial shows the affection of the <relevant> part of the body—either upper or lower.

[Ibn Sīnā], *On Urines* (version edited by John Zacharias Aktouarios), 45, ed. Lamagna (2017) 78.12–14[136]

Ἀπὸ δὲ τοῦ ἐπικρατοῦντος τόπου ἐν τῇ ἀμίδι, οἷον ἄνω ἢ κάτω ἢ μέσον, τὸ οἷον ὑπόστασις φαινόμενον, τὸν πάσχοντα τόπον ἑκάστου μορίου ἔχεις.
Depending on the main part of the <urine> vial, whether at the top or the bottom or in the middle, where the sediment appears, you can deduce the affected place in each part <of the human body>.

John Zacharias Aktouarios, *On Urines*, 3.12.8, ed. Ideler (1842) II.65.24–6

. . . ὥσπερ αὖ ἐπὶ τῶν ἐναιωρουμένων περὶ τὰ ἀνάλογα τοῦ σώματος μέρη τοῦ παντός ἐν οὔροις διαστήματος ἀναλογοῦντος τῷ τοῦ σώματος διαστήματι.
. . . as the suspended parts correspond to specific parts of the body, the regions in the urine <vial> correspond to the regions of the body.

---

lung diseases, the third to the intestines, and the fourth to urogenital diseases and the lower parts of the body. The same notion is briefly presented in the Byzantine uroscopic treatise ascribed to Ibn Sīnā (see Table 2.5).[137] This idea is found neither in Ibn Sīnā's *Canon of Medicine* (*Kitāb al-Qānūn fī al-Ṭibb*) nor in Isḥāq al-Isrāʾīlī's *Book of Urine* (*Kitāb al-Bawl*) and it should be considered of Salernitan origin.

[135] Later in his account Maurus identifies the first (upper) region with the 'crown', here 'circulus': *Rules on Urines* (*Regulae Urinarum*), ed. Renzi (1854) 41.18–20: 'Prima regio dicitur circulus. Secunda superficies seu corpus aereum. Tertia perforatio seu substantia. Quarta fundus.'

[136] See also, [Ibn Sīnā], *On Urines* (version edited by John Zacharias Aktouarios), 19, ed. Lamagna (2017) 53.21–31.

[137] [Ibn Sīnā], *On Urines* (brief version), 20, ed. Ideler (1842) II.293.10–12; and [Ibn Sīnā], *On Urines* (version edited by John Zacharias Aktouarios), 19 and 45, ed. Lamagna (2017) 53.21–5 and 78.12–14. The similarities between John's work and the treatise attributed to Ibn Sīnā in relation to this particular aspect have been noted by Lamagna (2011: 29–31) and (2017: 119–20). See also Lamagna (2017: 126), who informs us that in some manuscripts of the version edited by John there is a diagram in which the names of various parts of the body are placed beside different areas of the urine vial. The diagram was not included in Lamagna's edition.

There is no surviving Greek translation of Maurus' treatise or evidence to suggest such a venture was ever attempted. John's active involvement as an editor of a revised version of the Greek treatise ascribed to Ibn Sīnā, most probably in the early years of his career and before the completion of his *On Urines*,[138] indicates that this notion must have been introduced to John's work through this treatise.[139] This conclusion is corroborated by the fact that another urinary characteristic which is discussed in detail by John,[140] that is the so-called 'crown' (*stephanē*)—referring to a crown that is differentiated from the rest of the urinary liquid since it appears in different colours forming a circle around the periphery of the vial—is actually the central focus of the treatise ascribed to Ibn Sīnā.[141] Crowns were not mentioned in Theophilos or any other earlier Byzantine treatise on the topic. Interestingly, Maurus of Salerno and Gilles de Corbeil each provide a brief account of the subject.[142] Consequently, it is not impossible that the Greek treatise ascribed to Ibn Sīnā might have been a translation of a Pseudo-Avicennic Latin work on the subject and perhaps the product of blending Arabic and Latin contributions on the subject through one or more intermediary stages.[143]

The introduction, discussion, and practical application of the theory of analogies between the vial and the human body in John's treatise are something new in Byzantine uroscopy. John's most original contribution is the introduction and detailed definition of the various sub-areas in the urine vial. One might expect that John would have provided the precise correspondence of each sub-area to specific parts of the human body. The failure to do so should not be put down to lack of confidence on John's part, who even devoted special clinical reports to emphasizing the importance of the new theory in prognosis and stressed the significance of its application to his readers. John's model offered a better idea of the upper and lower limits of each of the three traditional areas, thus enabling his reader to make precise judgments in

[138] On John's involvement in the edition of this treatise, see Chapter 1, Section 4.2.6.

[139] John does not make use of direct quotations from the treatise ascribed to Ibn Sīnā in his *On Urines*. Unlike in the *Medical Epitome* (see Chapter 5, Section 5) in which John acknowledged the use of non-Greek sources, he does not refer to any foreign source in his *On Urines*. This is perhaps due to the nature of the work, which does not consist of excerpts from earlier authors, as was the case with the *Medical Epitome*, which is a compilation. Furthermore, it is worth noting that John generally abstains from referring to his sources by name throughout his corpus, except in cases where he suggested a special passage or work to his readers, for example, something from Galen's corpus (see n. 42, above; and cf. Chapter 5, p. 158).

[140] John devotes special chapters to crowns: JZA, *On Urines*, 1.19, 3.14, 5.5, and 6.16, ed. Ideler (1842) II.26.33–28.4, II.67.31–12, II.118.28–119.9, and II.170.1–171.10.

[141] For references, see n. 22. See also Lamagna (2017: 11–12).

[142] Maurus of Salerno, *Rules on Urines* (*Regulae Urinarum*), ed. Renzi (1854) 41.21–4; Gilles de Corbeil, *On Urines*, 220–34, ed. Kliegel (1972) 44.

[143] A presumed Latin origin of the text is also suggested by the fact that Ibn Sīnā's name appears in the title of the various versions of the work in Greek transliteration of the Latin or medieval Italian version of his name. On this, see the discussion in Chapter 1, n. 223.

debatable cases where, for example, a certain particle might be somewhere between the points of suspension and cloud.

3. CONCLUSION

This close examination of John's *On Urines* has produced a number of findings concerning his intellectual and medical activity in early-fourteenth-century Constantinople. The work was certainly written for experts, who could spend considerable time studying the various details provided. John endeavoured to elevate the examination of urine to equal status with that of the examination of the pulse by producing an exhaustive account of the topic, which had not hitherto received the treatment it deserved. His treatment of so many different urinary characteristics in diagnosing and prognosticating the disease equipped future physicians in a way that had never happened before.

By Byzantine standards in relation to medical literature the work is certainly original in a variety of ways. Unlike, for example, the first four books of the *Medical Epitome*, which lacks John's all-pervasive authorial presence, here he is eager to show that he has something to say about all the available uroscopic theories. For example, we have seen him tell his readers how to distinguish the saffron-yellow colour, guiding them step by step and using concrete examples from daily life. Accounts of various features relating to the examination of urine are often accompanied with didactic material marked by the use of special terms, such as *paradeigma* (example) and *historia* (case history),[144] which help to explain certain aspects of the text using knowledge connected with his practical experience.

The work follows a symmetrical and straightforward structure as regards its contents, providing a clear division of the material according to diagnosis, aetiology, and prognosis. This not only shows John's desire to assist contemporary physicians in their examination of a patient's urine, but it is also indicative of John's inquiring spirit in evaluating his records in a systematic way. As in the case of his *On Psychic Pneuma*, John shows traditional theories on human physiology, which had remained undisputed for centuries (in this case the phases of human digestion), being critically examined and supplemented by his own ideas.

The use of the graduated urine vial is certainly John's greatest innovation. He comes up with a much more detailed approach than his predecessors, which clearly helps future physicians to get a more accurate idea of the new theory in Byzantine uroscopy of the analogies between particular locations in

[144] On *historia*, see Chapter 3, Section 2.1.

the urine vial and the organs of the human body. Not unlike with pharmacology, where a considerable transfer of knowledge can be seen in John's *Medical Epitome* as a result of the introduction of Arabic material (as I discuss in Chapter 5), here, too, John was influenced by a text coming from outside Byzantium, the Greek uroscopic treatise ascribed to Ibn Sīnā. However, in this case the precise route through which this text reached Byzantium is not entirely clear.

3

On Urines

The Physician and His Patients

> When an individual plays a part he implicitly requests his observers to take seriously the impression that is fostered before them. They are asked to believe that the character they see actually possesses the attributes he appears to possess, that the task he performs will have the consequences that are implicitly claimed for it, and that, in general, matters are what they appear to be.
>
> Erving Goffman, *The Presentation of Self in Everyday Life* (1959: 28)

John makes a significant effort in his *On Urines* to connect theory with practice. His extensive uroscopic treatise is characterized by his consistent enthusiasm for presenting original observations. At some points, he deems it necessary to substantiate his material with detailed reports of his medical visits, thus providing a vivid picture of medical practice. In presenting his clinical accounts John has a dual role. He is a practising physician, and thus the central character in the story, but also a 'chronicler', i.e. he constructs a narrative based on the patient's history and the physician's performance. This chapter focuses on the relationship between physician and patient, as depicted by John,[1] taking into consideration factors such as medical expertise and the patient's response. I will also be paying particular attention to narratological features that John may have used to construct his encounters, and thus impress his readers and attract their attention.

But how can we visualize medical practice by means of clinical narratives? As Erving Goffman has suggested (see above), social behaviour involves the way an individual performs in society.[2] In order to fulfil certain expectations a person has to consider his social reality, his presence in the social group(s) he belongs to. Consequently, there is an interaction between the performer and

[1] It is worth stressing that all the details are seen from John's perspective and the veracity of his account cannot be checked with other sources.

[2] Goffman (1959: 28–82).

Innovation in Byzantine Medicine: The Writings of John Zacharias Aktouarios (c.1275–c.1330). Petros Bouras-Vallianatos, Oxford University Press (2020). © Petros Bouras-Vallianatos.
DOI: 10.1093/oso/9780198850687.001.0001

other individuals, a mutual influence upon one another's actions. In the case of John, we can imagine a physician interacting with patients, and thus giving a performance. This performance is about the practice of medicine, the way that a physician and a patient approach each other and their developing interaction. The growing intimacy represents several steps in an ascending scale of confidence; confidence that gives the practitioner credibility, something which is ideally appraised by his audience. Therefore, we can consider an internal audience related to John's immediate actions and consisting of his patients and other characters who might be present. We can also assume a further external, physically absent, audience, as discussed in Chapter 2, consisting of his readers, fellow physicians. With regard to John's clinical accounts, we may also consider intellectuals from John's circle, scholars, who might or might not include medicine among their wide range of interests. In fact, these accounts could be read separately and with no prior knowledge of uroscopy. They could function as didactic content for readers with specialist knowledge, while at the same time they could be used as self-promotional material to impress the specialist and non-specialist alike with the physician's skills in diagnosing, prognostication, and his self-proclaimed ability to treat his patients most successfully.

1. CLINICAL NARRATIVES IN HISTORY

Even nowadays physicians communicate their clinical knowledge by providing an account of physical events related to an individual's medical condition.[3] The accounts could be used as educational reading matter, and thus stimulate practising physicians' awareness of and reflections on certain cases.[4] The earliest known example of medical case histories[5] is attested around the fifth to fourth century BC in the seven books of the Hippocratic *Epidemics*.[6] These vary in form

[3] On the development of medical records in contemporary medicine, see Reiser (1986). On narrative in contemporary medicine, see Kleinman (1988); Good (1994); Epstein (1995); Frank (1995); Mattingly (1991); Brody (2003); and Charon (2006). See also the introductory essay by Class (2014) of a recent edited volume dealing with new approaches to the evaluation of medical case histories.

[4] On medical narrative and medical training, see Hunter (1991); and DelVecchio Good (1995).

[5] I call the ancient and medieval clinical narratives 'case histories', although they do not share the detailed, formal format of modern case histories.

[6] There are a few studies of the history of case histories from antiquity to medieval times; see Temkin (1929); Laín Entralgo (1950); and Böhm, Köhler, and Thome (1978). See also the recent edited volume by Petridou and Thumiger (2016). For an introduction to *Epidemics*, in particular, see Laín Entralgo (1950: 17–47); Langholf (1990); Álvarez-Millán (1999: 21–7); Mattern (2008: 28–31); and Thumiger (2016). For a detailed study of the various groups and their dating, see Deichgräber (1971). On patients in the *Epidemics*, see Jouanna (1999: 112–25) and Thumiger

and structure and are traditionally divided into three subgroups: a) books one and three; b) books two, four, and six; and c) books five and seven. The first group consists of forty-two clinical accounts, which are characterized by a tendency to present symptoms—the most common being acute fever—in strict chronological order and in connection with geographical and climatological data. The author assumes the role of an anonymous observer in the narrative and the focus is clearly on the patient, for whom a name is usually provided. We can identify a constant concern on the part of the author to provide details on turning points and critical days. In the second group, we are sometimes aware of the presence of the physician in reporting his actions, although he does not have a central role. The author gives information on diagnosis, prognosis, and therapy, underlining the seat of a disease. In the last group, especially in book seven, there are examples reporting the physician's effectiveness in treating his patients where the author uses the first-person singular. The *Epidemics* on the whole seem to have functioned as teaching tools or aides-memoire, providing young physicians with useful details on how to diagnose and make a prognosis, which will help them build a reputation.

After the Hippocratic examples, case histories are rarely found in other authors apart from Galen. We know from mentions in Galenic works that Erasistratos (*c.*315–*c.*240 BC) produced some accounts, which are now lost in the original Greek.[7] The same applies to Rufus of Ephesos' (*fl.* AD 100) examples, which only survive in Arabic translation.[8] In this version, which contains twenty-one case histories altogether, the author is no longer an anonymous observer. We can see a strong first-person singular or even plural, 'we', denoting the active participation of the physician. Rufus is presenting himself as very successful in treating his patients; although four of the twenty-two patients died, this is explained by the author as the outcome of non-compliance with his advice or erroneous recommendations by other physicians. Furthermore, there is a strong emphasis on a patient's history or anamnesis, but, unlike in the

(2018); on female patients, see Hanson (1989); and King (1998: 54–74); on slaves, see Kudlien (1968a: 14–25); on women and slaves, see Demand (1998). For a prosopography of the patients, see Deichgräber (1982). See also the recent studies by Wee (2016) and Webster (2016).

[7] Two of these examples are cited in Galen's, *On Bloodletting against the Erasistrateans in Rome*, 3, ed. Kühn (1826), XI.200–1 and XI.206–9. On these accounts in the context of ancient case histories, see Mattern (2008: 31, and 215–16, n. 104).

[8] The text with German translation and commentary is published by Ullmann (1978). See also Álvarez-Millán (1999: 27–30), who discusses various features of Rufus' accounts. No Greek version survived into the early Middle Ages and John does not seem to be aware of Rufus' accounts. There are about fifteen more cases in Rufus' surviving works; see Ullmann (1978: 17–18). See also Letts (2016), who has recently examined the importance of questioning the patient as featured in Rufus' *Medical Questions*.

Epidemics, no details are provided on the season or the weather conditions at the time of treatment.[9]

Later on, in the second century AD, Galen included more than 300 case histories scattered in his work, providing an enormous set of data about his medical activity.[10] He does not produce a separate work with case histories like earlier authors, but he employs the case history in his attempt to illustrate how medical theory could be applied in daily practice. His accounts combine details of diagnosis and prognosis entailing narratological features; the result often gives an air of rhetorical performance, which is a common trait of the highly competitive environment of Rome in the second century AD and the Second Sophistic, the leading intellectual current of this period.[11] Galen often describes an intense contest with other physicians and always ends up presenting himself as the most effective practitioner.

For almost twelve centuries, between Galen and John, we do not have other recorded examples of medical case histories in the Greek language.[12] Although Byzantine physicians produced very useful practical handbooks, which were circulated in a large number of manuscripts, they do not seem interested in writing down their experiences in such a way.[13] However, in a different context and a scientifically highly developed society, authors writing in Arabic showed a considerable interest in recording clinical data. Although there are occasional instances of case histories incorporated into medical treatises, the

[9] On diagnosis and treatment in Rufus' case histories, see Thomssen and Probst (1994: 1266–90).

[10] For an introduction to Galenic case histories, see García Ballester (1995); and Lloyd (2009). See also Mattern (2008), who provides a comprehensive study of the entire group of Galenic case histories. In particular, on Galen's young patients, see Gourevitch (2001).

[11] See von Staden (1995) and Gleason (2009), who discuss Galenic rhetoric in presenting his anatomical treatises. See also Debru (1996) and Mattern (1999), who gives an insight into medical performances in Imperial Rome.

[12] Two case histories dealing with horses by Theomnestos (*fl.* early fourth century AD) survive in the Byzantine compilation of veterinary medicine, the *Hippiatrica*. See McCabe (2007: 186–91). There are also four very brief examples in the uroscopic treatise ascribed to Ibn Sīnā, in the version edited by John. [Ibn Sīnā], *On Urines*, 16, 26, ed. Lamagna (2017) 48.11–17 (no. 1), 48.17–25 (no. 2), 60.5–7 (no. 3), 60.7–15 (no. 4) On this treatise, see the discussion in Chapter 1, Section 4.2.6. According to Lamagna (2017: 118), the first one is not found in the earlier version of the text by Christodoulos and is perhaps an addition by John. In the absence of a critical edition for all surviving versions of this treatise, which could help us clarify John's actual involvement, I shall not discuss these examples here. Lastly, one should note that there are a large number of surviving accounts of Christian miracles in which we can sometimes see a detailed description of patients' symptoms and clinical conditions, but these accounts were not written by physicians and they mainly aimed to emphasize the miraculous cures. For an introduction, see Efthymiadis (2014).

[13] Alexander of Tralles, who shows a constant awareness of the need to provide recommendations refined by his rich clinical experience, includes some references to patients, usually in a short phrase confirming the validity of his pharmacological recipes. However, these examples cannot be considered case histories. For example, see Alexander of Tralles, *Therapeutics*, 1.15, ed. Puschmann (1878) I.551.17–25.

most common example takes the form of short working notes on efficient therapeutic agents applied to patients. These were sometimes recorded by students, as in the case of al-Rāzī's (d. *c*.925) *The Book of Experiences* or *Casebook* (*Kitāb al-Tajārib*), which contains an amazing 900 cases.[14] Al-Rāzī is shown treating his patients and is usually presented using the third-person singular. There are no remarkable cases of prognosis and the diagnosis is usually implicit. The therapeutic observations seem to serve as a teaching tool for the instruction of young physicians rather than for self-promotion.

At the end of the thirteenth century, in the West, the first *consilia* were introduced (*consilia* is the plural of *consilium* meaning 'advice'). These usually take the form of written recommendation in abbreviated form from experienced physicians.[15] For example, Taddeo degli Alderotti (*c*.1215–95), a pioneer physician and the founder of academic medical training in Bologna, left 185 *consilia* of which over a hundred contain just a simple recipe.[16] Surgery is very rarely recommended except for the usual techniques of phlebotomy or cauterization. Even the longest *consilia* do not refer to the patient's day-to-day history nor do they provide details on the progress of the disease as in Hippocratic or Galenic case histories, although sometimes we find details about the patient's symptoms. Their main role is to recommend appropriate methods of diagnosis and some well-tested medicament to trainee physicians in the early stages of their career, or in Taddeo's case to provide an academic handbook with useful 'tips' for medical students. Although Taddeo and his circle were contemporaries of John's, it does not seem that these kinds of premodern clinical records had any direct influence on the Byzantine world. The same applies to those accounts from the Islamic medical tradition, which did not circulate in Greek translation, although other Arabic works were translated into Greek.[17]

It is no coincidence that the reappearance of the genre in the Greek-speaking world occurred in early Palaiologan Byzantium. As has already been discussed in Chapter 1, the period was marked by a rich intellectual activity and the production of works written in classicizing Greek. Scholars participated in intellectual gatherings, *theatra*, presenting their works and debating on various subjects.[18] Niels Gaul has coined the term 'late Byzantine

[14] On al-Rāzī's clinical accounts, see Álvarez-Millán (1999: 33–42); Álvarez-Millán (2000); Pormann and Savage-Smith (2007: 115–19); and Álvarez-Millán (2015). See also Koetschet (2016: 231–8), who provides some examples of mental patients in case histories from the medieval Islamic world. On the genre of the case history in the medieval Islamic medical tradition, see Álvarez-Millán (2010).

[15] On medieval Latin *consilia*, see Laín Entralgo (1950: 65–104); and Agrimi (1994).

[16] For Taddeo degli Alderotti's *consilia* and his students, see Siraisi (1981: 269–302).

[17] See the discussion in Chapter 5, nn. 13–15.

[18] See Gaul (2018: 233), who argues that *theatra* also functioned as social spaces that were intended to bring intellectuals together with the aristocracy 'by means of patronage and social inclusion'.

sophistic', which describes scholarly activity in the period by analogy to the intellectual movement of the Second Sophistic.[19] Consequently, the Galenic case histories, a distinctive product of a period, which presented significant parallels to John's era, constituted the ideal model for John's case histories.

2. JOHN'S CASE HISTORIES

2.1 Introducing a clinical narrative

John's work *On Urines* includes a total of eleven case histories involving twelve patients altogether (see Table 3.1).[20] The majority of them (seven) are situated in the books on prognosis, while two can be found in the books on diagnosis and another two are embedded in the books on aetiology. Each of them forms an integral part of the relevant chapter's contents, usually appearing in the middle or towards the end. In two cases, a set of two clinical accounts appear in the same chapter.[21] The case histories are not of equal length: some are short, comprising just a few lines, while others are quite long, extending to up to three printed pages. In some cases, we can see a detailed account of a patient's medical condition, while at other times the account is short, giving only essential details on the colour of the urine followed by a brief diagnostic or prognostic statement.

However, all case histories share common features, which allow us to study them as a distinct category of material. They are all narrated in the past tense and John is an eyewitness present in every case, even when he describes the involvement of other physicians. Thus, all the case histories constitute examples of his personal experience relating to contemporary patients. John does not follow a strict chronological approach and there is no systematic attempt to locate his cases in time and space, as in the majority of the Hippocratic clinical accounts. Furthermore, there is no regular mention of crises and critical days, and his nosological data is limited. All patients mentioned remain anonymous. The main focus is on diagnosis and prognosis by means of uroscopy. There are, nonetheless, occasional brief references to therapeutic advice. In all cases, John presents himself in true Galenic fashion, as the most capable physician in attendance and his advice as the most beneficial for the patient. When a patient dies, it is either due to the severity

[19] Gaul (2011).

[20] John's case histories were briefly summarized by Kourousis (1980/2: 270–5) and Hohlweg (1983: 308–9).

[21] Case histories nos. 6 and 7 are part of chapter twelve of the sixth book, the first book on prognosis. Also, case histories nos. 8 and 9 constitute parts of chapter thirteen of the same book.

Table 3.1. List of John's case histories

Case no. [Reference to the edition]	Patient	Problem	John's involvement	Patient's response	Other characters involved	Place of medical activity
1 [*On Urines*, 2.19.14–28, ed. Ideler (1842) II.50.26–52.1]	Male (*therapeuomenos*).	Unspecified.	John suggests drug treatment.	Patient refuses to swallow the drug.	Attendant (*therapōn*); and friend (*tina tōn filōn*). Attendant is diagnosed (examination of urines).	Unspecified.
2 [*On Urines*, 3.10.5–10, ed. Ideler (1842) II.62.29–63.13]	Two females (*gynē, nosousēs, algousēs*).	Spontaneous 'wound-like' fatigue (*helkōdē kopon automaton*) / Chronic pains in joints (*harmonias algousēs*).	John diagnoses patients (examination of urines). He treats the first patient suggesting a particular diet. He suggests drug treatment to the second patient.	The second patient refuses to swallow the drug.		Unspecified.
3 [*On Urines*, 4.9.5–12, ed. Ideler (1842) II.92.9–93.3]	Male adolescent (*meirax*).	Stomach pain (*gastēr enyxen*).	John diagnoses patient (examination of urines, blood, and excrement).			Unspecified.
4 [*On Urines*, 4.12.23–6, ed. Ideler (1842) II.95.34–96.9]	Male (*anthrōpos*).	Strong pains in kidneys (*algēsas tous nephrous*).	John diagnoses patient (examination of urines and blood) and suggests treatment by using warming agents.			*Iatreion*.
5 [*On Urines*, 6.7.3–17, ed. Ideler (1842) II.154.31–156.11]	Male acquaintance (*asthenēs, anthrōpos, gnōrimos*).	Accumulation of bilious humour (*cholōdē chymon*), jaundice (*ikteros*).	John diagnoses, prognosticates (examination of urines), and treats the patient suggesting an appropriate diet.	Patient shows some lack of faith in physicians.		Patient visited the physician's place of work.

(*continued*)

Table 3.1. Continued

Case no. [Reference to the edition]	Patient	Problem	John's involvement	Patient's response	Other characters involved	Place of medical activity
6 [*On Urines*, 6.12.11–24, ed. Ideler (1842) II.162.17–163.27]	Male adolescent (*meirax, kamnōn*).	Fever (*pyretois*), diarrhoea (*gastrorroiais*).	John prognosticates patient (examination of urines, pulse, and blood). The patient dies.		One of the visiting physicians suggests a treatment by means of venesection (*tis tōn ekeise thamizontōn iatrōn*).	Unspecified.
7 [*On Urines*, 6.12.26–32, ed. Ideler (1842) II.163.28–164.11]	Male (*anthrōpos*).	Dropsy [?] (*hydaleos kai exōdēkōs*).	John prognosticates patient (examination of urines) and suggests a particular diet.	The patient is persuaded.		Patient visited the physician's place of work.
8 [*On Urines*, 6.13.5–14, ed. Ideler (1842) II.165.9–166.16]	Female (*anthrōpos, gynē, kamnousa*).	Pain in the hypochondrium (*hypochondria … algēdonos*).	John prognosticates patient (examination of urines) and suggests treatment using purgatives.	The patient at first refuses to accept the use of purgatives. Later, she agrees, as a result of the advice of the most notable physician.	Other physicians: a Syrian physician (*Syros iatros*) suggests a strong purgative and one of the most notable doctors (*axiologoterōn tē technē*) diagnoses *hypochondrismos*.	Unspecified.
9 [*On Urines*, 6.13.17–23, ed. Ideler (1842) II.166.24–167.5]	Male acquaintance (*anthrōpos, pyressōn, kamnōn, gnōrimos*).	Fever, affection of parotid glands (*parōtides*).	John prognosticates patient (examination of urines).			Unspecified. The patient is confined to bed.

10 [*On Urines*, 7.13.7–26, ed. Ideler (1842) II.181.11–183.12]	Wealthy female (*gynē tis tōn malakōn kai plousiōn*).	Blood around the womb (*athroizomenou men peri tēn mētran tou haimatos*).	John prognosticates patient (examination of urines and pulse). The patient dies.		Other physicians (*tōn ekeise thamizontōn/ thamizousin iatrois*), women (*gynaixi*), and husband (*anēr).*	Unspecified. The patient is confined to bed from the fifth month onwards.
11 [*On Urines*, 7.15.12–25, ed. Ideler (1842) II.186.6–187.4]	Male acquaintance (*anthrōpos, gerōn, gnōrimos*).	Fever (*epyresse, pyretos*), cough (*bēx*).	John prognosticates patient (examination of urines, pulse, sputum, and excrement).			Patient's house [?]. The patient was lying supine.

of the disease or the erroneous treatment given by other physicians. Finally, as in Galen's treatises, the case histories do not constitute an independent work, but they are part of medical argument to provide support for a particular theoretical exposition.

John is conscious of the special nature of these accounts as distinct elements of discourse in his work. He employs a variety of ways to introduce his case histories. For example, he may use the term *historia* (inquiry/written account) or a past form of the verb *diēgeomai* (to set out in detail/narrate) in connection with *horaō* (to see) or simply a past form of the verbs *horaō* and *theaomai* (to behold/to observe). As regards the former case, the Greek term *historia*, which essentially means 'research', had been used as early as the fifth century BC by the Greek historian Herodotus (*c*.484–25 BC) to signify learning or knowledge obtained by 'inquiry' with regards to the Persian wars.[22] In tracing the occurrence of the term *historia* in a medical context, it is quite remarkable that the term does not appear in medical sense in the Hippocratic *Epidemics*. The term must have had special importance for the physicians of the ancient Empiric sect, who considered experience the primary source of medical knowledge. However, since no work by members of the sect survives intact, we only know of their writings from short fragments.[23] Galen's use of the term is very limited; there are only two instances in connection with a case history that might indicate its usefulness to his readers. John's usage of the term echoes that of Galen (see Table 3.2).[24]

As can be seen from the examples in Table 3.2, the term *historia* functions as an emphatic pointer, which is intended to engage the reader's attention, usually as a preparation for a more important piece of information to follow.[25] For example:

[22] Herodotus, *Histories*, 1.1, ed. Legrand (1932) I.13: '*Ἡροδότου Θουρίου ἱστορίης ἀπόδεξις ἥδε*...' For a critical commentary on Herodotus' proem, see Krischer (1965: 159–67); and Nagy (1987: 175–84).

[23] See, for example, Galen, *Outline of Empiricism*, ed. Deichgräber (1965) 66–9. On Empiricism and the employment of the term *historia*, see Deichgräber (1965: 298–301); and von Staden (1975: 190). For the re-employment of the term in early modern medicine, see Pomata (2005: 122–37).

[24] There are four examples where the use of the word *historia* indicates the beginning of the narrative: JZA, *On Urines*, 6.12.26, 6.13.17, 7.13.7, and 7.15.12, ed. Ideler (1842) II.163.29, II.166.26, II.181.13, and II.186.6. In the rest of the cases, the term appears twice at the end of the case history and once in the middle of the story: JZA, *On Urines*, 3.10.10, 7.13.26, and 7.13.21, ed. Ideler (1842) II.63.11, II.183.9, and II.182.33.

[25] The special role of the case histories in John's texts is also attested in various manuscripts, such as Parisinus gr. 2270 (fourteenth century), Florentinus Laurentianus gr. plut. 75.11 (AD 1411/12), Londiniensis Wellcomensis MS.MSL.52 (fifteenth century), and Parisinus gr. 2304 (fourteenth century), in which the scribe indicated the beginning of case histories by inscribing the term '*ἱστορία*' in the margins. In Parisinus gr. 2304, for example, there are relevant annotations in red ink in the margin in six out of the eleven case histories on ff. 32v, 58v, 99v, 100v, 108r, and 110v.

Theory: '...and the colour of the urine already seems over reddish and almost becomes even more red.'
Introduction to case history: 'But in order to provide my account with some kind of grace, and at the same time to make my speech trustworthy, let us introduce this case history too, which will benefit my account...'
Case history: 'One woman from the soft and rich...was in danger of becoming distressed at the idea of having an only child.'[26]

Table 3.2. Examples of the use of forms of *historia* in Galen's and John's case histories

Galen	John
On Anatomical Procedures, 7.13, ed. Kühn (1821) II.632.5 = ed. Garofalo (2000) 459.16: ...*διὰ γὰρ τὸ χρήσιμον τῆς ἱστορίας*... ...for the usefulness of the case history...	*On Urines*, 6.12.26, ed. Ideler (1842) II.163.29–30: *Ἐπεὶ δέ τινας εἰκὸς ποθεῖν εἰδέναι καὶ τοιαύτην ἱστορίαν ἑτέραν, καὶ ταῦτα προσεπιθήσω τῷ λόγῳ*... Since some people might reasonably wish to learn about another such case history, I will add these to my account...
On Affected Parts, 4.8, ed. Kühn (1824) VIII.266.11–12: ...*βέλτιον οὖν ἔδοξέ μοι καὶ ταῦθ' ὑμῖν ἱστορῆσαι.* ...I thought it useful to tell you of these case histories.	*On Urines*, 6.13.17, ed. Ideler (1842) II.166.26–7: ...*καὶ προσθήσω κἀπὶ τούτων ἱστορίαν ἑτέραν σαφηνείας τινὰ τῶν λεγομένων ἕνεκεν.* ...I shall add to what I have said another case history in order to ensure the clarity of my exposition.
	On Urines, 7.13.7, ed. Ideler (1842) II.181.12–13: ...*καὶ ταύτην ἐπιθήσωμεν τὴν ἱστορίαν τῷ λόγῳ λυσιτελοῦσαν.* ...let us introduce this case history, too, which will benefit my account.
	On Urines 7.15.12, ed. Ideler (1842) II.186.5–6: ...*ἀλλὰ κἀνταῦθα θεὶς τῷ λόγῳ ἱστορίαν προσήκουσαν ἐφ' ἕτερα τῷ λόγῳ τρέψομαι.* ...after adding a suitable case history at this point, I will turn to another subject.

[26] JZA, *On Urines*, 7.13.6–8, ed. Ideler (1842) II.181.9–19: '...*τὸ χρῶμα ἤδη τοῦ οὔρου πρός γε τὸ ὑπέρυθρον καὶ ἔτι τὸ ἐρυθρὸν πρόεισιν. Ἀλλ' ἵνα τῷ μὲν λόγῳ χάρις τις ᾖ μεταβαλλομένῳ, πίστις δ' οὐκ ὀλίγη τῶν λεγομένων, καὶ ταύτην ἐπιθήσωμεν τὴν ἱστορίαν τῷ λόγῳ λυσιτελοῦσαν*... *Γυνή τις τῶν μαλακῶν καὶ πλουσίων*... *αὐτῆς δὲ κινδυνευούσης ὑφ' ἑνὶ μόνῳ παιδὶ τὰς ἐλπίδας ἐν ἀπρούπτῳ σαλεύειν.*'

The introductory sentence serves as an intermediary between the theory and the case history. John gives his typical account, in this case of the various kinds of urine related to uterine affections. Then he admits honestly that he is citing a specific case in order to give credence to his writings. The use of the word *historia* at the beginning of a case history marks its role as a transitional step between the theoretical and the clinical details. John expands his narration by embedding a text, which deals with everyday practice.

A similar process can also be identified at the end of many case histories. For example, in the previous case, John concludes by referring to his account, using the word *historia* once again:

> The <specifics> of the case history were more or less as stated. And from now on you should be clearly and precisely informed that so much blood accumulated around the womb transmits its colour to the urine due to the proximity <between the two>.[27]

He insists on the usefulness of his case history and concludes with this main point in order to make its connection with the context of the chapter clearer. It marks the end of a pattern that is indicated by the outcome of his clinical test, and confirms the correctness of his uroscopic theories. Furthermore, the use of the second-person singular address maintains a certain degree of intimacy between the narrator and the reader. Consequently, it can also give a didactic tone to John's words.[28]

At other times, John launches a case history by simply saying, *heōrakōs*/*heōraka* ('having seen/I saw') and *tetheametha* ('I beheld/observed') or *heōrakōs* followed by *diēgēsasthai* or *diēgēsaimēn* ('having seen...to narrate/I would narrate') or *memnēmai idōn* ('I remember having seen').[29] Examples of these related verbs had sometimes been used in the past by Galen in introducing his case histories.[30] John's employment of these terms resembles

[27] JZA, *On Urines*, 7.13.26, ed. Ideler (1842) II.183.9–12: '*Τὰ μὲν οὖν τῆς ἱστορίας οὕτως πως εἶχε· σὺ δ' ἀκριβῶς ἐντεῦθεν πυθόμενος ἴσθι σαφῶς, ὡς λόγῳ τῆς ἐγγύτητος μετέδωκε τοῦ χρώματος τὸ περὶ τὴν μήτραν ἀθροισθὲν τόσον αἷμα τοῖς οὔροις.*'

[28] See also the final sentence in case history no. 4, in which the didactic tone is heightened through the use of the infinitives *skeptesthai* and *manthanein*, JZA, *On Urines*, 4.12.27, ed. Ideler (1842) II.96.10–12: '*Ὑμῖν δὲ θέμις τὰ τοιαῦτα σκέπτεσθαι καὶ μανθάνειν ἔχειν*...' ('It is fair for you to be able to consider and learn these <theories>...'). See also Chapter 2, n. 59.

[29] In two cases the verb *diēgeomai* is used in connection with *horaō*: JZA, *On Urines*, 2.19.14 and 6.7.3, ed. Ideler (1842) II.50.27–8 and II.154.32. The verb *horaō* is used in connection with *mimnēskō* three times: JZA, *On Urines*, 4.9.5, 4.12.22, and 6.13.5, ed. Ideler (1842) II.92.10, II.95.34, and II.165.9–10. The verb *horaō* and *theaomai* are used once each: JZA, *On Urines*, 3.10.5 and 6.12.10, ed. Ideler (1842) II.62.30 and II.162.17–18, respectively.

[30] See, for example, see Galen, *On Affected Parts*, 3.11, ed. Kühn (1824) VIII.194.4–5: '*καὶ τοῦτ' ἐθεασάμην*...'; *Therapeutic Method*, 10.3, ed. Kühn (1825) X.671.6: '*Καί σοι διηγήσομαι τοιοῦτον ἄῤῥωστον*...'; *Therapeutic Method*, 12.7, ed. Kühn (1825) X.856.16–17: '*ὧν ἤδη μνημονεύσω δυοῖν ἢ τριῶν οὐ πρὸ πολλοῦ θεραπευθέντων*...'; and *Commentary on Hippocrates' 'Prorrhetics'*, 3.120, ed. Kühn (1825) XVI.771.18 = ed. Diels (1915) 139.7: '*εἶδον οὖν ἅπαξ*...' For more examples, see Mattern (2008: 37–43; 218–21, nn. 129–30, 139–40; and 234, n. 38).

that of Galen, although we cannot identify any further textual similarities. As in the case of the *historia*, they are part of an introductory sentence functioning as a connecting link between theory and case history. For example: 'And having seen in the past the same things [i.e. urine indicating jaundice] happening to an acquaintance, it is fitting to narrate them now.'[31] We can see it as an alternative way of engaging his readers. It is a different way of framing his experiences. John has a clear plan of how to display his material appropriately. It is worth giving an example from the modern world. A manual of surgery containing videos with operations would be more likely to attract and retain the attention of trainee physicians rather than one with printed images. Thus, any book puts across its ideas to its intended audience. In an analogous vein, John wants to give his reader the impression that he had been an eyewitness and could thus assume the authority of first-hand experience. A specialized audience consisting of contemporary physicians and people with considerable medical knowledge would have been impressed to receive this contemporary clinical data.

The idea of observation and its importance for the reader is encapsulated in sentences such as: 'I remember having seen something like this in an adolescent.'[32] In this case, John emphasizes once again that he has observed what he narrates, but in addition he stresses the act of recall. The practice of narrating a case history involves a process of retaining and recalling facts and impressions.[33] For a reader the way they see a text is immediately changed. The theoretical details give way to real entities, the characters in a case history.

2.2 Characters

The main characters in a case history are John and his patients, although occasionally other contemporary physicians feature, too. At times, a patient's relative is also present. Furthermore, in one case there is a person who seems to be John's attendant. In presenting the characters, I would like to examine the use of the various terms employed to describe them, and also how John chooses to narrate them.

The physician's perspective is mostly given through a powerful first-person narrative. John usually represents himself as making an observation or reporting

[31] JZA, *On Urines*, 6.7.3, ed. Ideler (1842) II.154.31–2: '*Καί ποτε αὐτὸς ἐπί τινος γνωρίμου τὰ παραπλήσια ἑωρακὼς νῦν ἂν διηγησαίμην κατὰ καιρόν.*'

[32] JZA, *On Urines*, 4.9.5, ed. Ideler (1842) II.92.9–10: '*Ἐγώ γε μὴν ἐπί τινος μείρακος τοιοῦτον τι μέμνημαι ἰδών.*' See also Chapter 2, n. 60.

[33] Psychologists often call the recollection of episodes from an individual's life 'autobiographical memory'. For an overview of the various ideas concerning autobiographical memory, see Brewer (1996). On the reconstruction of autobiographical information in the process of narration, see Barclay (1996). On Galen and autobiographical memory, see Mattern (2008: 43–7).

his thoughts and medical actions. For example: 'When I saw these <signs> and having been persuaded . . . ' or even more decisively: 'When I saw him still in a healthy condition, although his urine was suddenly giving the impression that he suffered from a most severe sickness . . . '.[34] Sometimes, he chooses to use the first-person plural, 'we'. For example: 'So we decided that the patient should follow a diet <to help> his digestive capacity . . . '.[35]

The narration usually shifts from the first-person to the third-person singular, in order to present the patient's medical condition. This does not have the clear structure of a scientific report. The details, as regards various symptoms, are usually scattered throughout his narration. The focus is clearly on the careful examination of the urine, while other information, including the pulse rate, sometimes plays a supplementary role. For example:

> . . . it is not long ago that I have seen something of that sort <happening to> an adolescent. He was in a good state as regards the strength and the size of his body and he consumed many and various kinds of food without following any specific diet. For the adolescent <belonged to> the group of people having a voracious appetite, and he constantly suffered from fevers and diarrhoea, and although he experienced these repeatedly, he was eventually freed of this terrible condition. But once, when he suffered from fever, having been attacked by an extraordinary putrefaction <of humours>, he invited me <to treat him> showing confidence in the <suggested> treatment.[36]

The passage describes the patient's lifestyle, diet, and age, and gives details of his clinical condition. This description constitutes the patient's history immediately before John became involved. The story is directly followed by an examination of the urine that was carried out on an almost daily basis.

The patient might be a woman or man, an adolescent or an elderly person. John uses a variety of terms that may all be translated as 'patient' in English. He refers to his patients as *asthenēs, arrōstos, kamnōn/kamnousa, nosousa* and *paschōn*, thus denoting someone who is ill.[37] He also frequently uses the term

[34] JZA, *On Urines*, 4.12.26, ed. Ideler (1842) II.96.7–8: '*Ἐγὼ μὲν οὖν ταῦτα ἰδών τε καὶ πυθόμενος . . .*'; and *On Urines*, 6.7.11, ed. Ideler (1842) II.155.17–20: '*Ἐγὼ δὲ τὸ μὲν τοιαῦτα οὖρα προΐεσθαι ἐξαίφνης αὐτὸν μὲν ὁρῶν ἔτι ὑγιῆ περιϊόντα, ἐκεῖνα δ' εἰδὼς ἐπὶ χειρίστοις νοσήμασι φαινόμενα . . .*'

[35] JZA, *On Urines*, 6.12.31, ed. Ideler (1842) II.164.6–7: '*Ἔδοξε οὖν ἡμῖν ἐπὶ ἀρρώστῳ ἔτι τῇ πεπτικῇ δύναμει ἐκδεδιητῆσθαι τὸν ἄνθρωπον . . .*'

[36] JZA, *On Urines*, 6.12.11–13, ed. Ideler (1842) II.162.17–24: '*. . . οἷόν τι κἀπί τινος οὐ πάνυ πρῴην ἑώρακα μειρακίου. Εὖ μὲν γὰρ οὗτος εἶχεν ῥώμης τε καὶ μεγέθους σώματος, πλείοσι δὲ καὶ διαφόροις χρώμενος βρώμασιν ἀδιαιτήτως. Τῶν ἀδδηφάγων καὶ γὰρ ἦν ὁ μείραξ, συνεχῶς ἡλίσκετο πυρετοῖς καὶ γαστρορροίαις ἐπὶ τούτοις περιπίπτων, ἀπηλλάττετο του δεινοῦ. Ἀλλά ποτε περιπεσὼν πυρετῷ ὑπ' ἐξαισίας ἀναφθέντι σήψεως ἐμέ τε μετεκαλεῖτο καὶ τὴν θεραπείαν ἐπίστευε.*'

[37] John uses the term *asthenēs* and *arrōstos* once each: JZA, *On Urines*, 6.7.14 and 6.12.31, ed. Ideler (1842) II.155.33 and II.164.6. He employs the term *kamnōn/ousa* six times: JZA, *On Urines*, 6.12.14, 6.12.24, 6.13.7, 6.13.10, 6.13.12, and 6.13.14, ed. Ideler (1842) II.162.26, II.163.25, II.165.16, II.165.33, II.166.6–7, and II.166.14. Finally, the term *nosousēs* and *paschōn* appear twice and once respectively: JZA, *On Urines*, 3.10.5, 3.10.8, and 6.7.14, ed. Ideler (1842) II.62.31,

anthrōpos ('person'), which could refer to either a male or a female patient.[38] A female patient can also be called merely a *gynē* ('woman').[39] In total, female patients appear in three case histories.

Occasionally, there are words with special connotations in the immediate context. For example, the masculine form of the present participle of the verb *pyressō* ('to be feverish'), that is *pyressōn*, indicates a man suffering from heavy fever.[40] The term is only used twice, although cases of fever are reported elsewhere, too. John uses the participle to express a dramatic change in the condition of a patient, that is a deterioration that reaches its climax, when he states that he '... was relieving in bed his physical needs'.[41] In a similar vein, the term *algousa* is only used when John wants to denote chronic pain of a female patient, thus indicating certain special ongoing characteristics of a patient's condition.[42] Furthermore, *therapeuomenos* ('one who receives treatment'), the passive participle of the verb *therapeuō* ('to heal') refers to a case where John's own therapeutic recommendation plays a central role.[43] This particular account begins by presenting the patient as rejecting a certain medicament. Thus, the use of the term *therapeuomenos* emphasizes the treatment as a process, and indicates its particular significance for the rest of the story.

Although John does not give us precise ages for his patients, he occasionally designates them with words that provide an approximate notion of how old they were. Thus, he uses the noun *meirax* ('lad' or 'adolescent') twice probably to refer to a boy in his late teens,[44] while one patient is called *gerōn* ('old man').[45] When John uses the term *gnōrimos* ('acquaintance'), he emphasizes his familiarity with the patients.[46] Moreover, it is worth mentioning that no indication of a patient's profession is given. Nevertheless, there are cases where we find information regarding their social background. This sort of

II.63.3, and II.155.29. On the use of various terms in Galenic case histories, see Mattern (2008: 98–119). It is worth noting that there is no case history dealing with slaves in John's work.

[38] The term is used nine times for male patients and twice for females: JZA, *On Urines*, 2.19.17, 2.19.18, 4.9.12, 4.12.24, 6.7.14, 6.8.17, 6.12.24, 6.12.31, 6.13.22, 6.13.11, and 7.13.25, ed. Ideler (1842) II.51.3, II.51.9, II.92.34–5, II.96.5, II.155.35, II.156.8, II.163.26–7, II.164.7, II.167.2, II.165.35, and II.183.7–8.

[39] JZA, *On Urines*, 3.10.5, 3.10.10, 6.13.5, 7.13.8, 7.13.13, 7.13.16, and 7.13.21, ed. Ideler (1842) II.62.30, II.63.8, II.165.10, II.181.14, II.181.30, II.182.2, and II.182.22.

[40] JZA, *On Urines*, 6.13.18 and 7.15.15, ed. Ideler (1842) II.166.28 and II.186.16.

[41] JZA, *On Urines*, 6.13.19, ed. Ideler (1842) II.166.31–2: '... *ἐπὶ κλίνης τὰς φυσικὰς ἀνάγκας ἐπλήρου.*'

[42] JZA, *On Urines*, 3.10.5, ed. Ideler (1842) II.62.31–2. For a list of various terms denoting and characterizing various qualities of pain in Greek medical literature with a special focus on Galen, see Siegel (1976: 205).

[43] JZA, *On Urines*, 2.19.16, ed. Ideler (1842) II.50.37.

[44] JZA, *On Urines*, 4.9.5, 6.12.11, and 6.12.12, ed. Ideler (1842) II.92.10, II.162.17–18, and II.162.20–1.

[45] JZA, *On Urines*, 7.15.13 and 7.15.19, ed. Ideler (1842) II.186.7 and II.186.27.

[46] JZA, *On Urines*, 6.7.3, 6.7.4, and 7.15.13, ed. Ideler (1842) II.154.31, II.154.33, and II.186.7.

information is provided either by adverbs indicative of origin such as *agroikōs* or *agrothen* ('coming from the countryside'), or adjectives denoting socio-economic status, such as *plousios* ('wealthy').[47] Such social distinctions among patients, as we will see later, are sometimes important for the patients' own assessment of John's medical advice and performance.

We can also see a number of other characters appearing in a small number of other cases. John mentions the presence of an attendant or servant (*therapōn*), who follows him in one of his case histories.[48] This person's voice and actions are relayed in the third-person singular and he appears to have some knowledge of the efficacy of drugs, which could be seen as the result of his experience in assisting John or perhaps even other physicians in the past.[49] The attendant is also called *pais*, a noun that sometimes denotes a servant in ancient and medieval Greek literature.[50] In this case, it might be seen as an indication of age showing that the attendant is quite young. In the same case history, there is also a mention of one of John's friends (*tina tōn philōn*) to whom the attendant was sent, without offering any further details.[51]

Moreover, John attests the presence of other physicians in three case histories always using indirect speech in reporting their recommendations.[52] He may refer to a group of physicians as *thamizontes iatroi* ('frequenting physicians') or simply to one physician, *iatros*.[53] In one case, the physician's response is associated with that of some other people, *anthrōpoi*, probably assistants who happened to be there: 'when the physician (*iatros*) saw this—and the rest of the people (*anthrōpoi*) who were around the patient—they tried to treat the bloody parts...'[54] In addition to physicians, in one case John mentions the presence of the husband of one of his female patients (*tō te autēs andri*) appearing to attend the physicians and expressing the hope that his

[47] A term signifying an origin in the countryside is used twice: JZA, *On Urines*, 3.10.10 and 6.12.28, ed. Ideler (1842) II.63.9 (in this case, Ideler's edition reads wrongly '*ἀγροικῶς*' instead of the correctly accented version '*ἀγροίκως*') and II.163.33. A female patient is characterized as wealthy: JZA, *On Urines*, 7.13.8, ed. Ideler (1842) II.181.15.

[48] JZA, *On Urines*, 2.19.14, 2.19.18, and 2.19.20, ed. Ideler (1842) II.50.27–8, II.51.10, and II.51.14. There is another case where the text reads erroneously '*θεραπών*' instead of the correctly accented version '*θεράπων*': JZA, *On Urines*, 2.19.15, ed. Ideler (1842) II.50.31. See Miller (2017: 259), who has recently translated the term as 'pharmacist assistant' with reference to John's relevant case history, although there is no associated evidence in John's text to support such a specific role. See also the discussion of this case history (no. 1) in Section 2.4, below.

[49] JZA, *On Urines*, 2.19.15, ed. Ideler (1842) II.50.30–2.

[50] JZA, *On Urines*, 2.19.26, ed. Ideler (1842) II.51.30. LSJ s.v. *παῖς*, III, in relation to condition, *slave*, *servant*, *man* or *maid* (of all ages). See also Kriaras s.v. *παις*, 4.

[51] JZA, *On Urines*, 2.19.20, ed. Ideler (1842) II.51.15.

[52] See case history nos. 6, 8, and 10.

[53] JZA, *On Urines*, 6.12.23, 6.13.5–7, 6.13.12–13, 7.13.20, and 7.13.24, ed. Ideler (1842) II.163.19–20, II.165.9–18, II.166.3–12, II.182.16–19, and II.183.1–3.

[54] JZA, *On Urines*, 6.13.7, ed. Ideler (1842) II.165.15–18: '*Τοῦτο ἑωρακὼς ὅ τε ἰατρὸς καὶ οἱ περὶ τὴν κάμνουσαν ἄνθρωποι ἱστᾶν τε ἐπεχείρησαν τὰ αἱματώδη ἐκεῖνα...*'

wife's health would improve.[55] Finally, in the same case history, John refers to some women (*gynaixi*) whom the female patient had asked for help.[56] He does not provide any further identification, so we cannot identify any other characteristics of this contemporary group, although we should not exclude the possibility that they may have been folk practitioners.[57]

2.3 Place, time, and seasons

There are only a few scattered details on place in John's case histories, and thus it is impossible to reconstruct his working environment and daily timetable.[58] In most cases, John is shown visiting or leaving the place where the patient is, but no particular term is used to denote it. John's arrival at a place is once described by the use of the verb *aphikneomai* ('to arrive at'). For example, he states: 'I arrived and saw him, since he happened to be a neighbour and a very good man.'[59] He does not give any information about any particular medical facilities or other physicians who may have treated this particular patient before, and the only detail in respect of the space in which the consultation takes place is that the patient was lying supine.[60] Perhaps John is referring to a house call.[61] Another time, John is called (*metaklētheis*) to examine an adolescent and reports: 'that was the third day, when I was called to go in and the patient was relatively unwell.'[62] Later on, in the same case, referring to the presence of other physicians he gives a vague indication by using an indefinite adverb of place, *ekeise thamizontōn*, meaning 'the physicians who used to come there often' or 'frequenting physicians'.[63] The latter implies a place in which several physicians worked on a rotating basis to ensure the care of an individual patient, which could perhaps suggest the working environment of a Byzantine *xenōn*.

[55] JZA, *On Urines*, 7.13.24, ed. Ideler (1842) II.183.2–3.

[56] JZA, *On Urines*, 7.13.11, ed. Ideler (1842) II.181.23–5.

[57] The text does not imply the presence of those women at the birth itself, thus making their identification as midwives less certain.

[58] For example, see Horstmanshoff (1995: 84–8), who managed to provide an outline of Galen's daily timetable.

[59] JZA, *On Urines*, 7.15.13, ed. Ideler (1842) II.186.9–10: '*ἐγὼ δ' ἰδεῖν αὐτὸν ἀφικόμην, γείτονά τε ὄντα καὶ ἄλλως ἀγαθὸν τὸν ἄνθρωπον τυγχάνοντα.*'

[60] JZA, *On Urines*, 7.15.14, ed. Ideler (1842) II.186.11.

[61] Cf. case no. 5, in which John refers to his patient as 'spending the day in the house (*peri ta oikeia*)', but this reference cannot be directly connected with John's activity. JZA, *On Urines*, 6.7.11, ed. Ideler (1842) II.155.21–2.

[62] JZA, *On Urines*, 6.12.14, ed. Ideler (1842) II.162.24–6: '*Τρίτη μὲν οὖν ἦν ἐκείνῳ, καθ' ἣν ἐγὼ μετακληθεὶς εἰσήκειν καὶ ὁ κάμνων οὐ μετρίως εἶχε.*'

[63] JZA, *On Urines*, 6.12.23, ed. Ideler (1842) II.163.19: '... *τῶν ἐκεῖσε θαμιζόντων ἰατρῶν* ...'. The same expression is also used twice in one more case, *On Urines*, 7.13.20 and 7.13.24, ed. Ideler (1842) II.182.18 and II.183.3: '... *τῶν ἐκεῖσε θαμιζόντων* ...' and '... *τοῖς θαμίζουσιν ἰατροῖς*', respectively.

In two cases the patient appears to bring John a sample of urine and the text suggests that the patient visited the physician's place of work, but again there is no specific term used to define it: '…and he brought to us in the morning a urine vial…',[64] and 'He came to us from the countryside bringing a urine vial…'[65] The patient in both cases does not seem to spend a long time there or stay overnight with John. In the second case, having correctly diagnosed the patient's disease, John decides to recommend an appropriate diet to the patient, who left (*ōcheto*) after agreeing to this.[66] A term for the physician's location is clearly given only once when John names a place where he used to receive and examine patients: 'I remember having seen something of the sort in the *iatreion* which I was frequenting. Someone came bringing a urine vial…'[67] In this case, the patient does not suffer from any serious disease and specific details on treatment or the nature of the *iatreion* are not provided. Furthermore, there is no indication of other medical staff being present at the *iatreion* or any description of the space or its topography.

The term *iatreion* is not found in any other fourteenth-century Byzantine sources in the same context. Scholars have connected John's mention of it with references from the twelfth-century *Typikon* of the Pantokrator *xenōn* at Constantinople, and thus concluded that John is referring to a Byzantine *xenōn*.[68] It is worth noting, however, that in the *Typikon* of the Pantokrator, the term has a variety of uses. It is employed twice in order to indicate the hours of operation of the *iatreion*, which in this case refers to the entire *xenōn*;[69] twice in order to denote the medical staff, and only once to specify a particular space, that is the women's ward.[70] Furthermore, this term is not found

[64] JZA, *On Urines*, 6.7.12, ed. Ideler (1842) II.155.24: '…*κομίζει μὲν ἡμῖν ἕωθεν ἀμίδα*…'

[65] JZA, *On Urines*, 6.12.28, ed. Ideler (1842) II.163.32–4: '*Ἧκέ τις ἀγρόθεν εἰς ἡμᾶς ἀμίδα φέρων*…'

[66] JZA, *On Urines*, 6.12.32, ed. Ideler (1842) II.164.10.

[67] JZA, *On Urines*, 4.12.22–3, ed. Ideler (1842) II.95.34–5: '*Ἐγώ γε μὴν και τι τοιοῦτον μέμνημαι ἰδὼν περὶ τὸ ἰατρεῖον θαμίζων. Ἧκέ τις ἀμίδα κομίζων*…'

[68] Kourousis (1980/2: 273–4); Hohlweg (1983: 309); and Hohlweg (1984: 125–6). Cf. Stathakopoulos (2013a: 28–9), who considers the *iatreion* a clinic for ambulant treatment. In particular, Kourousis, in order to strengthen his argument, uses a reference from *Miracle* 30 of Sts Cosmas and Damian to '*τὸ ἰατρεῖον τοῦ ξενῶνος*', ed. Dübner (1907) 174.29. However, this particular phrase survives only in two manuscripts dated to the eleventh (Parisinus gr. 1519) and twelfth (Oxoniensis Bodleianus Clarkianus 50) century; for a description of the manuscripts, see Dübner (1907: 13–15). Thus, we can establish an eleventh-century *terminus ante quem*, which does not coincide with John's period. See Csepregi (2002), who provides a critical study on the miracles.

[69] *Typikon of Pantokrator*, 1000 and 1256, ed. Gautier (1972) 89 and 103. In a similar context the term is also attested in a letter by the well-known Komnenian intellectual John Tzetzes (*c.*1110–after 1160) addressed to the *nosokomos* (infirmarian) of the *iatreion* of the Monastery of Pantokrator, *Epistle* 81, ed. Leone (1972) 121.1–26: '*τῷ νοσοκόμῳ τοῦ ἰατρείου τοῦ Παντοκράτορος*'. The letter does not offer any information on the function of the *xenōn*, but deals with the dating of Galen's lifetime.

[70] See in relevant order, *Typikon of Pantokrator*, 1167, 1373, and 1070, ed. Gautier (1972) 99, 111, and 93. Cf. Volk (1983: 152–92).

in the *Typikon* of the late-thirteenth-century Lips *xenōn* in Constantinople, which is also the only extant *xenōn* foundation charter apart from that of the Pantokrator.[71] On the one hand, we cannot exclude the possibility that the term *iatreion* refers to a place within a Constantinopolitan *xenōn* or a *xenōn* itself. However, it should be noted that there is no surviving evidence to suggest John had a definite affiliation with any *xenōn*. On the other hand, bearing in mind that, *pace* the views of some earlier scholars, there is no consistent use of the term *iatreion* in Byzantine sources, we should not reject out of hand the idea that John's *iatreion* might have had a private character,[72] i.e. been somewhere John examined patients and offered treatment, where the patients were not confined to bed.

Having examined the scarce evidence on John's locus of medical activity, I will turn to the discussion of time and its particular function in John's narrative structure. We can observe a system for recording medical time in cases where John thought that it was crucial in presenting his material. First of all, we can identify the use of indefinite terms, which could give a vague notion of time rather than specific chronological details. For example, we sometimes observe words such as *pote* ('once/at some time'),[73] *epeidēper* ('when'),[74] or the somewhat more straightforward *enanchos* ('recently'). The last can have a particular place in John's case histories as regards the administration of drugs. For example: 'When I saw this, I thought that a lot of matter had been excreted from the heaviest parts of the body as a result of the drug recently given <to her> . . .'[75] By using this word, John attempts to emphasize the immediate action of a particular drug. He might not provide the exact length of time, but he gives an easily memorable indicator for those interested in similar situations.

Sometimes time occupies an even more important place in the narrative structure, especially in cases dealing with the gradual worsening of a patient's condition. In case history no. 6 John is called to treat the patient on the third day after the onset of a severe disease; the patient suffers from putrefaction of humours (*sēpsei tōn chymōn*).[76] The background narrative of the patient's critical condition is followed by a first indication of time, which is employed in order to show that the physician's ability to help is clearly limited due to the late call-out. John then proceeds to one of his most detailed descriptions of a

[71] On the Lips *xenōn*, see Chapter 1, n. 122.

[72] No specific term is used in surviving, edited sources to denote a physician's private practice in late Byzantium. However, it is worth noting that the term *iatreion* (the Latin equivalent is *taberna medica*) was used to signify a physician's home or surgery in the ancient and early Byzantine world. See LSJ, s.v. *ἰατρεῖον*; Harig (1971: 179–88); and Andorlini (2007: 406–8).

[73] JZA, *On Urines*, 6.12.13, ed. Ideler (1842) II.162.23.

[74] JZA, *On Urines*, 2.19.26, ed. Ideler (1842) II.51.29.

[75] JZA, *On Urines*, 6.13.10, ed. Ideler (1842) II.165.25–8: '*Ἐγὼ μὲν οὖν ταῦθ' ὁρῶν ἐστοχαζόμην ἀπό γε τοῦ δοθέντος ἔναγχος φαρμάκου ταύτῃ οὐ μετρίαν ὕλην ἀποσπαθεῖσαν τῶν βαρυτέρων τοῦ σώματος* . . .' See also JZA, *On Urines*, 2.19.24, ed. Ideler (1842) II.51.24.

[76] JZA, *On Urines*, 6.12.11–24, ed. Ideler (1842) II.162.17–163.27.

patient's clinical presentation; the greater part concerns uroscopy. On the fourth day the bladder had swollen up to such a degree that the patient was not able to urinate. On the sixth day, the patient died as a result of an extraordinary spasm. In recording the particular day John successfully presents the progress of the illness. Time becomes a tool which helps the narrator to explain the causes of disease, based on the examination of urine. Each day also pinpoints step by step the physician's response to a patient's medical condition, helping John's audience to understand better the specifics of medical examination and performance as regards the pattern and timing of disease.

As we have seen in Chapter 2 on John's uroscopic theory, prognosis is clearly a distinct process. Thus, one might expect that John would not have hesitated to provide his patients with a precise prognostication as regards time. However, this is not the case, with John giving an exact time only once.[77] The time frame of prognosis is usually implied indirectly in the description of a disease's progress. A central role in these cases is assigned to the times at which patients present specific signs. This is emphatically demonstrated in the case of a female patient suffering from a womb condition (case history no. 10).[78] In this sole instance John follows a rigorous month-by-month account reporting the patient's clinical presentation and signs in strict chronological order.

John appears to have visited the woman quite often as someone involved in the woman's treatment, although other physicians examined her as well. The descriptions of the woman's condition in the second, third, and fourth months are quite short, whereas in the fifth month John reports that it was at this point that he found out the woman's disease. He presents himself as examining the patient, taking her pulse and checking her urine. The patient's clinical presentation is supplied in the woman's voice: 'I addressed her and asked how she felt and then I took her pulse. She consented and replied in a very faint voice. <Her> pulse was very weak and irregular...'[79] This is followed by emphatic imagery: 'Her colour was like pomegranate peel, and almost acquiring the colour of those having jaundice...'[80] John provides laconic accounts for the next two months and the patient, unable to recover, finally dies. The crucial point in the worsening of the woman's condition is in the fifth month, when the patient was confined to bed.[81] John manages to identify the disease and

[77] In this case he prognosticates the imminent death of a patient who is an old acquaintance, providing an expected timeframe of three days; JZA, *On Urines*, 7.15.18, ed. Ideler (1842) II.186.25–6.

[78] JZA, *On Urines*, *On Urines*, 7.13.7–26, ed. Ideler (1842) II.181.11–183.12.

[79] JZA, *On Urines*, 7.13.17–18, ed. Ideler (1842) II.182.4–7: '*Προσαγορεύσας δ' ἠρόμην τε ὅπως ἔχει καὶ τοῦ σφυγμοῦ ἡπτόμην. ἡ δ' ὑπισχνᾷ μὲν καὶ λεπτῇ πάνυ τῇ φωνῇ ἀπεκρίνατο. Σφυγμοὶ δὲ οἱ πάνυ λεπτοὶ καὶ ἀνώμαλοι ἦσαν...*'

[80] JZA, *On Urines*, 7.13.18, ed. Ideler (1842) II.182.8–9: '*Χροιὰ δὲ σιδιοειδὴς καὶ πρὸς τὸ τῶν ἰκτεριώντων οἷον ἀπεστραμμένη χρῶμα...*'

[81] JZA, *On Urines*, 7.13.18, ed. Ideler (1842) II.182.4.

predicts its severity. The description reaches a peak, at which point the viewer perceives a dramatic moment in the narrative flow. John gives this impression by using time to frame physician–patient episodes of interaction.

Finally, the connection of humours with qualities and seasons was a central aspect of ancient humoral medicine and remained a prominent theory in Byzantium as well.[82] The subject can be found in some of John's case histories. In one case, John wants to show that some urine, which has the colour of red wine (*oinōpon*) from an adolescent patient is connected with the extreme heating of the patient's blood. This was actually the result of the very hot weather at the time and the exposure to the sun (*hēliokaias*). In order to emphasize this, John states that it happened around the rise of the Dog Star (*peri Kynos epitolēn*), which occurs towards the end of July,[83] which is indeed a hot and dry period of the year in the northern hemisphere.[84] In another example, John refers to the production of dark grey urine (*phaion*) in wintertime (*cheimerios men hē hōra*) and suggests a therapy using warming agents.[85] If not as comprehensive in its approach as the Hippocratic *katastaseis*, which provided detailed climatological data in connection with certain geographical regions, these examples still show John's constant awareness of the need to occasionally include such key factors in his aetiology.

2.4 Physician–patient encounters

My analysis will focus first on one of the longest, most detailed, and best developed case histories (no. 5). This is in book six, in the chapter focusing on the prognosis of blue (*kyanōn*) urine, resulting from the dispersal (*diaphoras*) of the accumulated yellow bile (*cholēs*) in the liver, which according to John indicates incipient jaundice (*ikteron*).[86] John states:

> It was wintertime and my acquaintance to whom I referred had been badly treated by someone... He spent most of the days without food, and even when it was necessary to take some food, he preferred mostly pickled or salted <foodstuffs>... It was in his nature to set himself against people who were opposed to him, and to be in anguish for fear of suffering greatly. For these reasons, he passed

[82] See the discussion in Chapter 1, Section 1.1.

[83] JZA, *On Urines*, 4.8.4–5, ed. Ideler (1842) II.92.2–14.

[84] Interestingly, the days under the Dog Star (Sirius) are connected with severe cases of fever in Galenic case histories: *Therapeutic Method*, 8.2 and 10.5, ed. Kühn (1825) X.537.13–16 and X.688.1–4. See also Mattern (2008: 62–3, and 230, n. 53).

[85] JZA, *On Urines*, 4.12.25–7, ed. Ideler (1842) II.96.5–12. John indicates that it is wintertime in another two cases: JZA, *On Urines*, 6.7.4 and 7.15.19, ed. Ideler (1842) II.154.32–3 and II.186.27–8.

[86] JZA, *On Urines*, 6.7.1, ed. Ideler (1842) II.154.20–4. See also Theophilos, *On Urines*, 6, ed. Ideler (1841) I.267.15–17, who states that blue (*kyanoun*) urine indicates jaundice (*ikterikōn oura*) and is connected with the corruption of yellow bile (*cholēs xanthēs*).

> the night sleepless and his body became dry and short of sleep. It was in his nature that in the past, too, he had consumed gifts of bad food, as he gave us to understand... All these things gathered that bilious humour, which was removed through his urine. When, by chance, he saw an unusual colour in his urine, he realized that there was some kind of irregularity and he told me about it and asked me to find out the cause.[87]

At this point in the narrative John has not yet become actively involved. We can see that the patient is the most highly developed character. He appears as John's acquaintance and as someone who had failed to follow a proper diet all his life. This seems to be the main reason for his sickness. We are not informed of any symptom, such as pain, which features in some other cases, and the first instance of physician–patient communication is concerned exclusively with the nature of the urine. An observation made by the patient suffices to present himself before the physician. Even someone without any particular medical knowledge can attest the power of urine as a mirror of the internal condition of the body. The physician-narrator provides the background and nature of the disease by employing technical language (e.g. *cholōdē chymon*). In this way he opens a channel of communication with his specialized audience, who are expected to perceive those aspects of common professional interest. John then proceeds:

> When I saw him still in a healthy condition, although his urine was suddenly giving the impression that he suffered from a most severe sickness, I asked him to show me the vial with his urine the following day. I then left; he spent the day in his house without food. When the night came, he lay down having eaten only a small portion of food, and brought to us in the morning a vial with blue urine like that of a jaundiced patient.[88] And he thought that he was without fever. Prediction: if he does not take proper care, he will suffer from jaundice. The <patient> remained calm on the first day... The next day thinking to himself that he was not suffering from anything severe... he dismissed us, claiming that we know nothing and he ate thicker foodstuffs and drunk wine. But before night the humour started moving and was getting warm and the man was highly distressed and, acknowledging our good judgment, he then invited us and he entrusted his

[87] JZA, *On Urines*, 6.7.4–10, ed. Ideler (1842) II.154.32–155.17: '*Ὥρα μὲν ἦν χειμῶνος καὶ ὁ ῥηθεὶς ἡμέτερος γνώριμος τὰ μέγιστα ὑπό τινος ἀδικούμενος... Τὰς πλείους δ' ἄσιτος διημέρευε, κἂν ποτε αὐτὸν ἐδέησεν ἅψασθαι βρώματος, τῶν δριμυτέρων ἢ ταρίχων τὸ πλέον ἐτύγχανεν... εἰκὸς δ' ἐκεῖνον διαμάχεσθαι μὲν πρὸς τοὺς ἐναντίους, ἀδημονεῖν δ' ἐφ' ἑαυτοῦ ὡς τὰ μέγιστα ζημιωθῆναι δεδιότα. Ἠγρύπνει οὖν διὰ ταῦτα καὶ ἄλλως δέ οἱ τὸ σῶμα αὐχμηρὸν ἐτύγχανεν καὶ βραχύυπνον. Εἰκός γε μὴν καὶ πρότερον φαύλων αὐτὸν βρωμάτων χρήσασθαι προσφοραῖς, ὡς ἐδίδου οἴεσθαι... Ταῦτα δὴ ταῦτα πάντα τὸν χολώδη χυμὸν ἐκεῖνον συνήθροισαν ἤδη δὲ καὶ δι' οὔρου οὗτος ἐξεκενοῦτο. Ἐπεὶ δ' ἐκεῖνος τύχῃ τινὶ τὰ οὖρα ἑωράκει μὴ κατὰ φύσιν ἰόντα τῷ χρώματι, καί τινος βραχείας τῆς ἀνωμαλίας ᾔσθετο, ἐμοί τε τὸ πρᾶγμα ἐξήγγειλε, καὶ τὴν αἰτίαν μαθεῖν ἐπυνθάνετο.*'

[88] Ideler's edition erroneously reads '*ἰκτερώντων*' rather than '*ἰκτεριώντων*', which is the correct spelling. Cf. JZA, *On Urines*, 7.13.18, ed. Ideler (1842) II.182.9; *Medical Epitome*, 1.27, ed. Ideler (1842) II.377.25; and *On Psychic Pneuma*, 1.12.8, ed. Ideler (1841) I.333.21.

> salvation to us. According to my judgment, I taught him with words that he should not show disbelief to the physicians that command him, and, knowing that the bilious humour was not in much excess, I told him to abstain from thicker food and the wine. Following a leaner diet...he was freed from the disease...[89]

The patient constitutes the direct audience of the physician's performance. He perceives the physician's actions as a symbolic transformation of a visible sign (the colour of urine) into a verbal pronouncement (prognosis) through the examination of the urine.[90] The physician appears before his patient using the interpretive power of uroscopy in an attempt to get the patient's attention and communicate the severity of his condition. An actor attempts to persuade his/her audience through a variety of gestures. The audience responds according to their background and familiarity with the skill of the actor. In our case the patient consistently refuses to accept the physician's prognosis, which takes the form of advice. The patient's denial can only result in the aggravation of his problem. The reciprocal character of the physician–patient interaction is emphatically attested by the patient being presented as having entrusted his 'salvation' (*sōtērian*) to the physician. This capitulation can be interpreted as an act of repentance, which indicates the patient's reliance on the physician's assistance despite his initial rejection thereof. The physician's prognosis and the subsequent usefulness of uroscopy is confirmed in the end. The patient is now persuaded to follow a specific, healthy diet, and is ultimately successfully treated. The developing intimacy between the patient and the physician, which follows the dramatic climax of the patient's suffering, concludes with the physician's exhortation to the patient not to mistrust doctors again.[91]

[89] JZA, *On Urines*, 6.7.11–17, ed. Ideler (1842) II.155.17–156.7: '*Ἐγὼ δὲ τὸ μὲν τοιαῦτα οὖρα προΐεσθαι ἐξαίφνης αὐτὸν μὲν ὁρῶν ἔτι ὑγιῆ περιϊόντα, ἐκεῖνα δ' εἰδὼς ἐπὶ χειρίστοις νοσήμασι φαινόμενα, καὶ δὴ λέξας ἐπ' ἀμίδος τὴν ἐπιοῦσαν δείξειν τὸ οὖρον, ἐγὼ μὲν ἀπηλλαττόμην, αὐτὸς δὲ καὶ εἰσαῦθις περὶ τὰ οἰκεῖα διέτριβε διημερεύσας ἄσιτος. Ἐπεὶ δὲ νυκτὸς μὲν ἧκε, βραχέος δὲ τοῦ σιτίου γευσάμενος ἔκειτο, κομίζει μὲν ἡμῖν ἕωθεν ἀμίδα κυανᾶ οὖρα ἔχουσαν καὶ οἷα τὰ τῶν ἰκτερώντων, αὐτὸς δὲ ᾤετο ἔτι ἀπύρεκτος τελεῖν. Πρόρρησις, εἰ μὴ φυλάξαιτο ἰκτέρῳ περιπεσεῖν. ὁ δὲ τὴν πρώτην φυλαττόμενος ἀτάραχος ἔμενεν... Τὴν μετ' αὐτὴν δὲ σκοπῶν ἑαυτὸν μηδέν τι δεινὸν πάσχοντα... ἡμᾶς μὲν εἴασεν ὡς μηδὲν δῆθεν εἰδότας φάμενος, αὐτὸς δὲ ἐγεύσατο μὲν τροφῆς παχυτέρας, οἶνον δ' ἀσθενῆ ἐπέπιε, καὶ οὔπω νὺξ ἦν καὶ ὁ χυμὸς ἐκεκίνητο καὶ διετεθέρμαστο καὶ ταραχή τις οὐκ ὀλίγη τὸν ἄνθρωπον κατέσχε καὶ ἡμᾶς τότε συνεὶς εὖ κρίνοντας μετεκαλεῖτό τε καὶ τὴν σωτηρίαν ἐπίστευεν. Ἐγὼ δὲ ἐκεῖνον μὲν λόγοις ὡς ἐδόκουν παιδεύσας μὴ ἀπιστεῖν ἰατροῖς προστάσσουσι, συνεὶς δὲ μὴ ἐπὶ πολὺ ἐξῆφθαι τὸν χολώδη χυμὸν τοῦτον παραφυλάξασθαι μὲν ἔφην τὰ παχύτερα βρώματα καὶ τὸν οἶνον. Διαιτήσας δὲ λεπτότερᾳ διαίτῃ... καὶ τοῦ νοσήματος ἀπαλλαγέντος...*'

[90] On healing 'gestures' as part of ancient rhetoric and, in particular, on Latin medical literature, see the collection of essays by Gaide and Biville (2003). On the popularity of the urine vial and the associated 'gestures' in the Middle Ages, see Moulinier-Brogi (2012: 77–92).

[91] The same motive is also found in another case history (no. 8) where a female patient initially refuses to receive a purgative suggested by John. She finally takes the drug on the advice of a notable contemporary physician. See n. 123, below.

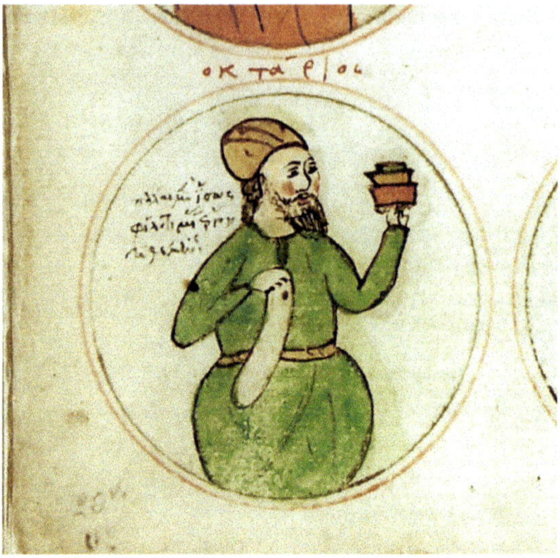

Figure 3.1. The miniature shows John holding a urine vial with an inscribed motto derived from the opening phrase of his work *On Urines*.[92] Bononiensis 3632 (mid fifteenth century), f. 20v.

At the same time, the physician-narrator retains a didactic tone in presenting his intervention in respect of this individual. By giving a protreptic air to his prognosis he engages more actively with his external audience. It suggests a concern to provide useful data, which might fulfil contemporary needs. Physicians/readers who could prognosticate accurately seemed more reliable and strengthened their position vis-à-vis those following other healing practices.[93] Later on, John embeds in his account a statement in connection with the practice of medicine, his art. In particular, we can see the physician, urging his patient to trust a physician's opinion. Thus we may consider a metalevel where the physician, who in the meantime has taken on the role of a skilful raconteur, communicates his experiences in a 'seminar' attended by professional colleagues. John uses a particular event in order to introduce his ideas about his art or the social group he belongs to, in his attempts to build a relationship with his readers. This is a metatextual element used by John as a rhetorical device in an account of medical events; a device, in this case with

[92] The text above the miniature reads: 'οκτάριος', which is found in various manuscripts instead of the usual 'ἀκτουάριος', and is a vernacular version of the same term. See also Chapter 1, n. 154. The phrase on the right-hand side reads: 'πάλαι μὲν ἴσως φιλοτιμίας ἔργον τιθέμενος', which coincides with the introductory phrase of John's work: *On Urines*, 1.pr.1, ed. Ideler (1842) II.3.1.

[93] The importance of prognosis in the patient-physician encounter had been a significant issue of the healing processes already in the Hippocratic treatises. See, for example, [Hippocrates], *Prognostic*, 1, ed. Littré (1840) II.110.1–6 = ed. Jouanna (2013) 1.1–2.2.

ethical connotations, which John uses so as to communicate with his audience at another level in an attempt to transmit his knowledge.[94]

To return to the role of uroscopy within the context of physician–patient communication, it may be useful to focus on some other examples, which can give a more precise image of this interaction. In one of the cases (no. 7), in which John seems to receive a patient at his workplace,[95] the case history starts by showing the patient himself bringing a urine vial with him from the countryside. Although the patient is not an expert in interpreting urinary signs, he identifies the use of sign-equipment, in this case the urine vial, in order to make the physician aware of his clinical condition. The physician proceeds immediately to the examination of the urine:

> ...if I have to describe them by giving an example, they seemed like clouds which, since the sun never turns <towards them> nor shines on them, seem naturally dense and abnormal in their colour. The man who carried the urine vial was dropsical and swollen up and said that he was going to suffer from a serious disease, which did indeed beset him... So we decided that the patient should follow a diet <to help> his digestive capacity... And, having been persuaded that he ought to follow that diet, he left.[96]

A quick observation of the patient's urine is followed by a description of the patient's clinical presentation, which gives John the opportunity to attest signs of excessive accumulation of water in the patient's body. However, after John's initial comments on the urine, we hear the patient's perspective on his sickness. The patient's statement is probably uttered before the examination of the urine by John. He confirms John's implied prognosis and point outs the reliability of his uroscopic method. The patient appears aware of his condition and feels some familiarity with the physician. Having been persuaded by the physician's performance in identifying the development of the disease, the patient willingly agrees to follow the physician's therapeutic advice concerning his diet. The patient's compliance is related to his impression of the physician's proficiency in dealing with the disease by skilfully articulating technical characteristics.

[94] When I use terms with the prefix 'meta-', I am mainly referring to the way the treatment of medical elements in John has implications for how the text itself may influence the reader on a more abstract level of perception. On this, see Jordanova (2006: 56–8, 228). On metatext in ancient Greek literature, see Danielewicz (2001) and Xenophontos (2016), who examine the cases of Greek lyric poetry and Plutarch respectively.

[95] See my discussion in Section 2.3.

[96] JZA, *On Urines*, 6.12.29–32, ed. Ideler (1842) II.163.37–164.10: '...*εἰ δεῖ παραδειγματίσαι τὸν λόγον νέφεσιν ἐῴκεσαν, ἃ μήτε πάμπαν ἀπεστραμμένου τοῦ ἡλίου μήτε καταφωτιζομένου, πυκνὰ δὲ καθ' αὑτὰ πεφυκότα καὶ τῇ χροιᾷ ἀνώμαλα φαίνεται. Οὗτος δ' αὖ ὁ τὴν ἀμίδα ἔχων ὑδάλεος ἦν καεί ἐξωδηκώς, ἔφασκε δὲ προνενοσηκέναι νόσον οὐ μετρίαν... εἰς τοῦτο τοῦ πάθους γέγονεν. Ἔδοξε οὖν ἡμῖν ἐπὶ ἀρρώστῳ ἔτι τῇ πεπτικῇ δυνάμει ἐκδεδιητῆσθαι τὸν ἄνθρωπον... Καὶ δὴ τότε μὲν ᾗ κεχρῆσθαι ἐχρῆν διαίτῃ πυθόμενος ᾤχετο.*'

On another level, the educational dimension of John's words is indicated by his providing an appropriate simile about urine's morphological features, as a form of example (*paradeigmatisai*, 'to give an example').[97] The colour of the urine is compared to the appearance of clouds that are not illuminated by the sun's light. A complicated case is simplified by giving it noticeable characteristics from daily life. John is trying to clarify his identification, but also to show the value of learning in recognizing urinary characteristics correctly. The audience, through his use of visualization techniques for hard-to-spot or obscure theoretical details, receives a detectable and coherent answer to its supposed inquiries. The simile takes the role of a didactic device in the general context of the narrator–reader communication.[98]

Furthermore, by using the first-person plural (*hēmin*), the physician-narrator manages to radiate an air of communal response to the disease.[99] The author appears aware of his readers' presence, giving the impression that they are all acting as a group. Ultimately, John addresses his readers at the very end of this case history in an attempt to keep communicating with them:

> And you who are excellent in these matters and who know so well that the very thick urine is bad, you should add these predictions to the above-mentioned as fitting, looking at the natural capacity, and the change of the consistency and the colour <of urine>.[100]

John praises his reader's ability to distinguish various types of urine and the associated prognoses, and thus in so doing he employs the second-person singular (*sy*), which denotes an implied reciprocal 'non-direct' interaction. John's expectations that his readers will approve his medical advice are elegantly imposed upon them through the notion of trust that he establishes in his relation with them. He gives an apophthegmatic air to his sayings, which takes the form of prudent advice. It can be seen as a memorable tip, which will help the physician-reader give an appropriate performance in a similar case.

The next two cases (nos. 1 and 2) to be examined involve a patient's negative response to the suggested therapy.[101] In the first case, which is in

[97] On the use of examples (*paradeigmata*) and their didactic role in John's *On Urines*, see Chapter 2, Section 2.1.

[98] The use of similes as a didactic tool was common in Greek and Roman literature, see Morgan (1998: 262–70). See also, JZA, *On Urines*, 3.6.3–5, ed. Ideler (1842) II.58.24–59.4. We can also observe some similes in John's treatise on pneuma. See, for example, JZA, *On Psychic Pneuma*, 1.2.8–10 and 1.19.10, ed. Ideler (1841) I.317.9–16 and I.347.20–3.

[99] On the use of the first-person plural in John's *On Urines*, see Chapter 2, Section 2.1.

[100] JZA, *On Urines*, 6.12.33, ed. Ideler (1842) II.164.12–16: '*Σύ γε μὴν ὁ περὶ τὰ τοιαῦτα σπουδαῖος οὕτω πάνυ φαῦλα συνιὼν τὰ σφόδρα παχέα οὖρα καὶ τὰ ἐπὶ τούτοις ὡς εἰκὸς ἐπιτίθει προρρήσεις εἴς τε τὴν φυσικὴν ἀφορῶν δύναμιν καὶ εἰς τὴν τῶν συστάσεών τε καὶ χρωμάτων μεταβολήν.*'

[101] A similar motive is also common in various Galenic case histories; see Mattern (2008: 145–9).

the chapter on diagnosis and is based on the identification of dark grey (*phaiōn*), livid (*pelidnōn*), and black (*melanōn*) urine, John appears to prepare a lozenge, which is called 'bitter' (*pikros*).[102] Later on, under certain circumstances the lozenge was mixed with *oxymeli*, a mixture of vinegar and honey, which only made it taste even more bitter, as can be seen in the following case:

> Taking this drug in my hands—I think it was the bitter lozenge—I mixed it with as much *oxymeli* as I considered enough, and added warm water to it, in order to make it more liquid and easy to swallow, and then I gave it to the patient to drink. He took the cup and pressed his lips firmly against it, and he felt that the drug was disgusting, for it was very bitter indeed; but since he was a man in all other respects proud and profound, and with regard to the provision of drugs disobedient and intractable, since he wanted to tease us and test how easy it was to vomit it . . .[103]

Swallowing a pill is a hard task for many patients even in modern societies. We can clearly see here that John attempts to provide his patient with an easier-to-swallow version of the lozenge in the form of a potion, thus giving us an insight into his active involvement with his patient's case and his eagerness to persuade him. In the case (see no. 5 above) of the patient who followed an inappropriate diet, I showed how the display of a particular colour in urine could aid a physician's attempts to provide a prognosis for a disease and finally induce the patient to comply with the exigencies of a particular therapy. Similarly, the active involvement of the physician in the preparation of a medicament could enhance the level of trust the patient showed towards the physician. By shifting his narration from the first-person to the third-person singular, John ultimately points up the patient's reluctance to take the medicine and demonstrates that there was no point in further urging him in that direction. Afterwards, as we shall see below, John decides to give this drug to his attendant.

However, before we examine the case of the attendant, it is worth providing a brief discussion of another similar case history (no. 2). This is part of the

[102] In the unedited fifth book of his *Medical Epitome*, John provides a recipe for the 'bitter' lozenge, which most probably derives its name from the bitter almonds that constituted its main ingredient, and gave it its bitter taste. JZA, *Medical Epitome*, 5, Vindobonensis med. gr. 17, f. 120v, ll. 13–14: '*Τροχίσκος ὁ πικρὸς πρὸς στομαχικούς· ἡπατικούς· σπληνικούς· ἰκτερικούς· σελινόσπερμα· ἄσαρ· ἀψίνθιον· ἄνισον· ἀμύγδαλα πικρά, ἀνὰ οὐγγ α΄·*'; ed. Mathys (1556) II.340.10–13.

[103] JZA, *On Urines*, 2.19.16–17, ed. Ideler (1842) II.50.33–51.8: '*Καὶ τοίνυν μετὰ χεῖρας αὐτὸ λαβὼν τὸ φάρμακον–τροχίσκον δὲ ἦν ὁ πικρὸς οἶμαι–προσεπέμιξα τούτῳ καὶ ὀξυμέλιτος ὅσον ἀρκεῖν ἐνόμισα, προσενέχεον δὲ καὶ ὕδατος ζέοντος, ἵνα ὑγρότερόν τε ἅμα καὶ εὐκατάποτον εἴη τὸ φάρμακον καὶ τῷ θεραπευομένῳ πιεῖν παρέσχον. Ὁ δὲ λαβὼν τὴν κύλικα καὶ τοῖς χείλεσι προσερείσας, ἐπεί τινος ᾔσθετο τοῦ φαρμάκου ἀηδείας πικροῦ μὲν αὐτοῦ καὶ δηλονότι τυγχάνοντος, ἀλλὰ δὴ καὶ τοῦ ἀνθρώπου τἆλλα μὲν ἀγερώχου καὶ ἐμβριθοῦς, πάνυ δὲ περὶ τὰς προσφορὰς τῶν φαρμάκων ἀγεννοῦς καὶ οὐκ εὐαγώγου, προσπαῖξαι μέν τι καὶ αὐτὸς βουλόμενος, ἐλέγξαι δὲ καὶ τὸ εὐεμὲς ἐκείνου . . .*'

chapter dealing with diagnosis based on the examination of urine containing a combination of various kinds of particles (*symmemigmenōn paryphistamenōn*). The two female patients involved in this case were suffering from spontaneous fatigue and chronic pain in joints respectively.[104] John proceeds to examine the urine of the first patient, observing bran-like (*pityrois*) particles, whereas most of the urinary liquid is fulvous (*pyrrō*) in colour.[105] The other patient has thinner (*leptotera*) particles and most of the liquid is white (*leukon*).[106] John omits any reference to the patient's initial response to his diagnosis or prognosis and proceeds directly to the therapeutic advice:

> For the <first> female patient suffering from spontaneous fatigue, she was saved from the disease having followed the diet we <recommended>. The other one was not persuaded[107] to drink the drug we gave her in order to treat the disease... as she did not happen to know the name of the drug, she would not drink it. For the woman was in all other respects like a peasant. I abandoned her and left and I do not know what happened to her... so you may learn how beneficial the precise examination of urine normally is.[108]

The first woman follows the recommended diet and recovers, while the second refuses to take a certain drug. Although John does not name or specify the medicine, he reports the woman's emphatic refusal, a fact he ascribes to her ignorance. There is no attempt to reason with her in order to convince her to follow the recommended treatment and he simply explains that the woman was from the countryside. If we compare the case of the female patient with the aforementioned cases (nos. 1 and 5) of the male patients, we can see that John does not show the same degree of patience here. Furthermore, it seems that patients without experience of medical assistance, patients who were deemed ignorant as a result of their sociocultural background, were reluctant to seek or follow medical advice, which seemed strange to them or simply unfamiliar. Finally, by stepping back from the narration of the history and

[104] JZA, *On Urines*, 3.10.5, ed. Ideler (1842) II.62.25–32.
[105] JZA, *On Urines*, 3.10.6, ed. Ideler (1842) II.62.32–5.
[106] JZA, *On Urines*, 3.10.7, ed. Ideler (1842) II.62.35–63.3.
[107] The original in JZA, *On Urines*, 3.10.8, ed. Ideler (1842) II.63.3–6 reads: '*ἡ δ' ἑτέρα φάρμακον μέντοι ὑφ' ἡμῶν πεπωκέναι πέπειστο λυσιτελῆσον τῷ πάθει.*' However, the addition of '*οὐ*' (not) before '*πέπειστο*' is necessitated by the context. The previous sentence refers to a female patient who followed the suggested treatment, whereas the next sentence comes as a contrast to this if one considers the presence of '*μέντοι*' and its close association to '*δέ*' (which contradicts the previous '*μέν*'). Furthermore, in the next two sentences, it is clearly stated that the woman was not persuaded to drink the drug.
[108] JZA, *On Urines*, 3.10.8–10, ed. Ideler (1842) II.63.3–13: '*Ἀλλ' ἡ μὲν τὸν αὐτόματον τόπον νοσοῦσα ὑφ' ἡμῶν διαιτηθεῖσα τοῦ πάθους ἀπήλλακται· ἡ δ' ἑτέρα φάρμακον μέντοι ὑφ' ἡμῶν πεπωκέναι πέπειστο λυσιτελῆσον τῷ πάθει... οὔπω γάρ τοι ἔτυχε καὶ ὄνομα πυθομένη φαρμάκου, μή τοιγε ἐπεπώκει. Ἦν γὰρ ἡ γυνὴ καὶ τἆλλα ἀγροικῶς ἐσταλμένη· ἐγὼ μὲν ταύτην παρεὶς ᾠχόμην, ὅ, τι δὲ οἱ γέγονεν ἀγνοῶ... ἀλλ' ἵν' ὑμεῖς εἰδῆτε, ὁπόσον εἴωθε λυσιτελεῖν ἐπίσκεψις ἀκριβὴς τῶν οὔρων.*' See n. 47, above.

returning to his readers with an emphatic comment, John impresses upon them the importance of the accurate examination of urine.

We gain an even more lively sense of John's practices in referring to the case (no. 1) where he offers the patient's drug to his attendant, after the former has refused to take it. The attendant does not seem ill but in persuading him to drink it, John says that the drug will help his body.[109] He easily accepts John's suggestion and is immediately transformed into a test case. The experimental character of John's advice is further substantiated by the fact that the attendant is urged to run as fast as he can to deliver a message to one of John's friends, thereby covering a distance of around thirty *stadia*, the equivalent of three and a half modern land miles.[110] John is attempting to get him as tired as possible. Sometime thereafter the first signs of the drug's effect are traceable. Consequently, the interaction between the physician and the attendant becomes more and more active:

> When his urine became infected and appeared black in colour, he announced this terrible thing to me, and because he could not find the cause for this, he was extremely vexed by it. The next day I told him to show me the urine vial, so he did and asked me to find out what was going to happen, being terrified lest he should die suddenly of neglect. And first of all I was surprised, because I had forgotten which drug I had previously given him; and I did not observe either a quartan fever rising up in him or melancholy, but was only watching that his mixture was well balanced and to what degree it was inclined to the black humour... And when I at last remembered the drug, I realized <what had happened>, I smiled, and I encouraged the young man to be brave because nothing terrible was going to happen... the next day the urine was dark grey and the day after it changed to the natural <colour>.[111]

The attendant's body excretes black urine, which makes him worry and ask for the physician's help. The attendant appears familiar with uroscopy and allows John to examine his urine. The developing interaction is based on the power of interpreting the signs of the urine, which arouses the attendant's

[109] JZA, *On Urines*, 2.19.18–19, ed. Ideler (1842) II.51.8–13. In this instance John wants to emphasize to his readers that some purgative drugs (*ryptikou*) may cause the production of black urine, although this is not necessarily connected with an ongoing affection: JZA, *On Urines*, 2.19.13, ed. Ideler (1842) II.50.22–6.

[110] JZA, *On Urines*, 2.19.20–1, ed. Ideler (1842) II.51.13–18. On Byzantine *stadion*, see Silbach (1970: 282).

[111] JZA, *On Urines*, 2.19.22–7, ed. Ideler (1842) II.51.18–34: '*Ἐπεὶ δὲ εἰς οὖρον αὐτὸν ἠρέθισεν ἰέναι, μέλαν δὲ οἱ ἐπεφάνη, ἐμοί τε ἤγγειλε τὸ δεινὸν καὶ τὴν αἰτίαν ἀγνοῶν οὐ μετρίως ἤσχαλεν. Ἐπ' ἀμίδα τοίνυν φήσας αὐτὸν τὴν ἐπιοῦσαν δεῖξαι, οὕτω τε ἐποίει καὶ ἐλιπάρει τὸ ἀποβησόμενον μαθεῖν δεδιώς, μή πη λάθῃ θανὼν αἰφνίδιον. Κἀγὼ μὲν ἐθαύμαζον πρῶτον ἐπιλαθόμενος τοῦ δοθέντος φαρμάκου οἱ ἔναγχος, μήτε τεταρταῖον αὐτῷ σκοπῶν ἐμφύντα μήτε μελαγχολίαν, μόνον δὲ τὴν κρᾶσιν ὁρῶν εἰς οἷον εὔκρατον ῥέπουσαν χυμὸν μέλανα... Ἐπειδήπερ δὲ ἀπεμνήσθην τοῦ φαρμάκου, ἐδάην τε καὶ ἐγέλασα καὶ τὸν παῖδα θαρρεῖν ἐκέλευσα, ὡς μηδενὸς αὐτῷ προσδοκωμένου δεινοῦ... ἀλλὰ τὴν ἐπιοῦσαν φαιὸν φανέν, τὴν μετὰ αὐτὴν ἐνήλλακται πρὸς τὸ κατὰ φύσιν χωρῆσαν.*'

interest. The procedure of testing continues over the next couple of days with John exhorting the attendant to show courage. There is no evidence of non-compliance in this case and the attendant seems to recognize the physician's expertise in correctly identifying the urine when the latter regains gradually its natural colour.

John's exposition in this case is self-consciously rhetorical, combining certain narrative techniques. He starts by pretending that he is unaware of the drug's effect with the sole aim of setting out a test demonstration of the effects of this particular drug. This rhetorical *recusatio*, which does not seem to correspond to reality, plays a dual role in his text: first, it gives John the appearance of a modest speaker, and hence makes his narration more easily palatable to his audience, who can only be persuaded of the correctness of what he is saying if he can ensure their willingness to hear him (*captatio benevolentiae*); secondly, it drives the unfolding of the subsequent narration, as it gives John the opportunity to continue dissimulating. This time he supposedly does not remember that he had provided the drug; and after a differential diagnosis[112]—by his references to alternative candidates, in this case quartan fever and melancholy, that can cause the same result as the administered drug and which it could be helpful to eliminate as possible factors in the condition—his final discovery seems all the more significant and unique, given that it purportedly came about accidentally. The change in the colour of the urine becomes the vehicle through which John attempts to reverse the initial impression he has given of ignorance without presenting himself as being in the indefensible position of having lied. At the same time, by having deliberately delayed revealing the results of his test, John underlines its effectiveness.

Finally, the physician-narrator, using his creative strategy of engagement with his audience, relays a crucial recommendation:

> The urine would not have been coloured at the beginning if his tiredness had not contributed so much, so that the drug was distributed so easily on the one hand, and it carried away the developing and increasing matter on the other hand. One should keep each of these things in mind and observe those things which occur either as an outcome of drugs, that is if they remove a humour of this kind, or due to food or drinks that are stained with colours similar <to the colour of the humour>.[113]

[112] On John's particular interest in differential diagnosis, this time for eye diseases, see Chapter 4, Section 4.2.

[113] JZA, *On Urines*, 2.19.28–9, ed. Ideler (1842) II.51.35–52.5: '*Τάχα δ' ἂν τὴν ἀρχὴν οὐκ ἐχρώσθη τὰ οὖρα, εἰ μὴ καὶ ὁ κόπος τὰ μέγιστα συνεβάλλετο, διαδοθέντος μὲν οὕτω ῥᾳδίως τοῦ φαρμάκου, ἐσπασαμένου δὲ τὴν ὕλην ἀκμάζουσάν τε καὶ πλήθουσαν. Ταῦτά τοι δεῖ τούτων ἑκάστου μεμνημένον καὶ τὰ ἐπισυμβαίνοντα σκοπεῖν εἴτ' ἐκ φαρμάκων εἴη δηλαδὴ τοιοῦτον χυμὸν κενούντων εἴτ' ἐκ τροφῶν καὶ πωμάτων παραπλησίως χρωσθέντων χρώματι.*'

The reference to physical weakness supplements the causation John has given and underlines the use of somatic factors in understanding the distribution and effectiveness of drugs. The conclusion of the case history is marked by the explicit use of the element of memory. John highlights the recollection of medical information, by advising his readers to keep in mind the suggestions he has given them, while at the same time striving to retain their attention. Memory now takes a metatextual twist, as it reveals the author's expectation that his audience will remember his medical work and his contribution when faced with similar cases.

2.5 The contest

The last issue worth discussing relates to cases where other physicians are present. There are three instances in which John appears to challenge his colleagues' recommendations.[114] In the first example, the case history (no. 6) starts as usual with John providing the patient's anamnesis. In this case, the young male patient suffers from a urinary disease related to the bladder, which causes fevers and diarrhoea.[115] According to John, this is connected with the patient's bad diet and voracious appetite. John is finally called out (*metaklētheis eisēkein*) and proceeds to make a physical examination. He appears to take the patient's pulse and diagnose the ongoing fever.[116] The next part is dedicated to uroscopy with a very long and detailed description of the urine. However, in this case, in the presence of other physicians, a comparison of the various diagnoses makes the narration even more intriguing:

> I saw in the vial that the urine was quite thick... and varied and weird in colour... I was astonished and I had the suspicion that the humours were hugely putrefied or more precisely some sort of decomposition of the humours was happening, as someone once said when he saw the urine... The next day... even some parts of mortified blood were expelled through the nostrils and also through the pharynx, but when one of those physicians who used to come often saw this, he cut the vein although it was not fitting... When the fourth day came and the urine stopped completely, the bladder was swollen up, having become inflated with urine that had no way out; on the sixth day the patient was convulsed by an extraordinary spasm... and the patient died.[117]

[114] These are case histories nos. 6, 8, and 10. The term 'agonistic' has been used by Mattern (2008: 69–72) in order to describe Galen's rivalries with other physicians. Cf. König (2005: 263–5).

[115] JZA, *On Urines*, 6.12.11–12, ed. Ideler (1842) II.162.18–22.

[116] JZA, *On Urines*, 6.12.13–15, ed. Ideler (1842) II.162.22–8.

[117] JZA, *On Urines*, 6.12.16–24, ed. Ideler (1842) II.162.28-.163.27: Ἐπὶ τούτοις ἀμίδα ἑωρακὼς πολὺ μὲν τὸ πάχος ἔχουσαν... καὶ τὸ χρῶμα ποίκιλόν τε καὶ ἀλλόκοτον... ἐθαύμασα καὶ πολλὴν τὴν τῶν χυμῶν διαφθορὰν ὑπονοεῖν ἐπῄει μοι, ἢ τό γε ἀληθέστερον ἀναστοιχείωσίν τινα

John's initial diagnosis of putrefaction of the patient's humours is later confirmed by the patient's worsening health. In this case he shows no interest in transmitting the patient's voice, but vividly presents another physician's actions. John has no hesitation in arguing against the venesection performed by the other physician, who was unable to prevent the patient's death. There is no indication of an actual oral debate with the other physician. John is only interested in presenting his superiority as an outcome of his technical mastery in interpreting the patient's urine.

In the next two cases to note the presence of other physicians, it seems that John was in the early stages of his professional career.[118] In the first example (no. 8), which is in the chapter on prognosis based on the place of a particle in the urine vial,[119] a female patient appears to have drunk a purgative, which had been prepared by a Syrian physician, presumably a foreign doctor who happened to be practising in Constantinople.[120] However, the drug offers only a temporary purgation and, because of its strong action, causes severe abdominal pain. The physician tries to alleviate the pain and ultimately the woman believes that she has fully recovered.[121] Up until then John has not been involved in the patient's treatment and appears to be a passive observer, commenting on another physician's advice, as well as on the patient's response. However, immediately after he actively engages with the patient, he describes her urine and stresses the patient's reactions:

> Her urine was warm and thick... and it would have been better to proceed to a purgation using a clyster, but I could not persuade her because she was scared... After a short while, when her condition became worse, she called one of the most notable physicians and he arrived and pronounced that the affection of the patient was *hypochondrismos*[122]... he [i.e. one of the most notable physicians] persuaded her to accept the purgative drug and said that she could not otherwise be relieved from the pains that possessed her unless she complied with the advice of those who knew very well how to make judgments on diseases... she was

τῶν χυμῶν εἶπέ τις ἰδὼν τὰ οὖρα... Ἡ δὲ ἐπιοῦσα... αἵματος δὲ τεμμάχια ἤδη νενεκρωθέντος διά τε τοῦ μυκτῆρος πέμπεσθαι καὶ διὰ τοῦ φάρυγγος ἐξωθεῖσθαι, ἀλλὰ τοῦτο μὲν ἰδών τις τῶν ἐκεῖσε θαμιζόντων ἰατρῶν φλέβα ἔτεμεν μηδὲν ὂν προσῆκον... Ἐπεὶ δὲ ἤδη τετάρτη μὲν ἦν, ἀφ' ἧς τὰ οὖρα ἐπέσχετο, ἡ δὲ κύστις ἐξῴδηκε, πλείονος ἀθροισθέντος οὔρου καὶ μὴ χώραν εἰς ἔξοδον ἔχοντος, ἕκτη τε ἤδη ἦν καὶ σπασμὸς ἐξαίσιος ἐντεῦθεν εἶχε τὸν κάμνοντα... συναπῄει... ὁ ἄνθρωπος'.

[118] See also the discussion on the dating of John's corpus in Chapter 1, Section 4.2.1.

[119] On the notion of analogies between parts of the human body and the place of particles in the urines vial, see Chapter 2, Section 2.7.

[120] The term used by John is '*Σύρος*'. Kourousis (1984/8: 140) suggests that this might be the young Syrian physician, who was introduced to the Emperor Andronikos II around 1299–1300 by the scholar Maximos Planoudes. See Maximos Planoudes, *Epistle* 12, ed. Leone (1991) 27.18–20.

[121] JZA, *On Urines*, 6.13.5–8, ed. Ideler (1842) II.165.9–21.

[122] A disease related to the hypochondrium, i.e. the soft parts of the body below the cartilage and above the navel. On hypochondrium (Gr. *hypochondrion*), see Leven (2005b).

persuaded and she drank the drug, which purged her mildly, and she was freed from her terrible pains.[123]

The patient does not seem to trust John's advice because she is afraid, and perhaps on account of his youth. Various other symptoms develop and the patient's condition gradually deteriorates. Later on, one of the most notable doctors is called out, which tends to support the assumption that John was not well established at this point. The woman, relying on the second physician's diagnosis, agrees to receive the suggested purgative, which ultimately freed her from the pain. It is clear that patients who could afford to consult more than one doctor did not hesitate to do so.[124] Although we do not have John performing a healing 'gesture' himself, the presence of the 'most notable physician' functions as an evident symbol of professionalism and trustworthiness for the patient and, thus, as a central element of the persuasion process.

In the second case (no. 10), where John discusses a gynaecological problem related to the accumulation of blood around the womb, he is eager to state his lack of specialist knowledge on the topic: '...and then I was not able to diagnose easily the affection, and I turned to some brief medical books...'[125] Despite the fact that he claims to be quite inexperienced, after consulting appropriate medical treatises he manages to foresee the severity of the woman's disease, primarily through the correct interpretation of the uroscopic examination; in this case he identified the presence of red particles like coarse meal (*erythra kai krimnōdē*) located in the lower part of the urine vial.[126] He is not involved in the woman's treatment and even makes caustic reference to the hope given her by the other physicians, although he himself seems to have already foreseen the patient's death.[127]

Although John does not manage to gain the patients' trust and they do not at first rely on his therapeutic advice, he is eager to share his viewpoint with his audience. The main way he demonstrates his abilities to his readers is through identifying the patient's problem and predicting the course of the disease. The

[123] JZA, *On Urines*, 6.13.9–14, ed. Ideler (1842) II.165.21–166.16: '*Οὖρα ταύτῃ ὅτὲ μὲν θερμὰ καὶ παχέα... οὖν ἢ κατὰ κλύσμα δεῖσθαι ταύτην καθάρσεως οὔτ' ἔπειθον δέος οὐκ ὀλίγον ἔχουσαν... Ἐπεὶ δὲ μετ' οὐ πολύν τινα τὸν χρόνον ἐπὶ τὰ χείρω φερομένη τῶν ἀξιολογωτέρων τινὰ τῇ τέχνῃ μετεκαλεῖτο ἄνθρωπον, κἀκεῖνος εἴξαις ταῖς ἀξιώσεσιν καὶ ἀφικόμενος ᾠήθη εἰς ὑποχονδρισμοῦ περιπεσεῖν τὴν κάμνουσαν πάθος... τὴν τοῦ καθαρτηρίου ἔπειθε προσφορὰν φαρμάκου, καὶ μὴ ἂν ἄλλως ἔφασκεν ἀπηλλάχθαι τὸν κατεχόντων ἀλγεινῶν, εἰ μὴ ταῖς ὑποθήκαις ἐνδοίη τῶν εὖ κρίνειν εἰδότων νοσήματα... ἐπείσθη τε ἡ κάμνουσα καὶ μετρίως καθαῖρον ἐπιπιοῦσα φάρμακον τῶν λυπούντων αὐτὴν δεινῶν ἀπηλλάττετο.*'

[124] In case history no. 10, John hints at the wealthy background of his female patient: JZA, *On Urines*, 7.13.8, ed. Ideler (1842) II.181.14–15.

[125] JZA, *On Urines*, 7.13.20, ed. Ideler (1842) II.182.16–18: '*... καὶ τότε μὴν οὐχ οἷός τε ἦν ῥᾳδίως διαγνῶναι τὸ πάθος πάνυ προσομιλήσας βραχείαις βίβλοις ἰατρῶν...*'; and *On Urines*, 7.13.21, ed. Ideler (1842) II.182.19–20, in which John specifies that he looked at books 'on female affections' (*peri gynaikeiōn pathōn*).

[126] JZA, *On Urines*, 7.13.19 and 7.13.21, ed. Ideler (1842) II.182.12–16 and II.182.21–34.

[127] JZA, *On Urines*, 7.13.24, ed. Ideler (1842) II.183.1–3.

narration reaches a dramatic climax either with the patient's recovery or death. By imagining John's performance, his audience is convinced by the author's self-confidence in affirming his opposition to the prognostications of others. Finally, in his constant attempts to keep his specialized audience interested, John does not hesitate to refer to his consultation of medical handbooks, where necessary. This could have a metatextual function for his readers, with John impressing upon his medical audience the need to look at relevant textbooks when dealing with unfamiliar situations.

3. CONCLUSION

Although we cannot exclude the possibility that John's case histories may be partly the product of literary construction, they were certainly written by a practising physician, who knew how to present and narrate the interaction between physician and patient in a colourful fashion. Following the Galenic model of embedding narratives within a technical treatise rather than composing a separate collection of accounts, John provides distinct sections in his *On Urines*, where he recounts his clinical experience with his patients. His narration is informed by his medical knowledge, his perceptions, and his social relationships. Although there is scant evidence to reconstruct exact details of John's workplace, we can see patients calling for the physician's advice or visiting him in his own professional space.

The key element in these accounts is the medical performance, which arises from the interaction between the physician and his patients and which reveals certain contemporary sociocultural features. John demonstrates his expertise through uroscopy, which constitutes the fundamental factor in the process of diagnosing and prognosticating a patient's condition, and exemplifies the physician's most efficient weapon against disease or any other physician's views. The visual aspect of the urine vial constitutes a recurrent element of symbolic significance, which helps the patients decipher the physician's actions and shows the physician's awareness of the need for individualized patient care. This process of individualization is articulated through a common 'language' of communication that may be adjusted according to the patient's needs and special characteristics, such as, for instance, the degree of John's familiarity with the individual patient, and the patient's background and experience of being treated by a professional physician. The physician's repeated success in dealing with disease not only functions as an index of his reputation, but also as a way of accounting for his noteworthy contribution to contemporary medicine through his treatise.

Having been drawn in by the narrator's rhetorical devices, the reader is transferred to the locus of medical activity. Subsequently, having gradually absorbed details taken from the primary narration, he is able to delve deeper into the practical value of these theoretical details, becoming an 'eyewitness' to a demonstration of healing. The observed becomes part of the performance and the observers are transformed into active practitioners by following the physician-narrator's advice, which has the characteristic of being worth remembering. As well as the explanatory and didactic role of John's account in supporting his theoretical details, there was also an intense desire on his part for professional self-aggrandizement in the eyes of his contemporaries, by reflecting the performance he gives in the various places of day-to-day medical activity. He is a physician and, at the same time, a scholar, who through his skilful account of his medical expertise attempts to attract attention. Bearing in mind that this is John's earliest medical work—whether or not these accounts were actually read by his non-medical contemporaries—it is only to be expected that his combined medical and writing expertise would have played an essential role in establishing himself in society and putting him in contact with other eminent Palaiologan scholars or even the Emperor, Andronikos II, himself.[128]

[128] Some parts from Sections 2.1, 2.2, 2.4, and 2.5, of this chapter, concerning the terminology used for patients and the patient's response, have been published elsewhere in the form of a brief chapter, Bouras-Vallianatos (2016c). Here they are embedded in revised form and in association with evidence from all the cases histories in John's *On Urines*.

4

Medical Epitome

A Handbook for *Philiatroi* ('Amateur Physicians')

> Moreover, in my opinion Alexander's love of the art of healing (*philiatrein*) was inculcated in him by Aristotle pre-eminently. For he was not only fond of the theory of medicine, but actually came to the aid of his friends when they were sick, and prescribed for them certain treatments and regimens, as one can gather from his letters.[1]
>
> Plutarch, *Life of Alexander the Great* 8.1

John's longest work, the *Medical Epitome*, has hitherto received very little scholarly attention, not least because a complete edition of the text is lacking.[2] The objective of this chapter is to present the structure of John's little-known work and clarify his sources. This will help us to contextualize the author's intentions with regard to the type of text he was producing. My aim is to place the treatise within the spectrum of ancient and Byzantine medical handbooks. The main focus will be on John's dependence on earlier approaches to diagnosis and treatment. I argue that the text is primarily written for *philiatroi* or non-expert readers: intellectuals who were deeply interested in medicine, but not practising physicians themselves. I will concentrate first on John's overall aims in writing his work and planning its structure; then I will explain his compilation methods in order to highlight the intellectual processes involved in selecting, adapting, and/or copying his sources. My analysis in this chapter focuses on the first four out of a total of six books, since pharmacology, which is treated in John's last two books, merits discussion in a separate chapter.[3]

[1] English translation by Perrin (1919: 243) slightly modified.

[2] See Chapter 1, Section 4.2.3, and Appendix 5, on the title of the work and the text which I use for the unedited books respectively.

[3] As we shall see in Chapter 5, the pharmacological part (books five and six) must have had a further specific use, that is to provide a much-needed revision of the subject, taking into account all the new material.

Innovation in Byzantine Medicine: The Writings of John Zacharias Aktouarios (c.1275–c.1330).
Petros Bouras-Vallianatos, Oxford University Press (2020).
DOI: 10.1093/oso/9780198850687.001.0001

1. TEXTS FOR AMATEUR PHYSICIANS (*PHILIATROI*) IN THE ANCIENT AND EARLY BYZANTINE WORLD

Before I focus on John's *Medical Epitome*, it is necessary to sketch in some background to the medical literature especially written for *philiatroi* ('friends/devotees of medicine' or 'amateur physicians') in the ancient and Byzantine worlds.[4] The concept of writing special medical works for the benefit of the layperson (*idiōtēs*) goes back to the Hippocratic corpus.[5] The earliest surviving medical work to attest the use of the term *philiatros* is Dioscorides' *De Materia Medica*:

> And we think that it is also useful to describe for *philiatroi* the preparation of composite wines, in order that this treatise should be comprehensive. Not that they [i.e. the wines] are used much or that it is necessary to use them, but rather so that I may in no way appear to have omitted anything. Some of them [i.e. the wines] are no trouble to make and are applied to <medicinal> uses, for instance, wines from quinces, pears, fruit of the carob tree, and even from myrtles.[6]

The term denotes a particular group of people, who are clearly not medical professionals, but able to prepare composite drugs, in this case various kinds of wines, by themselves. This is the only mention of the term in Dioscorides' work and there are no further explanatory details about the *philiatroi*. Dioscorides' reference may be explained as an attempt to reach a wider audience and thus to provide an easier way for non-specialists, too, to follow his text.[7] Although this is not a medical treatise for *philiatroi* per se, it is still noteworthy that a professional in the field was providing them with advice as early as the first century AD.

[4] LSJ, s.v. *φιλίατρος*: 'friend of the art of medicine'. On the concept, see Luchner (2004: 9–21). See also Nutton (1985: 31–4). Since it is difficult to translate the term in a modern sense, I use it in transliteration. On the importance of the concept of provision of medical education for the educated layman in the first/second century AD, see also Jori (2009), who discusses Plutarch's (before AD 50–after AD 120) *Prescriptions for Health*. A special work for the layman (*The Layman*) was written by the late-first-century AD Greek physician Rufus of Ephesos and survives only in some fragments in Arabic. On this, see Abou-Aly (1992: 43); and Nutton (2008: 154–5). Oribasios, *For Eunapios*, pr., ed. Raeder (1926) 318.4–7, reports that the work was already partly lost in his own day, i.e. second half of the fourth century AD. See also Hagedorn (2004).

[5] A prominent example is the *On Affections*. See Totelin (2018: 34–7) with references to earlier studies on this text. For evidence from the Roman Empire, see Draycott (2016).

[6] Dioscorides, *De Materia Medica*, 5.19.3, ed. Wellmann (1914) III.19.15–21: '*οὐκ ἄχρηστον δὲ ὑπογράψαι νομίζομεν πρὸς τὸ πλήρη τὴν ἱστορίαν τοῖς φιλιατροῦσι γενέσθαι καὶ τὴν τῶν ποικιλωτέρων οἴνων σκευασίαν, οὐχ ὅτι πολλὴ ἔστιν ἢ ἀναγκαία ἡ χρῆσις αὐτῶν ἀλλ' ἵνα κατὰ μηδὲν αὐτῶν ἐλλείπειν δοκῶμεν. εἰσὶ δὲ αὐτῶν ἔνιοι ἧττον περίεργοι καὶ πίπτοντες εἰς τὴν χρῆσιν, ὡς οἱ διὰ τῶν κυδωνίων καὶ ἀπίων καὶ κερατίων, ἔτι καὶ μύρτων σκευαζόμενοι*'. I use Beck's (2005: 343) English translation slightly modified.

[7] See van der Eijk (1997a: 88), who has convincingly argued that a certain treatise can address a variety of audiences at one and same time.

Galen tells us about the special characteristics of a certain *philiatros* in some of his treatises. He had dedicated some texts to certain friends, who had a particular interest in medicine.[8] For example, he wrote his *Therapeutics to Glaucon* as a result of a request from the contemporary philosopher Glaucon to 'sketch out . . . some general method of treatment'.[9] This work provides basic details on diagnosis and therapy in two books and it could be seen as a short medical handbook, unlike his substantially longer work the *Therapeutic Method*. From various references in the text, we can deduce that Glaucon was already familiar with Galenic texts on anatomy (*On Anatomical Procedures*) and drugs (*On the Capacities of Simple Drugs*) and was expected to start reading Galenic treatises on the pulse and the *On Mixtures*;[10] furthermore, he could most probably prepare some medicaments himself.[11] Other evidence shows that Glaucon was aware of Galen's recommendations for the treatment of cancerous swellings,[12] and was probably expected to be able to venesect.[13] In the epilogue of his work, Galen confirms that Glaucon was to take his book on an impending trip (*apodēmian soi makran*), just in case he encountered any medical problems.[14]

In his *On the Preservation of Health*, Galen provides more details about the group of *philiatroi*. It is striking that, although he clearly mentions that this book is primarily intended for physicians, he does not hesitate to provide extra information in particular passages, so as to be clear enough even for those with just an elementary knowledge of medicine:

> In this section I am not addressing the doctors but all those others, commonly called the *philiatroi*, who are in the first stages of learning, so as to train their way of thinking; for it is not necessary for those people to have studied my works on simple and compound drugs . . .[15]

[8] On Galen and his contemporary readers, see Johnson (2010: 74–97).

[9] Galen, *Therapeutics to Glaucon*, 1.1, ed. Kühn (1826) XI.1.9–2.1. English translation by Johnston (2016: 337). On Glaucon as a *philiatros*, seen through a detailed textual study of this specific Galenic treatise, see Peterson (1974: 25–46). On the audience of this particular work with references to earlier studies, see Bouras-Vallianatos (2018b: 180–3).

[10] Galen, *Therapeutics to Glaucon*, 2.8, 2.4, and 1.1, ed. Kühn (1826) XI.112.7, XI.99.15, and XI.5.11–13.

[11] Galen, *Therapeutics to Glaucon*, 2.2 and 2.9, ed. Kühn (1826) XI.81.7–10 and XI.124.10–13.

[12] Galen, *Therapeutics to Glaucon*, 2.12, ed. Kühn (1826) XI.143.7–8.

[13] Galen, *Therapeutics to Glaucon*, 1.12, 2.3, and 2.12, ed. Kühn (1826) XI.38.3–5, XI.84.7–8, and XI.142.14–16.

[14] Galen, *Therapeutics to Glaucon*, 2.13, ed. Kühn (1826) XI.145.12–14.

[15] Galen, *On the Preservation of Health*, 4.5, ed. Kühn (1823) VI.269.11–17 = ed. Koch (1923) 118.30–119.4: '*ἐν ἐκείνῃ μὲν γὰρ αὐτοῖς μόνοις διαλέγομαι τοῖς ἰατροῖς, ἐνταυθοῖ δὲ καὶ τοῖς ἄλλοις ἅπασιν, οὓς ὀνόματι κοινῷ προσαγορεύουσιν ἔνιοι φιλιάτρους, ἐν τοῖς πρώτοις δηλονότι μαθήμασι γεγονότας, ὡς γεγυμνάσθαι τὴν διάνοιαν. οὔκουν ἀναγκαῖόν ἐστι τοῖς τοιούτοις οὔτ' ἐν τῇ περὶ τῶν ἁπλῶν φαρμάκων οὔτ' ἐν τῇ περὶ συνθέσεως αὐτῶν γεγυμνάσθαι πραγματείᾳ . . .*' The quoted Greek text follows Koch's edition.

Later on, Galen further clarifies his intentions by showing a strong desire to teach the fundamentals on a particular subject:

> I am laying out general advice for all those reading this who have no professional knowledge in medicine but are not untrained in thinking.[16]

It is evident, therefore, that *philiatroi* were expected to be well-educated but not physicians, although they should possess a strong interest in medicine. Furthermore, it does not seem to be a requirement that they should prepare and administer drugs themselves or practise bloodletting, although this was an option, depending on the particular skills some of them developed, as we saw in the case of Glaucon.

A similar trend continued in later centuries, most prominently in the case of Oribasios, who wrote, among other works, a particular medical compilation for his friend, the 'sophist' Eunapios. In the *For Eunapios*, we find a similar approach to that of Galen's *Therapeutics to Glaucon*:

> From what you have told me in conversation, dearest and most eloquent Eunapios, it is clear that you are someone who wishes to know the simple and easily available remedies, so that when you are travelling in the countryside with no doctor being around, you can use them easily and effectively when facing things that happen unexpectedly... For those parts of the study of medicine that require considerable theoretical study and practical exercise belong to the expert only, but those that are easy to apply are available also to *philiatroi*. You have reached a level in the study of the art of medicine that is beyond what is suitable for *philiatroi*, and this will make it possible for you not only to help yourself and others in cases of illness, but also to make a judgment in most cases of disagreement between physicians and to choose what is best and most beneficial.[17]

Eunapios, like Glaucon, appears to be a *philiatros* for whom Oribasios writes a work with medical advice at his request in case there is no physician available. Eunapios, too, is well-equipped with the appropriate knowledge to treat himself or even others who happened to be with him. The most notable aspect, however, which expands our understanding of the group of *philiatroi*, is that Oribasios goes

[16] Galen, *On the Preservation of Health*, 6.14, ed. Kühn (1823) VI.449.5–7 = ed. Koch (1923) 197.2–4: '*κοινὴν δέ τινα συμβουλὴν ἅπασι τοῖς ταῦτα ἀναγνωσομένοις, ἰδιώταις μὲν τῆς ἰατρικῆς, οὐκ ἀγυμνάστοις δὲ τὸν λογισμόν, ὑποτίθημι τήνδε·*' The quoted Greek text follows Koch's edition.

[17] Oribasios, *For Eunapios*, pr., ed. Raeder (1926) 317.1–30: '*Ἐξ ὧν ἡμῖν διελέχθης, Εὐνάπιε κράτιστε καὶ λογιώτατε, δῆλος γέγονας ἰάσεις βουλόμενος ἐκμαθεῖν ὅσων οἷόντε νοσημάτων ἁπλᾶς καὶ εὐπορίστους, αἷς χρήσαιο ἂν ἔν τε ὁδοιπορίαις καὶ κατ' ἀγροὺς καὶ ὁπουδήποτε μὴ παρόντος ἰατροῦ, ῥᾳδίως καὶ ὠφελίμως τοῖς ἐξαίφνης προσπίπτουσιν ἀνθιστάμενος... τῶν γὰρ ἐν ἰατρικῇ πραγματείᾳ ὅσα μὲν ἱκανῆς δεῖται θεωρίας καὶ τῆς ἐπὶ τῶν ἔργων ἀσκήσεως, ταῦτα ἴδια τοῦ τεχνίτου μόνου, τὰ δ' εὐμεταχείριστα καὶ τοῖς φιλιατροῦσιν ἐφικτά· σὺ δὲ πλέον ἢ προσήκει τοῖς φιλιάτροις ἐπὶ τὴν θεωρίαν τῆς τέχνης ἐλήλυθας· τοσοῦτο ὑπάρξει σοι τὸ δύνασθαι μὴ μόνον ὠφελεῖν αὑτόν τε καὶ ἑτέρους ἔν τισι τῶν παθῶν, ἀλλὰ καὶ τὸ κρίνειν ἐπὶ τῶν μειζόνων τὴν τῶν ἰατρῶν διαφωνίαν αἱρεῖσθαί τε τὸ κρεῖττον καὶ ὠφελιμώτερον*'. I am using the English translation by van der Eijk (2010: 529–30).

a step further in representing his addressee as able to judge a physician's opinion where there is a disagreement, *diaphōnia*, between professionals.[18]

Although the term *philiatros* is not used in any medical work produced by Byzantine authors in later centuries, there are some notable cases from that period. In 1047, the polymath and statesman Michael Psellos (1018–*c.*1076) received the title of Consul of Philosophers, which refers to a sort of supervisor of higher education in the capital. Among his didactic works, he wrote a 1,375-line *Poem on Medicine.*[19] It starts by providing various medical terms, followed by a part on vegetal ingredients and basic details on pulse theory and uroscopy. Here, I cite an example from his advice on the examination of pulse:

> You should know the first ten categories of the pulse;
> swift, slow, and balanced in terms of time,
> which is actually the number of motions.
> And so the swift pulse occurs for a short period of time...
> Frequent or sparse is the seventh category;
> for as the artery moves in this way
> <there is a> twofold motion from opposing directions...
> The next one is the tenth and last category;
> it is the result of the aforementioned uneven pulse,
> the pulse that you could call 'ordered',
> while the other one is more properly called 'disordered'...
> <and> in between them is one called 'balanced'.[20]

The text aims to provide a summary of some basic aspects of medicine in an easily memorable form and is written for a non-specialist audience. At the same time, Psellos writes other didactic works on medicine, including short poems on parts of the human body and stones,[21] and sends letters on specific

[18] On the *diaphōnia*, see van der Eijk (2010: 531).

[19] See Volk (1990: 52–102), who provides a paraphrase of the poem in German accompanied by some comments on specific terms. See Hohlweg (1988), who discusses Psellos' sources. For a discussion of its didactic role, see Hörandner (2012: 61), who argues that it is addressed to an 'educated circle'. See also Bouras-Vallianatos (2015d), who discusses a new fragmentary witness of the text.

[20] Michael Psellos, *Poem on Medicine*, 283–421, ed. Westerink (1992) 200–4:

> Σφυγμῶν γένη γίνωσκε τῶν πρώτων δέκα·
> ταχύν, βραδύν, σύμμετρον ὡς πρὸς τὸν χρόνον,
> οὗτος ἀριθμός ἐστι τῶν κινουμένων.
> ταχὺς μὲν οὖν πέφυκεν ὃς βραχεῖ χρόνῳ...
> Ὁ πυκνὸς ἠδ' ἀραιὸς ἕβδομον γένος·
> κινουμένης γὰρ ὧδε τῆς ἀρτηρίας
> διπλῆν κίνησιν ἐξ ἐναντιωτάτων...
> Δέκατον ἄλλο καὶ τελευταῖον γένος,
> ἀνωμάλου γέννημα τοῦ λελεγμένου,
> οὗ τὸν μὲν εἴποις τὸν σφυγμὸν τεταγμένον,
> τὸν ἄλλον αὖ ἄτακτον ἀκριβεῖ λόγῳ...
> μέσος τίς ἐστι σύμμετρος κεκλημένος·

[21] Michael Psellos, *Names of the Limbs of the Human Body*, ed. Westerink (1992) 428–9; and *On the Properties of Stones*, ed. Duffy (1992) 116–19.

aspects of medicine to his friends and students, who having probably already taken tutorials on the subject, wanted to improve their knowledge in other areas.[22]

Moreover, there are two brief late Byzantine medical texts, which serve as an elementary introduction to the examination of blood and urine respectively and which are presented in most manuscripts under the name of Nikephoros Blemmydes.[23] These are written in sacred forms, i.e. stichera and canon, that combine mnemonic techniques and belong to a group of didactic poems that emerged in Byzantium in the later period for purposes other than the liturgy.[24] Both Psellos and Blemmydes led advanced educational programmes in Constantinople and Ephesos (Empire of Nicaea), which—combined with the very basic nature of the information contained in these texts—suggest that they were used to instruct Byzantine intellectuals, thus enabling them to cope with fundamental aspects of medical theory and terminology.

2. JOHN'S PROEM: PURPOSE AND AUDIENCE

In the early 1980s, in the sole modern study dealing briefly with John's *Medical Epitome*, Armin Hohlweg says among other things:

> It is not a collection of popular medicine, but a work written for doctors by a doctor, and indeed by a doctor who possessed a great deal of practical experience. This is clear from his own opinions, prescriptions, evaluations of medicines of others, as well as from a whole series of personal assertions.[25]

Although Hohlweg is right to highlight the absence of folk medicine from John's work, nevertheless his overall statement about the work having been written especially for physicians is, as we will see later on, certainly misleading and to a large extent not based on an assessment of the entire work, but just on the last two books on pharmacology. Before I attempt to respond to his assertions, I will start by concentrating on the proem of John's *Medical Epitome*.

[22] Among these, we can see letters written in various circumstances in order to provide short tutorials to his friends on various matters, such as the production and nature of cheese [Michael Psellos, *Epistle* 206, ed. Kurtz and Drexl (1941) II.235.25–238.15] or on the description and properties of the chestnut [Michael Psellos, *Epistle* 236, ed. Kurtz and Drexl (1941) II.286.15–287.10]. For a summary of these two letters, see Jeffreys (2017: 264, 279).

[23] On Blemmydes, see Chapter 1, n. 48.

[24] The text on urines has been edited by Ideler (1842) II.318–22. Both texts have been edited by Kousis (1944b) 59–63. On Byzantine parahymnography, with a focus on these medical hymns, see Mitsakis (1990: 47–52). In some manuscripts authorship is ascribed to Maximos Planoudes, a well-known early Palaiologan teacher and scholar in Constantinople. I am currently preparing a critical edition, English translation, and commentary of the texts in collaboration with Dimitrios Skrekas.

[25] Hohlweg (1984: 132) [originally published in German (1983: 321)].

Proems are traditionally ideal places from which to collect information about the author's aims, motivations, and self-fashioning. John starts his work by setting out his objectives:

> When you were sent on an embassy on behalf of our nation to the Hyperborean Scythians, after our most excellent, divine, and wise Emperor so decided, you did not consider that you should be deprived of our help. But on the contrary you wished to be accompanied by our own art, so that in case your health encountered any problems, you could be consoled by considering the words of this brief[26] book. It seemed to me such an easy task to make an improvised draft of this sublime and excellent art with brief words for you... These things, as you yourself know, my excellent friend, I have postponed many times... anyway I decided to compose this book and offer it to you as some sort of advice... this essay will be the unique reminder of a precious friendship... you know that I have often encouraged you to be initiated into the 'secrets' of the art, seeing that you were so naturally disposed to learn everything about it...[27]

The *Medical Epitome* was written for Alexios Apokaukos to take on his diplomatic mission.[28] Several aspects are reminiscent, for example, of Oribasios' project for Eunapios. Although Apokaukos is neither a philosopher nor a physician, he is, like Eunapios, a well-educated person with a strong interest in medicine.[29] John praises his patron's inclination towards medical science, in the same way Oribasios lauds the prior medical knowledge already

[26] The term *brachysyllabou* is attested in a similar context in other Palaiologan authors; see, for example, Constantine Akropolites, *Epistle* 2, ed. Romano (1991) 109.1–3: '*Καὶ τίς ἂν με δεόντως οὐκ αἰτιάσαιτο ἐς τοσοῦτον περιιδόντα τὸν φίλτατόν μοι ἐκ παιδὸς Ἄγγελον, ὡς μηδὲ βραχυσυλλάβου γράμματος ἀξιῶσαι μηδὲ ψιλὴν στεῖλαι τὴν προσαγόρευσιν;*' In a medical context, Hippocrates' name is traditionally combined with brevity of sayings; see, for example, Galen, *On Hippocrates' 'Fractures'*, 3.4, ed. Kühn (1830) XVIIIb.540.5; and John of Alexandria, *Commentary on Hippocrates' 'On the Nature of the Child'*, 1, ed. Bell et al (1997) 132.27. See also n. 42, below, for all terms in connection with brevity in John's work.

[27] JZA, *Medical Epitome*, 1.pr., ed. Ideler (1842) II.353.8–354.24: '*Ἐπειδὴ σοι εἰς τὴν ὑπὲρ τοῦ γένους ἡμῶν στελλομένῳ πρεσβείαν ἐπὶ τοὺς ὑπερβορείους Σκύθας, οὕτω δὴ τοῦ παντ' ἀρίστου καὶ θείου καὶ σοφοῦ ἡμῶν αὐτοκράτορος κρίναντος, μηδὲ τῆς ἀφ' ἡμῶν σοι δεῖν ἐδόκει ἐπικουρίας λείπεσθαι, ἀλλά τι καὶ τῆς ἡμετέρας σοι συναφικέσθαι τέχνης, ὡς ἂν εἴ τι τῶν ἐκ τοῦ πεφυκότος συναντῴη ἀνιαρὸν εἰς ὑγίειαν, ἔχῃς παραμυθεῖσθαι, προσέχων τοῖς τῆς βραχυσυλλάβου ταυτησὶ δέλτου γράμμασιν, ἔργον μὲν ἐδόκει μοι ῥᾳδίως οὕτω καὶ ἐπὶ βραχέσι ῥήμασιν αὐτὴν δὴ τὴν μεγίστην καὶ ἀρίστην ὑποσχεδιάζειν σοι τέχνην... ταῦτά τοι ὡς οἶσθα καὶ σύ, φίλων ἄριστε, ἀνεβαλλόμην πολλάκις ἀξιωθεὶς τὸν λόγον... ἀμέλει καὶ ἔδοξέ μοι τουτὶ τὸ βιβλίον συντάξασθαι καὶ ὡς ἐν ὑποθήκης τρόπῳ ἐκδοῦναί σοι... μόνον εἴη τουτὶ τὸ γράμμα ἀκριβοῦς φιλίας ὑπόμνημα... οἶσθα δὲ καὶ ὡς πολλάκις τὰ τῆς τέχνης προὐτρεψάμην μυηθῆναι ὄργια, οὕτως εὐφυῶς ἔχοντά σε περὶ ταύτην καταμαθών...*'

[28] John had probably managed to finish only the first book of his work before Apokaukos' departure. See JZA, *On Psychic Pneuma*, 2.15.9, ed. Ideler (1841) I.380.11–14. See also the discussion in Chapter 1, Section 4.2.1, in which I also refer to Apokaukos' embassy.

[29] Apokaukos was educated in Constantinople by the eminent teacher Theodore Hyrtakenos (*fl.* early fourteenth century). See Hyrtakenos' letter to Apokaukos, *Epistle* 69, ed. Karpozilos and Fatouros (2017) 248–52. On Hyrtakenos' educational activity in the capital, see Constantinides (1982: 93–5). On his pupils, see Karpozilos (1990: 289).

acquired by his dedicatee, which allows him to consult medical handbooks. Apokaukos, in particular, commissioned two full-page parchment illustrations in a manuscript of Hippocrates' work (Parisinus gr. 2144) that he owned, in which he had himself depicted (on one folio) in dialogue with Hippocrates (who is depicted facing him on the other folio). In the verse text Hippocrates appears to praise Apokaukos' intellectual capacity and also his natural disposition for medical learning, while Apokaukos in his turn applauds Hippocrates' wisdom and refers to the fact that his reading of Hippocratic works had helped him broaden his knowledge of medicine.[30]

The second notable aspect in John's proem is that his work provides a manual that could be carried by a traveller who might wish to treat himself. In his *On Psychic Pneuma*, John reconfirms that Apokaukos will be able to diagnose and treat himself or others by consulting his *Medical Epitome*, while on his diplomatic mission:

> The *prokathēmenos* of the imperial *koitōn*,[31] who was sent on an embassy to the Hyperborean Scythians, considered that I should write a book for him, so that he would be able to identify and diagnose the diseases in a reasonable manner, and provide treatment to those having been diagnosed...[32]

The concept of providing a handbook for the non-expert to take on a trip has already been described above with regard to Glaucon and Eunapios.[33]

[30] On Apokaukos' manuscript of Hippocrates' works, see Munitiz (1996), who provides an edition and English translation of the dialogue; and Makris (2005).

[31] Note that in this case John does not refer to Apokaukos using the rank of *parakoimōmenos*, the office which he held from 1321, but rather calls him *prokathēmenos*. I have checked the vast majority of the manuscripts of the *On Psychic Pneuma* and they all retain the word *prokathēmenos*. The *prokathēmenos* is a much lower-ranking office and is found in sixtieth place in the fourteenth-century list by Pseudo-Kodinos compared to the *parakoimōmenos* which comes in the fifteenth place. See the relevant list in Macrides, Munitiz, and Angelov (2013: 455–64). No other source reports that Apokaukos ever held the office of *prokathēmenos*. Before his appointment to the office of *parakoimōmenos*, we know that he was appointed to the office of *domestikos* of the Western themes around 1320 (*PLP* 1180), which is a lower office compared to that of *prokathēmenos*. Thus, even if we take John's reference at face value and consider that Apokaukos held the office of *prokathēmenos* between 1320 and 1321, it would only indicate a slightly earlier probable starting point (i.e. *c.*1320–1) for the composition of the *Medical Epitome*. See also Chapter 1, Section 4.2.1.

[32] JZA, *On Psychic Pneuma*, 2.15.9, ed. Ideler (1841) I.380.6–11: '*τῷ γάρ τοι προκαθημένῳ τοῦ βασιλικοῦ κοιτῶνος εἰς πρεσβείαν στελλομένῳ ἐπὶ τοὺς ὑπερβορείους Σκύθας, ἀξιώσαντί με ἐκδοῦναί οἱ βιβλίον, ὅπως ἂν ἔχῃ μετρίως περὶ νοσημάτων κρίνειν τε καὶ διαγινώσκειν, καὶ θεραπείας ἐπάγειν τοῖς διαγινωσκομένοις...*'

[33] The concept also appears in the Pseudo-Galenic *On Procurable Drugs*, 1.pr, ed. Kühn (1827) XIV.311–12, which was intended to serve those who were travelling, and, in particular, those spending time in the countryside or in deserted places. Galen also seems to have written a book *On Procurable Drugs*, as the Pergamene physician confirms in his *On the Capacities of Foodstuffs*, 2.46, ed. Kühn (1823) VI.634.12–13 = ed. Wilkins (2013) 155.2–3, but it does not survive. The work was already lost by Oribasios' own time; see Oribasios, *For Eunapios*, pr., ed. Raeder (1926) 317.35–6.

John's aim in writing the *Medical Epitome* seems also to reflect current trends. It was, in fact, in this period that the Greek translation of the *Ephodia tou Apodēmountos*[34] (Ar. *Zād al-Musāfir wa-Qūt al-Ḥāḍir/Provisions for the Traveller and Nourishment for the Sedentary*/Lat. *Viaticum*) by Ibn al-Jazzār (*fl.* tenth century)—originally an Arabic medical text composed specifically for travellers—was enjoying considerable popularity, as the number of surviving codices from the period confirms.[35] John's awareness of this particular work can be deduced by his using it as one of his sources in composing the pharmacological part of the *Medical Epitome.*[36]

John appropriates an earlier concept,[37] particularly prominent in the field of medical writings, that of providing written advice for the *philiatros* or the non-expert, and adapts it to his own intellectual environment.[38] In the introduction to book four, we can even see John's attempt to highlight his aim of reaching the widest possible audience. He states:

> ... since we have set down the method according to the medical art, but we have not treated everything yet, only the first three books, which we have presented in abridged form; and because they will not be easily accessible to those with less

[34] '*Ἐφόδια τοῦ Ἀποδημοῦντος*' ('Provisions for the Traveller'). We do not know exactly where this translation was made. The earliest surviving manuscripts originate in southern Italy or Sicily, i.e. Vaticanus gr. 300 (AD 1130/40) and Parisinus gr. 2311 (twelfth/thirteenth century). On the dating and origin of the two manuscripts, see Lucà (1993: 36–63) and Canart (1978: 146) respectively. The date of the first manuscript (1130/40) gives a *terminus ante quem* for the Greek translation of the work. In the vast majority of the manuscripts the translation is attributed to a certain *prōtasēkrētis* or *asēkrētis* Constantine of Reggio [see Bouras-Vallanatos (forthcoming: n. 114)]. The Greek text remains unedited; some chapters were published by Daremberg and Ruelle (1879) 582–96. Book seven, on fevers, was partly published by Bernard (1749) 1–306. For an introduction to the Greek translation, see Touwaide (2008b); and Congourdeau (2012: 226–30). For some observations on the textual transmission of the Greek translation, see Daremberg (1853: 65–76); and Gabrielli (1905: 29–50). The most recent study of the Greek translation is by Miguet (2017). The Arabic text has been published by Suwaysī et al. (1999), based on a nineteenth-century copy of the text. For a critical edition and English translation of book six and seven, see Bos (1997) and (2000; 2015) respectively. Although the original Arabic, and also the Greek and the Latin title of the work, refer to a traveller's manual, there is a debate as to whether it was actually used for this purpose; see Schipperges (1955: 65); and Bos (1993: 296–7). See also Miguet (2017: 59–74, 76–7).

[35] There are in total forty-four extant manuscripts, including excerpting ones, according to the most recent estimate by Miguet (2017: 85). There are only two manuscripts dating to before the fourteenth century (see n. 34, above), while the rest were copied from the fourteenth to the eighteenth century. See also Costomiris (1891: 101–4); and the list on *Pinakes: Textes et manuscrits grecs*, at http://pinakes.irht.cnrs.fr/notices/oeuvre/13334/ (accessed 20 July 2018). See also Chapter 5, n. 53.

[36] See Chapter 5, Section 4.1.

[37] In using the term 'appropriates' here, I am following Hardwick's (2003: 9–10) definition: 'Appropriation: taking an ancient image or text and using it to sanction subsequent ideas or practices (explicitly or implicitly)'.

[38] In addition to Apokaukos, Joseph Rhakendytes can be considered another *philiatros*; see Chapter 6, n. 25, and Section 5.1, n. 94, below. On John's contacts with the contemporary intellectual community, see Chapter 1, Section 4.1.

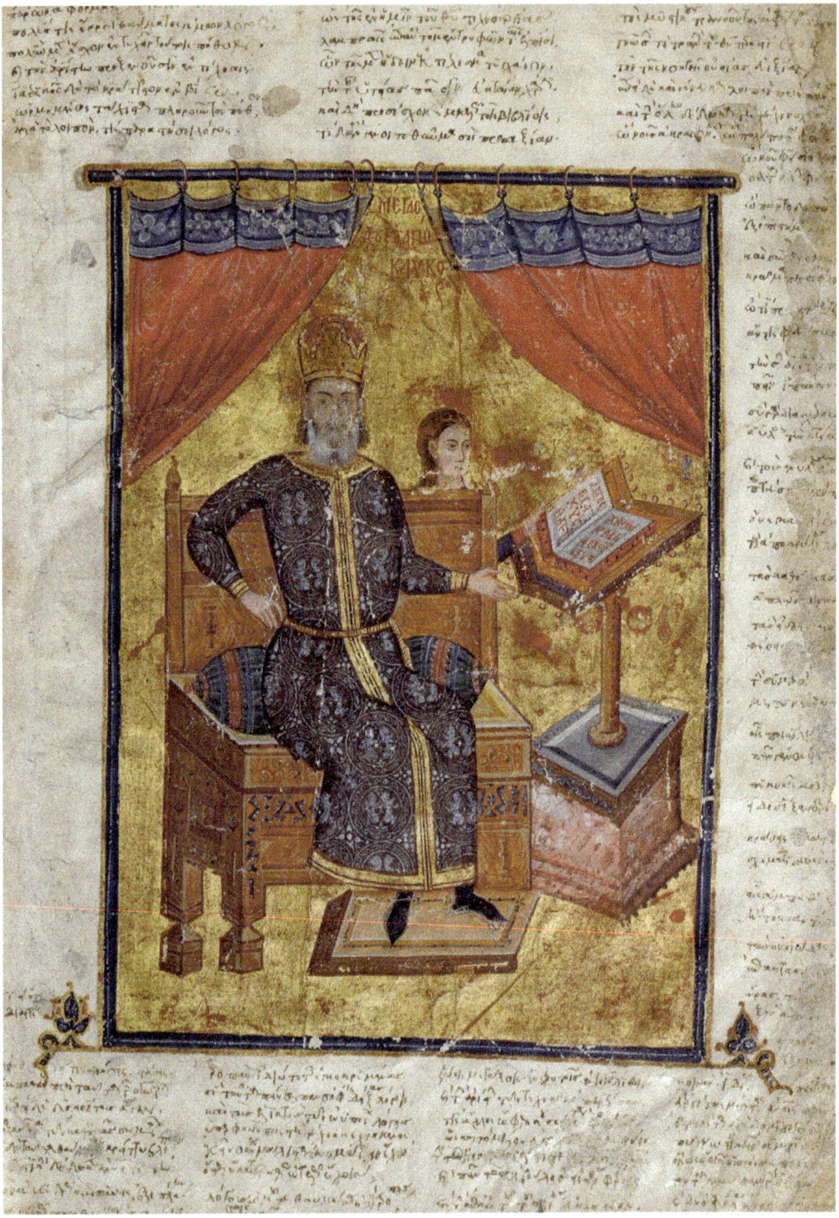

Figure 4.1. The portrait of Alexios Apokaukos in Parisinus gr. 2144, containing the Works of Hippocrates. In the margins a eulogy in sixty-five dodecasyllable verses praises Hippocrates and stresses Apokaukos' personal passion for medicine.[39] Parisinus gr. 2144 (first half of the fourteenth century), f. 11r.

[39] Apokaukos is designated as *megas doux* in the parchment bifolium containing his and Hippocrates' portraits. Apokaukos received this title in 1341 and died in 1345.

experience, we have already added a fourth book in addition to the three aforementioned books.[40]

The use of the word *apeiroteros* ('most inexperienced'/'most unskilled') is applied here specifically to those not having enough experience in medical practice. In contrast, for example, to his highly specialized work *On Urines*, where he gives an extensive treatment of a particular topic,[41] in this case we can see John's awareness of providing a work that could appeal to a non-specialist audience. This should not be perceived as an attempt to popularize medical knowledge, but rather above all to provide a quick-reference vade mecum of practical and well-chosen data for the contemporary *philiatros*. This does not necessarily mean that the work would not be useful to physicians interested in John's medical advice, too; rather, it shows that John wants to communicate information in such a way that non-expert readers would be equally able to access his work in its entirety and, at the same time, assess and evaluate John's contribution to his area of expertise.

3. STRUCTURE

The *Medical Epitome* is characterized by *brachylogia*[42] ('brevity'), which is intended to make John's work easily accessible. We noticed that brevity was emphasized already in the proem. This characteristic is evident at both the micro and macro level in the work. Individual chapters usually cover a few lines in a printed edition or about half a folio in manuscripts. In total, the work is about 135,000 words long, which is two thirds the size of Paul of Aegina's

[40] JZA, *Medical Epitome*, 4, Vindobonensis med. gr. 17, f. 76r, ll. 15–18: '…*ἐπεὶ τοίνυν καὶ ἡμεῖς τὴν κατὰ τὴν ἰατρικὴν προστησάμενοι μέθοδον, οὔπω τὸ πᾶν διελάβομεν, ἤδη τριῶν ἠνυσμένων λόγων· καὶ ταῦτα συντετμημένως τὰ κατ' αὐτὴν διεξιόντες, καὶ ὡς οὐκ ἂν γε τοῖς ἀπειροτέροις ἁρμόσειεν, ἤδη καὶ τέταρτον τοῖς προρρηθεῖσι τρισὶ λόγοις προστίθεμεν·*'; ed. Mathys (1556) II.214.8–14.

[41] On the audience for John's *On Urines*, see Chapter 2, Section 2.1.

[42] John uses a variety of terms to denote brevity in his *Medical Epitome*, for example, 1.4, 2.41, ed. Ideler (1842) II.359.19, II.463.25: '*βραχυλογία*'; *Medical Epitome*, 1.31, 1.56, 2.3, ed. Ideler (1842) II.381.30, 415.37, II.440.6: '*βραχυλογεῖν*'; *Medical Epitome*, 1.pr, ed. Ideler (1842) II.353.15: '*βραχυσύλλαβος*'; *Medical Epitome*, 1.33, ed. Ideler (1842) II.384.9: '*συντομία*'. See also a reference from the unedited book five in Chapter 5, n. 39. On brevity in medical literature, see, for example, Paul of Aegina, *Epitome*, pr., ed. Heiberg (1921) I.3.9: '*συντόμοις τε καὶ συνεκδήμοις*', whose primary purpose was the writing of an abridged medical compilation for quick reference. John also refers to the abridged nature of his account by using the adverb *syntetmēmenōs* ('in abridged form') (see LSJ, s.v. *συντέμνω*, 'to cut down/to speak briefly'). See, for example, n. 40, above, and JZA, *Medical Epitome*, 3, Vindobonensis med. gr. 17, f. 55r, ll. 11–13: '*νυνὶ περὶ θεραπευτικῶν μεθόδων διειληφέναι ὅσον οἷόν τε ἀσφαλῶς τὲ ἅμα καὶ συντετμημένως προτεθυμήμεθα·*'; ed. Mathys (1556) II.154.1–4.

Epitome, and much shorter than, for example, Aetios of Amida's *Tetrabiblos*, which consisted of sixteen books of about 30,000 words each. On the other hand, it is almost three times the length of Oribasios' *For Eunapios* and six times longer than Galen's *Therapeutics to Glaucon*. The fact that the text was substantially longer than Oribasios' and Galen's books produced specifically for *philiatroi* can be explained, as we will see in the next chapter, by the extended nature of John's section on pharmacology, which amounts to around 65,000 words (half of the *Medical Epitome*).[43]

John is eager to show that, although brevity is key, where there is a need for elaboration he will provide it in order to be sufficiently clear to his readers. Thus, for example, in the chapter on the diagnosis of brain affections, he writes:

> Since we have already talked about the brain itself... let us now give an account of what is appropriate, so that the book will be complete and reliable in all respects, otherwise brevity eliminates clarity.[44]

Among John's central sources in the first four books is Paul of Aegina's *Epitome* (see Tables 4.2 and 4.3, below).[45] Although John does not follow exactly the same structure as Paul of Aegina in arranging his books, we can discern obvious similarities with Paul's functional model. Thus, for example, John, like Paul (in books three and four),[46] consciously divides the diseases into two main groups, by following an *a capite ad calcem* order: a) those affecting internal (*entos*) organs of the body, such as the heart, lungs, and liver; and b) those affecting the external (*ektos*) parts of the body and the sense organs. He states:

[43] The estimation of the length of John's work is based on the transcription of the complete work from Vindobonensis med. gr. 17. The length given for the other medical works comes from the relevant word count for each work provided by *Thesaurus Linguae Graecae*, at http://stephanus.tlg.uci.edu/ (accessed 18 August 2018).

[44] JZA, *Medical Epitome*, 1.33, ed. Ideler (1842) II.384.5–9: '*Ἐπεὶ δὲ καὶ εἰς αὐτὸν κατέστημεν τὸν ἐγκέφαλον... τὰ δέοντα ἐξαγγείλωμεν, ὡς διὰ πάντων ὁ λόγος ἔχοι τὸ ἄρτιόν τε καὶ ἀσφαλές, εἰ καὶ ἄλλως ἡ συντομία ἀφαιρεῖται τὸ εὐκρινές.*'

[45] The use of Paul of Aegina's *Epitome* as one of the main sources of John's work (in books one and two) has been briefly underlined by Karpozilos (2008). In turn *Therapeutics to Glaucon* is one of Paul of Aegina's main Galenic sources. For a study of Galen's *Therapeutics to Glaucon* as a source of early Byzantine medical handbooks, see Bouras-Vallianatos (2018b: 194–7).

[46] Paul of Aegina's work is structured in seven books as follows: hygiene and dietetics (book one); diagnosis and therapy of fevers (book two); diagnosis and therapy of affections of the internal organs and sense organs in *a capite ad calcem* order (book three); diagnosis and therapy of affections of the external parts of the body (book four); on venomous animals and poisons (book five); surgery including invasive techniques (book six); simple and composite drugs (book seven). See, for example, Paul of Aegina, *Epitome*, pr. and 4.pr, ed. Heiberg (1921) I.4.32 and I.315.1–3: '*Ἐν τῶ τετάρτῳ περὶ τῶν ἐκτὸς τοῦ σώματος...*' and '*Ἐν τούτῳ τῷ βιβλίῳ τετάρτῳ τῆς ὅλης ὑπάρχοντι πραγματείας περὶ τῶν ἀορίστως τε καὶ σποράδην ἐκτὸς μάλιστα τοῦ σώματος γινομένων παθῶν ὁ λόγος ἐστίν.*'

> First, one must talk about the internal <affections>; those which naturally affect the head and the other internal parts. Then about <the affections> that occur on the outside <of the body>.[47]

However, John goes a step further than Paul by providing a clear distinction between diagnosis and therapeutics devoting separate books to each.[48] Furthermore, as you can see in Table 4.1, there is a clear correspondence between the diagnostic details in the first two books and the therapeutic details in book four, which enhances the consultation of the work.

John follows what is in effect a practical, general-to-specific approach, dividing his work into three main sections. Thus the first section consists of books one and two, and deals mainly with the diagnosis of various affections. In particular, book one gives introductory details on human physiology and humoral pathology, thus providing the necessary basic background to terms and physiological functions, followed by a long presentation on sphygmology. Next comes uroscopy, which is treated in just a few pages unlike the extensive treatise in his *On Urines*, and John makes clear to his readers that for more details they should consult the corresponding work.[49] The second half of the book deals with the diagnosis of internal affections in an *a capite ad calcem* order.

Table 4.1. Summary of contents of John's *Medical Epitome*, Books One–Four

Diagnosis	General Therapeutics
Book One (first part): General introduction on physiology, humoral pathology, sphygmology, and uroscopy.	**Book Three:** Phlebotomy and other non-invasive techniques, leeches; baths and exercise; dietetics.
Book One (second part): Diagnosis of affections of the internal parts of the body in *a capite ad calcem* order.	**Book Four (first part):** Therapy of affections of the internal parts of the body in *a capite ad calcem* order.
Book Two: Diagnosis of affections of the outer parts of the body and sense organs in *a capite ad calcem* order.	**Book Four (second part):** Therapy of affections of the external parts of the body and sense organs in *a capite ad calcem* order.

[47] JZA, *Medical Epitome*, 4, Vindobonensis med. gr. 17, f. 76v, ll. 19–21: '*πρότερον μὲν περὶ τῶν ἐντὸς ῥητέον· ὅσα κατά τε τὴν κεφαλὴν καὶ τὰ λοιπὰ σπλάγχνα συνίστασθαι πέφυκεν· ἔπειτα καὶ περὶ τῶν κατὰ τὴν ἐκτὸς ἐπιφάνειαν φαινομένων·*'; ed. Mathys (1556) II.215.24–9.

[48] This is emphasized in several cases by John. See, for example, the following excerpt from the introduction to book three, before he starts the discussion of his therapeutics: JZA, *Medical Epitome*, 3, Vindobonensis med. gr. 17, f. 55r, ll. 6–9: '*…χρεὼν ἂν εἴη ἐξασκεῖν ἡμᾶς τὸ διαγινώσκειν πρότερον· εἶθ' οὕτως τὸ κατὰ μέθοδον θεραπεύειν· καὶ τοίνυν ἐν τοῖν πρὸ τούτου δυοῖν βιβλίοιν φθάσαντες διὰ βραχέων διαλαβεῖν περὶ διαγνώσεως ….*' ('…it is necessary for us to perform the diagnosis first; then in this way to treat according to the method. The manner of diagnosis is discussed briefly in the two preceding books…'); ed. Mathys (1556) II.153.20–6. The particular attention John pays to the diagnosis of disease and the clear distinction he makes between different medical processes is also an important aspect of his *On Urines*, see Chapter 2, Section 2.2.

[49] JZA, *Medical Epitome*, 1.26–32, ed. Ideler (1842) II.375.11–384.3.

The second book provides a long discussion on fevers, crises, and critical days followed by an *a capite ad calcem* presentation of external affections with a special focus on skin affections. Books three and four concentrate on therapeutics. The former gives details on various methods of humoral evacuation. It starts with a presentation of phlebotomy and arteriotomy, and continues with the use of leeches and clysters. The second part of this book focuses on dietetics with special provision for the therapy of various kinds of fevers in addition to general information about bathing[50] and exercise. Book four provides details on the therapy of affections, listed in the same order as that given in the first two books. Thus the first part deals with internal affections and the second with external ones. Here we can see a holistic therapeutic approach, including recommendations on phlebotomy, baths, exercise, diet, and drugs. As regards the use of medicines, John usually refers to simple or composite drugs only by name; details on the preparation and special use of drugs are given in books five and six. Book five is structured according to the various kinds of drugs, while book six addresses the subject mainly in an *a capite ad calcem* order.

4. JOHN'S CONTENTS AND SOURCES: DIAGNOSIS

The *Medical Epitome*, in contrast to the much more original *On Urines* or a substantial part of the first book of John's *On Psychic Pneuma*, is a compilation from earlier sources on the subject. John follows the well-established Byzantine tradition of composing works by copying parts from other authors' books.[51] In the field of medical literature, this is particularly evident in the composition of early Byzantine medical works.[52] By critically comparing the compilation techniques of Oribasios, Aetios of Amida, and Paul of Aegina in one of his recent studies, Philip van der Eijk makes interesting points on the crucial role of these authors in the preservation and transmission of Graeco-Roman medical ideas.[53] He was the first to show convincingly and emphatically that their works should not be considered mere copies of pre-existing

[50] The chapter on bathing has been edited by Teza (1903/4: 312–14).

[51] On compilation literature in a variety of genres in Byzantium, see the case of the Macedonian compilations discussed by Holmes (2010).

[52] For an introduction to early Byzantine medical compilations, see the discussion in Chapter 1, Section 1.2.

[53] Van der Eijk (2010). See also van der Eijk's (1999) article on the role of Caelius Aurelianus (fifth century AD) as a doxographer of Soranus and Sideras (1974), who provides a comparative study of the excerpting techniques of Oribasios and Aetios of Amida. Early Byzantine medical handbooks are also important because they retain passages from ancient authors otherwise lost; see, for example, Mavroudis (2000: 212–27), who provides a list of extracts from Archigenes which survive solely in early Byzantine medical works.

material, but that they were based on a careful selection of sources related to the authors' professional expertise and target audience. More importantly, this thought-provoking approach opens up new ways to research other Byzantine medical compilations, which have been neglected by the vast majority of the modern scholarly community.

In attempting to get a better idea of John's use of earlier material, I have divided my study into two main parts, diagnosis and therapy, corresponding to John's division of his work. I first concentrate on books one and two, from which I shall present three case studies. The particular sections for each of the case studies have not been selected randomly, but each of them, as we will see below, shows special characteristics, which will provide important insights into John's method of compilation. Furthermore, they represent equally the two main topics of the first two books, i.e. general diagnostic techniques and the diagnosis of specific affections. The first case study will focus on John's discussion of the theory of pulse; then I will move on to the chapter on the diagnosis of eye affections; and, finally, to the diagnosis of scirrhus. In discussing John's sources, I will not give the texts in tables of parallel columns; instead, I will follow van der Eijk's methodology and give the Greek text followed by an English translation as *Lesetext*, which will provide a better overview of John's appropriation of earlier sources, and will permit us to evaluate his contribution.

Table 4.2. Overview of John's sources, *Medical Epitome*, Books One & Two[54]

Book One	Source
Physiology (mixtures, natural capacities, and activities).	Synopsis from Galen's *On Mixtures*; synopsis from John's *On Psychic Pneuma*; and excerpts from unidentified source.
Sphygmology.	Excerpts from Galen's works on the pulse.
Uroscopy.	Synopsis from John's *On Urines*.
Diagnosis of affections of the internal parts.	Excerpts from Paul of Aegina's *Epitome*, book three.
Book Two	
Diagnosis of affections of the outer part of the body and sense organs.	Excerpts from Paul of Aegina's *Epitome*, books three and four.

[54] This table and the next one (4.2), showing John's sources in the *Medical Epitome*, are not intended to provide an exhaustive reference to John's use of earlier works, but to give the modern reader an idea of the variety of material that I have managed to identify. A complete list of John's sources will be made available in the *apparatus fontium* of my prospective *editio princeps* of John's *Medical Epitome*.

4.1 Case study 1: Sphygmology

The first example is related to two of John's chapters dealing with the pulse in book one. John is excerpting from Galen's *On the Causes of the Pulse.*[55] The printed text is by Galen; the underlined parts are those copied by John, while those in bold are John's additions.

Galen, *On the Causes of the Pulse*, 4.6–7, ed. Kühn (1825) IX.161.10–165.1; JZA, ***Medical Epitome***, 1.24–5, ed. Ideler (1842) II.374.4–375.10:

(***κδʹ. Περὶ τῶν κατὰ τὰς ὀδύνας καὶ φλεγμονὰς σφυγμῶν***)

(161) ...*Ἄλγημα δὲ τὸ τρέπον τοὺς σφυγμούς· τρέπει δὲ ἢ τὸ ἰσχυρὸν* (***σφοδρόν***), *ἢ ἐν κυρίοις*[56]*μορίοις, ὡς καὶ ἡ φλεγμονή· μικρὸν μὲν ὂν ἔτι καὶ ἀρχόμενον μείζονα καὶ σφοδρότερον καὶ ὠκύτερον καὶ πυκνότερον τὸν σφυγμὸν ἐργάζεται, αὐξηθὲν δὲ καὶ ἰσχυρὸν πάνυ γενόμενον, ὡς ἀδικεῖν ἤδη τὸν ζωτικὸν τόνον, μικρότερον* (***καὶ ἀμυδρότερον***) *καὶ ταχὺν καὶ πυκνόν. καὶ ὅσῳ ἂν ἐγχρονίζῃ μᾶλλον, ἢ σφοδρότερος γίνηται, τῶν εἰρημένων ἕκαστον ἐπιτείνει. τὸ δὲ ἤδη διαλῦον τὴν δύναμιν καὶ* (162) *εἰς ἀμυδρότητα καὶ μικρότητα καὶ τάχους ψευδῆ φαντασίαν, καὶ ὑπερβάλλουσαν πυκνότητα τὴν τροπὴν ἐργάζεται. Ὥσπερ ἐπὶ τῶν ἄλλων ἁπάντων τῶν λυπούντων, οὕτω καὶ τῶν ἀλγημάτων ἡ δύναμις ἐπεγείρειν πέφυκεν ἑαυτὴν καὶ διαμάχεσθαι καὶ διωθεῖσθαι πᾶν τὸ διοχλοῦν, ὅθεν εὐλόγως εἰς μέγεθος καὶ τάχος καὶ σφοδρότητα τρέπει τοὺς σφυγμούς... Φλεγμονῆς σφυγμὸς ὁ μὲν κοινὸς ἁπάσης οἷον ἐμπρίων ἐστὶν, ὡς δοκεῖν τὸ μέν τι διεστάλθαι τῆς ἀρτηρίας, τὸ δὲ μή, σκληροτέρας δηλονότι φαινομένης αὐτῆς. ἔχει δέ τι καὶ κλονῶδες ὁ σφυγμὸς οὗτος. καὶταχὺς* (163) *μέν ἐστι καὶ πυκνὸς, οὐκ ἀεὶ δὲ μέγας. ὁ δὲ ἴδιος ἑκάστης ὁ μὲν τῆς ἀρχομένης μείζων τοῦ κατὰ φύσιν καὶ σφοδρότερος καὶ ὠκύτερος καὶ πυκνότερος. ὁ δ᾽ αὐξανομένης ἔτι ταῦτά γε προσαυξάνει πάντα, καὶ σαφῶς τε ἤδη σκληρότερός ἐστι καὶ κλονωδέστερος· τῆς δ᾽ ἀκμαζούσης σαφέστερος μὲν ἔτι καὶ σκληρότερος καὶ κλονωδέστερος, μικρότερος δὲ ἢ πρόσθεν, οὐ μὴν ἀμυδρότερός γε, πλὴν εἰ μὴ ὑπὲρ τὴν δύναμιν εἴη τὸ πάθος. ἀλλὰ καὶ πυκνότατος*(***-τερος***) *γίνεται καὶ ταχύς· εἰ δ᾽ ἱκανῶς χρονίζοι καὶ ἤδη σκληρύνοιτο σκιρρωδῶς, πρὸς τοῖς εἰρημένοις ἰσχνότης σφυγμοῦ καὶ σκληρότης* (***πυκνότης***) (***προσ-***)*γίνεται. ταῦτ᾽ ἐπὶ τῆς τὸν ἐν ὅλῳ τῷ*

[55] It is worth noting that Galen's account constitutes an extended version of his corresponding section in the *On the Pulse for Beginners*, 12, ed. Kühn (1824) VIII.474.5–477.1. The account *On the Pulse for Beginners* is longer than John's, but shorter than that in the *On the Causes of the Pulse*. It omits the same long passage as John does in chapter 24 (starting from '*Ὥσπερ ἐπὶ τῶν ἄλλων...*'), but it retains the passage corresponding to John's long omission in chapter 25. By looking at other instances, it is clear that John copied from the *On the Causes of the Pulse*. See, for example, JZA, 1.23, ed. Ideler (1842) I.373.32–5 [corresponding exactly to Galen, 4.3, *On the Causes of the Pulse*, ed. Kühn (1825) IX.159.10–14], which retains an extra sentence that is not found in the *On the Pulse for Beginners*, 12, ed. Kühn (1824) VIII.473.15–16. On the textual relationship between the two aforementioned Galenic treatises on the pulse, see Asper (2007: 329–33).

[56] Ideler's edition, here retains '*καιρίοις*'.

ζώῳ σφυγμὸν τρεπούσης φλεγμονῆς, ἢ διὰ τὸ μέγεθος, ἢ διὰ τὸ κύριον τοῦ μέρους ἐν ᾧ συνέστη. τῆς δὲ μὴ συγκινούσης τὸ πᾶν ὅ γ' ἐν τῷ φλεγμαίνοντι μέρει σφυγμὸς οἷος εἴρηται.

(***κε'. Περὶ τῶν κατὰ τὰς διαφορὰς τῶν μορίων ἀλλοιουμένων σφυγμῶν***)
ἐπιτείνεται δὲ καὶ ἀνίεται τῶν εἰρημένων ἕκαστον ἢ παρὰ τὸ ποσὸν τῆς φλεγμονῆς, ἢ (***καὶ***) *παρὰ τὴν αὐτοῦ τοῦ φλεγμαίνοντος ὀργάνου φύσιν. τὰ μὲν γὰρ νευρωδέστερα μέρη σκληροτέρους καὶ μᾶλλον ἐμπρίοντας καὶ μικροτέρους τοὺς σφυγμοὺς ἐργάζεται, τὰ δὲ φλεβωδέστερα καὶ ἀρτηριωδέστερα τοὺς ἐναντίους.* (164) *αὐτῶν δὲ τούτων μείζων ὁ ἐν τοῖς ἀρτηριώδεσι καὶ ῥᾳδίως ἀνώμαλος καὶ ἄτακτος γενόμενος. δῆλον οὖν ἤδη καὶ ὁ τῶν τὸ ἧπαρ φλεγμαινόντων σφυγμός, οἷος ἂν εἴη* (***ὁποῖος ἔσται***)*, καὶ ὁ τῶν τὸν σπλῆνα, καὶ ὁ τῶν τοὺς νεφρούς, ἢ τὴν* (***καὶ***) *κύστιν, ἢ τὸ κῶλον, ἢ τὴν* (***τε καὶ***) *γαστέρα, καὶ* (***ὁ τῶν***) *πλευριτικῶν καὶ περιπνευμονικῶν καὶ πάντων ἁπλῶς εἰπεῖν ὧν τῇ τοῦ μέρους φλεγμονῇ πυρετὸς ἕπεται, πλὴν ὅσα διὰ τὴν τῶν συμπτωμάτων φύσιν τῶν τε ἐξ ἀνάγκης ἑπομένων αὐτοῖς καὶ τῶν κατὰ τύχην συνδραμόντων, ὡς ἂν ἕκαστον τρέπειν δύνηται. καὶ τὸν σφυγμὸν ἐπὶ τοσοῦτον ἀλλοιοῦσθαι συμβήσεται, μικτῆς τροπῆς ἐν αὐτῷ γινομένης τῆς τε κατὰ τὸν λόγον τῆς φλεγμονῆς, καὶ ἣν ἡ τοῦ τόπου φύσις, ἢ τοῦ παρόντος συμπτώματος ἐργάζεται. σπασθῆναι μὲν γὰρ τοῖς τὰς φρένας φλεγμαίνουσιν ἕτοιμον, πνιγῆναι δὲ τοῖς τὸν πνεύμονα, συγκοπῆναι δὲ τοῖς τὸ στόμα τῆς γαστρός, ἀτροφῆσαι δὲ τοῖς τὸ ἧπαρ, ἀπεπτῆσαι δὲ τοῖς τὴν κοιλίαν, ἐπισχεθῆναι δὲ τὰ οὖρα τοῖς τοὺς νεφρούς. καὶ τὰ μὲν αἰσθητικώτερα μέρη καὶ διὰ τὰς ὀδύνας τρέπει τοὺς σφυγμούς· τὰ δὲ ἀναισθητότερα κατὰ* (165) *τὴν διάθεσιν μόνην.* (***ἀλλ' ἐπειδή σοι καὶ τὴν περὶ τῶν σφυγμῶν, ὡς οἷόν τε διὰ βραχέων ἐξεθέμεθα μέθοδον, ἔχοις γὰρ ἂν ἐντεῦθεν καὶ τὰ μὴ ῥηθέντα συνιδεῖν, ἀγχίνους ὢν καὶ περὶ τοιαύτην θεωρίαν δεικνύμενος σχετικῶς, δέον ἂν εἴη ἐπιθεῖναί σοι μετὰ τοῦτο τὸν περὶ τῶν οὔρων λόγον, τὰ μέγιστά σοι συνοίσοντα.***

κς'. Περὶ τῶν ἀπὸ τῶν οὔρων σημαινομένων . . .)

(24. **On pulse concerning pains and inflammations**)[57]

(161) . . . Pain of the sort that alters the pulse—and this happens in the case of severe pain or pain in the main parts—acts in the same way as inflammation. In the early stages, when it is still small, it renders the pulse fairly large, vigorous, swift, and frequent; once it has become larger and more severe, so that it harms the vital tension, it makes the pulse smaller, (**fainter,**) swift, and frequent. And in cases where it remains for a long time and becomes more vigorous, each of these features is intensified. Pain that actually dissolves the capacity (162) brings about a change to faintness, smallness, a false impression of swiftness, and excessive frequency. As in all

[57] For those parts of the text that are the same as Galen's *On the Pulse for Beginners*, I use Singer's (1997: 335–7) English translation slightly modified. I have also benefited from the Spanish translation of Galen's *On the Causes of the Pulse* by Pino Campos (2019).

other cases of suffering, so too with physical pain the capacity naturally raises itself in order to fight and reject everything that disturbs it, hence it changes the pulse appropriately in size, swiftness, and vigour... The pulse that is common to all cases of inflammation has a saw-like quality: the artery—which of course takes on a hard appearance—appears to be partially dilated and partially not. And this pulse is also somewhat tremulous. It is also swift (163) and frequent, but not always large. The features specific to different cases are as follows. In the early stages it is more vigorous, swift, and frequent than the norm; as it grows, these features increase, and at the same time it becomes definitely harder and more tremulous. It is most clearly perceptible as both harder and more tremulous, but now smaller than before, although not fainter, except in cases where the illness exceeds the patient's capacity; but it also becomes more frequent and swift. Where it remains for a long period, and the hardness reaches a point similar to that of indurations, thinness, and hardness (**frequency**) of pulse may be added to the above features. These things come about in cases of inflammation that change the pulse of the organism as a whole, either because of the size of the inflammation or because of the importance of the part affected. Where the whole organism is not affected, the pulse will be as already described, but confined to the part in question.

(25. On the difference in pulse related to altered parts)

And each of the above features is intensified or eased according to the degree of inflammation and the nature of the organ that it affects. The parts with more nerves in them, for example, give rise to harder, more saw-like, smaller pulse. The parts with more vein or artery have the opposite effect, (164) those with more artery having the larger pulse of the two, which is also liable to become uneven and disordered. It should by now be clear what will be the nature of pulse in those suffering from inflammation in the liver, in the spleen, or in the kidneys, bladder, colon, and stomach, but also in those suffering from pleurisy, peripneumonia, or any other disease in which a fever follows from the inflammation of a single part; except that there are additional phenomena due to the nature of the symptoms that are necessary consequences of these complaints, and to random, accidental features. To the extent that these latter phenomena are causes of change they too will affect the pulse; and so its alteration will be a 'mixed' one, arising from the characteristics of inflammation itself, from the nature of the part affected and from that of the symptom present. Inflammation of the midriff, for example, may lead to spasms; inflammation of the lungs to suffocation; of the mouth of the stomach to stoppages; of the liver to lack of nourishment; of the stomach to lack of digestion; of the kidneys to retention of urine. The parts with more sense perception affect the pulse because of the pain experienced; those with less affect it by virtue (165) of their own state

alone. But now that we have presented to you the method on pulse as briefly as possible, you are from now on able to perceive the things that have not been told, since you are shrewd and the relevant theory has already been pointed out to you. After this, it is fitting to provide you with the account on urine, which will assist you greatly.
(26. On those <things> indicated by the urine)...

John offers quite an extensive treatment of sphygmology compared to other topics dealt with in the first book, devoting seventeen out of the fifty-seven chapters of his first book to it.[58] The chapters provided above constitute the last section of this part, before he gives a short account (in seven chapters) of the diagnosis of disease using urine.[59] John does not name his source, as is his wont throughout his corpus.[60] He eliminates almost half the Galenic text in both chapters. Whether long or short, in all cases the omissions correspond to further explanations, exceptions, and extraordinary cases connected with phenomena arising from a combination of causes. John is fully aware of the contents of the Galenic passage. He does not simply copy his source-text, but he also provides a more elementary, condensed version. He divides the Galenic text into chapters and supplements its titles, which could be seen as providing a user-friendly reference tool.[61] It is noteworthy that in the end, he introduced a short piece of advice for his reader, who is addressed in the second-person singular.[62] John mentions once more the brevity of his writing; at the same time, in his attempt to keep up a certain level of communication with his reader, he praises the latter's medical abilities and informs him about the next set of details to follow. In this way, the non-expert reader is also given some reassurance that he will be able to use specific advice when he faces a corresponding medical condition.

4.2 Case study 2: Diagnosis of eye affections

In the second example, I focus on John's discussion of the diagnosis of eye affections. The passage is particularly interesting, since it shows that John

[58] JZA, *Medical Epitome*, 1.9–24, ed. Ideler (1842) II.362.32–375.10.

[59] JZA, *Medical Epitome*, 1.26–32, ed. Ideler (1842) II.375.11–384.3.

[60] See also Chapter 2, n. 139. Cf. Chapter 5, n. 59.

[61] This has been noted, for example, in relation to Oribasios by van der Eijk (2010: 528). See also De Lucia (1999: 483, n. 20) and MacLachlan (2006: 116), who both consider Oribasios' titles original to the text.

[62] There are lots of cases where John chooses a second-person singular to address his reader; see, for example, JZA, *Medical Epitome*, 1.32, 2.3, and 2.10, ed. Ideler (1842) II.384.2–3, II.436.31–6, and II.450.8–9. He also sometimes uses a second-person singular imperative of the verb *manthanō* (to learn) in stressing the didactic value of his advice: JZA, *Medical Epitome*, 1.17, 2.1, and 2.5, ed. Ideler (1842) II.368.8, II.423.35, and II.441.9. See also Chapter 2, n. 59, and Chapter 3, n. 28.

supplements his sources whenever he has something useful to add. In this case, John excerpts from Paul of Aegina's *Epitome*. The printed text is by Paul of Aegina; the underlined parts are those copied by John, while those in bold are John's additions.

Paul of Aegina, *Epitome*, 3.22.8–25, ed. Heiberg (1921) I.174.26–181.25;[63] JZA, ***Medical Epitome***, 2.7, ed. Ideler (1842) II.445.15–447.14:

(174) 8. *Πρὸς ἐμφυσήματα κνησμώδη καὶ ψωροφθαλμίας.*
. . . (***ὥσπερ καὶ ἡ ψωροφθαλμία τῆς ξηροφθαλμίας διαφέρει***) *ἡ δὲ* (***μὲν γὰρ***) *ψωροφθαλμία κνησμώδης τοῦ βλεφάρου* (***αἴσθησις***) *ψωρίασις δι' ἁλμυρὸν* (***γινομένη φλέγμα . . . ἡ δὲ ξηροφθαλμία δυσκινησία τῶν ὀφθαλμῶν μετὰ πόνου χωρίς τινος ὑγρότητος ἐκρεούσης***) *καὶ νιτρῶδες ὑγρὸν γιγνομένη . . .*

(175) 9. *Περὶ σκληροφθαλίας καὶ ξηροφθαλμίας.*
Ἡ μὲν σκληροφθαλμία σκληρότης καὶ δυσκινησία ἐστὶ τοῦ ὀφθαλμοῦ μετὰ πόνου καὶ ἐρεύθους χωρὶς ὑγρασίας . . . ἡ δὲ ξηροφθαλμία κνησμώδης ἐστὶ τῶν ὀφθαλμῶν διάθεσις χωρὶς ῥεύματος . . .

(176) 12. *Περὶ τραχώματος.*
Τὸ μὲν (***δὲ***) *τράχωμα τραχύτης ἐστὶ τῶν ἔνδον τοῦ βλεφάρου* (***μερῶν***), *ἡ* (***ἐπιταθὲν***) *δὲ τούτων ἐπίτασις, ὥστε καὶ οἷον* (***ὡς καὶ***) *ἐντομὰς* (***δοκεῖν***) *ἔχειν, σύκωσις καλεῖται,* (***ἐγ-***)*χρονίσασα δὲ καὶ* (***αὐτή, ὥστε καὶ***) *τυλωθεῖσα*(***-ῆναι***) *τύλωσις*(***-ος***) *ὀνομάζεται . . .*

13. *Περὶ χαλαζίων.*
(***τούτων δὲ διαφέρει τὸ***) *Χαλάζιόν ἐστιν ἀργοῦ ὑγροῦ* (***τινος***) *σύστασις* (***ὂν***) *κατὰ τὸ βλέφαρον . . .*

(177) 14. *Περὶ κριθῆς.*
(***τὴν δὲ οὕτω καλουμένην***) *Κριθή*(*ν*) (***πάντως οὐκ ἀγνοεῖς***) *ἐστιν ἀποστημάτιον κατὰ τὸν τοῦ βλεφάρου ταρσὸν* (***τι οὖσαν***) *ἐπίμηκες . . .*

15. *Πρὸς φθεῖρας τοὺς ἐν τοῖς βλεφάροις.*
Ἐκκαθάραντας πρότερον τοὺς φθεῖρας δεῖ θαλάσσῃ προσκλύζειν χλιαρᾷ . . .
(***Ὅτι δὲ φθειριῶσι τὰ βλέφαρα, καὶ τὸ ἐξ αὐτῶν πάθος διασημαίνει, φθειρίασις λεγόμενον. καὶ αὗται δὲ τοῖς ἀκριβῶς ὁρῶσι ζῶσαί τε καὶ κινούμεναι φαίνονται.***)

(181) 25. *Περὶ πτερυγίων.*
(***τοῖς τῶν ὀφθαλμῶν δὲ πάθεσι καὶ***) *Τὸ πτερύγιον* (***συγκαταλεγόμενον***) *νευρώδης ἐστὶν τοῦ ἐπιπεφυκότος ὑμένος ὑπεροχὴ ἐκφυομένη μὲν ἀπὸ τοῦ κανθοῦ, προϊοῦσα δὲ μέχρι* (***αὐ***)*τῆς στεφάνης* (***χωρεῖ***)*· ὅταν δὲ* (***ἄν γε μὴ***) *ὑπεραυξηθῇ*(***-ὲν τὸ πτερύγιον τύχῃ***), *καὶ τὴν κόρην* (***αὐτὴν***) *καλύπτει* (***ἐπικαλύπτοι καὶ τοῦ ὁρᾷν κωλύει***). *τὰ μὲν οὖν μεγάλα καὶ χρόνια τῶν πτερυγίων διὰ μόνης χειρουργίας ἐκτέμνεται . . .*

[63] For a commentary on Paul of Aegina's section on eye affections, see Adams (1844: I.426–32).

(174) 8. On ocular itchy emphysema and psorophthalmia.[64]

. . . (**but just like psorophthalmia differs from xerophthalmia**) but psorophthalmia is an itchy eruption of the eyelid, arising from a saltish (**phlegm . . . however, xerophthalmia is <a condition involving> difficulty in moving the eyes accompanied by pain and no moisture**) and nitrous liquid . . .

(175) 9. On sclerophthalmia and xerophthalmia.
Sclerophthalmia is a hardness of the eye and difficulty in moving accompanied by pain, and redness, without moisture . . . Xerophthalmia is an itchy condition of the eyes without rheum . . .

(176) 12. On trachoma.
Trachoma is a roughness of the inner (**parts of the**) eyelid; an increase in intensity will give the appearance of clefts, which is called sycosis. When it becomes chronic and callused, it is called tylosis . . .

13. On chalazia.
Chalazion (**differs from these**), in that it is an accumulation of stationary (**some sort of**) liquid in the eyelid . . .

(177) 14. On stye.
(**In any case you cannot be ignorant of the so-called**) Stye, (**since it**) is an elongated abscess on the tarsus of the eyelid . . .
15. On lice in the eyelids. Having firstly cleared away the lice, it is needful to wash the part with tepid seawater . . .
(**When the eyelids have lice, and the affection from them is clearly indicated, it is called pediculosis; and to those who watch these creatures closely, they appear to be alive and moving**).

(181) 25. On pterygia.[65]

(**Among the eye affections is also the**) Pterygium (**which**) is a sinewy projection of the conjuctival membrane beginning at the canthus and proceeding to the rim of the cornea; if (**by chance**) the pterygium overgrows, it may cover the pupil itself (**thus hindering the vision**). And so the large and chronic pterygia are removed only through a surgical operation . . .

John starts his chapter on diagnosis of eye affections by giving brief details on the function of vision. In particular, he points out the importance of the optic

[64] For Paul of Aegina's text, I use my own translation. I benefited from the relevant parts of Adams' (1844–7) English translation.

[65] Savage-Smith (1984: 184–5) states that John's source for the section on pterygium is the Pseudo-Galenic *On Procurable Drugs*, 2.4, ed. Kühn (1827) XIV.410.14–17. As is shown in the extended example presented here, John most probably excerpted from Paul of Aegina, since he also followed Paul's arrangement of the eye conditions. Furthermore, Paul's text is the main source of the remaining part of his books one and two (see also nn. 45 and 73, above and below, respectively). The similarity of John's account of this particular eye condition to the Pseudo-Galenic treatise is either due to Paul of Aegina's dependence on that text or vice versa.

nerve, which is the conduit for the luminous (*augoeides*) pneuma. Any lack of distribution of this particular pneuma due to an ongoing *dyskrasia* or the accumulation of a thick humour is the reason for reduced sight or loss of vision.[66] John presents his ideas very briefly here, as they are discussed in detail in his *On Psychic Pneuma*.[67] The rest of the chapter discusses various affections following the same order as in Paul of Aegina's section on ophthalmology.

John takes a step further by including instances of differential diagnosis in cases where multiple alternatives are possible.[68] This is a method which essentially helps the physicians in eliminating possible candidate diagnoses, and hence in administering the right treatment to their patients. In particular, in the first case, John is eager to point out the difference between psorophthalmia and xerophthalmia by using the verb *diaferō* ('to be different') and providing extra explanatory material.[69] The second case is more complicated since, for the diagnosis of chalazion, we have three alternative possibilities, namely trachoma, sycosis, and tylosis. Here John does not provide new details on how to differentiate between these affections, but supplements Paul's text once more with the verb *diaferō* ('to be different').[70] The word functions as a pointer to the reader, who might have to deal with a similar situation in the future. For it is particularly important to provide details which could help a non-physician to identify an eye affection, which might seem confusingly similar to something else in the absence of a professional physician. Finally, it could likewise help a non-medic to judge between medical opinions where there was a disagreement, a notable feature of the sort of literature that was intended to be used by *philiatroi*.

4.3 Case study 3: Diagnosis of scirrhus

The third example concentrates on the diagnosis of scirrhus. The printed text is by Paul of Aegina; the underlined parts are those copied by John, while those in bold are John's additions.

Paul of Aegina, *Epitome*, 4.32, ed. Heiberg (1921) I.353.1–8;[71]
JZA, ***Medical Epitome***, 2.38, ed. Ideler (1842) II.461.25–462.2:

[66] JZA, *Medical Epitome*, 2.6, ed. Ideler (1842) II.443.26–34. See also Chapter 6, Section 5.

[67] JZA, *On Psychic Pneuma*, 1.8–9, ed. Ideler (1841) I.327.1–329.30.

[68] His interest in differential diagnosis has already been noticed in connection with his *On Urines* in Chapter 3, p. 98.

[69] On psorophthalmia and xerophthalmia in ancient and Byzantine medical sources, see Magnus (1901: 518–20); and Marganne (1994: 135–9).

[70] We can see further cases attesting John's interest in providing details about differential diagnosis; see, for example, John's discussion on the diagnosis of fetid polyp: JZA, *Medical Epitome*, 2.10, ed. Ideler (1842) II.450.8–13.

[71] For a commentary on Paul of Aegina's chapter on scirrhus, see Adams (1846: II.90–1).

(353) 32. Περὶ σκίρρων. (λη´. **Περὶ σκίρρου.**)
Ὁ μὲν (**δὲ**) ἀκριβὴς σκίρρος ὄγκος ἐστὶν παρὰ φύσιν ἀναίσθητός τε καὶ σκληρός, ὁ δὲ οὐκ ἀκριβὴς δυσαίσθητος· (**ἐκπέφευγε δὲ τὸν ἀκριβῆ ὁ μετρίως αἰσθανόμενος·**) καὶ (**ἀλλ᾽**) ὁ μὲν ἀναίσθητος (**ἤδη και**) ἀνίατος, (**ᾧ γὰρ μὴ ἐπαΐειν τῶν ἐπιτιθεμένων φαρμάκων πέφυκε, τίς ἂν ἐκεῖθεν βοηθείας προσδοκηθείη ἐλπίς; κατὰ τοσοῦτον δὲ ἐλπιστέοι οἱ αἰσθανόμενοι, καθ᾽ ὅσον μετειλήφασι καὶ αἰσθήσεως**) ὁ δὲ δυσαίσθητος οὐκ ἀνίατος μέν, οὐ μὴν εὐίατος· γίνεται(**-ονται δ᾽ ἅπαντες**) γὰρ ὑπὸ γλίσχρου καὶ παχέος χυμοῦ δυσλύτως (**δυσαποσπάστως**) ἐμπλαττομένου τοῖς σκιρρουμένοις μορίοις. ἐνίοτε μὲν οὖν εὐθὺς ἐξ ἀρχῆς συνίσταταί τε καὶ αὔξεται, (**συνίστανται δὲ τὴν ἀρχήν, ἐνίοτε μὲν ἐξ αὐτομάτου τοιούτου τινὸς χυμοῦ τῷ τυχόντι προσερεισθέντος μορίῳ·**) τὰ πολλὰ (**πολλάκις**) δὲ (**καὶ**) ὑπὸ (**ἀμαθίας**) τῶν ἰατρῶν κατασκευάζεται ψυξάντων τε καὶ στυψάντων σφοδρῶς ἐρυσιπέλατά τε καὶ φλεγμονάς (**τοῦ προσήκοντος πέρα**).

(353) 32. On scirrhuses. (**38. On scirrhus.**)
Genuine scirrhus is an unnatural swelling, insensible, and hard; but the non-genuine is scarcely sensible. (**however, the scirrhus that is mildly sensed flees the consequences of the genuine one**); but that which is insensible is (**actually**) incurable. (**for it is naturally made so as not to perceive the applied medicines; can one expect any hope of help? But the sensed <scirrhuses> may retain hope in so far as they are sensed**). However, the one which is scarcely sensible is not incurable, and yet it is not easily curable; for (**all kinds**) are made of gluey and thick humour, which is fixed on the hardened parts, so that it is difficult to remove. Sometimes <the scirrhus> might be created from the very start and then increases; (**the scirrhus is created at the start, and sometimes when some similar humour might itself be accumulated spontaneously in a certain part**) but several times is created by the physicians' (**ignorance**) when they apply extremely (**more than required**) cooling and astringent <medicines> to erysipelas and inflammations.

Paul of Aegina uses Galen's *Therapeutics of Glaucon* as his source for this passage.[72] John excerpts from Paul's text, as the overall presentation and order of affections in his work confirms.[73] It is worth noting that a text actually composed by Galen for the *philiatros* Glaucon was reused by John through the intermediary of Paul almost eleven centuries later. John sometimes changes

[72] Galen, *Therapeutics to Glaucon*, 2.6, ed. Kühn (1826) XI.103.13–104.4. For a discussion of scirrhus in Galen's *Therapeutics to Glaucon*, see Peterson (1974: 68–9, 90–1). On the role of early Byzantine medical authors in regulating access to the Galenic corpus in Byzantium, see Bouras-Vallianatos (2019: 94–8).

[73] John's chapter is followed by discussion of diagnosis of scrofula. Exactly the same order is followed by Paul of Aegina; see Paul of Aegina, *Epitome*, 4.32–4, ed. Heiberg (1921) I.353–5. See also below where I show that the therapeutic advice on scirrhus is based on Paul of Aegina's account.

the structure, but he keeps the meaning of the original source, as in the cases of incurable insensible scirrhus, or in discussing the aetiology for the formation of scirrhus. In the former, he supplements the text with a rhetorical question, emphasizing its untreatable nature. In contrast to the previous cases discussed, here John does not attempt to omit a specific part or considerably condense a passage from an earlier source, but retains the sense of the Galenic account as it was originally composed specifically for Glaucon.

5. JOHN'S CONTENTS AND SOURCES: THERAPY

An even clearer view of John's prospective audience can be obtained by studying his compiling methods in books three and four, which constitute the general therapeutic part of his work. First, I examine John's recommendations on surgery, since it is the first therapeutic agent presented in book three. Then I proceed to an examination of two particular parts of book four, which are his chapters on the treatment of eye affections and scirrhus corresponding to the sections already discussed in the first part of this chapter and thus making a convenient comparison.

5.1 Surgery

No extensive surgical manuals were produced in the middle and late Byzantine period providing details of operations as, for example, in book six of Paul of

Table 4.3. Overview of John's sources, *Medical Epitome*, Books Three & Four

Book Three	Source
Phlebotomy and other non-invasive techniques.	Synopsis from Galen's *On Treatment by Bloodletting*; and excerpts from unidentified source.
Simple purgative drugs.	Excerpts from unidentified source.
Baths and exercise.	Excerpts from unidentified source.
Dietetics.	Synopsis from book two of John's *On Psychic Pneuma*; excerpts from Paul of Aegina's *Epitome*, book one; and excerpts from unidentified source.
Book Four	
Therapy of affections of the internal organs in *a capite ad calcem* order.	Excerpts from Paul of Aegina's *Epitome*, book three.
Therapy of affections of the external parts of the body and organs of sense.	Excerpts from Paul of Aegina's *Epitome*, books three and four.

Aegina's *Epitome*,[74] and we have very little evidence for the performance of invasive surgery in this period. For example, we are aware of a spectacular operation during the reign of Constantine VII (sole r. 945–59) in which two Siamese twins, connected at the upper abdomen, were separated after one of them had died, thus confirming some surgical activity at least in the capital.[75] Later on, in the *Typikon* of the Pantokrator *xenōn* (AD 1136) in Constantinople, there is a mention of a part-time specialist in hernia surgery (*kēlotomos*),[76] but there has been no archaeological excavation of any Constantinopolitan *xenōn*, which could provide more data about the medical instruments used for the performance of surgery in these places.[77]

John's surgery-related advice is mainly restricted to an account of various techniques of bloodletting.[78] The relevant section in book three is not very long, and John does not seem to be following any earlier source as closely as he had done in the first part of his book. He mainly provides a summary of

[74] Paul of Aegina, *Epitome*, 6, ed. Heiberg (1924) 42–183. There is only some brief advice given in Leo the Physician's (ninth[?] century) *Synopsis of Medicine*, in which he names about forty operations and almost fifteen surgical instruments. On this text, which was edited by Ermerins (1840) 80–197, see Bliquez (1999).

[75] Pentogalos and Lascaratos (1984). See also the case of a certain Niketas, about whose life we have no details, who commissioned the production of an illustrated manuscript in the tenth century, Florentinus Laurentianus gr. plut. 74.7, depicting various orthopaedic operations. On this codex, see the edited volume by Bernabò (2010). The codex consists of a collection of excerpts from Greek treatises on the subject by Hippocratic authors, Apollonius of Citium, Rufus of Ephesos, Galen, and Soranus. A later note confirms that it was once owned by a Byzantine *nosokomeion* (infirmary[?]), but the manuscript shows very little evidence of actual use. The *monokondylion* on f. 407v is lacunose and reads: '[. . .] *παρὸν* [. . .]*βλίον ὑπάρχει τοῦ* [. . .] *τοῦ νοσοκομείου τῶν* [. . .] *ἔχει δὲ φύλλα* [. . .]*κόσια εἴκοσι πέντε μηνὶ Μαΐῳ* [. . .] *ἰνδικτιῶνος ἕκτης*'. See Speranzi (2010: 13, n. 6), who explains that in the literature it is mistakenly assumed that the note refers to the Constantinopolitan *xenōn* of Forty Martyrs due to an unsubstantiated reconstruction of the text by Cocchi (1754: 41–2) as '[. . .] *τοῦ νοσοκομείου τῶν μ΄ μαρτύρων. ἔχει δὲ* [. . .]'. Furthermore, we are aware of lists of medical instruments surviving in two codices, Florentinus Laurentianus gr. plut. 74.2 (eleventh century) and Bononiensis 3632 (mid fifteenth century), contain eighty-nine and sixty-five entries respectively. The text in Laurentianus is available in an edition by Schöne (1903). The list in Bononiensis has been edited by Fischer (1987: 30–1). These lists may not be directly connected with medical practice, but they indicate a certain awareness of the field in Byzantium. On surgical instruments dated to the Byzantine period, see Bliquez (1984).

[76] *Typikon Pantokrator*, 1271–82, ed. Gautier (1974) 105. In the same passage, there is also mention of the responsibilities of the 'sharpener', *akonētēs*, who was to keep all the surgical instruments used by the physicians clean. On the Pantokrator *xenōn*, see Chapter 1, n. 124. It should be pointed out that in the ancient world, even among professional physicians, certain practitioners would have had a particular specialty in surgery. See Jackson (2003), who discusses the excavated house of a Greek surgeon in Rimini dated to the second half of the second century AD.

[77] Furthermore, in the few edited examples of *iatrosophia* and the so-called *xenōnika* (texts associated with Byzantine *xenōnes*), one finds only some limited examples of venesection. For references to phlebotomy in the *xenōnika*, see Bennett (2003) 334.42–4 and 335.47. See also in John Archiatros' *iatrosophion*, N.37 and N.108, ed. Zipser (2009) 86.17–21 and 120.16–7.

[78] John also omits any reference to wounds, except for a short chapter on the diagnosis of skin ulcers; see JZA, *Medical Epitome*, 2.41, ed. Ideler (1842) II.462.24–463.35.

Galenic ideas.[79] John starts by indicating spring as the most appropriate season for the performance of phlebotomy, which according to Galen is the best time of the year for prophylactic venesection.[80] He then continues his account by indicating phlebotomy to remove excess blood from a particular part of the body, but also notes that it could help to remove other humours in excess.[81] In some cases, he suggests the use of revulsion (*antispasis*) in order to divert blood from a particular part of the body, as in the case of genitourinary affections.[82] Then, he proceeds to a discussion of the various kinds of phlebotomy according to the parts of the body and relates them to diseases. John gives an account of the following parts, where it is appropriate to cut a vein, including the tongue (*glōtta*), lips (*cheilē*), gum (*oula*), ears (*ōta*), forehead (*metōpon*), temple (*krotaphos*), throat (*trachēlos*), elbow (*ankōn*), shoulder (*ōmos*), thumb (*megas daktylos*), ring finger (*paramesos*), small finger (*mikros daktylos*), and feet (*podes*).[83] He also includes a short passage on arteriotomy, which is only indicated in certain cases, e.g. extremely bad headaches and toothache, where it might be particularly efficient.[84] Finally, he provides a separate chapter on the use of leeches.[85] In the subsequent chapters, and, in particular, in his *a capite ad calcem* presentation of diseases

[79] For Galen's recommendations on bloodletting, see Brain (1986), who provides an introduction, English translation, and commentary of the relevant Galenic works.

[80] JZA, *Medical Epitome*, 3, Vindobonensis med. gr. 17, f. 55v, ll. 20–1: '*χρηστέον τοίνυν φλεβοτομίας, ἐπί τε πλήθει καὶ σήψει θερμοτέρων χυμῶν· ἐν ὥρᾳ μάλιστα μὲν ἔαρος·*'; ed. Mathys (1556) II.156.4–7. On Galenic advice for prophylactic venesection in spring, see Galen, *On Treatment by Bloodletting*, 7, ed. Kühn (1826) XI.270–1.

[81] JZA, *Medical Epitome*, 3, Vindobonensis med. gr. 17, f. 56r, ll. 18–21: '*εἰδέναι γάρ τοι χρὴ ὡς οὐ μόνον ὅταν ἀκραιφνὲς τὸ πλεονάζον αἷμα ἢ ταῖς φλεβοτομίαις κεχρήμεθα, ἀλλὰ καὶ ὁπόταν μετ' αὐτοῦ καὶ ἕτεροι χυμοὶ χολώδεις ἢ ὀρρώδεις ἢ τινὲς τοιοῦτοι ὦσι πλεονάζοντες· ἐκεῖ μὲν γὰρ τῷ κενῶσθαι* (E: *κεκενῶσθαι*) *τὸ λυποῦν λυσιτελοῦσα ὤφθη ἡ φλεβοτομία·*'; ed. Mathys (1556) II.157.16–23.

[82] For example, JZA, *Medical Epitome*, 3, Vindobonensis med. gr. 17, f. 57v, ll. 22-58r, l.1: '*τῶν γε μὴν γεννητικῶν κατά τι φλεγμαινόντων μορίων, ἐπί τε γυναικῶν ὡσαύτως καὶ ἀνδρῶν τὰς πρὸς τῷ ἀγκῶνι τέμνειν ἄμεινον ἀντισπῶντας καὶ μὴ καθέλκοντας ἐπὶ τὰ πεπονθότα μέρη τοὺς χυμούς· εἰ μήπου τῷ χρόνῳ στηριχθέντων τῶν χυμῶν, ἄμεινον ἀπὸ τῶν ποδῶν τὸ αἷμα ἀφαιρεῖν δόξειε· πλανωμένων γὰρ ἔτι τῶν χυμῶν, ἄμεινον κεχρῆσθαι ταῖς ἀντισπάσεσι . . .*'; ed. Mathys (1556) II.161.10–30. For an introduction to revulsion, see Brain (1986: 13–14).

[83] Each part of the body is connected with particular affections. For example, John suggests cutting the veins of the tongue for those suffering from uvula and tonsil affections. JZA, *Medical Epitome*, 3, Vindobonensis med. gr. 17, f. 57v, ll. 3–4: '*τέμνομεν δὲ καὶ τὰς ὑπὸ τὴν γλῶτταν φλέβας, ἐπὶ τῶν κατὰ τὸν γαργαρεῶνα τὲ καὶ ἀντιάδας παθῶν·*'; ed. Mathys (1556) II.160.21–5.

[84] JZA, *Medical Epitome*, 3, Vindobonensis med. gr. 17, f. 58r, ll. 1–11: '*ἀρτηρίας δε τέμνειν, λυσιτελὲς μὲν ἐνίοτε δοκεῖ· τῶν ἐργωδεστάτων δὲ πέφυκεν . . . κἀντεῦθεν αἵ τε ἰσχυραὶ κεφαλαῖαι καὶ ὀδονταλγίαι·*'; ed. Mathys (1556) II.162.4–23. The technique is also suggested by Paul of Aegina as an ultimate measure against severe headaches and migraines; see Paul of Aegina, *Epitome*, 3.5.7, ed. Heiberg (1921) I.143.22–4.

[85] JZA, *Medical Epitome*, 3, Vindobonensis med. gr. 17, f. 58v, ll. 16–18: '*Περὶ χρήσεως βδελλῶν: βδέλλαις δὲ κεχρήμεθα . . . ἂν μορίων τεθῶσι τὰ δήγματα ἐπάγουσαι βδάλλουσι τὸ πέριξ αἷμα·*'; ed. Mathys (1556) II.164.6–10.

in book four, John's instructions on the appropriateness of bloodletting appear with great frequency.

However, we can see a limited number of cases in book four where John refers to invasive procedures:

I. 'The fistula which goes deep ... it is not fitting to perform a surgical operation,'[86]

II. 'Some people try to heal enterocele and omental hernia using just external plasters. And some people manage to heal when the affection is still in a mild condition. In the majority of cases, they are healed only through the performance of surgery, since this happens to be one of the worst diseases, and endangers many patients.'[87]

III. 'The ectropion caused by growth of flesh is remedied either by surgical operation or by the administration of drugs causing purgation.'[88]

IV. 'On pterygia, we can say only these things, that the large and chronic ones are only cured by surgical operation.'[89]

V. 'The sebaceous tumour is only cured through the performance of surgery; it does not rot and it cannot be dispersed.'[90]

VI. 'If it [i.e. a certain kind of ulcer] reaches the bone, it is impossible to heal it without performing surgery.'[91]

In the first case, although John mentions the performance of surgery for chronic and very deep fistulae, he does not recommend this technique. Examples III and IV deal with ophthalmological conditions, and at least in one case (i.e. chronic pterygium) surgery is recommended as the sole remedy. But John does not go further and provide details of the operation. Similarly, in the last two cases, he suggests surgery as the only effective treatment without

86 JZA, *Medical Epitome*, 4, Vindobonensis med. gr. 17, f. 91v, l. 25-f. 92r, l. 1: '*τὴν εἰς βάθος δὲ προβαίνουσαν σύριγγα ... μὴ δ' ἐγχειρεῖν προσήκει·*'; ed. Mathys (1556) II.258.13–16.

87 JZA, *Medical Epitome*, 4, Vindobonensis med. gr. 17, f. 97v, l. 24-f. 98r, l. 2: '*ἐντεροκήλην δὲ ἢ ἐπιπλοκήλην, πειρῶνται μέν τινες καὶ μόνοις τοῖς ἔξωθεν ἐπιθέμασιν ἰᾶσθαι· καί γε ἔνιοι ἐπιτυγχάνουσιν ἔτι μετρίου τοῦ πάθους τυγχάνοντος· οἱ πλείους δὲ καὶ ταύτας χειρουργίαις ἰῶνται· ὅτι δὲ τῶν δυσχερῶν καὶ τοῦτο τυγχάνει, καὶ πολλοῖς ἐνίοτε κίνδυνον ἐπήγαγεν·*'; ed. Mathys (1556) II.274.30–275.6.

88 JZA, *Medical Epitome*, 4, Vindobonensis med. gr. 17, f. 102r, ll. 19–21: '*τό γε μὴν ἐκτρόπιον δι' ὕπερ σάρκωσιν γινόμενον, ἢ χειρουργίᾳ καταστέλλεται, ἢ τοῖς καθαίρουσι φαρμάκοις·*'; ed. Mathys (1556) II.286.23–6.

89 JZA, *Medical Epitome*, 4, Vindobonensis med. gr. 17, f. 103v, ll. 13–15: '*περὶ δὲ πτερυγίων τοσοῦτον ἔνεστιν εἰπεῖν ὡς τὰ μὲν μεγάλα καὶ χρόνια, χειρουργίᾳ ἰᾶται·*'; ed. Mathys (1556) II.291.5–7.

90 JZA, *Medical Epitome*, 4, Vindobonensis med. gr. 17, f. 110v, ll. 4–5: '*τὸ δὲ στεάτωμα, διὰ τῆς χειρουργίας μόνης θεραπεύεται· μήτε σαπῆναι μήτε διαφορηθῆναι δυνάμενον·*'; ed. Mathys (1556) II.311.1–2.

91 JZA, *Medical Epitome*, 4, Vindobonensis med. gr. 17, f. 111v, ll. 15–16: '*εἰ μὲν οὖν εἰς ὀστοῦν καταλήγει, τῶν ἀδυνάτων ἄνευ χειρουργίας ἰαθῆναι·*'; ed. Mathys (1556) II.314.25–6.

any further explanatory data. Both cases deal with the removal of external protuberances, in the former of a sebaceous tumour and in the latter an extremely deep ulcer extending to the bone.

The most extraordinary example, that is number II, is connected with various cases of hernia. Although John reports the effectiveness of surgical operations and even emphasizes the severity of the disease, once again no further information is included in his statement. Hernia operations were popular in early Byzantium, judging not only from the meticulous accounts given by Paul of Aegina,[92] but also from the large number of accounts in healing miracles performed at the sanctuary of St Artemios.[93] The absence of accounts of invasive operations in John's work does not necessarily suggest a corresponding lack of interest in, or actual performance of, such surgical techniques by John or other physicians in late Byzantium; it could be related to the nature of his text. Since the work is designed to appeal to *philiatroi*, who could not themselves perform surgery, such information would not be of use. The references are probably given in cases where other kinds of treatment were not effective, so that they could have a view on possible alternatives. It is important to note that the topic was also omitted from the relevant treatises by Galen and Oribasios, probably because it was considered too advanced for an audience consisting of *philiatroi*.

One might still wonder why John includes such details on bloodletting techniques. However, *philiatroi*, who were the intended readers of these accounts, were probably able to perform bloodletting where necessary, as a reference from John's work *On Psychic Pneuma* attests. Referring to a previous conversation with his friend Joseph Rhakendytes or the Philosopher, John states:

> ... you spent a great deal of time searching for the cause. Then, you cut your vein driven by the affection, and when you saw the corrupted blood, you discovered the cause and you announced it to us.[94]

Joseph had tried to find out the cause of an ongoing *dyskrasia* through an examination of the blood. Although not a physician himself, he is very interested in medicine, as is also attested by the dedication of John's *On Psychic Pneuma* to him.[95]

[92] See, for example, the extremely detailed description by Paul of Aegina on the enterocele operation in his *Epitome*, 6.65, ed. Heiberg (1924) II.107.22–110.3. See also Geroulanos (2005: 129–30); and Lascaratos, Tsiamis, and Kostakis (2003).

[93] See the study by Alwis (2012), who provides an interpretation of miracle narratives concerning hernias in the light of early Byzantine medical literature.

[94] JZA, *On Psychic Pneuma*, 1.20.9, ed. Ideler (1841) I.348.34–349.1: '... *καθὰ δὴ τὸν ἅπαντα διετέλεις χρόνον, καὶ τὴν αἰτίαν ἐζήτεις. φλέβα δὲ τεμὼν δι' ὃ κατήπειγε τότε πάθος, ἐπεὶ διεφθορὸς αἷμα τεθέασαι, ᾗ τὴν αἰτίαν ἐμάνθανες, καὶ κοινὸν ἡμῖν ἐποιοῦ τὸν λόγον.*'

[95] John's *On Psychic Pneuma* was also included in some of the manuscripts of Joseph's *Synopsis Variarum Disciplinarum*. See Chapter 6, nn. 21–2.

5.2 Treatment of eye affections and scirrhus

In contrast to my study in the first part of this chapter, I will present both chapters in the same section, since John follows a similar approach in adopting Paul of Aegina's text. Here, I print the therapeutic section of Paul of Aegina's text; the underlined parts are those copied by John,[96] while those in bold are John's additions.

Paul of Aegina, *Epitome*, 3.22.12-25, ed. Heiberg (1921) I.176.15–181.31; JZA, ***Medical Epitome***, 4, Vindobonensis med. gr. 17, f. 102v, l. 6–f. 103v, l. 17; ed. Mathys (1556) II.287.13–291.11:

(176) 12. *Περὶ τραχώματος.*
...(**τράχωμα δὲ καὶ σύκωσις καὶ τύλος τὰ αὐτὰ τῷ γένει τυγχάνοντα, διαφέροντα δ' ἀλλήλων τῷ χρόνῳ καὶ τῇ δύναμει**) κολλουρίοις (**θεραπεύεται**) μὲν οὖν χρηστέον τῷ τε δι' οἴνου καὶ τῷ διὰ τῶν δύο λίθων καὶ αὐτῷ τῷ αἱματίτῃ λίθῳ δι' ὕδατος πλυθέντι καθ' ὑποβολὴν (**γὰρ**) ὑποσμήχοντα τὸ βλέφαρον· καὶ τὸ ἁρμάτιον δὲ μετ' ὀλίγου τοῦ κυκναρίου ἢ (**καὶ τὸ**) διακρόκου πρὸς τούτοις καὶ ταῖς ψωροφθαλμίαις ἁρμόζει (**ταῖς**) χωρὶς ἑλκώσεως ἐκστρεφομένου τοῦ βλεφάρου ἐπιχριόμενον. εἰ δὲ σκληρὸς (**μικρὸς**) ὢν ὁ τύλος μὴ τούτοις εἴκοι, ἐκστρέψαντες τὸ βλέφαρον ξέσομεν διὰ κισήρεως ἢ σηπέας ὀστράκου ἢ φύλλων συκῆς ἢ καὶ διὰ τοῦ ὀργάνου τοῦ βλεφαροξύστου καλουμένου.

13. *Περὶ χαλαζίων.*
...(**τὸ δὲ χαλάζιον**) ἀμμωνιακὸν ὄξει λειώσας ἅμα χαλβάνῃ χρῖε· (**δεῖ γὰρ ὧδε τῶν μαλακτικῶν καὶ διαφορητικῶν...**) ποιεῖ δὲ καὶ ἅμα κηρωτῇ καὶ τερεβινθίνῃ ἀναλαμβανομένῃ.

(177) 14. *Περὶ κριθῆς.*
...(**τὴν δ' οὕτω καλουμένην κριθὴν**) δεῖ οὖν αὐτὸ κηρῷ λευκῷ πυριᾶν ἢ μυίας τὴν κεφαλὴν ἀποβαλόντα τῷ λοιπῷ (**ταύτης**) σώματι παρατρίβειν(**-οντες, τὸ πάθος θεραπεύομεν**) ἢ (**ἔνιοι δὲ καὶ**) κριθῶν ἀποβρέγματι καταντλεῖν(**-οῦντες βοηθοῦσι· κριθαῖς κριθὰς ἐκκρούοντες·**).

15. *Πρὸς φθεῖρας τοὺς ἐν τοῖς βλεφάροις.*
Ἐκκαθάραντας πρότερον τοὺς φθεῖρας δεῖ (**φθειριάσεως δ' ἐνοχλούσης, πρῶτον μὲν δεῖ τὰς φθείρας ἐκκαθᾶραι· εἶτα**) θαλάσσῃ προσκλύζειν (**ἀποκλύσαι**) χλιαρᾷ, εἶτα (**κἄπειθ' οὕτως**) προσάπτεσθαι τοῦ ταρσοῦ τῷ ὑπογεγραμμένῳ φαρμάκῳ· στυπτηρίας σχιστῆς μ^ϵ β', σταφίδος ἀγρίας μ^ϵ α'· λείοις χρῶ...

(181) 25. *Περὶ πτερυγίων.*
...(**περὶ δὲ πτερυγίων τοσοῦτον ἔνεστιν εἰπεῖν ὡς**) τὰ μὲν οὖν μεγάλα καὶ χρόνια τῶν πτερυγίων διὰ μόνης χειρουργίας(**ᾳ**) ἐκτέμνεται (**ἰᾶται**)· τὰ δὲ νεώτερα καὶ σύμμετρα τῷ μεγέθει καὶ τὰ σμηκτικὰ τῶν βοηθημάτων, οἷα τὰ τραχωματικά

[96] In the absence of an edition of John's text, I have provided transcriptions of the relevant parts in Appendix 4.

τέ ἐστι καὶ λευκωματικά, δαπανᾷ. ἐν ἁπλοῖς μὲν οὖν (**ὁποῖον ὁ**) *χαλκὸς* (*ὁ*) *κεκαυμένος ἢ χάλκανθον ἅμα χοιρείᾳ χολῇ καλῶς ποιεῖ, δραστικώτερον δὲ τοῦτο· χαλκάνθου μέρος α´, κόμμεως μέρος <ʿ· οἴνῳ ἐκλειοῦντες ἐγχρίομεν ἢ καὶ κολλούρια πλάσσομεν· τινὲς δὲ χολὴν αἰγὸς* (**ἅμα**) *μέλιτι μίξαντες ἐγχρίουσιν.*

(176) 12. On trachoma.

. . . (**trachoma, sycosis, and tylosis happen to be of the same kind, but they differ from each other as regards their duration and severity**) and so (**are cured by**) one must use collyria; the one made of wine and the other one made of the two stones; and the eyelid should be rubbed with the haematite and washed with much water accordingly. The eyesalve called *harmation* together with a small quantity of that one called *kyknarion*, or (**and**) that one made of saffron should be used for these [i.e. trachoma, sycosis, and tylosis], and are also fitting for the cure of psorophthalmia without ulceration, when they are anointed on the everted eyelid. But if the callus is hard (**small**) and is not similar to these things, having turned the eyelid out and rubbing it down with the pumice stone, or the shell of the cuttlefish or fig leaves or by the surgical instrument called *blepharoxyston*.

13. On chalazia.

. . . (**the chalazion**) mass ammoniac with vinegar and anoint it with galbanum. (**for it is necessary to use emollient and discutient medicines . . .**) It is also efficient to apply cerate and turpentine.

(177) 14. On stye.

. . . (**the so-called stye**) It is necessary to foment it with white wax or, after throwing away the head of a fly to rub it with the rest of its body (**in this way we cure the affection**) or (**and some others**) wash it with an infusion made of barley (**and it helps; so the stye is got rid of <by using> barley**).

15. On lice in the eyelids.

Having first cleared away the lice (**someone troubled by pediculosis should first clear the lice; then**) wash with tepid seawater and apply the following medicine on the tarsus: two parts of cloven alum, one part of stavesacre; mass and use . . .

(181) 25. On pterygia.

. . . (**On pterygia, we can say only these things, that**) the large and chronic ones are only (**cured**) extirpated by surgical operation. However, the most recent ones and symmetrical in size may be cured by purgative medicines, like those used against trachoma and leucoma. Among the simple medicines (**such as**) burnt copper, and copper sulphate with gall of swine cure well. But the following medicine is stronger: one part of copper sulphate, half part of gum, wine, and anoint with it or mash as we make collyria; some people mix the gall of goat with honey and anoint with it.

Paul of Aegina, *Epitome*, 4.32, ed. Heiberg (1921) I.353.8–354.2;

JZA, ***Medical Epitome***, 4, Vindobonensis med. gr. 17, f. 110r, ll. 16–23; ed. Mathys (1556) II.310.4–17:

(353) 32. *Περὶ σκίρρων.* (***Περὶ σκίρρου***)

…(**Ὁ δὲ ἀκριβὴς σκίρρος, ἀνίατος. ἤδη ὢν ἀναίσθητος, καὶ μὴ φαρμάκοις εἴκων. ὁ δὲ ἕτερος οὐκ εὐίατος, μετρίαν ἔχων αἴσθησιν. διαφορητικοῖς οὖν ἅμα καὶ μαλακτικοῖς οὗτοι θεραπεύονται**) *ἐὰν μὲν οὖν τις τὰ ἰσχυρῶς διαφοροῦντα τοῖς σκιρρουμένοις σώμασιν προσφέρῃ φάρμακα, σαφῆ μείωσιν ἐργασάμενος τοῦ σκίρρου χρόνῳ βραχεῖ τὸ λοιπὸν τοῦ πάθους λείψανον ἀνίατον ἐργάσεται τῆς μὲν λεπτοτέρας ὑγρότητος διαφορηθείσης, τῆς δὲ λοιπῆς ἀποξηρανθείσης καὶ οἷον λιθώδους γεγενημένης. χρὴ τοίνυν τὸ διαφορητικὸν φάρμακον ἔχειν τι καὶ μαλακτικὸν ἄνευ τοῦ θερμαίνειν τε καὶ ξηραίνειν ἰσχυρῶς· τοιοῦτοι δέ εἰσιν* (**ὁποῖα οἵ τε**) *μυελοί τε σύμπαντες καὶ μᾶλλον ὁ ἐλάφειός τε καὶ μόσχειος,* (**καὶ τὰ**) *στεάτων*(**-έατα καὶ μᾶλλον τῶν ἀγρίων ζῴων**) *δὲ τό τε λεόντειον καὶ τὸ τῆς παρδάλεως καὶ τὸ τῶν ἄρκων, εἶτα τῶν ταύρων, ἐν δὲ τοῖς ὀρνέοις τό τε χήνειον καὶ τὸ τῆς ἀλεκτορίδος καὶ φασιανικόν, ξηρότερόν τε τὸ τῶν αἰγῶν τε καὶ τράγων, ἔτι τε πρὸς τούτοις ἀμμωνιακὸν θυμίαμα καὶ βδέλλιον, μάλιστα τὸ Σκυθικόν, καὶ στύραξ ὁ ὑγρότερός τε καὶ λιπαρὸς καὶ ἡ Αἰγυπτία μαστίχη* (**καὶ ταῦτα μέν, ἐν τοῖς κατὰ πᾶν τὸ σῶμα σκίρροις ἐπιτίθεται**). *ἐπὶ μὲν οὖν τῶν ἄλλων μορίων σκιρρωθέντων ἑκάστῳ τε τούτων κατ' ἰδίαν χρηστέον καὶ τοῖς ἐξ αὐτῶν συντιθεμένοις φαρμάκοις· ἐπὶ δὲ τῶν τενόντων καὶ συνδέσμων* (**πεπονθότων**) *ὄξει δριμυτάτῳ δεῖ σβεννύειν προπυρωθέντα λίθον, εἰ μὲν οἷόν τε, τὸν πυρίτην, εἰ δὲ μή, τὸν γοῦν* (**ἢ**) *μυλίτην, ἐφ' οὗ τὸ πεπονθὸς μόριον χρὴ διακινεῖν, ὅπως* (**καὶ**) *τὸν ἀναφερόμενον ἀτμὸν δέχοιτο*(**-εσθαι τῷ πεπονθότι μορίῳ**), *καὶ μετὰ τοῦτο πάλιν τὸ μαλακτικὸν ἐπιτιθέναι φάρμακον* (**ἀμοιβηδὸν ταῦτα ποιοῦντα μέχρι τελείας λύσεως.**) *ἐλαίῳ τε μὴν λεπτομερεῖ ἀπ' ἀρχῆς, οὐχ ὕδατι, τὸ μόριον καταντλεῖν ἄχρι παντὸς ἑκάστης ἡμέρας, ἐναφέψοντας ἐνίοτε τῷ ἐλαίῳ καὶ τῆς ἀλθαίας τὴν ῥίζαν ἢ τοῦ ἀγρίου σικύου· λουτροῦ δὲ τὸ παράπαν ἀφεκτέον αὐτοὺς ἢ γοῦν τοῦ συχνοῦ. μετρίως δὲ τοῦ σκίρρου μαλαχθέντος ἀμμωνιακὸν τὸ λιπαρώτατον διέντες ὄξει δριμυτάτῳ καταχρίομεν τὸ* (354) *μόριον ἄχρι συχνῶν ἡμερῶν· μεθ' ἃς πάλιν τῷ μαλακτικῷ χρηστέον προσειληφότι χαλβάνης τε καὶ ὀποπάνακος καὶ τῶν λιπαρωτάτων·*

(353) 32. On scirrhuses. (**On scirrhus**)

…(**The genuine scirrhus is incurable, since it is insensible and is not cured by medicines. The other one [i.e. the non-genuine] is not easy to cure and is mildly sensible; and so these are cured by emollient and discutient medicines**) if one applies strong discutient medicines to indurations of the body, one can achieve a clear reduction in the size of the scirrhus in a short time, but what is left of the induration will stay in an incurable condition because the thin moisture is dissipated or the rest of it becomes dry and hard as stone. For it is necessary to use a discutient medicine, which has also a certain degree of emollient quality, and without warming it or getting it

> extremely dry. There are all kinds of (**such as**) marrows and, in particular, that of a deer or a calf, and (**above all**) the fat (**of wild animals**) of a lion, or a leopard, or of bears, or of bulls, and among birds, that of geese, or of cocks, or of pheasants; however, that of female and male goats is drier. Furthermore, to these may be added, ammoniac incense, bdellium, and, in particular, the Scythian one, and storax, the most humid and fat one, and Egyptian mastic (**and these can be applied on scirrhuses in any part of the body**). To all other indurated parts of the body, these medicines are useful when applied individually or in the form of composite medicines; but for (**affected**) tendons and ligaments it is necessary to apply a heated stone together with the strongest vinegar, and if possible use pyrites, if not, then use (**or**) lapis molaris. Thus, the affected part is to be moved in order to (**and**) receive the aforementioned vapour and after this apply again the emollient medicine (**and do these things alternatively until the scirrhus is dissolved.**) Then anoint the part with a thin oil, and not water, once every single day, and sometimes one may mix the oil with the root of marshmallows or of wild cucumber. The patients should abstain completely from bathing or at least from frequent use of it. And when the scirrhus is mildly softened, the softest ammoniac should be dissolved in the strongest vinegar and anointed on the part (354) for several days; afterwards it is necessary to apply emollient medicines such as the fattest galbanum and opopanax.

John clearly follows a selective technique in adopting Paul's text. The first noticeable characteristic of his text is that he provides a short introductory phrase for each affection, which in the case of trachoma confirms his great interest in the differential diagnosis of eye affections (see Section 4.2, above). In this case, John uses the present participle of the verb *diaferō*, that is *diaferonta*, to make clear that the duration and severity of the condition are the main factors in identifying the possible alternatives. In the case of the treatment of scirrhus, his addition is quite long and almost identical to the introductory part of his diagnostic exposition on the affection concerned (see Section 4.3, above). This is probably John's way of reintroducing this particular affection to his reader, in case he has failed to read the diagnostic part in advance.

As regards the actual therapeutic part, it is remarkable that in the case of the therapy of trachoma, although he uses Paul's text in its entirety, he does not include the reference to a rather specialized surgical instrument, the *blepharoxyston*.[97] The instrument, which is something like an eyelid lancet, is used for the removal of calluses and would certainly be unfamiliar to non-practising physicians. John's decision not to include this instrument, as

[97] On the particular instrument, see Geroulanos (2007: 131); and Bliquez (2015: 139). Cf. Magnus (1901: 623).

in the case of other surgical operations explained above, corresponds to his audience's abilities and expectations.

In the process of further condensing Paul's text, we can see that the dietetic and pharmacological advice is massively diminished. In particular, in the case of scirrhus, John does not hesitate to omit lots of explanatory data. For example, he prefers not to refer to lions or leopards, and simply mentions a group of wild animals, probably reflecting the difficulty of finding and purchasing parts of these animals in fourteenth-century Byzantium. In another instance, in referring to the suggested treatment of affected tendons and ligaments, he includes only information about the application of a heated stone and of emollient drugs, thus completely omitting the next steps in Paul's account. However, John supplements the text with some brief advice indicating that the suggested therapy should be applied repeatedly until the scirrhus was cured. In this case, we can see a process of refinement of the original, probably reflecting John's personal experience and his desire to provide a pertinent account of effective material.[98]

6. CONCLUSION

John's *Medical Epitome* belongs to the genre of 'encyclopedic' medical handbooks written throughout the Byzantine period. I have shown that the text was not primarily written for doctors, as scholarly consensus suggests. On the contrary, it is mainly addressed to the non-expert with a strong interest in medicine, allowing them to easily access information on the subject. It is a project on a larger scale than the similar ones by Galen, (*Therapeutics to Glaucon*), and Oribasios (*For Eunapios*), but certainly on a smaller scale than the early Byzantine handbooks by Oribasios (*Medical Collections*), Aetios of Amida (*Tetrabiblos*), and Paul of Aegina (*Epitome*), although the latter ones were not written for *philiatroi*, but for physicians.

A study of his compilation methods has shown that John should not be considered a mechanical copy-paster, but a careful compiler who knew how to make the best possible selection for his readers. As succinct as possible and at the same time useful and effective, each piece of advice is planned to suit the needs of his dedicatee, Alexios Apokaukos, and by extension those of any contemporary *philiatros*. The lack of details on invasive operations is not fortuitous, but can be explained by the fact that they were not expected to be performed by his target readership. The first

[98] See Chapter 5, Section 3, where I show how John's personal experience in selecting his material is central to the pharmacological section of the text.

four books of the *Medical Epitome* certainly do not contain the most interesting medical material in John's corpus, but seem to draw, at least in part, on John's own insights, as is, for example, demonstrated in the way he supplements his source-text with his own knowledge and perspective on particular topics such as differential diagnosis.

5

Medical Epitome

Assembling Pharmacological Knowledge in Late Byzantium

This chapter deals with the last two books of John's *Medical Epitome*, which focus on pharmacology. This is undoubtedly the most interesting part of his work. In contrast to the diagnostic parts and the various therapeutic methods provided in the first four books, John uses a more eclectic approach in selecting his sources here. He also shows a dynamic adaptation of new material, including recently introduced oriental[1] substances and recipes for composite drugs. To make a comparison with the world of art, in shaping a piece of stone a conventional sculptor cuts away at the surface until the stone takes the desired shape. This process can involve further stages in which the artist scrapes away various portions to adapt the artefact to the requirements of his audience. In a different approach to the visual arts, an artist who creates artefacts consisting of various objects put together, the so-called assemblage (see Figure 5.1), produces something not entirely new but nevertheless gives a fresh perspective adjusted to a new environment.[2]

In John's case, the ancient and early Byzantine sources he relies on in his first four books constitute the basis upon which he composes his own work, adapting and condensing his material according to the needs of his non-specialist audience. On the other hand, the pharmacological part of the work, although it involves a comparable process of excerpting and abbreviating is, unlike the first four books, composed of a wider variety of sources, including

[1] I prefer to use the term oriental to denote substances originating from the Middle and Far East rather than exotic, which might refer more generally to something foreign or tropical. The term has been used with reference to the import of spices from Asia to the Mediterranean by David Jacoby; see, for example, Jacoby (1998: 113) and (2016: 196).

[2] In a similar vein, the term 'assemblage' has recently been applied in a literary context by Johndan Johnson-Eilola and Stuart Selber (2007) to the process in which texts may be 'built primarily and explicitly from existing texts in order to solve a writing or communication problem in a new context'.

Innovation in Byzantine Medicine: The Writings of John Zacharias Aktouarios (c.1275–c.1330). Petros Bouras-Vallianatos, Oxford University Press (2020).
DOI: 10.1093/oso/9780198850687.001.0001

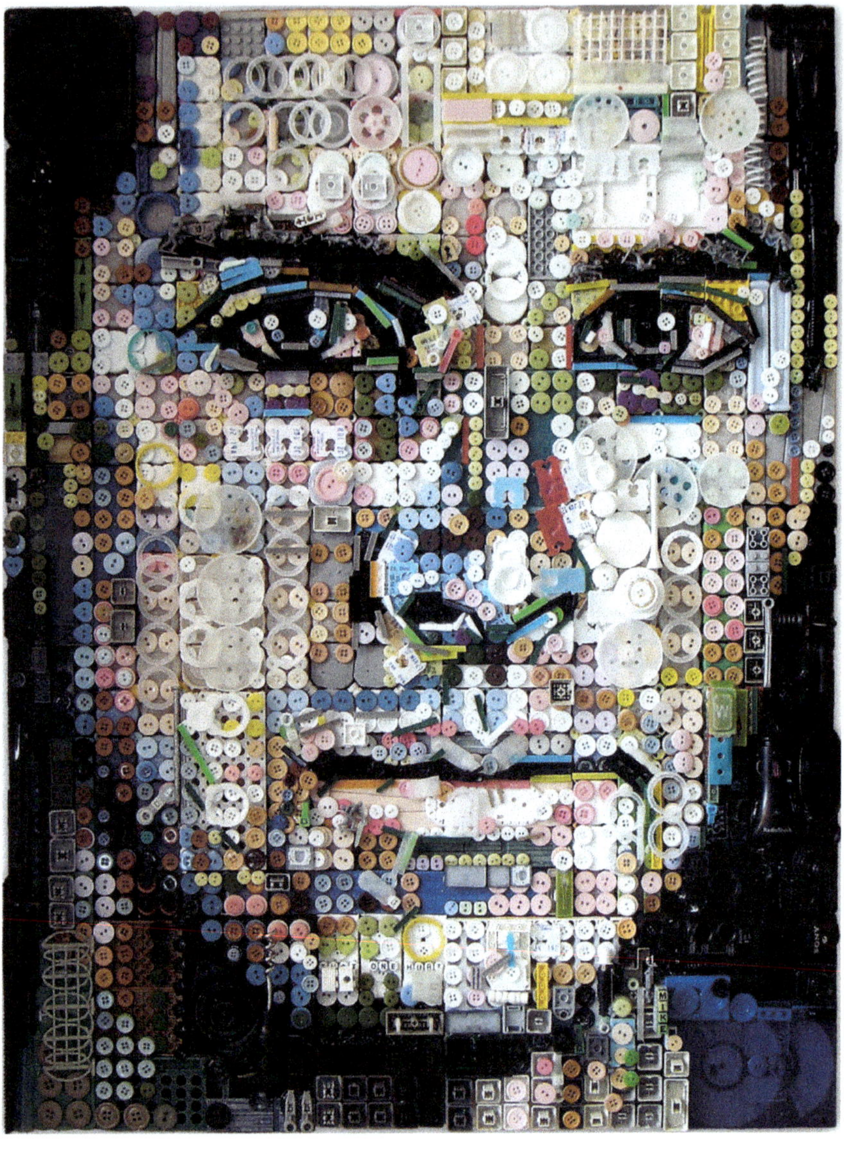

Figure 5.1. Zac Freeman (b. 1972). Assemblage series: Mike. An impressionistic two-dimensional face made up of a collection of buttons, bottle tops, pen barrels, bread tags, office equipment, telephones (and any other three-dimensional scrap plastic objects).
© Woolff Gallery, London.

both earlier Greek sources and foreign ones in translation. Furthermore, here we find explicit mentions of John's practical experience, which he used to help him refine his selection of sources and assemble his material.

John's pharmacological project could be seen as an attempt to both assist and impress his non-expert readers by responding to recent developments in the field. At the same time, he creates a much-needed wholesale revision of the subject, which could also appeal to contemporary practising physicians and be used independently.[3] For example, the vast majority of the contents of his first four books could be accessed by contemporary physicians through other well-circulated handbooks, such as Paul of Aegina's *Epitome*, which is the main source for the greater part of them. On the other hand, John is the sole late Byzantine author to provide an up-to-date summary (in the form of books five and six of his *Medical Epitome*) of the accumulated ancient pharmacological knowledge, which had been passed down to Byzantium and supplemented and/or transformed century by century. Informed and expanded by wider medieval developments in the field, it presents a fresh pharmacological assemblage, attuned to contemporary reality.

Since the pharmacological section is still unedited in Greek, I would first like to outline its structure and show the underlying concepts behind it. Then I will discuss John's experience and his selection of recipes. Special consideration will also be given to the newly introduced foreign material, since this will assist us in evaluating the impact of transcultural influence in the field of medicine in late Byzantium and more generally the cross-cultural encounters of Byzantium with the Islamic world. In the meantime, it is essential to give an overview of late Byzantine pharmacological texts, which will help us to understand and evaluate John's contribution more thoroughly.

1. PHARMACOLOGICAL MANUALS IN LATE BYZANTIUM: BEYOND THE GRAECO-ROMAN BACKGROUND

The field of pharmacology constituted the most pre-eminent and productive area of late Byzantine medical literature. There were four main Greek pharmacological texts that influenced Byzantine authors substantially: Dioscorides' (*fl.* AD 65) *De Materia Medica*, which gives a detailed description of more than a thousand substances, and Galen's treatises *On the Capacities of Simple Drugs*, *On the Composition of Drugs According to Places*, and *On the Composition of Drugs According to Kind*.[4] Galen provided the scientific background to Byzantine pharmacology with a system of classification of single drugs by allotting each substance certain primary qualities (dry, moist, warm, cool) and ranking their strength on a scale from one (weakest) to four (strongest). The complicated Galenic system relating to the course of action of drugs did not

[3] See n. 136, below.

[4] On Dioscoridean and Galenic pharmacology, see Riddle (1985) and Vogt (2008) respectively.

often find practical application, and, in particular, with regard to the composite drugs where Galen himself failed to apply.[5] Classical works continued to be copied and used by Byzantine physicians into the late Byzantine period.[6] Furthermore, early Byzantine medical compilations by authors such as Oribasios, Aetios of Amida, and Paul of Aegina, and the tenth-century practical handbook by Theophanes Chrysobalantes, which inter alia included various chapters or entire books devoted to the discussion of simple and composite drugs and provided abridged versions of classical knowledge, also remained in circulation in the later periods.[7]

The period from the eleventh century onwards was increasingly marked by the introduction of Arabic medical lore,[8] leading to the dissemination of knowledge on the medicinal use of new, oriental substances, such as myrobalan and sandalwood, as well as innovative pharmaceutical dosage forms, such as syrups and juleps. Perhaps the earliest example is Symeon Seth's *Treatise on the Capacities of Foodstuffs*, which was written for the Emperor Michael VII Doukas (r. 1071–8).[9] This is an alphabetical collection listing the properties of 183 different kinds of aliments and is based on earlier Greek (mainly Galen) and Arabic sources, as Symeon admits in his proem when he refers to Persian (*Persōn*), Hagarene (*Agarēnōn*),—a term used in Byzantine literature to denote Arabs or more generally Muslims[10]—and Indian (*Indōn*) sources.[11] We can see an effort on Symeon's part to introduce new knowledge about the origins and other characteristics, such as the degree of qualitative intensity, of ingredients which had never before been described in detail in any Byzantine treatise, e.g. ambergris (*ampar*), camphor (*kaphoura*), and musk (*moschos*).[12]

[5] Vogt (2008: 314). For the Galenic and Arabic views, see Riddle (1985: 168–76) and Chipman (2019) respectively. See also the study by Pormann (2011), who discusses the reception of Greek scientific pharmacology by Arab authors such as al-Kindī (d. 873), who even proposed a system to calculate degrees of intensity in compound drugs.

[6] On the Greek manuscripts of Dioscorides, see Diels (1906: II.29–31; 1908: 48), and the studies by Touwaide (2003) and Cronier (2006). For an inventory of Galenic manuscripts of the relevant treatises, see Diels (1905: I.96–8).

[7] For example, in the case of Paul of Aegina's *Epitome*, there are more than forty surviving manuscripts produced in the fourteenth and fifteenth centuries; see Diels (1906: II.77–81; 1908: 62) and the updated list on *Pinakes: Textes et manuscrits grecs*, at http://pinakes.irht.cnrs.fr/notices/oeuvre/6215/ (accessed 30 July 2018).

[8] See also Chapter 1, n. 35.

[9] Symeon Seth, *Treatise on the Capacities of Foodstuffs*, ed. Langkavel (1868). The edition does not consider all the available manuscripts of the work. For a study of the textual tradition, see Helmreich (1913).

[10] See *ODB*, s. v. Arabs.

[11] Symeon Seth, *Treatise on the Capacities of Foodstuffs*, pr., ed. Langkavel (1868) 1.1–3.

[12] Symeon Seth, *Treatise on the Capacities of Foodstuffs*, ed. Langkavel (1868) 26.1–14, 58.19–59.9, 66.20–67.20. In the only available study of the text, Harig (1967) showed that a large number of the details that are not found in earlier Greek or early Byzantine medical literature originated from the medieval Arabic medical literature.

The most extensive and well-circulated Arabic text in Greek translation is certainly the *Ephodia tou Apodēmountos* (*Zād al-Musāfir wa-Qūt al-Ḥāḍir*/*Provisions for the Traveller and Nourishment for the Sedentary*/Lat. *Viaticum*) of Ibn al-Jazzār, which had been written by 1130/40 and played a major role in the promotion of Arabic pharmacological lore in Byzantium.[13] The work is divided into seven books and provides an *a capite ad calcem* list of diseases with great emphasis on therapeutic recommendations and pharmacology. Furthermore, we can see Greek translations of Persian antidotaries, such as those by George-Gregory Chioniades[14] and Constantine Melitiniotes, an otherwise unknown physician from Constantinople.[15]

Meanwhile, overland trade, including that in ingredients from Asia and the Far East, was further facilitated during the thirteenth and fourteenth centuries due to the more stable conditions brought about by the Mongol conquests across Eurasia that resulted in what is often called the 'Pax Mongolica'.[16] At the same time, we can attest the production of works, including the pharmacological part of John's *Medical Epitome*, incorporating the newly introduced material and thus depicting current trends. A work which deserves to be given special attention is the *Dynameron* by the so-called Nicholas Myrepsos.[17] The oldest surviving manuscript, i.e. Parisinus gr. 2243, dated to 1339, presents the text arranged alphabetically

[13] See Chapter 4, nn. 34–5. See also the brief case study by Touwaide (2013). The Greek translation circulated in the wider area of southern Italy and Sicily by the early twelfth century. This area played an important role in the exchange of medical knowledge between Greeks and Arabs. On interactions between Greek and Arabic speakers in southern Italy and Sicily with a particular focus on medical texts, see Pormann (2003); Zipser (2003/4); and Mavroudi (2008).

[14] The work consists of around 240 recipes and remains unedited. It survives complete in two manuscripts, i.e. Venetus Marcianus gr. V.8 (coll. 1334) (fourteenth century), ff. 138r–156r, and Matritensis Vitr. 26–1 (fourteenth century), ff. 281v–300v. The title in Venetus Marcianus gr. V.8 reads: '*Ἀντίδοτοι ἐκ Περσίας κομισθεῖσαι καὶ ἐξ ἑλληνισθεῖσαι· παρὰ τοῦ Χιονιάδη κυροῦ Γεωργίου.*' ('Antidotes from Persia, brought and translated into Greek by *kyr* George Chioniades'). There are also one fragmentary and one excerpting manuscript, Mediolanensis Ambrosianus gr. 693 (Q 94 sup.) (fifteenth/sixteenth century), ff. 336r–347r, and Scorialensis T.II.14 (fifteenth century), ff. 183v–185r, respectively. On this work in the framework of late Byzantine pharmacology, see Bouras-Vallianatos (forthcoming).

[15] This antidotary has been edited by Kousis (1939b: 210–17) and consists of around fifty-three recipes. It survives in two manuscripts, i.e. Parisinus gr. 2194 (fifteenth century), ff. 400v–404v and Berolinensis Phillippicus gr. 1562 (sixteenth century), ff. 80r–88r. The title in Parisinus gr. 2194 reads: '*Αὗται αἱ ἀντίδοται ἐμεταγλωττίσθησαν ἐκ τῶν Περσῶν εἰς τὴν Ἑλλάδα παρὰ Κωνσταντίνου ἰατροῦ τοῦ Μελιτινιώτου ἐκ Κωνσταντινουπόλεως.*' ('These antidotes translated from Persian into Greek by the physician Constantine Melitiniotes from Constantinople'). Constantine (*PLP* 17855) is probably a member of the well-known Byzantine family of Meliteniotes, and he should not be confused with the homonymous (*PLP* 17856) unionist archdeacon and friend of Patriarch John XI Bekkos (1275–82). Cf. Mioni (1972: 262), Schönauer (1996: 8–10).

[16] On the significant stimulus given to trade in the Mongol Empire, see Biran (2015: 550–3).

[17] The text has been recently edited by Valiakos (2019). It also available through an early Latin translation by Fuchs (1549). On the author of the *Dynameron*, see Chapter 1, n. 156; and Bouras-Vallianatos (forthcoming: nn. 172–5). See Ieraci Bio (2007: 288–90), who has pointed to some references in the work which suggest a date close to the end of the thirteenth century.

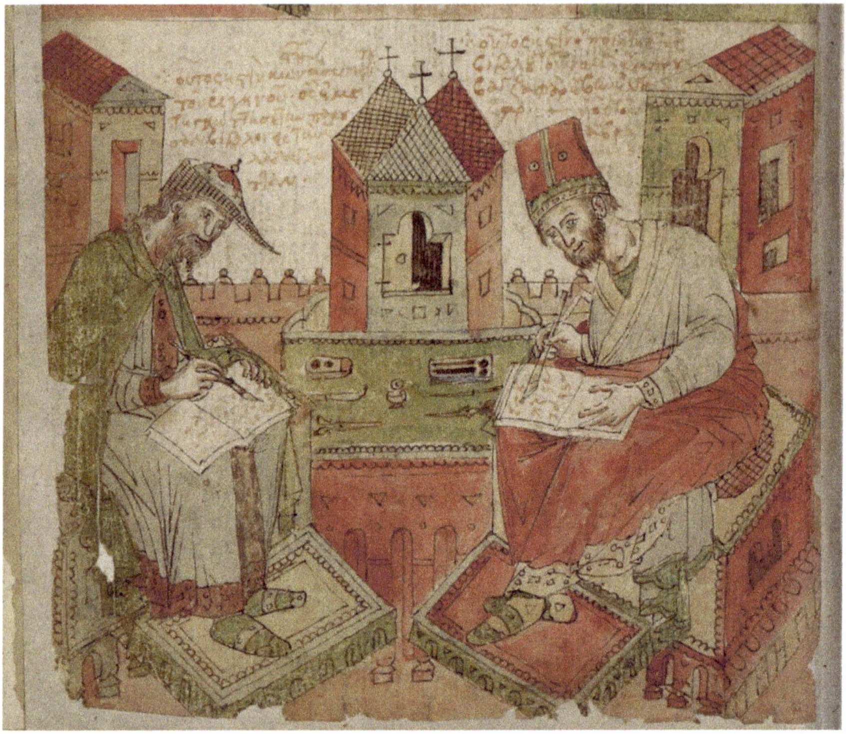

Figure 5.2. Left: Constantine of Reggio, the Greek translator. Right: Ibn al-Jazzār, the Arab author of *Zād al-Musāfir wa-Qūt al-Ḥāḍir*. Matritensis Vitr. 26-1 (fourteenth century), f. Vv.

in twenty-four classes according to the various kinds of drugs and consists of *c.*2,650 recipes, making it the most extensive medieval Greek work on the topic. There are consistent references to newly available oriental ingredients and dosage forms in the *Dynameron*.[18] The compiler used earlier Greek sources, such as Galen and Metrodora.[19] Furthermore, there are many words of Latin provenance in transliteration but also various mentions of contemporary Latin language attesting to the considerable influence of the medieval Latin medical tradition.[20] Moreover, one of the sources seems to be the Latin *Antidotarium Magnum*,[21] which perhaps suggests the compiler

[18] See nn. 98, 120, and 128, below. [19] Ieraci Bio (2007: 298–302).

[20] Ieraci Bio (2007: 291); and Hohlweg (1991).

[21] Some examples have been cited by Ieraci Bio (2007: 292–4) and (2017: 306–7). Cf. Lutz (1963). I had the chance to compare the section on antidotes with a transcription (kindly offered to me by Kathleen Walker-Meikle) of the *Antidotarium Magnum* (based on Londiniensis Wellcomensis MS.MSL.138, early twelfth century) and I discovered a large number of borrowings.

of the *Dynameron* was capable of dealing with Latin sources in the original. Overall, the *Dynameron* could be seen as the first Byzantine pharmacopoeia which aimed to systematize the composition of drugs. It is not a list of official recipes aimed at regulating pharmaceutical activity as in the case of the *Ricettario Fiorentino*, the first European pharmacopoeia which was published in Florence in 1499,[22] but it offers a reference manual of standardized recipes.

Finally, a combination of traditional Byzantine sources with an increasing number of references to oriental *materia medica* is evidenced in various collections of recipes or *iatrosophia*, some of them anonymous or sometimes written in vernacular versions.[23] The recipes are either arranged in an *a capite ad calcem* order or according to the kind of drug involved, so that they can be easily consulted in daily practice. There are also a large number of short, anonymous glossaries including technical terms, most commonly pharmacological substances, produced for the convenience of Greek readers. A synonym for the relevant Greek word is found in foreign languages, e.g. Arabic, medieval Latin, Ottoman Turkish, and given in transliteration, showing great concern to become acquainted with new data.[24]

[22] *Ricettario Fiorentino* (1499). On this, see Colapinto (1993).

[23] Perhaps, the earliest surviving collection of recipes is that by Philip Xeros (active in southern Italy in the early twelfth century) and the otherwise unknown physician Euphemios of Sicily. It survives in Parisinus gr. 2194 (fifteenth century), ff. 454r–464v. The title reads as follows: '*Βιβλίον περιέχον συνθέσεις συναχθὲν καὶ πειραθὲν παρὰ Εὐφημίου Σικελοῦ τοῦ θαυμασιωτάτου· καὶ Φιλίππου Ξηροῦ τοῦ Ῥιγινοῦ, τῶν θαυμασίων ἰατρῶν*' ('Book containing recipes compiled and tested by the most marvellous Euphemios of Sicily and Philip Xeros of Reggio, both among the marvellous physicians'). For the medical activity of the members of the Xeros family, see Ieraci Bio (2006). Another surviving example is by a certain Jew called Benjamin, which survives in Venetus Marcianus gr. V.8 (coll. 1334) (fourteenth century), ff. 158v–165v, Mediolanensis Ambrosianus gr. 693 (Q 94 sup.), ff. 349r–364r (fifteenth/sixteenth century), and Vaticanus gr. 282 (fifteenth century), ff. 437v–442v. The title in Vaticanus gr. 282 reads: '*Ἑτέραι σκευασίαι κοκκίων· ζουλαπίων· ἐμπλάστρων· συντεθεῖσαι εἰς τὴν Ἑλλάδα παρὰ ἰουδαίου Βενιαμίν*' ('Further recipes for pills, juleps, and plasters composed in Greek by Benjamin the Jew'). I am currently working on the edition and English translation of both collections. See also John Archiatros' *iatrosophion* edited by Zipser (2009) and her recent study on the text (2018). Zipser (2009: 33–7) has suggested a *terminus post quem* around 1209 for the later version, which presents several vernacular elements. See also Stathakopoulos (2011), who provides more evidence in favour of a date before 1200 for the early version of the text. In this group, we may also include the so-called *xenōnika*, which contain lists of recipes related to the practice of medicine in Byzantine *xenōnes*. See Bennett's monograph (2017). A preliminary edition of some examples is available in Bennett's thesis (2003: 331–439).

[24] See, for example, those glossaries edited by Delatte (1939) II.394–417, II.428–50. On Byzantine botanical lexicography, see Stannard (1971: 168–87). See also Touwaide (1999: 211–28), who provides a preliminary list of manuscripts containing such glossaries. Perhaps the earliest example in Greek, surviving in Oxoniensis Bodleianus Holkhamicus gr. 112 (olim. 289) (AD 1100–23), has been edited by Bouras-Vallianatos (2018a).

2. STRUCTURE OF JOHN'S PHARMACOLOGY

John lists his recipes of composite drugs in book five following an order based on the various kinds of drugs (mainly orally administered medicines,[25] e.g. potions, lozenges). Later on, in book six, he gives special emphasis to the various drugs applied to the external parts of the body in an *a capite ad calcem* order. However, there are some exceptions, as, for example, the fact that a structure based on drug types is also partially adopted in book six, i.e. the final chapters (e.g. plasters, pessaries, oils),[26] which is potentially confusing for readers, as can also be seen in two branches of the textual tradition. In fact, a considerable number of manuscripts copy the second part of book six immediately after book five.[27] Moreover, one particular group of manuscripts copies the first part of book six between books three and four.[28]

In Table 5.1, I present a reconstruction of the order of the thematic units in books five and six based on a study of the manuscripts and John's

Table 5.1. Outline of contents of John's *Medical Epitome*, Books Five & Six

Book Five	Book Six
	Part I
Proem	Proem
Potions on fevers	On affections of the surface of the head
Juleps and syrups	On head affections
Lozenges and pills	On ear affections
Antidotes	On nasal affections
Wines	On eye affections
Simple purgatives	On facial affections
Composite purgatives (oral drugs, nasal drugs, externally applied drugs)	On oral affections
	On skin affections and ulcers
Poisons (animal, vegetal, and mineral ingredients)	**Part II**
	Plasters
	Pessaries
	Oils
	Venomous animals

[25] There are, however, a few exceptions, as in the case of composite purgatives, in which John also includes nasal drugs and externally applied drugs, such as ointments.

[26] Further confusion may have been caused by the fact that the category of pessaries, which mainly comprises composite drugs for various gynaecological affections, was discussed in book six, although in the diagnostic part gynaecological affections were grouped with the affections of the internal parts of the body. In particular, the chapter dealing with the diagnosis of the affections of the womb (56) comes at the end of book one in between the diagnosis for intestinal hernia (55) and the chapter on sweats (57), JZA, *Medical Epitome*, 2.55–7, ed. Ideler (1842) II.412–16.

[27] See Groups II and III in Appendix 5, Table App.1.

[28] This is Group III in Appendix 5, Table App.1.

statements. The most complete account of his contents, which also helps us to clarify the inconsistent structure of book six, is provided in the proem of the same book:

> In the previous book [i.e. book five] I considered it right to mention those <drugs> in advance, all those which if taken internally are beneficial: antidotes, and the so-called juleps, and some other composite liquid drugs, and in addition the purgative drugs... In the remaining and last book [i.e. book six], I will put together those externally applied for the various affections of the parts of the body, and those that are suited to the entire surface of the body: ointments... and differently prepared oils, plasters... We will begin this account with the affections of the surface of head.[29]

John ends his passage by referring to the content of chapter one of book six focusing on affections related to the head, thus initiating his *a capite ad calcem* arrangement.[30] Later on, at the end of the first part of book six, after dealing with the various drugs for skin ulcers, he adds a couple of sentences:

> ... so now we will take the account further by discussing the emollients and the rest of the drugs. In addition to these, we will give an account of the preparation of oils and unguents; and so in all respects, this account would be complete.[31]

By providing a linking sentence, John attempts to connect the two differently arranged parts of book six. Afterwards, he starts his account with treatments using plasters and so on.

[29] JZA, *Medical Epitome*, 6, Vindobonensis med. gr. 17, f. 167r, l. 26-f. 167v, l. 13: '*ὅθεν ἐν μὲν τῷ πρὸ τούτου λόγῳ, ἐκείνων ἔκρινα δεῖν πρότερον μνημονεῦσαι, ὅσα ἐντὸς λαμβανόμενα, ὠφελεῖ· ἀντίδοτοι δὲ καὶ τὰ καλούμενα ζουλάπια· ἅτινα* (here I follow E: *καί τινα*) *ἕτερα συντεθειμένα ὑγρὰ φάρμακα· καὶ προσέτι τὰ καθαίροντα τῶν φαρμάκων...ἐν τῷ λειπομένῳ δέ, τούτῳ καὶ ὑστάτῳ λόγῳ ἀποταμιεύεται, ὅσα ἔξωθεν προσφέρεται ἔν τε τοῖς κατὰ μέρος τοῦ σώματος παθήμασι καὶ ἐν τοῖς καθ' ὅλην τὴν ἐπιφάνειαν τοῦ σώματος προσήκουσιν· ἀλοιφαί...καὶ ἔλαια διαφόρως σκευαζόμενα· ἔμπλαστροι...ἀρχὴν τῆς ὑποθέσεως, τὰ περὶ τὴν ἐπιφάνειαν τῆς κεφαλῆς θέμενοι πάθη·*'; ed. Mathys (1556) II.433.21–434.9.

[30] Here John is mostly referring to affections of the external parts of the body. There is one notable exception in the chapter on head affections, in which drugs applied externally for headaches and migraines are also included. JZA, *Medical Epitome*, 6, Vindobonensis med. gr. 17, f. 177v, ll. 16–22: '*Ἀλλὰ τὰ μὲν κατὰ τῆς* (E: *κατὰ τὴν τῆς*) *κεφαλῆς ἐπιφάνειαν πάθη, ταῦτα καὶ οὕτω θεραπευτέον· ἐπεὶ δὲ τῷ καταλόγῳ τῶν ἔξωθεν ἐπιτιθεμένων ἅπτεται ἡ ὑπόθεσις καὶ τῶν κατὰ τὰ ἐντὸς παθημάτων, ἅτε καὶ μέχρι τοῦ βάθους ἐνίοτε τῶν ἔξωθεν ἐπιτιθεμένων ἐξικνουμένων, φέρε καὶ ἐπὶ τῶν καθ' ὁποίαν δήτινα διάθεσιν κεφαλαλγούντων τὰ διὰ τῆς ἔξωθεν ἐπιθέσεως βοηθοῦντα εἴπωμεν·*'; ed. Mathys (1556) II.458.9–17.

[31] JZA, *Medical Epitome*, 6, Vindobonensis med. gr. 17, f. 210r, ll. 9–11: '*...εἶθ' οὕτως ἐπὶ τὰ μαλάγματα καὶ τὰ λοιπὰ τὸν λόγον προάξομεν φάρμακα· ἐπὶ δὲ τούτοις τὴν τῶν ἐλαίων τε καὶ μύρων ἐκθησόμεθα μέθοδον· ὡς ἂν ἐν πᾶσιν ἄρτιος ὁ λόγος τελοίη.*'; ed. Mathys (1556) II.526.6–10.

Each group of recipes might be quite short, just a couple of folia, or very long, as for example in the case of antidotes, which is about twenty folia long.[32] The vast majority of the content concentrates on the preparation of composite drugs.[33] The recipes may be just a few lines long or quite extensive, as, for example, in the case of theriac.[34] The structure of each recipe follows the classical and Byzantine model for composite drugs, which is basically divided into five parts. Here I present a typical example from book five, which refers to a certain pill prescribed for breathing difficulties (the division by lines is mine):

<Pill> of native sulphur
for those suffering from difficulty of breathing:
anise, native sulphur, three ounces of each; incense of ammoniac, castoreum,[35] black cumin, four drachmas of each;
dissolve them into water and make pills;
and give one <pill> with three *kyathoi* of *oxymeli*.[36,37]

Thus we can see the following distinct categories of data provided: a) title, which might also include details on the origin of the particular recipe; b) indication, usually listing various ailments; c) the actual list of substances together with posological details; d) the method of preparation, which may include several stages; e) details on the administration of the particular medicament including dosage.[38] The latter part varies greatly from recipe to recipe. It may sometimes be omitted or can even be more detailed, referring to the particular days of each week on which the relevant drug had to be given to the patient.

[32] JZA, *Medical Epitome*, 5, Vindobonensis med. gr. 17, ff. 122r, l. 10–141r, l. 18; ed. Mathys (1556) II.342.6–375.

[33] The most notable exceptions are the parts on simple purgatives, poisons, and venomous animals. See, JZA, *Medical Epitome*, 5, Vindobonensis med. gr. 17, ff. 144v, l. 12–149v, l. 14; *Medical Epitome*, 5, Vindobonensis med. gr. 17, ff. 161v, l. 14–167r, l. 18; and *Medical Epitome*, 6, Vindobonensis med. gr. 17, ff. 239r, l. 2–242v, l. 25; ed. Mathys (1556) II.379.15–392.12; II.416.18–432; and II.553.8–563.

[34] JZA, *Medical Epitome*, 6, Vindobonensis med. gr. 17, ff. 122r, l. 11–123r, l. 23; ed. Mathys (1556) II.342.7–345.24. On theriac, see Boudon-Millot (2010: 261–70).

[35] A secretion from the beaver.

[36] Mixture of vinegar and honey.

[37] JZA, *Medical Epitome*, 5, Vindobonensis med. gr. 17, f. 140v, ll. 11–14: '*τὸ διὰ θείου ἀπείρου* (E: *ἀπύρου*) *δυσπνοϊκοῖς· ἀνίσου· θείου ἀπύρου, ἀνὰ οὐγγ. γ′· ἀμμωνιακοῦ θυμιάματος· καστορίου· μελανθίου· ἀνὰ < δ′· ὕδατι διαλύσας, ποίει καταπότια· καὶ δίδου ἓν δι' ὀξομέλιτος* (E: *ὀξυμέλιτος*) *κυάθων γ′*.'; ed. Mathys (1556) II.374.5–11.

[38] The first four parts of the recipe may be also referred to in Greek as *prographē*, *epangelia*, *synthesis*, *skeuasia*. The Greek words correspond to terms used by Galen to name parts of his recipes. John does not use these terms. They were never used consistently by Greek and Byzantine authors and have been derived from a detailed study of Galen's pharmacology by Fabricius (1972: 24–30); see also Marganne (2006: 65–6).

3. EXPERIENCE

John gives an outline of his intentions in compiling his pharmacology in the proem to book five, in which he is eager to demonstrate that his experience has played an important role in the writing of this particular section of his *Medical Epitome*. It should just be noted that there is no mention of *peira* ('experience') or any cognate in this context in the first four books. Thus John states:

> The exposition of the four previous books has already become available to you. This is the fifth book of the entire work, which includes the composition of drugs... for this needs to be expressed in a brief account... And so having been selected from old books, the recipes for composite drugs will be added to this book... each of the <recipes> is tested by means of experience...[39]

First, we should note the common element with his approach in the first part of his work, i.e. the desire to provide a short account.[40] In fact, as we will see, John manages to use a considerable number of sources by excerpting specific passages from each of them and finally composing a much shorter version than is to be found in any other ancient or Byzantine examples of pharmacological works.[41] Even more striking is John's use of special terms in describing his selection process, using, for example, the word *eklegenta*, aorist passive participle of the verb *eklegō* ('to pick out/select').[42] John then goes a step further, informing his readers that *peira* is the main tool he relies on in the

[39] JZA, *Medical Epitome*, 5, Vindobonensis med. gr. 17, f. 112v, ll.3–16: '*Ἤδη σοι καὶ τὸν ἐπὶ τοῖς τέτταρσι βιβλίοις* (E: *Ἐπὶ τοῖς προεκτεθεῖσι τέσσαρσι βιβλίοις*) *ἐπιτίθεμεν λόγον· ὃς πέμπτος τῆς ὅλης πραγματείας ἐστί· συμπεριειληφὼς δὲ τὴν περὶ τῶν φαρμάκων σύνθεσιν... τοῦτο γὰρ πάνυ βραχέος λόγου δεῖται... οὐκοῦν τὰ μέν, τῶν συντιθεμένων φαρμάκων, ἐκ παλαιῶν βιβλίων ἐκλεγέντα, τῷ βιβλίῳ προστεθήσεται... ἕκαστα δὲ τῇ πείρᾳ βασανιζόμενα...*'; ed. Mathys (1556) II.317.6–318.6.

[40] See Chapter 4, n. 42; and n. 68, below.

[41] To give an example, John's pharmacology is about 65,000 words, which is one fourth the size of Galen's two works on composite drugs (*On the Composition of Drugs According to Places* and *On the Composition of Drugs According to Kind*). As for the contemporary *Dynameron* attributed to Nicholas Myrepsos, the section devoted to antidotes contains almost five hundred different recipes whereas in John's corresponding section there are about ninety. On this section, see n. 32, above. For the list of antidotes in the *Dynameron*, see Parisinus gr. 2243, ff. 11v–99r; and Valiakos (2019) 3–225. This part is also available through the early Latin edition by Fuchs (1549) 1–150.

[42] We can also observe references to cognates of the verb *ἐρανίζω* ('to collect/gather/bring together') in connection with the inclusion of particular recipes. See, for example, JZA, *Medical Epitome*, 5, Vindobonensis med. gr. 17, f. 167r, ll. 15–16: '*... ἔξεστι κἀκεῖθεν ἐρανίζεσθαι τὰ πρὸς τοὺς ἐνισταμένους κινδύνους χρήσιμα·*'; and *Medical Epitome*, 6, f. 167r, ll. 22–3: '*... μὴ καὶ ἀπὸ τούτων ἐρανίσασθαι τὰ χρησιμώτερα·*'; ed. Mathys (1556) II.432.13–4 and II.433.15–6 respectively. The term is also used in book three, in which John states that some parts on dietetics have been excerpted from his *On Psychic Pneuma*. JZA, *Medical Epitome*, 3, Vindobonensis med. gr. 17, f. 63r, ll. 16–19: '*... καὶ τοίνυν εἴρηται μὲν καὶ πρότερον περὶ τούτων, ἔν οἷς περὶ τοῦ ψυχικοῦ πνεύματος διεξείημεν* (E: *διεξῄειμεν*)*· τὸ γὰρ τοι δεύτερον βιβλίον μικροῦ δεῖν τὸν πάντα σκοπὸν ἐμπεριείληφε τῆς ὑγιεινῆς πραγματείας· κἀκεῖθεν ἔξεστι, ταῦτ' ἐρανίζεσθαι·*'; ed. Mathys (1556) II.177.16–21.

process of selection.[43] The use of experience as an instrument of testing the capacity and effectiveness of drugs is exemplified by authors in antiquity, most notably Galen himself.[44] Later on, for example, in Alexander of Tralles' work, written in the second half of the sixth century, clinical experience is used to check the efficacy of past medicaments, and also to modify earlier recipes or introduce new medicines.[45] As we can see in Table 5.2, John's wording recalls

Table 5.2. Examples of the use of the word *peira* in Galen's and John's pharmacology

Galen	John Zacharias Aktouarios
On the Composition of Drugs According to Places, 1.2, ed. Kühn (1826) XII.393.2–3: . . . *τὰ δ' ὑφ' ἡμῶν αὐτῶν διὰ μακρᾶς πείρας βεβασανισμένα* . . . . . . the <recipes of composite drugs> that have been tested by us by means of long experience . . .	*Medical Epitome*, 5, Vindobonensis med. gr. 17, f. 112v, l. 16; ed. Mathys (1556) II.318.5–6: . . . *ἕκαστα δὲ τῇ πεῖρᾳ βασανιζόμενα* . . . . . . each of the <recipes> is tested by means of experience . . .
On the Composition of Drugs According to Kind, 2.1, ed. Kühn (1827) XIII.459.11–12: . . . *βέλτιον μὲν οὖν ἐστι τοῖς διὰ τῆς πείρας ἤδη βεβασανισμένοις χρῆσθαι* . . . . . . and so it is better to use <those drugs> which have already been tested by means of experience . . .	*Medical Epitome*, 6, Vindobonensis med. gr. 17, f. 167v, ll.18–20; ed. Mathys (1556) II.434.16–21: *Νυνὶ μόνα παραγράψαντες τὰ φάρμακα, ὅσα ἐκ διαφόρων βίβλων ἐρανισάμεθα, ἢ ἀγράφῳ πείρᾳ παρελάβομεν, ἢ καὶ αὐτοὶ δοκιμάσαντες ἔγνωμεν*[46] *χρήσιμα* . . . Now we will only give an account of the drugs that we gathered from various sources or that we collected by means of unwritten experience, and even those we considered useful after testing them . . .
On the Composition of Drugs According to Kind, 4.5, ed. Kühn (1827) XIII.708.1–2: . . . *πολλά γε τοιαῦτα διὰ πείρας μακρᾶς βεβασανισμένα γραφήσεται.* . . . many of these <recipes>, which have been tested by means of long experience, will be recorded <in this book>.	
On the Composition of Drugs According to Kind, 7.11, ed. Kühn (1827) XIII.1009.10–11: *Ὥσπερ οὖν εἴωθα τοῖς πρεσβυτέροις διὰ μακρᾶς πείρας βεβασανισμένα γράφειν* . . . And so just like the elder physicians, I used to write down <recipes> which I have tested by means of long experience . . .	

[43] See also John's references to *peira* in his *On Urines*, Chapter 2, n. 55.

[44] Fabricius (1972: 41–3, 50–1). Vogt (2008: 314–15). Van der Eijk (1997b: 39–40) rightly emphasizes that the 'straightforward . . . expressed belief that something—a statement or claim, an issue, idea or notion—may be in need of qualification by means of experience' should not be confused with Galen's particular notion of 'qualified experience' (*diōrismenē peira*). On the latter, see van der Eijk (1997b: 40–55).

[45] Scarborough (1984: 226–8); and Bouras-Vallianatos (2014: 344–8).

[46] E reads '*εὕρομεν*' ('found').

Galenic phraseology, which is used in connection with the use of a certain composite drug or group of them.

An even more insightful comment is explicitly made in the part introducing juleps and syrups:

> . . . here the drugs [i.e. juleps and syrups] are set out, those which have been taken from Greek medical books and those from barbarian works that have been translated into the Greek language. Furthermore, those <drugs> that have been composed by us; and some others that we happened to hear about and which we have tested.[47]

In this passage and also the second example in Table 5.2, we can see the use of the first-person plural either in the form of a personal pronoun or a verb, in an attempt by John to give a personal touch to communicating his expert pharmacological knowledge and to engage the reader's attention when referring to a significant set of details.[48] It reveals John's expectations of demonstrating the quality of his therapeutic advice by establishing his authority on the subject and providing his own perspective as an experienced practising physician,[49] and not merely a compiler of medical writings. In addition to the intriguing reference to his non-Greek, barbarian sources, which will be discussed below, John does not hesitate to refer to recipes, some of which had been composed by him as well as those that he had happened to hear about. In the second example (Table 5.2), there is also a reference by John to 'unwritten experience', *agraphō peira*, which implies the inclusion of oral recipes in his work.[50] It is not possible to determine which are the 'unwritten' and/or 'personal' recipes. Nevertheless, it is to be expected that an active, practising physician such as John would personally test the greater part of the recipes he suggested and make his own modifications to some of them as a result of his many contact hours with patients.[51]

[47] JZA, *Medical Epitome*, 5, Vindobonensis med. gr. 17, f. 116r, ll. 21–4: '. . . *ἐκτεθήσεται δὲ τὰ φάρμακα τὰ μέν, ἐξ' ἑλληνίδων ἰατρικῶν βίβλων· τὰ δ' αὖ ἐκμετενεχθεισῶν εἰς ἑλληνίδα γλῶτταν βαρβάρων βίβλων· τὰ δ' αὖ καὶ ὑφ' ἡμῶν αὐτῶν συντεθέντα· ἔνια δὲ καὶ ἐκ τοῦ παρατυχόντος ἀκουσθέντα καὶ δοκιμασθέντα·*'; ~ed. Mathys (1556) II.329.7–10.

[48] See also Section 4.2, below, in which John uses the first-person plural ('*πεποιήκαμεν προσδιορισμούς . . .*') in stating that he had tested the drugs that he included in his *Medical Epitome*. See also Chapter 2, Section 2.1, for the use of first-person singular and plural statements in his *On Urines*.

[49] See Totelin (2012: 308–10), who shows how Galen constructs his authority in his pharmacological works by use of first-person statements. Galen's pharmacological works are also largely based on the works of earlier authors. See Fabricius (1972: 180–205); and Guardasole (2015).

[50] On the concept of the transmission of oral recipes in ancient pharmacological works, see the study provided by Totelin (2009: 21–64), who discusses examples from Hippocratic recipes.

[51] An interesting case of a process involving modifications of a certain recipe is reported by John in one of his case histories in JZA, *On Urines*, 2.19.14–28, Ideler (1842) II.50.26–52.1. See also the discussion of this in Chapter 3, Section 2.4.

4. JOHN'S PHARMACOLOGICAL SOURCES

4.1 Book five

To provide a convenient starting point for the identification and discussion of John's pharmacological sources, I will start by analysing book five. The first example (see Table 5.3) is related to composite purgative drugs from book five, which presents an interesting case of combining earlier Greek sources with Arabic ones in translation. Unlike in Chapter 4 where I preferred to set out the texts in a *Lesetext* structure, in this instance, due to the absence of an edition for many of John's sources, the texts will be provided in transcription in tables of parallel columns. Similarities between the various texts will be underlined.[52] I give the page numbers in the primary sources or the folio numbers for manuscripts in bold. The beginning and ending of each recipe in all sources will be marked by two asterisks: '**'.

The first obvious point to be made after looking at the three recipes provided is that they combine at least two different sources, the *Ephodia tou Apodēmountos*[53] for recipes A and B and Aetios of Amida's *Tetrabiblos* for recipe C. The next notable feature is the actual rearrangement of the order of the recipes in John's text. The *Ephodia tou Apodēmountos* follows a 'head to toe' order, and thus recipe A (Vaticanus gr. 300, f. 204r), which relates to the treatment of gout, comes towards the end of the original text, while recipe B (Vaticanus gr. 300, f. 145v) for stomach affections, involving an extremely popular purgative in the medieval Islamic medical tradition, i.e. the so-called *triphyllos* or *tryphera* (Ar. *iṭrīful*),[54] is discussed earlier in the

[52] Posological information on individual ingredients may vary greatly even among manuscripts of the same work.

[53] I use the earliest surviving manuscript of the work, i.e. Vaticanus gr. 300. On this manuscript, see Chapter 4, n. 34. I am aware that this manuscript lacks several chapters of books one and two; for preliminary notes on the relationship between the Greek version of the text in Vaticanus gr. 300 and other surviving manuscripts, see Duffy (1997: 15, nn. 1–3); Ieraci Bio (1989: 221–8); Lucà (2012: 579–84); and Miguet (2017: 85–7). Note that Vaticanus gr. 300 preserves several peculiar readings, e.g. '*ὠφέλημος*' instead of '*ὠφέλιμος*', '*μοιροβάλαν*' instead of '*μυροβάλανον*' or '*δαμασόνιον*' instead of '*δαμασώνιον*', and '*καλλοπίζουσι*' instead of '*καλλωπίζουσι*'. I have also checked these particular recipes in two more manuscripts of the *Ephodia*. The second earliest surviving manuscript, Parisinus gr. 2311 (twelfth/thirteenth century) does not preserve Recipe A (and some other recipes at the end of book six), but preserves Recipe B (f. 136v, l. 4–f. 137r, l. 2), omitting just a brief phrase (i.e. '*σίνφη . . . ἀγάλοχον*'). Vindobonensis med. gr. 30 (AD 1315) preserves both recipes without any omissions (Recipe A: f. 362v, l. 16–f. 363r, l. 3; Recipe B: f. 278r, l. 3–f. 287v, l. 12). Lastly, it is worth noting that both recipes are part of the original text: Ibn al-Jazzār, *Zād al-Musāfir wa-Qūt al-Ḥāḍir*, 4.19 and 6.20, ed. Suwaysī et al. (1999) I.376–8 and ed. Bos (1997) 230–2.

[54] John refers only to the lesser (*mikra*) *tryphera*. Authors writing in Arabic mention recipes of a lesser and a greater *tryphera*. In the *Ephodia tou Apodēmountos,* we find both recipes one after the other. On the *tryphera* in the Islamic medical tradition, see Levey (1973: 83–6); and Lev (2013: 511–15).

Table 5.3. Sources of John's composite purgatives

Number of sample recipe followed by its name in John's work	John's source	John Zacharias Aktouarios, *Medical Epitome*, Book Five
A Royal pill for gout	... καὶ διαίτης· ἐπεὶ ὠφέλημος ἐστιν. ** στήλη ὠφέλημος εἰς ποδαλγίαν λαμβάνεται δὲ ἐν παντὶ καιρῷ, ἁρμόζει δὲ τοῖς βασιλεῦσιν· ἡ σύνθεσις: λαβὼν μοιροβάλανον ξανθόν, τὸν φλοιὸν λέγει καὶ δαμασόνιον τὸ πελίλητζ· καὶ ἔμλετζ· καὶ ζινζίβερ, ἀνὰ τεσσάρων ἐξαγ.· ὀρίγανον, ἑπτὰ ἐξαγ.· κάψικον ἰνδικὸν δύο ἐξαγ.· ἑρμοδάκτυλον λευκὸν ἓν καὶ εἴκοσι ἐξαγ.· παινί[Δ] δώδεκα ἐξαγ.· βδέλλυον πέντε καίδεκα ἐξαγ.· κόψας σείσας, ζύμωσον μετὰ χυλοῦ στρύγχνου· καὶ γενήσονται κόκκοι καὶ ξήρανον ἐν σκιᾷ· καὶ ἅμα τοῦ γνῶναι ὀδύνην τὸν νοσοῦντα πρὸ βρώσεως ἢ μετὰ τὴν βρῶσιν λαμβανέτω ἐξ αὐτῶν δύο ἐξαγ. μετὰ ὕδατος θερμοῦ· ἢ μετ' οἴνου καὶ καιρόν, μὴ τήρη: ** σύνθεσις ... *Ephodia tou Apodēmountos*, 6.20, Vaticanus gr. 300, f. 204r, l. 14–f. 204v, l. 1.	... καὶ ποίησον κοκκία· ἡ δόσις <′ β′: ** ἕτερον εἰς ποδαλγίαν τὸ βασιλικόν· λαβὼν μυροβάλανον ξανθόν· δαμασώνιον· ἔμπλιτζι· καὶ ζιγγίβερ, ἀνὰ (ἐξαγ.) δ′· ὀρίγανον, (ἐξαγ.) ζ′· κάψικον, (ἐξαγ.) β′· ἑρμοδάκτυλον λευκὸν (ἐξαγ.) κ′· πενίδια, (ἐξαγ.) ιβ′· βδέλλιον, (ἐξαγ.) ιε′· κόψας σήσας ζύμωσον μετὰ χυλοῦ στρύχνου, καὶ ποίει κοκκία· καὶ ἅμα τῷ γνῶναι ὀδύνην τὸν νοσοῦντα, πρὸ βρώσεως ἢ μετὰ βρῶσιν λαμβανέτω (ἐξαγ.) β′· μεθ' ὕδατος θερμοῦ ἢ οἴνου: ** ζουλάπιον καθαῖρον χολὴν ξανθὴν ... Vindobonensis med. gr. 17, f. 152r, l. 25–f. 152v, l. 5; ed. Mathys (1556) II.399.21–30.
B Small *triphyllos*	... ἢ μετὰ ὕδατος πρασσίου: ** ἐν τούτοις στήλη τῆς μικρᾶς τρυφερᾶς, ὠφελοῦσα εἰς τὰς ἐσωχάδας καὶ εἰς πόνον στομάχου καὶ ἀδυναμίαν αὐτοῦ, ἀπὸ τοῦ πλήθους τῆς ὑγρότητος· καὶ φυλάττει τὴν ὑγείαν, ἀποπέμπεται δὲ εἰς χρῆσιν πλῆθος ἀρρωστιῶν· λαβὼν τὸν φλοιὸν τοῦ μυροβαλάνου τοῦ κέπουλι καὶ ἀντὶ τούτου εἰ θέλεις θὲς τὸ ἰνδικόν· καὶ πελίλιζ καὶ ἔμλεζ, ἀνὰ ἑνὸς μέρους· κόψας σείσας ἀνάμιγε μετὰ ῥοδελαίου καὶ φύρασον σὺν μέλιτι ἀπαφρισμένῳ· καὶ ἀπόθου εἰς κορούπιν λεῖον· ἡ δὲ πόσις ἐξ αὐτοῦ δύο ἐξαγ., μέχρι τριῶν μετὰ ὕδατος χλιαροῦ· αὕτη δὲ ἡ σύνθεσις τῆς μικρᾶς τρυφερᾶς τῆς ἐπαινετῆς εἰς τὴν κοινότητα τῶν ἰατρῶν καὶ τῶν ἐπισήμων, καὶ	... ποίει ζουλάπιον· ἡ δόσις, οὐγγ. α′· ἢ δύο: ** ἡ μικρὰ τρίφυλλος ἡ λεγομένη· ὠφελοῦσα εἰς ἐσωχάδας· εἰς πόνον στομάχου καὶ ἀδυναμίαν αὐτοῦ ἀπὸ ὑγρότητος· φυλάττει καὶ τὴν ὑγείαν· καὶ ἔστι εἰς ἄλλα τινὰ χρήσιμος· λαβὼν τὸν φλοιὸν τοῦ μυροβαλάνου· τοῦ κέπουλε· καὶ ἀντὶ τούτου εἰ θέλεις τὸ ἰνδικὸν μπελίλιζ καὶ ἔμπλιτζι ἀνὰ μέρος α′, κόψας σήσας, ἀνάμιγε (E: ἀνάμισγε) μετὰ ῥοδελαίου· καὶ φύρασον σὺν μέλιτι ἀπηφρισμένῳ· ἡ δόσις, (ἐξαγ.) β′ μέχρι (E: ἢ) γ′· μεθ' ὕδατος χλιαροῦ ὅστις βούλεται εἰς τελείαν ὠφέλειαν ἰέναι τῶν ἐσωχάδων τοῦ πόνου τοῦ ἀφεδρῶνος, προστιθέτω μέρος βδελλίου γλαυκοῦ· εἰδ' ὠφελῆσαι θέλει εἰς τὸ κενοῦν τὸ αἷμα, μέρος κομμιδίου προστιθέτω

(*continued*)

Table 5.3. Continued

Number of sample recipe followed by its name in John's work	John's source	John Zacharias Aktouarios, *Medical Epitome*, Book Five
	*ἔστιν εἰς αὐτοὺς γνωστὴ εἰς ὠφέλειαν· ὅστις δὲ βούλεται εἰς ἄκρως ὠφελείας τῶν ἐσωχάδων· καὶ πόνου τοῦ ἀφεδρῶνος· προσθήει εἰς αὐτὸν μέρος βδέλλυον γλαυκόν· εἰ δὲ θέλει εἰς τὸν καθεύδοντα αἷμα, τιθέτω μέρος κομίδιν ἀραβικὸν πεφρυγμένον· καὶ μέρος μηρσυνόκοκκα πεφρυγμένα· εἰ δὲ καὶ θελήσεις, εἰς ὠφέλειαν τοῦ χαύνου στομάχου, καὶ τοῦ ἠτονημένου διόρθωσιν τῶν κάτω· πρόσθες μέρος ῥόδα καὶ μαστίχιν μέρος· καὶ ἥμισυ μέρους ἄνισον· καὶ ἥμισυ μέρους καρεόφυλλον· εἰ δέ που θελήσει ὁ παλμὸς τῆς καρδίας, προσθέσεις αὐτῷ ἀγάλοχον φημὶ ξαλαλώην μέρος, σίνφη, χώρα εἰς ἰνδίαν· ἢ πρόσθες ἰνδικὸν ἀγάλοχον· εἰ δὲ θέλεις ὠφελεῖν εἰς τὰς μελαγχολικὰς ἀρρωστίας, πρόσθες μέρος ἐπίθυμον· καὶ εἰ θέλεις κενῶσαι τὴν ἀπὸ τοῦ φλέγματος ὑγρότητα, πρόσθες ἀλυπίαν, φημὶ τούρβεθ λευκόν· εἰ δὲ θέλεις πρὸς ὄγκον πνευμάτων καὶ ἀπεψίαν καὶ πρόσθεσιν συνουσίας· ἐπίθες μέρος ζινζήβερ, καὶ μέρος γαλαγγᾶν καὶ σίτραζ τὸ ἰνδικὸν κάψικον· καὶ μακροπίπερ· καὶ λεπτοκιννάμωμον ἀνα ἡμίσεως μέρους· καὶ γίνεται παράξενον, τουτέστι θαυμαστόν· ἔνιοι δὲ τῶν ἰατρῶν καλλοπίζουσι τὴν χροιὰν τῆς τρυφερᾶς μετὰ κρόκου· καὶ ἔστιν ὠφέλιμος εἰς ἃ ἔφημεν: ** στήλη τῆς μεγάλης τρυφερᾶς…* *Ephodia tou Apodēmountos*, 4.19, Vaticanus gr. 300, f. 145v, l. 3–f. 146r, l. 10.	*πεφρυγμένου· εἰς δὲ ὠφέλειαν τοῦ ἠτονημένου στομάχου καὶ διόρθωσιν τῶν κάτω προστιθέτω ῥόδων μέρος· καὶ μαστίχης μέρος· καὶ ἥμισυ μέρος ἀνίσου· καὶ ἥμισυ μέρος καρυοφύλλου· εἰς δὲ παλμὸν τὸν τῆς καρδίας, προστίθει* (E: *προστιθέτω*) *ξυλαλόην· εἰς δὲ τὰς μελαγχολικὰς ἀρρωστίας προστιθέτω μέρος ἐπιθύμου· εἰ δὲ θέλεις κενῶσαι φλέγμα προστίθει ἀλυπίαν ἤτοι τούρπετε λευκόν· πρὸς δὲ ὄγκον πνευμάτων καὶ ἀπεψίαν καὶ πρόσθεσιν συνουσίας· μέρος ζιγγίβερ· καὶ μέρος γαλαγγᾶν· καὶ σίστεζ τὸ ἰνδικὸν κάψικον· καὶ μακροπέπερι· λεπτοκινάμωμον, ἀνὰ* S″ *μέρος· καὶ γίνεται ἐπιτήδειον· ἔνιοι δὲ τῶν ἰατρῶν, καλλωπίζουσι τὴν χρόαν βάλλοντες καὶ κρόκον:* ** *ἡ ἱερὰ πικρὰ τοῦ γαληνοῦ ἡ διὰ τῆ ἀλόης σκευαζομένη…* Vindobonensis med. gr. 17, f. 152v, l. 14–f. 153r, l. 7; ed. Mathys (1556) II.400.1–27.
C Purgative plaster, the so-called *chezanankē*	*…λείου πάλιν μετὰ χολῆς μοσχείας, ὡς γλοιῶδες γενέσθαι καὶ ἐπίχεε τὰ τηκτὰ καὶ ἑνώσας, χρῶ, φησιν, ὡς παραδόξῳ.* ** *ἄλλη ἔμπλαστρος καθαρτικὴ ᾗ χρῶμαι,*	*…τοῦτο ἐπιτιθὲν καὶ κινῆσαν τὴν κοιλίαν, ἀναλαμβάνειν χρή:* ** *ἕτερος* (E: *ἑτέρα*) *ἔμπλαστρος καθαρτικὴ ἡ καλουμένη* (E: *λεγομένη*) *χεζανάγκη· αὕτη*

*καλουμένη χεζανάγκη, αὔτη ἐπιτιθεμένη τῷ ὀμφαλῷ, κινεῖ τὴν κάτω κοιλίαν· ἐπὶ δὲ τοῦ θώρακος καὶ τοῦ στομάχου ἐπιτιθεμένη ἔμετον κινεῖ, μέχρις οὗ ἄρη τὸ σπληνίον· ἔμμηνα δὲ ἄγει ταῖς γυναιξὶ καὶ ἔμβρυα φθείρει, κατὰ τοῦ ὑπογαστρίου καὶ τῆς ὀσφύος ἐπιτιθεμένη. ἡ δὲ σύνθεσις αὔτη. κόκκου κνιδίου < γ΄ λίθου ἀσίου < ι΄ ἐλλεβόρου λευκοῦ < δ΄ αἰγείου στέατος < ε΄ ἐλατηρίου < δ΄ τιθυμάλλου ὀποῦ < δ΄ ἀμόργης < ιβ΄ χολῆς ταυρείας < ιβ΄ ἀφρονίτρου < ε΄ θέρμων πικρῶν ἀλεύρου Γο β΄· ἀψινθίου κόμης < β΄· τὰ μὲν ἄλλα κόπτε καὶ σῆθε λεπτοτάτῳ κοσκίνῳ, ἔπειτα λείου ἐπιβαλὼν τὴν χολήν, εἶτα τὴν ἀμόργην καὶ τήξας τὸ στέαρ κατάχεε καὶ ἑνώσας χρῶ. ** ἐπομφάλιον καθαρτικόν. Τὸ αὐτὸ καὶ ἔμετον κινεῖ ἐπιτιθέμενον . . .*	*ἐπιτιθέμενη τῷ ὀμφαλῷ, κινεῖ τὴν κάτω κοιλίαν· ἐπὶ δὲ τοῦ θώρακος καὶ τοῦ στομάχου ἐπιτιθεμένη, ἔμετον κινεῖ μέχρι οὗ ἄρῃς τὸ σπληνίον· ἔμμηνά τε ἄγει ταῖς γυναιξί· καὶ ἔμβρυα φθείρει κατὰ τοῦ ὑπογαστρίου* (E: *ἐπιγαστρίου*) *καὶ τῆς ὀσφύος ἐπιτιθέμενη· ἡ δὲ σύνθεσις, ἔστιν αὔτη· κόκκου κνιδείου, < γ΄·λίθου ἀσίου, < β΄· ἑλεβόρου λευκοῦ, < δ΄· αἰγείου στέατος, < ε΄· ἐλατηρίου· τιθυμάλου ὀποῦ, ἀνὰ < δ΄· ἀμόργης, < β΄· χολῆς ταυρείας, οὐγγ.* (*E*: <) *β΄· ἀφονίτρου < ε΄· θέρμων πικρῶν ἀλεύρου, οὐγγ. β΄· ἀψινθίου κόμης, < β΄· τὰ μὲν ἄλλα, κόπτεται καὶ σήθεται ἔπειτα λείου ἐπιβαλὼν τὴν χολήν· εἶτα τὴν ἀμόργην· καὶ τήξας τὸ στέαρ, κατάχεε· καὶ ἑνώσας, χρῶ:* ** *ἕτερον ἐπίθεμα ἐπαγγελόμενον διὰ ῥινῶν αἷμα . . .*
Aetios of Amida, *Tetrabiblos*, 3.136, ed. Olivieri (1935) I.315.26–316.1.	Vindobonensis med. gr. 17, f. 157v, l. 17–f. 158r, l. 2; ed. Mathys (1556) II.410.1–18.

part devoted to gastrointestinal diseases. The same process is followed throughout the *Medical Epitome* (book five and the second part of book six) for individual recipes or groups of them coming from one or more authors. The only criterion in terms of listing is that the recipes should be defined in relation to the kind of drugs.

Table 5.4 provides a further useful example, focusing this time on the chapter on lozenges. In this case, John's recipes are almost identical with those in the unedited *Dynameron*,[55] which, in contrast to the *Ephodia tou Apodēmountos*, presents the recipes according to drug type. Despite the poor quality of the text and the different versions given for the names of some

[55] My access to the *Dynameron* is based on the earliest surviving manuscript of the work, i.e. Parisinus gr. 2243 (AD 1339) and the early printed Latin edition by Fuchs (1549). On Parisinus gr. 2243, see Mondrain (1999). Note that Parisinus gr. 2243 preserves some peculiar readings, e.g. '*ἀμύδου*' instead of '*ἀμύλου*', '*κύτρινον*' instead of '*κίτρινον*'. When the final manuscript of this book was already at an advanced stage of preparation, I was able to access Valiakos' edition (2019). I subsequently replaced my transcriptions from Parisinus gr. 2243 with the text of Valiakos' edition.

Table 5.4. Lozenge recipes in Myrepsos' and John's works

Number of sample recipe following the order and name in John's work	Nicholas Myrepsos, *Dynameron*, T.56–61, ed. Valiakos (2019) 1013.15–1015.13.	John Zacharias Aktouarios, *Medical Epitome*, 5, Vindobonensis med. gr. 17, f. 118v, l. 12–f. 119r, l. 1; ed. Mathys (1556) II.335.28–336.25.
A Lozenge of the Indian rhubarb	*. . . ζωμὸν τὸ ἀρκοῦν:* ** *τροχίσκος, ὁ διὰ ῥέου μπαρμπάρου· ὠφελεῖ, πρὸς ὑπόχονδριακούς, τοὺς ἐμπεπλησμένους ὕλην· ἡπατικούς· σπληνικούς· στόμαχον ἀτονούμενον, ἐν δυνάμει· ἔχει: ῥόδα· ἀψίνθιον· ῥέου βαρβάρου, ἀνὰ δράμ γ´· σπόδιον· στάχος· σχοίνου ἄνθος· λάκκα· εὐπατορίου ζωμόν, ἀνὰ δράμ α´· σάνδαλον κίτρινον· κρόκου· ξυλοκασίας· τετράγκανθον· μαστίχης· ἀνὰ σκρόπουλα β´· τρίψας ταῦτα πάντα καλῶς, ζύμωσον μετὰ χυλοῦ μαράθρου τὸ ἀρκοῦν καὶ πλάσσε τροχίσκους· ἐπὶ δὲ τῆς χρείας δίδου ἐξ αὐτῶν, μετὰ ἀποζέματος μαράθρου τὸ ἀρκοῦν· χρῶ.*** ***τροχίσκος, ὁ δι' ἀνίσου . . .*** ***τροχίσκος ὁ δι' ἀψινθίας . . .***	*. . . τῇ κράσει πέφυκε:* ** *τροχίσκος ὁ διὰ τοῦ ἰνδικοῦ ῥέου ὠφέλιμος εἰς ἔμφραξιν ἥπατος καὶ σπληνός· δυναμοῖ καὶ τὸν στόμαχον· ῥόδα ξηρά· ἀψίνθιον· ῥέον ἰνδικόν, ἀνὰ* (*ἐξαγ.*) *β´·* *σπόδιον· στάχος ἰνδικόν· σχινάνθος· λαχᾶν κεκαθαρισμένον· χυλὸν εὐπατωρίου, ἀνὰ* < *α´· σάνταλον κίτρινον· καὶ κρόκον· καὶ κασίας τὸ διπλοῦν· καὶ τραγακάνθης· μαστίχης ἀνὰ* (*ἐξαγ.*) s″· *κόψας σήσας, φύρασον μετὰ χυλοῦ τοῦ μαλάθρου· καὶ ποίει τροχίσκον· ποθήτωσαν μεθ' ὕδατος τοῦ λαχᾶν* (E: *λαχάνου*) *καὶ ὀξοσάχαρ:* **
B Lozenge of agrimony	** *τροχίσκος, ὁ δι' εὐπατορίου· ἐνὲς καλοῦσιν Ἰταλίᾳ γλῶσσῃ, ἰπιλατζιόνι· ὠφελεῖ πρὸς ἡπατικούς· σπληνικούς· στομαχικοὺς καὶ τοὺς μέλλοντας ἐν πάθει καχεξίας ἐμπεσεῖν· ἔχει: ἀψίνθιον· σχοίνου ἄνθος· ζωμὸν εὐπατορίου· ῥόδων· μαράθρου· μαστίχης, ἀνὰ δράμ γ´· ῥέου μπαρμπάρου· ἄνισον· τετράγκανθον· σάνδαλον κίτρινον· σπόδιον, ἀνὰ δράμ α´ καὶ ἥμισυ· τρίψας ταῦτα καλῶς, ζύμωσον, μετὰ ζωμοῦ ἀντιδίου τὸ ἀρκοῦν· καὶ πλάττε τροχίσκους· ἀνὰ ἐξάγ α´· καὶ λαβὼν δίδου ἐξ αὐτοῦ, μετὰ ἀντιδίου ζωμόν ἢ δροσάτου ὀξύνου τοῦ ἐπονομαζομένου ὀξυσάχαρ ἢ ὀξύνου ῥοϊδίου ζωμὸν καὶ οὕτως σκευάσας χρῶ.* ** ***τροχίσκος ὁ διὰ ῥόδων . . .***	** *ἕτερος δι' εὐπατωρίου· ὀνίνησιν εἰς ἧπαρ καὶ στόμαχον· καὶ ἀποφράττει τὰς ἐμπνευματώσεις· καὶ εἰς τὸ ῥίγος τοῦ* (E: *τὸ*) *ἀποφλέγματος πυρετοῦ· ἀψίνθιον· σχινάνθος· χυλὸν εὐπατωρίου· ῥόδα· μαλαθρόσπερμα καὶ μαστίχη· ἀνὰ δραχμὰς δ´· ἄνισον καὶ τραγάκανθαν λευκήν, ἀνὰ* <*´ β´· σάνταλον κίτρινον· καὶ σπόδιον· ἀνὰ* (*ἐξαγ.*) *α´· κόψας σήσας φύρασον μετὰ χυλοῦ ἰντύβων· καὶ ποίει τροχίσκους· ποθήτωσαν μεθ' ὕδατος τοῦ λαχᾶν καὶ ὀξυμέλιτος:***

C **Lozenge of *spodion* (ash)**	**τροχίσκος, ὁ διὰ σποδίου ἐπονομαζόμενος· ὠφελεῖ, πρὸς θέρμην ἥπατος· πυρετοὺς ὀξεῖς καὶ καυσώδεις· θαυμαστόν· ἔχει: ῥόδα, δράμ γ΄· σπόδιον· ἀνδράχνης σπέρμα· χυλὸν γλυκορίζου, ἀνὰ δράμ β΄· τετράγκανθον· ἀμύδου, ἀνὰ δράμαν α΄· σάχαρ, δραμ δ΄· τρίψας ταῦτα καλῶς, ζύμωσον μετὰ ψυλλίου τοῦ ζωμοῦ καὶ πλάττε τροχίσκους καὶ δίδου ἐπὶ τῆς χρείας· μετὰ ζωμοῦ τοῦ ψυλλίου**	** τροχίσκος ὁ διὰ τοῦ σποδίου· ὠφελῶν εἰς ὀξὺν πυρετόν· καὶ εἰς θερμότητα ἥπατος· καὶ εἰς τὴν δίψαν τὴν συνεχῆ· ῥόδα, (ἐξαγ.) δ΄· σπόδιον· ἀνδράχνης σπέρμα· χυλὸν γλυκυρίζης, ἀνὰ (ἐξαγ.) β΄· τραγάκανθαν λευκήν· καὶ ἄμυλον· ἀνὰ < α΄ s″· σάχαρ, (ἐξαγ.) β΄· φύρασον μετὰ χυλοῦ ψυλλίου· ἡ πόσις μεθ' ὕδατος τῶν ῥοῶν: **

substances—as in the case of Indian rhubarb,[56] described as 'barbarian' rhubarb in the *Dynameron*—a direct textual connection can be established, although we should not exclude the possibility that both the author of the *Dynameron* and John excerpted from a common source as yet unedited and unidentified.

4.2 First part of book six

As has already been noted above, the first part of book six is the only part in the pharmacology where John follows an *a capite ad calcem* order. The main source of this part is Galen's text *On the Composition of Drugs According to Places*, where the various drugs are presented in connection with the relevant part of the body. All the instances of first-person singular/plural are copied directly from Galen.[57] The names of other physicians provided by Galen are

[56] On various kinds of rhubarb used in medieval medicine, see Lev and Amar (2008: 259–61); and Foust (1994) on Chinese medicinal rhubarb. A glossary surviving in two manuscripts, Vindobonensis med. gr. 25 (second half of the fifteenth century) and Athous Iberiticus 182 (sixteenth century), refers to the origin of Indian rhubarb being either in India or Arabia, ed. Delatte (1939) II.357.1: '*ῥέον ἰνδικὸν τὸ ἀπὸ Ἰνδίας καὶ Ἀραβίας*'. A special control tax, the *garbellatura* (see n. 123, below), was levied on barbarian rhubarb (*ribarbero*) in fourteenth-century Constantinople, set at three carats per hundred pounds, which is the same as that paid for cubeb pepper, galangal, and aloe wood, according to Francesco Balducci Pegolotti, *La Pratica della Mercatura*, ed. Evans (1936) 44.30.

[57] For example, see the following Galenic statement on preparing a certain drug, *On the Composition of Drugs According to Places*, 1.2, ed. Kühn (1826) XII.421.8–10: '*. . . τὸ λάδανον ἐγὼ βρέξας ἐν οἴνῳ βραχεῖ ἐλείωσα τὸ στέαρ, τήξας ἐφ' ὕδατος ἀτμῷ, εἶτα τοῦ ὄνου τὸ μόριον ὀπτὸν ξύε . . .*', which occurs in almost identical form in John's text, *Medical Epitome*, 6, Vindobonensis med. gr. 17, f. 171v, ll. 9–11: '*. . . τὸ λάδανον ἐγὼ βρέξας ἐν οἴνῳ βραχεῖ ἐλείωσα τὸ στέαρ μίξας· εἶτα ὄνου τὸ μόριον ὀπτὸν ξύε . . .*'; ed. Mathys (1556) II.444.13–16.

cited here as well.[58] Furthermore, it should be pointed out that, although in the other parts of the *Medical Epitome* (and in his other works, i.e. *On Urines* and *On Psychic Pneuma*)[59] he never mentions his sources, here he does not hesitate to refer repeatedly to Galen briefly stating, for example: 'Galen says...', followed by a Galenic excerpt.[60] Together with some formulaic introductory phrases, this actually constitutes John's only intervention.

Below I present a passage from the drugs for nasal haemorrhage followed by the discussion of ophthalmic affections, which will help us to understand John's thoughts and writing methods in the first part of book six. The printed text is from Galen's text *On the Composition of Drugs According to Places*; the underlined parts are those copied by John, while those in bold are John's additions.

Galen, *On the Composition of Drugs According to Places*, 3.3 & 4.4, ed. Kühn (1826) XII.695.10–16 & 715.10–13;

JZA, *Medical Epitome*, 6, Vindobonensis med. gr. 17, f. 186r, l. 17–f. 186v, l. 25; ed. Mathys (1556) II.478.27–479.21:

(695) (***Πρὸς δὲ τὰς τῆς ῥινὸς αἱμορραγίας***)... *ἴσχαιμος ἡ μεγάλη. ♃ μίσυος κυπρίου < ζʹ. χαλκάνθου < ζʹ. φλοιοῦ πίτυος < δʹ. λεπίδος χαλκοῦ < δʹ. μάννης λιβάνου < δʹ. οἱ δὲ < ιεʹ. χαλκοῦ κεκαυμένου < ιεʹ. χαλκίτεως < ιεʹ. ἀσβέστου < ηʹ. οἱ δὲ < μʹ. γύψου πεφωγμένης < δʹ* (**ϵʹ**)*. οἱ δὲ < ηʹ. λείοις χρῶ.*[61] (***εἰς πᾶσαν αἱμορραγίαν.***) *ἴσχαιμος Ἀφρόδα. ♃ χαλκίτεως < στʹ. μάννης λιβάνου < βʹ. ῥητίνης τερμινθίνης φρυκτῆς < δʹ. οἱ δὲ γʹ. λείοις χρῶ*... (***Περὶ τῶν ἐν ὀφθαλμοῖς παθῶν· ὅσα τὲ καὶ δι᾽ ὁποίας αἰτίας συνίστανται, καὶ ὅπως ταῦτα διαγνωστέον, εἴρηται πρότερον· νυνὶ δὲ περὶ τῆς θεραπείας αὐτῶν καὶ οἷς χρηστέον φαρμάκοις ῥηθήσεται· τὰ ἀξιολογώτερα τοῖς τε καθ᾽ ἡμᾶς παλαιοῖς τε καὶ νεωτέροις ἕλλησι καὶ τῶν βαρβάρων τοῖς δοκιμωτάτοις· ὅσα εἰς ἡμᾶς ᾖ καὶ λυσιτελέστατα φάρμακα· ἐντεῦθεν οὖν ἀναλαβόντες τὸν λόγον, περὶ τῶν καθ᾽ ἕκαστα φαρμάκων φήσομεν· ὥσπερ καὶ ἐν ἄλλοις πεποιήκαμεν***

[58] For example, Galen is prescribing here a recipe from Archigenes: Galen, *On the Composition of Drugs According to Places*, 7.7, ed. Kühn (1826) XII.954.6–8: '*Ἀρχιγένης δὲ περὶ αὐτῶν οὕτως ἔγραψεν. Ἐπὶ δὲ τῶν λεγομένων ἐσχαρῶν ἰδίως συμφωνεῖ*...'. This passage occurs in identical form in John's text, *Medical Epitome*, 6, Vindobonensis med. gr. 17, f. 205v, ll. 8–9; ed. Mathys (1556) II.514.21–2: '*Ἀρχιγένης δέ, ἐπὶ τῶν λεγομένων ἐσχαρῶν· ἰδίως συμφωνεῖ*...'.

[59] See also Chapter 2, nn. 42 and 139.

[60] See the following passage: JZA, *Medical Epitome*, 6, Vindobonensis med. gr. 17, f. 168r, ll. 16–17: '...*ὅ γε μὴν Γαληνὸς φησὶ περὶ τοῦ πάθους τούτου διεξιών, ὡς ἐγὼ ἀεὶ διὰ τῆς ἱερᾶς ἐκάθηρα·*'; ed. Mathys (1856) II.435.25–7. The first part is John's introduction while the underlined part, which includes the first-person singular pronoun, is identical to Galen's text in *On the Composition of Drugs According to Places*, 1.2, ed. Kühn (1826) XII.382.13–14: '*ἐγὼ δ᾽ ἀεὶ διὰ τῆς ἱερᾶς ἐκάθηρα*...'.

[61] John's text reads as follows, *Medical Epitome*, 6, Vindobonensis med. gr. 17, f. 186v, l. 9–13: '*ἴσχαιμος ἡ μεγάλη μίσυος· χαλκάνθου, ἀνὰ < ζʹ· φλοιοῦ πίτυος· λεπίδος χαλκῷ* (E: *χαλκοῦ*)*· μάννης λιβάνου· ἀνὰ < δʹ· χαλκῷ* (E: *χαλκοῦ*) *κεκαυμένου· χαλκίτεως < ιεʹ· ἀσβέστου < ηʹ· οἱ δέ, μʹ· γύψου πεφρυγμένου, < ϵʹ· λείοις χρῶ·*'.

πρὸς διορισμοὺς (***E***: **προσδιορισμοὺς**) **τινὰς τῶν δοκιμωτάτων** (E: **τοῦ δοκιμωτάτου**) **τῶν πώποτε ἰατρῶν παλαιῶν τε καὶ νέων ἑλλήνων τὲ καὶ βαρβάρων· προεκτεθεικότες** (E: **προεκτεθεικότι**) **τῷ λόγῳ·**) (715) *φλεγμονῆς μὲν οὖν ἔτι κατὰ τὸν οφθαλμὸν* (**τῶν ὀφθαλμῶν**) *οὔσης ἢ καί τινος ὀδύνης, τὰ διὰ λιβανωτοῦ τε κολλύρια*(**-υρίου**) *καὶ τῶν πεπλυμμένων μεταλλικῶν καὶ τῶν ἀδήκτων χυλῶν*[62] *προσφέρεται*...

(695) (**On <therapeutic advice> for nasal haemorrhage**)... The great *ischaimos*: ♃ Cyprian copper ore, seven <; copper sulfate, seven <; bark of pine, four <; flake of copper, four <; powder of frankincense, four <‘; others <suggest> fifteen <; burned copper, fifteen <; rock alum, fifteen <; unslaked lime, eight <; others <suggest> forty <; roasted chalk, four (**five**) <; others <suggest> eight <; pound and use (**for any haemorrhage**). *Ischaimos Aphroda*: ♃ rock alum, six <; powder of frankincense, two <; turpentine, four <; other <suggest> three <; pound and use... (**On <drugs> for eye affections. It has already been said before how many the various <eye> affections are and from what sort of causes they arise, and how to diagnose them. Now, <an account> will be given of the therapy of these <affections> and the drugs which one must use, i.e. the most worthy of mention among our most notable ancient and recent Greek sources and the barbarian ones, and all those drugs which <seem> to us to give the best result. And so from now onwards let us talk about these particular drugs, just as in other cases, in exposing the account, we have undertaken some qualifications <for the drugs> of the most notable ancient and recent authors, both Greek and barbarian.**) (715) and so in the case of an eye inflammation which may be accompanied by some kind of pain, the collyria of frankincense, of threadbare metals, and of pungent juices, are given...

John includes Galen's recipe for the great *ischaimos* ('styptic')—an antihaemorrhagic agent—in his chapter on nasal haemorrhage, while he chooses not to copy the next one, which deals with the *ischaimos Aphroda*.[63] Then he provides a couple of introductory sentences. Afterwards he starts copying Galen again, having left out almost twenty pages in Kühn's edition of this particular Galenic treatise, in this case referring to some eye medicaments. Thus the whole process of condensing is based on minimizing the actual number of recipes.

[62] John's text reads as follows, *Medical Epitome*, 6, Vindobonensis med. gr. 17, f. 186v, ll. 23–5: '*φλεγμονῆς οὖν ἔτι κατὰ τῶν οφθαλμῶν οὔσης ἢ καί τινος ὀδύνης, διὰ λιβανωτοῦ κολλυρίου καὶ τῶν πεπλυμένων μεταλλικῶν τε καὶ ἀδήκτων χυλῶν·*'.

[63] Although John's presentation of his material shows that he follows Galen's *On the Composition of Drugs According to Places*, it is worth noting that both the recipe for the great *ischaimos* and that of the *ischaimos Aphroda* also appear in Galen's *On the Composition of Drugs According to Kind*, 5.13, ed. Kühn (1827) XIII.838.1–7. The fact that Galen sometimes presents the same recipes in both these works has been noted by other scholars in the past, including Vogt (2008: 311).

I selected this particular chapter because it is the only place in the first part of book six where John makes a statement about the sources of his recipes. In particular, John once again refers to barbarian, non-Greek sources, together with ancient and more recent Greek treatises. However, there is no sign of adopting any foreign material in his chapter on eye affections or any other chapter of the first part of book six. In other parts of his work, where he has referred to a non-Greek source, he clearly gives a good deal of such material, as we shall see in the next section of the present chapter. Perhaps John did not in the end manage to cover the external agents for eye affections in as much detail as he wanted and his unfulfilled promise to include some non-Greek material in this part, too, may indicate a partly unfinished project.[64]

5. JOHN'S FOREIGN SOURCES

Substances coming from faraway places, or which needed to be obtained by the physicians themselves to avoid adulteration, could be difficult to purchase and usually constituted the most precious items in their cabinets.[65] Running them a close second were various recipes for composite drugs combining a number of substances, which always excited physicians, who wanted not only to cure their patients with effective cures, but also with ones that differed from those of rival doctors. The recently discovered Galenic text, *Avoiding Distress*, presents, among other significant details, a vivid image of how ancient physicians thought about pharmacological material and provides important information on the availability of various substances and recipes in the ancient world.[66] In reporting his losses in the fire at the Temple of Peace in AD 192, Galen considered various quantities of drugs together with his medical instruments among the most valuable parts of his private collection.[67]

[64] We know that John's *Medical Epitome*, and in particular books 2–6, was his last known work. For a discussion of the dating of John's corpus, see Chapter 1, Section 4.2.1.

[65] See Galen, *On the Capacities of Simple Drugs*, 10.2 and 10.34, ed. Kühn (1826) XII.171.9–175.8 and XII.238.3–241.11, who reports his trips to Lemnos and Cyprus to get hold of Lemnian earth and copper sulphate respectively.

[66] See, for example, Galen, *Avoiding Distress*, 34–6, ed. Boudon-Millot, Jouanna, and Pietrobelli (2010) 12.8–20 = 15, ed. Kotzia and Sotiroudis (2010) 72.165–73.176, tr. Nutton (2014: 88–9): '[Teuthras] had obtained the parchments belonging to a doctor called Eumenes, who was himself also from Pergamum and was a particular connoisseur of many drugs among all doctors. These recipes had been collected in one place from all over the world during his travels before he settled in Rome until his death . . . If someone had a remarkable drug, I could get hold of it without difficulty by drawing on these collections and offering two or three similar ones in exchange.'

[67] Galen, *Avoiding Distress*, 2, ed. Boudon-Millot, Jouanna, and Pietrobelli (2010) 4.1–4 = 6, ed. Kotzia and Sotiroudis (2010) 67.24–8, informs his readers about the loss of his store of drugs and, in particular, a large quantity of theriac and cinnamon.

Although John does not provide evidence of any research trips or how he collected his recipes, he shows an awareness of other cultures and great interest in embellishing his medical cabinet. This material either involves sugar-based potions, such as julep and syrup, or recipes with systematic reference to newly introduced oriental substances. These are elements missing from ancient and earlier Byzantine medical works, and result from the gradual diffusion of Arabic pharmacological lore in Byzantium from the eleventh/twelfth century onwards.

Some of John's sources and also passages related to the origin of his sources have already been cited above. Another statement from his discussion on antidotes will help us to better contextualize his material:

> From now onwards we will give an account of the remaining antidotes. Those that have been composed by various ancient and more recent Greek authors as well as barbarian ones. I will not present all of them so as to avoid overextending this book. Thus I will refer only to those that seem to me more familiar or more useful and much more effective.[68]

We can see that John makes a distinction between Greek and non-Greek sources. For the Greek material John considers ancient works, but also more recent ones. Table 5.5 presents all the sources so far identified. Among the ancient sources Dioscorides and Galen must certainly be included. Early Byzantine authors, such as Aetios of Amida and Paul of Aegina, may be associated with his mentions of more recent Greek works. John uses the term *barbaros* ('barbarian') to refer to foreign authors and sources that have been provided in Greek translation.[69]

This distinction between Greeks (*Hellēnes*) or Byzantine Greeks (*Rhōmaioi*) and those living outside the Empire, i.e. 'barbarians' (*barbaroi*), was commonplace among Byzantine authors. Muslims were often designated 'barbarians', while sometimes even Christian Latins or Orthodox Bulgarians could be thus described.[70] John chose to use the generic label 'barbarian' to denote that they came from another culture. More explicitly, he uses the expression *barbarē phōnē* ('barbarian language') twice to refer to Greek terms derived

[68] JZA, *Medical Epitome*, 5, Vindobonensis med. gr. 17, f. 125v, l. 23–f. 126r, l. 1: '*ἐφεξεῖς* (E: *ἐφεξῆς*) *δὲ περὶ τῶν λοιπῶν ἐροῦμεν ἀντιδότων· ὅσαι διαφόροις παλαιοῖς καὶ νεωτέροις ἕλλησί τε βαρβάροις συνετέθησαν· οὐ πάσας δὲ ἐκθήσομαι εἰς μῆκος γὰρ οὐ μέτριον ἂν ἐπιταθείη τὸ βιβλίον· ἀλλ' ὅσαι μοι δοκοῦσι τούτων γνωριμώτεραι ἢ χρησιμώτεραι καὶ πολυχρηστότεραι·*'; ed. Mathys (1556) II.353.5–11.

[69] See the passage above (n. 47), in which John mentions that he had consulted 'barbarian' works in Greek translation. John refers to 'barbarian' authors/physicians two more times, see Section 4.2, above, and n. 72, below. There are also two explicit references to the 'barbarian' language, see nn. 72 and 101, below.

[70] On the term 'barbarian' to describe those living outside the Empire in a Byzantine context, see *ODB*, s.v. barbarians; and the recent discussion by Shukurov (2016: 28–37). See also Kaldellis (2007: 267–71); and Page (2008: 43–6). Kaldellis (2013: 82–183) also offers further examples from middle and late Byzantine literature.

Table 5.5. Overview of John's sources, *Medical Epitome*, Books Five & Six[71]

Book Five	
Potions on fevers	Many recipes common to Chariton's list of compound drugs, Parisinus gr 2240, ff. 18v–30r.
Juleps and syrups	Many recipes common to Chariton's list of compound drugs, Parisinus gr 2240, ff. 18v–30r.
Lozenges and pills	Excerpts from Galen's *On the Composition of Drugs According to Places*; many recipes common to the relevant part of the *Dynameron*, chapter T(lozenges); and excerpts from unidentified source(s).
Antidotes	Excerpts from Galen's *On Antidotes*; many recipes common to the relevant part of the *Dynameron*, chapter A(antidotes); and excerpts from unidentified source(s).
Wines	Excerpts from Dioscorides' *De Materia Medica*, book five.
Simple purgatives	Excerpts from Aetios of Amida's *Tetrabiblos*, book three; excerpts from unidentified source on oriental vegetal substances (e.g. various kinds of myrobalan).
Composite purgatives	Excerpts from Galen's *On the Composition of Drugs According to Places*; excerpts from Aetios of Amida's *Tetrabiblos*, book three; excerpts from the *Ephodia tou Apodēmountos*; and excerpts from unidentified source(s).
Poisons	Excerpts from Paul of Aegina's *Epitome*, book five.
Book Six	
On affections of the surface of the head	Excerpts from Galen's *On the Composition of Drugs According to Places.*
On head affections On ear affections On nasal affections On eye affections On facial affections On oral affections	
On skin affections and ulcers	Excerpts from Paul of Aegina's *Epitome*, book four.
Plasters	Excerpts from Galen's *On the Composition of Drugs According to Places* and *On the Composition of Drugs According to Kind*; and excerpts from Aetios of Amida's *Tetrabiblos*, book fifteen.
Pessaries	Excerpts from Aetios of Amida's *Tetrabiblos*, book sixteen; and excerpts from unidentified source(s).
Oils	Excerpts from Dioscorides' *De Materia Medica*, book one; and excerpts from Aetios of Amida's *Tetrabiblos*, book one.
Venomous animals	Excerpts from Paul of Aegina's *Epitome*, book five or excerpts from unidentified source(s).

[71] There is considerable variation in the recipes and their order in the manuscripts. This table does not aim to provide exhaustive identification of John's use of earlier works but to give the modern reader an idea of the variety of material that can be identified in the absence of an edition.

from Arabic,[72] thus confirming the origin of the foreign sources. The Greek translation of Ibn al-Jazzār's *Zād al-Musāfir wa-Qūt al-Ḥāḍir*, *Ephodia tou Apodēmountos*, is one of those 'barbarian', Arab sources mentioned by John. There are also parts from as yet unidentified literature, which may have been derived from no longer extant or unedited sources.

5.1 Sugar-based dosage forms

Before the introduction of sugar,[73] honey was used as a sweetener and preservative in composite drugs.[74] Honey or various mixtures of honey with water (*hydromeli* and *melikra(/ē)ton*), vinegar (*oxymeli*), wine (*oinomeli*), and less often with apple juice (*melimēlon*), juice of unripe grapes (*omphakomeli*), or juice of roses (*rhodomeli*)[75] could be administered on their own or used as a base for the preparation of composite drugs. Medical authors such as Dioscorides, Pliny the Elder (AD 23/24–79), and Galen refer to *sakchar*[*on*] in Greek or *sacc*[*h*]*aron* in Latin, which is perhaps the first reference in history to granulated sugar.[76] However, they show very little familiarity with this ingredient,

[72] The first is used to refer to the origin of the Greek terms used for syrups and juleps, see n. 101, below. The other is related to the various kinds of myrobalan (on myrobalans, see nn. 127–8, below). John states, *Medical Epitome*, 5, Vindobonensis med. gr. 17, f. 149r, ll. 2–5: 'τό τε μπελίλιζ [for the Arabic *balīlaj*]· τῇ βαρβάρῳ φωνῇ καλούμενον· καὶ τὸ ἔμπλιτζι [for the Arabic *ʾamlaj*]· ὅθεν καὶ τὰ πέντε ταῦτα μιγνύντες οἱ τῶν βαρβάρων ἰατροὶ σοφοί…'; ed. Mathys (1556) II.390.14–18. See Martínez Manzano (2015), who has interestingly shown that this passage from John's work has been inserted, at some point in the fourteenth century, in a branch of Dioscorides' *De Materia Medica* resulting in an interpolation in the ancient text that is evident even in the Aldine edition of 1499. In two cases, both parts of the as yet unidentified material in John's *Medical Epitome*, we can find the use of the term *latinos* (Latin). It is used with reference to a particular recipe and it does not relate to any of John's statements on barbarians. See JZA, *Medical Epitome*, 5, Vindobonensis med. gr. 17, f. 136r, l. 1: 'ἀντίδοτος ἡ διὰ καμερῶν κατὰ λατίνους· ποιεῖ δυσπνοϊκοῖς· ἀρτηριακοῖς·'; ed. Mathys (1556) II.367.23–4; and JZA, *Medical Epitome*, 5, Vindobonensis med. gr. 17, 5, f. 138v, ll. 14–17: 'εἴλιγμα πρὸς ἐπάνοδον ὑγρότητος…λέγεται παρὰ λατίνοις, ῥεσταυράτζις…'; ed. Mathys (1556) II.372.1–6.

[73] A substantially extended version of this section, including a detailed examination of the introduction and dissemination of sugar-based potions in Byzantium based on evidence from a wide variety of unpublished medieval Greek sources, is forthcoming in the form of an independent study. See Bouras-Vallianatos (forthcoming).

[74] On the medicinal uses of honey, see Balander (1993: 107–11).

[75] On these and other less common mixtures, such as *apomeli* (a mixture of honey and water), *thalassomeli* (a mixture of honey with sea water), or *melititēs* (a mixture of honey with wine), see, for example, Dioscorides 1.115 and 5.7–27, ed. Wellmann (1907) I.108.15–109.12 and (1914) III.11.15–22.8. For liquid dosage forms based on honey mixtures, see, for example, Galen, *On the Composition of Drugs According to Places*, 8.8, 9.1, and *passim*, ed. Kühn (1826) XIII.206.5–11, XIII.240.17–241.7. See also the *hydrorosaton*, a mixture of the juice of roses with water and honey, which appears in Oribasios, *Medical Collections*, 5.33, ed. Raeder (1928) I.1.152.5–9; Aetios of Amida, *Tetrabiblos*, 5.140, ed. Olivieri (1950) II.116.13–23; and Paul of Aegina, *Epitome*, 3.32, ed. Heiberg, (1924) II.332.17–18.

[76] On sugar in Greek and Latin medical authors, see Dalby (2003: 314–15). The Greek and Latin term is derived from the Sanskrit *śarkarā*; see LSJ, s.v. σάκχαρ. The first-century AD anonymous author of the *Periplus of the Red Sea*, 14, ed. Casson (1989) 58.7–16, most

which is described as a less sweet version of honey with laxative properties.[77] Galen's references were uncritically reproduced in the works of Oribasios and Paul of Aegina.[78]

Sugar cane was introduced from India to Persia, and its cultivation gradually spread throughout the Islamic East, especially from the seventh/eighth century onwards, a period in which the advancement of new refining techniques made granulated sugar more widely available.[79] Sugar became extremely popular as an excipient in liquid pharmaceutical dosage forms, mainly used as a preservative and also as a sweetener in order to alleviate the bitter taste of other ingredients. It is of higher purity than honey, thus a smaller quantity has a stronger preservative action;[80] it is also less susceptible to changes of temperature, ensuring greater homogeneity and better fluidity in the final product. Sugar is also available all year round unlike honey. The Islamic medical tradition is credited with the introduction and widespread distribution of various sugar-based, liquid, pharmaceutical dosage forms.[81] Among the most popular forms were juleps and syrups. The Arabic word *julāb* comes from the Persian *gul* (rose) and *āb* (water).[82] The original julep was made of

probably an Egyptian Greek merchant, who recounts his experiences in an attempt to provide a guide for traders, refers to *sakchari* as an export from the Indian port of Barygaza (modern Bharuch) to the Arabian Peninsula, although it is not clear whether he is referring to cane sugar or granulated sugar; cf. Warmington (1974: 208–10). On maritime trade routes from Asia to Europe in the early centuries AD, see Miller (1969: 119–52); and McLaughlin (2014: 73–94).

77 Dioscorides, *De Materia Medica*, 2.82, ed. Wellmann (1907) 1.167.4–9: 'there is a kind of solidified (*pepēgotos*) honey in India and Arabia Felix, that is called sugar (*sakcharon*), and is found in reeds, like in consistency to salt and brittle when broken between the teeth, as salt is'; Pliny the Elder, *The Natural History*, 12.32, ed. Ernout (1949) 29.16–20; Galen, *Therapeutic Method*, 9.4, ed. Kühn (1825) X.568.1; and Galen, *On the Capacities of Simple Drugs*, 7.9, ed. Kühn (1826) XII.71.2–9. On the debatable nature of Greek and Roman accounts of sugar, see Ouerfelli (2008: 15–19); and Sato (2015: 16–17). Cf. André (1981: 186, n. 2); and André and Filliozat (1986: 339, n. 3; and 360–1, n. 160), who argue that the early use of the word in Greek and Roman authors refers to what is usually called *tabasheer*, a white silicon accretion collected from the nodal joints of some species of bamboo.

78 Oribasios, *Medical Collections*, 15.1, ed. Raeder (1929) I.2.264.18–22; Paul of Aegina, *Epitome*, 7.3 and cf. 2.53, ed. Heiberg (1924) II.241.3–6 and (1921) I.122.1–4. It is worth noting that in Byzantine sources the term is mostly attested as *sachar*, following the ancient Greek *sakchar[on]* deriving from Sanskrit (see n. 76, above), but reflecting the vernacular pronunciation after the simplification of the consonant cluster (*κχ*/kch) to a single consonant (*χ*/ch).

79 Watson (1983: 24–30); Ouerfelli (2008: 19–24); and Sato (2015: 18–21).

80 The microbial cells of bacteria die in sugar solutions due to plasmolysis. On plasmolysis, see Ruhland (1955: 383–4). Sugar is still used nowadays for the preservation of jams and jellies.

81 Ouerfelli (2008: 503–21). On sugar-based potions in medieval Islamic medicine, see Levey (1973: 75–8); and Ouerfelli (2008: 549–67), who provides plenty of examples of sugar-based composite drugs from a large number of medieval Arabic and Latin sources.

82 Fellmann (1986: 201).

sugar, water, and rose water,[83] obtained by the distillation of roses.[84] An equally popular sugar-based potion of higher viscosity was syrup (Ar. *sharāb*), which contains more sugar (or occasionally honey, if sugar was not readily available),[85] water, and one or more kinds of fruit juices or extracts of flowers.[86]

By the tenth century sugar-cane cultivation had reached Syria, Palestine, and Egypt, gradually expanding to the large Mediterranean islands of Cyprus, Crete, Rhodes, and Sicily, and even Andalusia.[87] The earliest reference to a sugar-based potion in a medical context in Byzantine literature[88] is found in *Hippiatrica*.[89] The recipe belongs to recension B of the *Hippiatrica*, whose earliest witness, i.e. Berolinensis Phillippicus gr. 1538, dates to the tenth century and is connected with the imperial scriptorium of Constantine VII.[90] Anne McCabe has shown that, although the compilation was most probably first written down in the fifth/sixth century AD, the tenth-century re-edition includes notable mentions of oriental *materia medica* such as musk, ambergris, and galangal, which are not found in earlier medical texts.[91] The first Byzantine work to give a significant account of the role of sugar as a medicinal substance and its use in potions is the above-mentioned *Treatise on the Capacities of Foodstuffs* by Symeon Seth. A special chapter is also

[83] On distillation and the production of rose water in the medieval Islamic world, see al-Hassan and Hill (1992: 141–4); García-Sánchez (1998); and Sanagustin (2012).

[84] See, for example, the recipe by Ibn Sīnā, *The Canon of Medicine* (*Kitāb al-Qānūn fī al-Ṭibb*), 5.6, (1593) II.212, which consists of one *mann* (816 g) of sugar and four fluid ounces of water heated over a fire with the addition of two fluid ounces of rose water.

[85] Ouerfelli (2008: 553–4, n. 275; and cf. 558, n. 301). A small quantity of honey or lemon juice could sometimes be added to sugar-based potions in order to prevent recrystallization of the sugar; see examples of such recipes in Chipman (2010: 105–7).

[86] On syrups, see Fellmann (1986: 269–71). For examples of recipes, see the long list of 144 examples of syrups in al-Kūhīn al-ʿAṭṭār, *The Management of the* [*Pharmacist's*] *Shop* (*Minhāj al-Dukkān*), ed. al-ʿĀṣī (1992) 17ff; an English translation of the names of syrups accompanied by details of its indications and ingredients is provided by Chipman (2010: 185–96). Al-Kūhīn al-ʿAṭṭār aptly described pharmacy as 'the craft of perfume and syrups'; on this and the role of syrups in the practice of thirteenth- and fourteenth-century pharmacy in the Islamic world, see Chipman (2007).

[87] See the comprehensive study by Ouerfelli (2008: 31–140), with reference to earlier studies. For a brief overview, see Phillips (1986).

[88] Perhaps the earliest reference to a liquid concoction involving sugar is found in a non-medical Byzantine text, the so-called *Oneirokritikon* ascribed to Achmet, 195, ed. Drexl (1925) 150.21–3. This is a dream book which was put together by a Greek compiler at some point after 843 and before the late eleventh century, but most probably in the tenth century; see Mavroudi (2002: 1–5).

[89] *Hippiatrica Berolinensia*, 129.8, ed. Oder and Hoppe (1924) I.386.15–17.

[90] On the association of the Berolinensis Phillippicus gr. 1538 with the tenth-century imperial scriptorium, see Irigoin (1959: 177–81); see also Doyen-Higuet (2006: 68); McCabe (2007: 23–7); and Lazaris (2010: 133).

[91] McCabe (2007: 271–2); and McCabe (2009: 288–90). These mentions are mainly included in Appendix 7, which corresponds to the last folia of the Berolinensis Phillippicus gr. 1538 i.e. ff. 393v–394v, ed. Oder and Hoppe (1924) I.446.10–448.4.

devoted to julep (*zoulapion*).[92] He refers also to the administration of bugloss (*bouglōssou... zoulapion*), balm (*melissophyllou... zoulapion*), water lily (*nymphaiozoulapon*), and violet (*iozoulapon*) in the form of a julep in the chapters dealing with these vegetal substances, without providing any details about the preparation of these potions.[93] Interestingly, the text also provides the first mention in Byzantine literature of a simple mixture of vinegar and sugar (*oxysakchar*), which is the sugar-based equivalent of the potion known as *oxymeli* (vinegar with honey), which is well known in Greek and Byzantine medical literature.[94]

The *Ephodia tou Apodēmountos* is extremely important in the present case, as it was the first substantial medical handbook to provide consistent references to the use of sugar in medical preparations in the Greek language, and it contributed a great deal to promote the regular use of sugar and other oriental ingredients in Byzantine medical practice in subsequent centuries. In the *Ephodia*, in addition to direct references to sugar, we also find numerous references to named sugar-based potions such as *zoulabi(o)n* and *serabi(o)n* involving some special ingredient, for example, violet *zoulabion* or pomegranate *serabion*, and also to *oxysa(k)charon*. These may be used as composite drugs on their own or as a base for the administration of other ingredients.[95]

Sugar gradually became available in Byzantium and it was even included among the supplies of the *xenōn* of the Pantokrator monastery in Constantinople in the twelfth century.[96] It remained an expensive commodity right up until the fall of the Empire in the fifteenth century.[97] The first systematic list of sugar-based potions in a Greek work is found in the *Dynameron*.

92 Symeon Seth, *Treatise on the Capacities of Foodstuffs*, ed. Langkavel (1868) 41.5–13.

93 Symeon Seth, *Treatise on the Capacities of Foodstuffs*, ed. Langkavel (1868) 30.7, 66.17–19, 73.8–11, 48.1–3. Violet could also be administered in a form called *iosakchar*, which most probably denotes a lighter, less dense version of the violet julep. See Symeon Seth, *Treatise on the Capacities of Foodstuffs*, ed. Langkavel (1868) 48.1.

94 Symeon Seth, *Treatise on the Capacities of Foodstuffs*, ed. Langkavel, 46.2–4.

95 For a long list of references from the *Ephodia tou Apodēmountos*, see Bouras-Vallianatos (forthcoming: n. 119).

96 *Typikon* of the Pantokrator, 1106–11, ed. Gautier (1974) 95. Sugar also features in the supplies of a smaller institution (for the care of thirty-six elderly patients attended by only one doctor) attached to the monastery of the Virgin Mary Kosmosoteira (Saviour of the World), founded by John II's brother, Isaac Komnenos, in 1151/2 in the Thracian city of Bera (mod. Ferres). See *Typikon of Kosmosoteira*, 1120–2, ed. Papazoglou (2014) 93.

97 For example, Giacomo Badoer reports in his account book, *Libro dei Conti*, ed. Dorini and Bertelè (1956) 52.4–6, that around 1436 he bought a sugar syrup (*zucharo siropo*) and some more medicaments for his assistant, Antonio Bragadin, when he was ill, for two hyperpyra and twelve carats; the same price was paid to a barber to bleed him, while a nurse received one hyperpyron. On this, see Lefort (1998: 215). It is worth comparing this cost with, for example, the wage of a woman who gutted fish, which was approximately five hyperpyra per month according to Badoer, *Libro dei Conti*, ed. Dorini and Bertelè (1956) 116.6. The conversion of this wage to a monthly rate has been estimated by Morrisson and Cheynet (2002: 867).

The *Dynameron* includes fifteen recipes for sugar-based potions,[98] and sugar is also used as an ingredient in a large number of antidotes, although the possibility of replacing it with honey is mentioned throughout these recipes.[99] Chioniades' antidotary provides roughly twenty-nine recipes for juleps and other sugar-based potions.[100] The repeated references to juleps in Chioniades' recipe collection does not seem coincidental. Chioniades was aware of the importance of sugar in contemporary pharmacology and was probably attempting to attract the attention of his contemporaries by supplementing the Byzantine medical cabinet with recipes previously alien to it. However, the most extensive list of sugar-based potions is given by John.

In referring to syrups and julep in his introductory statement, John says: '...we call them syrup and julep in accordance with the barbarian language.'[101] Here, John refers explicitly to the Hellenized versions of julep and syrup as coming from a 'barbarian' language, thus pointing to the Arabic origin of these terms. He provides a long list of thirty-nine recipes (including juleps, syrups, and *oxosachara*) in three parts of book five, i.e. potions on fevers, juleps and syrups, and composite drugs (see Table 5.6),[102] thus giving paramount importance to the dissemination and widespread use of the new

[98] There are thirteen recipes for juleps and two more for rose-juleps. The names of each julep from the relevant table of contents in [Nicholas Myrepsos], *Dynameron*, *Z*(juleps) and P, ed. Valiakos (2019) 593 and 977, are as follows: '*α΄· ζουλάπιον πολυέψητον· τὸ καλούμενον ὑδροροσάτον: β΄· ζουλαπίου σκευασία, τοῦ ὑδροροσάτου τοῦ ἁπλοῦ: γ΄· ζουλαπίου σκευασία, τοῦ νενουφάρου δόκιμον: δ΄· ζουλάπιον, τὸ διὰ μελισσοβοτάνου, θαυμαστόν: ϵ΄· ζουλαπίου, τῶν ἴων σκευασία· πρὸς πυρετούς: στ΄· ζουλαπίου, σκευασία, διὰ τῶν μήλων· δόκιμον: ζ΄· ζουλαπίου τοῦ διὰ μήλων σκευασία, κρεῖττον: η΄· ζουλάπιον, τῶν ῥοϊδίων σκευασία, ἐπαινετή: θ΄· ζουλάπιον, τὸ διὰ τῶν μήλων· πρὸς διακαεῖς πυρετούς: ι΄· ζουλαπίου σκευασία, τοῦ διὰ ἀκαπνίου: ια΄· ζουλαπίου σκευασία, τοῦ δι' ὀξυφοινίκου: ιβ΄· ζουλαπίου σκευασία, τοῦ διὰ κυδωνίων· καλή: ιγ΄ ζουλαπίου σκευασία, τοῦ διὰ μύρτων·*' and '*θ΄· ῥοδοζουλαπίου σκευασία, πάνυ δόκιμος: ι΄· ῥοδοζουλαπίου, καθαρτικοῦ σκευασία.*'

[99] E.g. [Nicholas Myrepsos], *Dynameron*, A(antidotes).15, ed. Valiakos (2019) 34.7–11: '*Ἄλλη ἀθανασία· ἁρμόζουσα ἐπὶ πάντων, ὡς ἡ πρὸς ταύτης· ἔχει: κινναμώμου· κασίας, ἀνὰ ὁλκὰς ς΄· κρόκου· σμύρνης, ἀνὰ ὁλκὰς δ΄· κόστου, νάρδου Συριακοῦ, ἀκόρου, μαίου, ἀσάρου πετροσελίνου σπέρμα, πέπερι λευκόν, δαύκου Κρητικοῦ, σίνωνος ἀνὰ ὁλκὰς β΄· μέλιτος Ἀττικοῦ ἢ σάχαρ τὸ ἀρκοῦν ...*'.

[100] Given the large number of recipes in this case, I cite here only the *incipit* and *desinit*; the work lacks a table of contents. George-Gregory Chioniades, *Antidotes from Persia*, Venetus Marcianus gr. V.8 (coll. 1334), f. 146v, l. 25–f. 149r, l. 6: '*Ἀρχὴ τῶν ζουλαπίων καὶ τῶν ὑδροροσάτων καὶ τῶν ἀποζεμάτων+ α΄ ζουλάπιον...κθ΄ ἕτερον σκαντζιπὶν πρὸς καυσούμενον στόμαχον...καὶ διηθήσας...σάκχαρ τρά^μ ω΄· καὶ κρόκον τρά^μ α΄· καὶ ἕψε· καὶ δίδου τρά^μ κ΄ μεθ' ὕδατος ψυχροῦ:*'.

[101] JZA, *Medical Epitome*, 5, Vindobonensis med. gr. 17, f. 113r, ll. 1–2: '*...καὶ σεράπιον ἢ ζουλάπιν τῇ βαρβάρῳ φωνῇ καλοῦμεν·*'; ed. Mathys (1556) II.318.25–7. John refers once more to the 'barbarian' origin of the Greek term for these potions and he informs his reader that there is no consistent version of their name in Greek: *Medical Epitome*, 5, Vindobonensis med. gr. 17, f. 115v, ll. 23–4: '*...ἑψηθέντα σεράπια ἢ ζουλάπια· κάλει γὰρ ταῦτα ὅπως καὶ βούλει, βαρβάροις οὕτω καλούμενα ὀνόμασιν...*'; ed. Mathys (1556) II.327.24–6.

[102] It is worth mentioning that sugar is sometimes used as a sweetner for the preparation of lozenges. See, for example, Table 5.4, Recipe C.

Table 5.6. List of sugar-based potions in John's pharmacology, Book Five

Chapter Title	Titles of julep and syrup recipes
Potions on fevers Vindobonensis med. gr. 17, f. 113r, l. 16–f. 115v, l. 15; ed. Mathys (1556) II.319.22–321.7.	** *Περὶ ἰοζουλαπίου*: (On julep of violet.) ** *Νουφαροζούλαπον*: (Julep of water lily.) ** *Περὶ ὀξοσαχάριτος*: (On *oxosachar.*) ** *Ὀξοσάχαρ τὸ διὰ τῶν ῥιζῶν*: (On *oxosachar* of roots.) ** *Ἕτερον ὀξοσάχαρ τὸ διὰ τῶν κυδωνίων*: (On *oxosachar* of quince.) ** *Ῥοδοζούλαπον*: (Julep of rose.) ** *Σανταλοζούλαπον*: (Julep of sandalwood.) ** *Μηλοζούλαπον*: (Julep of apple.) ** *Δαμασκηνοζούλαπον*: (Julep of plum.) ** *Ζιζιφοζούλαπον*: (Julep of jujube.) ** *Ἀγουριδοζούλαπον*: (Julep of unripe grapes.)
Juleps and syrups Vindobonensis med. gr. 17, f. 116r, l. 26–f. 118r, l. 22; ~ed. Mathys (1556) II.329.16–335.17.	** *Περὶ ὀξοσαχάριτος*: (On *oxosachar.*) ** *Εἰς σπληνικούς· ἡπατικούς· καὶ στομαχικούς*: (<Julep> for those suffering from spleen, liver, and stomach affections.) ** *Σεράπιον τὸ δι᾽ ἀψινθίου* (Syrup of wormwood.) ** *Περὶ ζουλαπίων*: (On juleps.)[103] ** *Βηχικόν*: (<Julep> for coughs.) ** *Ἕτερον βηχικόν*: (Another <julep> for coughs.) ** *Ἕτερον ζουλάπιον εἰς θέρμην τοῦ ἥπατος*: (Another julep for heat in the liver.) ** *Ἕτερον ψυχρότερον τοῦ ῥηθέντος*: (Another <julep> colder than the previous one.) ** *Ἕτερον καταστέλλον τὰς ἀκρίτους καὶ ἀμέτρους ὁρμὰς τῆς χολῆς*: (Another <julep> reducing unceasing and immoderate flow of bile.) ** *Ἕτερον ἐφεκτικὸν τῶν ἀμέτρων δριμέων ῥευμάτων τῆς γαστρός*: (Another <julep> stopping immoderate and intense flux in the stomach.) ** *Ἕτερον εἰς αἵματα ὑπιόντα*: (Another <julep> when there is a casting out of blood.) ** *Εἰς ψύγματα* (E: *ψήγματα*) *τὰ ἐν τοῖς οὔροις φαινόμενα*: (<Julep> for small particles in the urine.) ** *Εἰς αἷμα καὶ πῦον ἀπό τε τῶν νεφρῶν καὶ τῆς κύστεως φερόμενον*: (<Julep> for blood and pus coming from the kidneys and bladder.) ** *Ἕτερον εἰς βῆχα . . .*: (Another <julep> for coughs . . .) ** *Ἕτερον εἰς παλμοὺς καρδίας· καὶ ἀναισθησίας*: (Another <julep> for heart beats and lack of sensation.) ** *Εἰς ἐποχὴν ἐμμήνων*: (<Julep> for the menses of women.) ** *Εἰς ἐμφράξεις τὲ καὶ ὄγκους τῶν σπλάγχνων καὶ πλανήτας πυρετούς*: (<Julep> for obstructions, tumours of internal parts of the body, and irregular fevers.)

[103] This title stands for the julep of roots '*τῶν ῥιζῶν*'.

Composite purgatives Vindobonensis med. gr. 17, f. 149v, l. 14–f. 152v, l. 14; ed. Mathys (1556) II.392.12–399.30.	** *Ζουλάπιον εἰς κένωσιν χολῆς ξανθῆς ζεούσης τε καὶ ἐκκαιούσης τὸν ἄνθρωπον*: (Julep for purging fiery yellow bile that burns someone.) ** *Εἰς ἧττον ζεούσης τε καὶ καιούσης*: (<Julep> for less fiery and burning <bile>.) ** *Εἰς φλέγματος*: (<Julep> for <purging> phlegm.) ** *Εἰς μελαγχολικοῦ χυμοῦ*: (<Julep> for <purging> melancholic [i.e. black] bile.) ** *Ἕτερον καθαρτικὸν ξανθῆς χολῆς καὶ μελαίνης*: (Another <julep> purging the yellow bile and the black bile.) ** *Ὀξοσάχαρ· εἰς ὀξεῖς πυρετούς*: (*Oxosachar* for acute fevers.) ** *Τὸ διὰ καπνίου εἰς ἔμφραξιν τοῦ ἥπατος*: (<*Oxosachar*> of the juice of celandine[104] for an obstruction in the liver.) ** *Ἕτερον εἰς ἔμφραξιν τοῦ ἥπατος*: (Another <*oxosachar*> for an obstruction in the liver.) ** *Ἕτερον ἀφέψημα λύον τὴν γαστέρα· καθαρτικὸν χυμῶν παντοίων*: (Another decoction for relieving the stomach; a purgative for all humours.) ** *Ζουλάπιον καθαῖρον χολὴν ξανθὴν καὶ μέλαιναν*: (Julep purging the yellow and the black bile.) ** *Ἕτερον καθαῖρον τὸν στόμαχον ἀπὸ χολῆς ξανθῆς*: (Another <julep> purging the stomach <affected by> yellow bile.)

forms. Although in John's pharmacology honey-based liquid drugs are still predominant, representing roughly twice as many as the sugar-based potions, the coexistence of sugar-based and honey-based forms confirms the decisive presence of Arabic drug lore in Byzantine pharmacology.[105] A better understanding of John's widespread adoption of Arabic pharmacological material can be shown by studying his references to oriental *materia medica* (see Section 5.2 below).

Meanwhile, a potential source for John's sugar-based potions is connected with the codex Parisinus gr. 2240. The manuscript was written in the sixteenth century by Jacob Diassorinos (d. 1563),[106] a Greek copyist from Rhodes, who was then working at the Royal Library of Fontainebleau in Paris. It contains medical works by unknown authors such as Chariton and well-known ones such as Rufus, Oribasios, and Paul of Aegina.[107] The

[104] Cf. Aetios of Amida, *Tetrabiblos*, 7.69, ed. Olivieri (1950) II.318.26–7: '*τὸν χυλὸν τῆς χελιδονίου καὶ καπνίου λεγομένης πόας*...'

[105] The popularity of sugar-based potions is also confirmed by the reference to a medicine made with sugar and roses for purging yellow bile in his *On Psychic Pneuma*, 2.12.4, ed. Ideler (1841) I.376.2–11, in which John otherwise makes very limited mention of composite medicines.

[106] *RGK* I.143, II.191, and III.241. On this scribe, see the recent thesis by García Bueno (2017: 332–5), who has dated the codex to approximately 1549–50.

[107] Omont (1888: II.219–20).

indefatigable, early-twentieth-century Greek medical historian Aristotelis Kousis (1872–1961) correctly identified the unpublished nature of the introductory treatise of the manuscript attributed to a certain Chariton, and edited a brief part of the text about lozenges,[108] without, however, pointing to any similarities with John's pharmacology.

The treatise by Chariton is thirty-nine folia long (ff. 1r–39v) and is entitled: 'On lozenges, pills, desiccative powders, and, in addition, juleps and clysters by Chariton'.[109] The name of the author, Chariton, is not associated with any known medical author or physician of the Byzantine period.[110] There is, however, a short introduction preceding the first recipe, which gives some details about the nature of the treatise:

> You can see in addition to these <recipes> the <account of the> composition on lozenges, pills, desiccative powders, and juleps, which are also called syrups (this is how the Egyptian physicians call them in the barbarian language), and some useful clysters, o Philip, most wise among the Asclepiads,[111] which I readily presented <to you>. Many of these have already been treated by the ancient <authors>, but they are scattered among their treatises . . . this treatise has been compiled by the use of many <sources> . . .[112]

Chariton's recipe book has been compiled at the request of an otherwise unknown physician called Philip.[113] The compiler refers to his recipes consisting of ancient and barbarian ones, including dosage forms similar to those mentioned by John. It is striking that he uses the same adjective as John does, i.e. *barbaros*, in referring to the origin of the terms for julep and syrup.

A comparative analysis of the contents of John's and Chariton's works shows that similar versions of a significant number of Chariton's recipes, especially for those devoted to juleps and syrups, can be found in John's work. For example, one of the most remarkable syrups in John's list (i.e. syrup of wormwood), containing several stages of refinement, is also present

[108] Kousis (1939a). The text edited by Kousis was recently republished with modern Greek translation and brief commentary by Taygetos (2013).

[109] Chariton, *Recipe Book*, Parisinus gr. 2240, f. 1r, ll. 1–2: '*Χαρίτωνος περὶ τροχίσκων, κόκκων τε καὶ ξηρίων, ἐν οἷς καὶ περὶ ζουλαπίων, καὶ κλυστήρων:*'.

[110] *PmBZ*, *PBW*, *PLP*, s.v. *Χαρίτων*, the vast majority of the entries refer to members of clergy.

[111] The term is used here to denote a group of physicians; cf. LSJ s.v. *ἀσκληπιάδης*: in pl. *ἀσκληπιάδαι*.

[112] Chariton, *Recipe Book*, Parisinus gr. 2240, f. 1r, ll. 3–11: '*Ἰδού σοι πρὸς τοῖς ἄλλοις καὶ τὴν περὶ τῶν τροχίσκων, κόκκων τε καὶ ξηρίων, ἔτι δὲ καὶ ζουλαπίων τῶν καὶ σεραβίων καλουμένων, οὕτω γὰρ βαρβάρῳ φωνῇ οἱ τῆς Αἰγύπτου κεκλήκασιν ἰατροί, καί τινων κλυστήρων ἀναγκαιοτάτων, σύνθεσιν εὐφυέστατε ἀσκληπιαδῶν προχειρίζομαι Φίλιππε· πολλὰ δὲ περὶ τούτων τοῖς ἀρχαίοις διαπεπόνηται, ἀλλὰ σποράδην ἐν ταῖς ἐκείνων πραγματείαις . . . ἡ δ' ἀνὰ χεῖρας πραγματεία ἐκ πολλῶν ἐρανισαμένη . . .*'

[113] The only well-known medieval Greek physician by the name of Philip is the southern Italian physician Philip Xeros from Reggio, who was involved in the commissioning of Vaticanus gr. 300, and who is also the co-author of an unedited recipe book. See Lucà (1993: 36–63) and n. 23, above.

Table 5.7. Syrup made of wormwood in Chariton's and John's works

Chariton, *Recipe Book*, Parisinus gr. 2240, f. 23r, l. 10–f. 23v, l. 12.	John Zacharias Aktouarios, *Medical Epitome*, 5, Vindobonensis med. gr. 17, f. 116v, l. 9–24; ed. Mathys (1556) II.330.6–29.
... ἔστι δὲ ἐπιτήδειον τὸ καθάρσιον ... ** σεράβιον τοῦ ἀψινθίου τὸ τέλειον, ὠφελοῦν πρὸς τὰς τοῦ ἥπατος ἀῤῥωστίας, καὶ τοῦ στομάχου, καὶ τὴν ἐκφλόγωσιν καὶ τὴν παχύτητα τοὺ σπληνός, καὶ πρὸς ἴκτερον τὸν γενόμενον ἀπὸ τῆς θερμασίας· καὶ πρὸς τὰ κωλυκὰ πνεύματα ἐξ αἰτίας θερμῆς· διευρύνει δὲ καὶ τὰς ἐμφράξεις, καὶ κινεῖ τὴν φύσιν, καὶ ἐξεεῖ τοὺς χυμοὺς δι᾽ οὔρων: λαβὼν ἀψινθίου σπέρμα < κ΄· καὶ σπέρμα κουσοῦθε· καὶ ἄνθη ἴων· καὶ γλυκύῤῥιζαν κεκαθαρισμένην τὴν ἐπιφάνειαν ἀνὰ < ι΄· ἀδίαντον, καὶ ῥίζαν σχινάνθης· καὶ πράσιον· καὶ μαραθρόσπερμα πλατύ· καὶ ἄνισον ἀνὰ < ε΄· στάχος ἰνδικόν· καὶ φύλλα εὐπατωρίου· καὶ φλοιὸν κασσίας· καὶ κόστον ἰνδικόν· καὶ σπέρμα σελίνου· καὶ φύλλα ἰνδικά· καλαμίνθην ποταμιαίαν ἀνὰ (ἑξαγ.) γ΄ β΄· ἑνώσας τὰ πάντα καὶ συνθλάσας, ἀπόβρεχε ἐν ὕδατι πάνυ θερμῷ λίτρ. η΄· καὶ κατάλειπε νυχθήμερον, καὶ ἕψησον ἐν μαλθακῷ πυρί, μέχρις ὅτου καταλειφθῇ τὸ ἥμισυ, καὶ τότε διύλισον καὶ ἀνθυπόστρεψον τὰ εἴδη ἐπὶ τοὺ πυρὸς μετὰ ς΄ λίτρ. ὕδατος καὶ ἕψησον ἕως οὗ καταντήσει εἰς δύο λίτρ. καὶ μαλάξας διύλισον· καὶ ἀνάμιγε μετὰ τοῦ πρώτου διυλίσματος· καὶ ἀναβιβάσας ἐπὶ πυρός, μετὰ γ΄ λίτρ. σάκχαρος σολομωνίου, ἕψησον ἕως οὗ γένηται εἰς σύστασιν τοὺ σεραβίου· ἡ πόσις ἐξ αὐτοῦ οὐγγ. α΄: ** σεράβιον τοῦ καπνοῦ ...	... βάλε εἰς πανίον καὶ βάλε ὅταν βράζῃ: ** σεράπιον τὸ δι᾽ ἀψινθίου ὠφελοῦν σὺν Θεῷ εἰς τὰς ἀρρωστίας τοῦ ἥπατος καὶ τοῦ στόμαχου καὶ τὴν ἐκφλόγωσιν καὶ παχύτητα τοῦ σπληνός· καὶ εἰς τὸν ἴκτερον τὸν γεννώμενον (E: γενόμενον) ἀπὸ τῆς θερμασίας· καὶ εἰς τὰ κωλικὰ πνεύματα τὰ γινόμενα ἐξ αἰτίας θερμοῦ· διευρύνει καὶ τὰς ἐμφράξεις· καὶ κενοῖ τὴν φύσαν, καὶ ἐξωθεῖ τοὺς χυμοὺς δι᾽ οὔρων: λαβὼν ἀψινθίου σπέρμα, < κ΄· σπέρμα κούσκουτε καὶ ἄνθη ἴων καὶ γλυκύριζον ἀνὰ < ι΄· ἀδίαντον· καὶ ῥίζαν σχινάνθους· καὶ πράσιον καὶ μαλαθρόσπερμα πλατὺ καὶ ἄνισον (E: ἄνησσον) ἀνὰ < ε΄· στάχος ἰνδικὸν καὶ φύλλα εὐπατωρίου· καὶ φλοιὸν κασίας (E: ξυλοκασίας)· καὶ κόστον ἰνδικόν· καὶ σελίνου σπέρμα· καὶ φύλλον ἰνδικόν· καὶ καλαμίνθην ποταμίαν ἀνὰ (ἑξαγ. β΄)· πάντα ἑνώσας καὶ συνθλάσας, ἀπόβρεχε εἰς ὕδωρ πάνυ θερμόν, λίτρ. ὀκτώ· καὶ κατάλιπεν νυχθήμερον· καὶ ἕψησον μετὰ μαλθακοῦ πυρός, ἕως οὗ λειφθῇ τὸ ἥμισυ· καὶ τότε σείρωσον καὶ ἀνθυπόστρεψον τὰ εἴδη ἐπὶ τοῦ πυρὸς μετὰ ἓξ λίτρ. ὕδατος· καὶ ἕψησον ἕως οὗ καταντήσῃ εἰς λίτρ. β΄· καὶ μαλάξας σείρωσον καὶ ἀναμίγνυε μετὰ τοῦ πρώτου ἀποσειρώματος ἀναβιβάσας ἐπὶ τοῦ πυρὸς μετὰ τριῶν λίτρ. σάχαρ, ἑψήσας μέχρι συστάσεως· ἡ δόσις (E: πόσις) ἐξ αὐτοῦ, οὐγγ. α΄· ** ἐνταῦθα στύλη (E: στήλη) ...

in Chariton's text (see Table 5.7). Bearing in mind that Chariton's collection is sometimes augmented with further recipes, we should most probably exclude the possibility that Chariton's treatise is an excerpted version of John's work. It seems that either John copied from Chariton's collection or both John and Chariton based their work on an as yet unedited, unidentified source.

5.2 Oriental *materia medica*

A more complete picture of John's oriental material could be given by focusing on the various ingredients (e.g. myrobalan, sandalwood, cubeb pepper, zedoary, galangal) used in his recipes, which attest to a systematic dissemination of substances previously very little used by Greek and early Byzantine authors, or completely unknown to them.[114] These are mostly native to India, China, and the Far East and knowledge of their medicinal use became available gradually in western Europe and Byzantium from the eleventh/twelfth century onwards in tandem with the widespread introduction of Arabic medical lore through translations into Latin, Greek, and Hebrew.[115] In Byzantium, in particular, they first appear systematically in the *Ephodia tou Apodēmountos*. Here I give some examples and, at the same time, by using evidence from non-medical sources, I will make some comments on the availability and cost of these substances in late Byzantium.

First, it is worth clarifying that there are lots of medicinal substances in John's work originating from Asia, which are commonly attested in Greek and early Byzantine authors, who were familiar with their uses and actions, and therefore I am not dealing with them here. For example, cinnamon (*kinnamōmon*), ginger (*zingiberi*), and pepper (*peperi*) had been traded in Europe since ancient times and their names had been systematized in the Greek language as far back as antiquity.[116] The last ingredient, pepper, gives us an opportunity to discuss another kind of pepper, which was unknown to early Byzantine authors. This is the so-called cubeb pepper (Ar. *kabāba* or *qūbība*), which appears in John's manuscripts as *koumpebe* or *koubebe*.[117] It is the fruit of a plant mainly grown in parts of tropical South East Asia, such as Java and Sumatra.[118] John refers to it as an ingredient of composite drugs for liver and stomach affections.[119] Cubeb pepper, for example, regularly appears in the *Dynameron* as an ingredient in various compound drugs,[120] and it appears

[114] On these oriental substances, see the recent survey by Amar and Lev (2017: 82–227). See also Amar, Lev, and Serri (2014), who argue that these ingredients became known to Arabs through the influence of the Ayuverdic medical tradition.

[115] For an overview of the various translation movements, see Glick (2005); and Touwaide (2010).

[116] See Dalby (2003: 87–8, 159, 254–5), who provides a brief overview of the use of these ingredients by ancient and early Byzantine authors. On cinnamon, in particular, see also Hardy and Totelin (2015: 97–8).

[117] On the Greek term, see Serikoff (2013: 107–8).

[118] On this and its use in medieval Islamic medicine, see Lev and Amar (2008: 393).

[119] See, for example, the following two recipes: JZA, *Medical Epitome*, 5, Vindobonensis med. gr. 17, f. 138r, l. 20–f. 138v, l. 3: '*ἀντίδοτος διάροδος ἡ διὰ τῶν λαχῶν· εἰς ἔμφραξιν ἥπατος καὶ ψυχρότητα καὶ σκληρότητα . . . στάχος ἰνδικόν· καρποβάλσαμον· ξυλοβάλσαμον . . . ῥέον ἰνδικόν . . . κάρυον ἰνδικόν . . . κουμπέβε . . .*', not in Mathys (1556); and *Medical Epitome*, 5, Vindobonensis med. gr. 17, f. 155r, ll. 10–19: '*κόκκοι στομαχικοί . . . ζαδούαρ* (E: *ζαδόαρ*)*· κουβέβε· μάκερ . . .*', ed. Mathys (1556) II.406.13–27.

[120] See, for example, the following recipe for an antidote for gout, [Nicholas Myrepsos], *Dynameron*, A(antidotes).80, ed. Valiakos (2019) 57.20–58.2: '*Ἄλλη δραγγαία λασατίβα· πρὸς ποδαλγικούς . . . σκαμωναίαν ὠμήν, οὔγγ ἥμισυ· ἄνισον· γαρόφαλα· ζιντζίβερι· μάκερ· κουμπέπες, ἀνὰ ἐξάγιον α΄ . . . ῥέου μπαρμπάρου, ἐξάγ β΄· σάχαρ . . . ἡ δόσις ἐξ αὐτῆς πρωί, ὅσον ἐξάγ. β΄ καὶ ἥμισυ ἢ γ΄ πρὸς δύναμιν· χρῶ.*'

occasionally in late Byzantine collections of recipes.[121] According to the Venetian businessman, diplomat, and geographer Marino Sanudo Torsello (*c.*1260–after 1343), cubeb pepper was considered a light if costly substance that reached the Mediterranean via Baghdad and Tabriz.[122] *La Pratica della Mercatura*, written by Francesco Balducci Pegolotti between 1335 and 1343, informs us that cubeb pepper (*cubebe*) was one of the main commodities in Constantinople's fourteenth-century spice trade and a special control tax, the *garbellatura*, was levied on it at three carats per hundred pounds, a considerably larger amount than the tax paid on regular pepper (*pepe*), i.e. one carat per hundredweight.[123]

Among the most popular medicinal substances in the wider medieval Mediterranean were the various kinds of myrobalan, referring to fruits of various species of trees, native to India, China, and South East Asia.[124] At least two kinds of myrobalan, the emblic and the belleric, passed through Red Sea ports between the first and the third centuries AD according to recent archaeological evidence,[125] but their medicinal use is not described by any ancient or early Byzantine author.[126] John refers to five different kinds: emblic (*emplitzi*, Ar. *ʾamlaj*), Indian (*indikon myrobalanon*, Ar. *halīlaj hindī*), chebulic (*kepoule*, Ar. *halīlaj kābulī*), belleric (*mpeliliz*, Ar. *balīlaj*), and yellow myrobalan (*chrysobalanos*, Ar. *halīlaj ʾaṣfar*).[127] Their use is attested in recipes in

[121] See, for example, three references in the collection of recipes of the late Byzantine physician Demetrios Pepagomenos, *Recipe Book*, ed. Capone Ciollaro (2003) 59.24, 66.7, 102.20.

[122] Jacoby (2008: 190).

[123] Francesco Balducci Pegolotti, *La Pratica della Mercatura*, ed. Evans (1936) 44.23–9. On this tax, see Morrisson (2012: 396). On the economic activity of Western merchants in the late Byzantine Constantinople, see Oikonomidès (1979: 35–52); and Matschke (2002: 789–806).

[124] On the plant and its uses in medieval Islamic medicine, see Lev and Amar (2008: 218–21).

[125] van der Veen and Morales (2015).

[126] The classical and early Byzantine use of the Greek term *myrobalanos* and *chrysobalanos*, which appears to be synonymous with *balanos myrepsikē* [see LSJ, s.v. *βάλανος μυρεψική*, *μυροβάλανος*, and *χρυσοβάλανος*; Aetios of Amida, *Tetrabiblos*, 1.58, ed. Olivieri (1935) I.45.14; and Ps.-Galen, *Plant Terms*, ed. Delatte (1939) II.387.2], referred either to the fruit of the Egyptian myrobalan, *Balanites aegyptiaca*, or to that of *Moringa peregrina*, not the fruit of trees of various species of the *Terminalia* genus. See also Dietrich (2012) and cf. Amar, Lev, and Serri (2014).

[127] See, for example, JZA, *Medical Epitome*, 5, Vindobonensis med. gr. 17, f. 151v, ll. 4–12: '*τὸ διὰ καπνίου εἰς τὴν ὑπέκκαυσιν τῆς ξανθῆς χολῆς καὶ ψώραν καὶ τραύματα· καὶ τὴν ἔμφραξιν τοῦ ἥπατος…φλοιὸν μυροβαλάνου τοῦ ξανθοῦ τοῦ κέπουλε· καὶ τοῦ ἰνδικοῦ· καὶ δαμασώνιον· τὸ μπελίλιζ· καὶ τὸ ἔμπλιτζι· καὶ ἄνθη ἴων· πολυπόδιον· καὶ ἀψίνθιον καὶ ἐπίθυμον, ἀνὰ οὐγγ. β′· ταῦτα συνθλασθήτωσαν καὶ ἀποβραχήτωσαν* (E: *ἀποβρεχέτωσαν*) *εἰς τὸ ὕδωρ τοῦ καπνίου νυχθήμερον· καὶ ἑψηθήτωσαν μέχρι λειφθῇ τὸ ἥμισυ· ἔπειτα διυλιθήτωσαν* (E: *διυλίσθωσαν*) *καὶ ἑψηθήτωσαν μέχρι συστάσεως μετὰ τοῦ σάχαρ· ἡ πόσις οὐγγ. β′· μετὰ σκαμμωνίας κοκκ. δ′·*'; ed. Mathys (1556) II.397.16–26. Furthermore, JZA, *Medical Epitome*, 5, Vindobonensis med. gr. 17, f. 151r, ll. 11–20: '*ἕτερον καθαρτικὸν ξανθῆς χολῆς καὶ μελαίνης· καὶ ὠμῶν χυμῶν· λεπτύνει καὶ τὸ αἷμα· ὅσα δὲ γαστέρας ὑπάγει… λαβὼν μυροβάλανα καὶ ξανθά· καὶ ἰνδικὸν καὶ μέλαν δαμασώνιον· καὶ χρυσοβάλανον· καὶ πιτυοῦσαν, ἀνὰ < ας′′· ἐπίθυμον κρητικόν· πολυπόδιον· ἴα, ἀνὰ < γ′· ῥόδα… σάχαρου οὐγγ. ας′′· κόψας σήσας, ἔχε ἐν ἀγγείῳ τὸ τρίμμα· ἡ δόσις, < γ′, ἢ δ′… δίδου μεθ' ὕδατος χλιαροῦ·*'; ed. Mathys (1556) II.396.16–397.1. See also n. 72, above, where John refers to five kinds of myrobalan ('*πέντε ταῦτα*'). The term *damasōnion* seems to be a synonym for

the *Ephodia tou Apodēmountos* and the *Dynameron*,[128] as well as some late Byzantine collections of recipes,[129] including *xenōnika* (manuals connected with Byzantine *xenōnes*).[130] Five different kinds of myrobalan are also attested in the fourteenth-century *Pratica della Mercatura*,[131] but none of the references is directly connected with Constantinople.

Nevertheless, this important witness, *Pratica della Mercatura*, provides evidence for other ingredients which were used by John and traded in Constantinople in the fourteenth century, including zedoary (*zettovare*), galangal (*galinga*),[132] and barbarian rhubarb (*ribarbero*),[133] alongside those already known since antiquity, such as cinnamon (*cannella*) and ginger (*giengiovo*).[134] Finally, it should be noted that some important medicinal substances could have been acquired directly from abroad through the mediation of some highly placed people in imperial circles. This is, for example, confirmed in a manuscript scholion which refers to the trip made to Egypt in January 1386 by some unnamed Byzantine at the behest of the Byzantine emperor (most probably, John V Palaiologos, r. 1341–76/1379–90/1390–1) in order to bring

myrobalanon in late Byzantine medical sources; see also the entries in the late Byzantine glossary edited by Thomson (1955) 147.43, 148.63, 150.84, 160.260. Cf. Langkavel (1866: 121, entry no. 236); and Serikoff (2013: 110). This should not be confused with the classical and early Byzantine use of the term referring to water plantain (see LSJ, s.v. *δαμασώνιον* and *ἄλισμα*).

[128] For the *Ephodia* see recipe B in Table 5.3. For the *Dynameron*, see A(antidotes).23, ed. Valiakos (2019) 37.12–38.9: '*Ἀντίδοτος ἡ ἀλκάνκαλι ... μυροβάλανον, κίτρινον· μυροβάλανον κέπουλιν· μυροβάλανον Ἰνδικόν, ἀνὰ δράμας ζʹ· ἀνδράχνης σπέρμα ... μυροβάλανον μπελίρικι καὶ ἔμπλικι ... ἢ μεθ' ὑδροροσάτου καὶ δίδου νῆστις χρῶ.*'

[129] E.g. Demetrios Pepagomenos, *Recipe Book*, ed. Capone Ciollaro (2003) 65.34, 106.3–4.

[130] The recipe is found in a a collection of recipes associated with the Mangana *xenōn* in Constantinople and was transcribed by Bennett (2003) 398.16–399.17. It survives in Vaticanus gr. 299 dated to the fourteenth century. It should, however, be assigned to the period before the fall of Constantinople to the Franks in 1204, since there is no evidence for the restoration of the Mangana *xenōn* in the Palaiologan period. See Chapter 1, n. 165.

[131] Francesco Balducci Pegolotti, *La Pratica della Mercatura*, ed. Evans (1936) 293.7, 294.17, 295.14, 295.18–19: 'belorigi', 'embrici', 'mirabolani conditi', 'mirabolani chieboli', 'mirabolani cetrini'.

[132] John refers to zedoary (Ar. *zadwār*) and galangal (Ar. *khūlanjān*) as *zado[/ou]ar* (see the recipe in n. 118) and *galangan* (see recipe B in Table 5.3) respectively. Some early references to both ingredients in editions of Aetios of Amida's *Tetrabiblos*, 1.131 and 11.13, ed. Olivieri (1935) I.66.13, I.66.24–5 and eds. Daremberg and Ruelle (1879) 575.31–6, are probably the result of the contaminated textual tradition of this text. On this, see also the example given by Garzya (1984: 255); and cf. Durak (2018: 215–16). It is worth mentioning that galangal [*Charter, Abbey of St Bertin* AD *867*, ed. Gysseling and Koch, (1950) I.68.11–12: '... et gallingar er cariofilo ...'] is attested among the ingredients that were supplied every year to the Abbey of St Bertin in northwest France according to a charter of 867, which is perhaps the earliest confirmed reference to this substance in a European source. On this, in the more general framework of the early medieval importation of oriental spices to western Europe, see McCormick (2001: 708–10).

[133] On this, see n. 56, above.

[134] Francesco Balducci Pegolotti, *La Pratica della Mercatura*, ed. Evans (1936) 44.21–30.

back some medicines,[135] a rare testimony to the importing of foreign substances to Byzantium. However, it is not certain whether these were destined for the palace itself or for wider consumption within Constantinople.

6. CONCLUSION

The examination of the last two books of John's *Medical Epitome* has revealed that the pharmacological part is compiled in a way that would not only have been likely to meet the standards expected by John's intellectual friends, but likewise have provided the most up-to-date and complete list of current drugs for contemporary physicians. In fact, the pharmacology became much more popular than the other books and had a wider reception including contemporary and later professional medical audiences.[136] The clear distinction between the general therapeutic part in books three and four and the composition of drugs in books five and six reveals contemporary interest in, and the advanced state of research into, the development of various methods for the preparation of drugs and the availability of new pharmacological material. Pharmacology was the most dynamic branch of Byzantine therapeutics and John wanted to show his personal involvement in adopting newly available material. Unlike in the first four books, John emphasizes here how experience had played a paramount role in the process of selecting the most valuable sources, and also served to highlight his authority on the subject. His project is not analogous in terms of length and overall aim with that of the author of the vast *Dynameron*, a work listing every single composite drug. John intended

[135] The scholion in Florentinus Laurentianus gr. plut. 28.16, f. 123r, was edited by Mercati (1926: 98, n. 1): '*ἔτους ͵ϛωϟδ' μηνὶ Ἰαννουαρίῳ α' κατὰ τὴν β' τρίωρον ἐγένετο ἔκλειψις Ἡλίου κατὰ τὸν Αἰγοκέρωτα, καὶ ὅλος ἐφάνη ἀμαυρός. καὶ ὄντος μοῦ ἐν Ἀλεξανδρείᾳ παρὰ τοῦ βασιλέως ἀπεσταλμένου ὠνῆς ἰατρικῶν εἰδῶν ἕνεκεν*...' The text was reproduced and translated into English by Pingree (1971: 199, 212): 'On January in the year 1385 at the second three-hour period there was an eclipse of the Sun in Capricorn, and the whole of it appeared darkened. As I was in Alexandria, having been sent by the emperor to buy medicines...' Pingree (1971: 199–200), in line with Mercati (1926: 97, n. 2), considered it an autograph scholion by one of the main copyists of the manuscript, the fourteenth-century astrologer John Abramios. Turyn (1972: I.247–8) and Tihon (1996: 273–4) believe that the scholion was not written by Abramios. Alexandria was an important port in the context of the middle-range trade in oriental spices in the Mediterranean. See Jacoby (1995).

[136] John's pharmacology influenced subsequent generations of physicians. See Chapter 7, nn. 14–15. There are also four surviving excerpting manuscripts of the *Medical Epitome*, which copy the last two books entirely or in part: Athous Iberiticus 151 (fifteenth century), Oxoniensis Bodleianus Laudianus gr. 62 (early sixteenth century), Parisinus gr. 2235 (sixteenth century), Vaticanus Palatinus gr. 370 (sixteenth century). Similarly, Ruelle (1539), the first translator of John's work into Latin, chose to publish only the pharmacological part, thus confirming its broader scope; the translation includes book five and the second part of book six. For more details on these manuscripts and the early printed editions, see Appendix 5.

specifically to collect those recipes that he considered most useful, according to his own practical experience.

The recently introduced oriental material is also the main aspect which differentiates John's handbook, in terms of content, from early Byzantine medical compilations or later ones by authors such as Theophanes Chrysobalantes. John occasionally uses the term 'barbarian' to indicate recipes coming from Arabic sources and, at the same time, advertise his awareness of wider Mediterranean advances in the field. He was the first medical author and practising physician to attain particularly eminent status, as is evidenced by his appointment to the office of *aktouarios* by Andronikos II, and, at the same time, to put together a powerful assemblage of data containing both classical and early Byzantine Greek material (e.g. Galen, Aetios of Amida, Paul of Aegina) and newly introduced Arabic pharmacological lore (e.g. *Ephodia tou Apodēmountos*). Although a definitive inventory of late Byzantine *albarelli* filled with oriental ingredients and available to physicians is hard to reconstruct for lack of archaeological data, it seems that many substances were imported, at least in Constantinople, in the fourteenth century, where the trade in spices was regulated by special control taxes.

6

On Psychic Pneuma

John's Advice on How To Lead a Healthy Life

> At that moment, I say most truly that the spirit of life (*spirito della vita*), which hath its dwelling in the secretest chamber of the heart, began to tremble so violently that the least pulses of my body shook therewith; and in trembling it said these words: *Ecce deus fortior me, qui veniens dominabitur michi.* At that moment the animate spirit (*spirito animale*), which dwelleth in the lofty chamber whither all the senses carry their perceptions, was filled with wonder, and speaking more especially unto the spirits of the eyes, said these words: *Apparuit jam beatitudo vestra.* At that moment the natural spirit (*spirito naturale*), which dwelleth there where our nourishment is administered, began to weep, and in weeping said these words: *Heu miser! quia frequenter impeditus ero deinceps.*[1]
>
> Dante Alighieri, *La Vita Nuova* 2

By the late thirteenth century, tripartite pneumatology was not only the mainstream medical approach to understanding human physiology in medieval medicine, but it gradually became so popular as to appear in non-medical contexts, such as the literature of courtly love. The Italian poet Dante Alighieri (*c.*1265–1321) was knowledgeable enough to locate the supposed origin of each pneuma in line with current views in the West. In fact, there was a variety of opinions in the western European, Byzantine, and Arabic traditions on how these pneumata were produced and distributed throughout the human body, and subsequently how essential physiological functions might be affected.

John's *On the Activities and Affections of the Psychic Pneuma and the Corresponding Regimen* is the most extensive medieval treatise dealing with pneuma and arguably one of the most original Byzantine medical works. This chapter presents a critical analysis of John's ideas on psychic pneuma and

[1] English translation by Rossetti (1904: 5–6).

Innovation in Byzantine Medicine: The Writings of John Zacharias Aktouarios (c.1275–c.1330). Petros Bouras-Vallianatos, Oxford University Press (2020). © Petros Bouras-Vallianatos.
DOI: 10.1093/oso/9780198850687.001.0001

other kinds of pneumata. I aim to show that John's significant advance involves the identification of four, rather than three, distinct pneumata and the correlation of each of them with two primary qualities. Consequently, he made a direct connection between the quality of pneuma and a person's daily regimen, including diet, physical exercise, bathing, and sleep. This chapter consists of six main sections. In the first three parts, I provide a brief introduction to the contents and audience of John's work and a discussion of John's conceptual framework with respect to the soul. The next deals with the formation of the various kinds of pneumata. The last two sections focus on the psychic pneuma and its dependence on bodily mixtures, accompanied by an analysis of John's model for the preservation of high-quality psychic pneuma through the regulation of various elements of the daily regimen.

1. CONTENTS

On Psychic Pneuma consists of two books, is seventy-four printed pages long, and was written in the late 1320s.[2] It is the most detailed, medieval treatment of medical pneumatology. As in the case of John's treatise *On Urines*, this is a work which shows a large degree of originality and limited use of verbatim quotations. Table 6.1 presents a brief synopsis of the contents of the work. The first book includes introductory sections on the soul, its capacities, and its connection to the body through the pneuma. These are followed by a detailed discussion of the production of the different kinds of pneumata. Finally, a significant part of the first book is devoted to the activities (*energeiai*) of the various kinds of pneumata, although the main focus is on the psychic pneuma and how problems with its distribution are connected to sensory impairment. The second book provides a detailed discussion on how modifying certain elements of one's daily regimen can help avoid the creation of harmful mixtures (*dyskrasiai*), thus ensuring physical and spiritual health; the vast majority of its contents focus on diet, including a long list of various foodstuffs and their qualities. Lastly, John provides brief chapters with diagnostic indications based on the examination of the pulse, urine, excrements, and other secretions. The work concludes with a useful synopsis in which John briefly presents the main concepts discussed throughout the treatise.

[2] See the discussion on dating in Chapter 1, Section 4.2.1.

Table 6.1. Summary of contents of John's *On Psychic Pneuma*

Book and reference to the edition	Contents of each thematic unit
Book 1 [ed. Ideler (1841) I.312–314.8]	Proem.
Book 1 [ed. Ideler (1841) I.314.9–321.25] 5 chapters	Discussion of the soul and its connection with the human body through the psychic pneuma; further details on the capacities of the soul.
Book 1 [ed. Ideler (1841) I.321.26–325.8] 1 chapter	The formation of the four pneumata.
Book 1 [ed. Ideler (1841) I.325.9–340.30, 344.7–349.37] 12 chapters	Different forms of psychic pneuma and its activities; further details on the role of the psychic pneuma in sense perception.
Book 1 [ed. Ideler (1841) I.340.31–341.36] 1 chapter	Activities of the natural pneuma.
Book 1 [ed. Ideler (1841) I.342.1–344.6] 1 chapter	Activities of the vital pneuma.
Book 2 [ed. Ideler (1841) I.350.1–22]	Proem.
Book 2 [ed. Ideler (1841) I.350.22–358.33, 375.24–376.37] 5 chapters	Human digestion and harmful mixtures (*dyskrasiai*).
Book 2 [ed. Ideler (1841) I.358.34–375.23] 7 chapters	List of various kinds of foodstuffs and their qualities, including other elements of the daily regimen, such as exercise and bathing.
Book 2 [ed. Ideler (1841) I.377.1–382.19] 4 chapters	Details of the diagnosis of bodily mixtures and humoral imbalances through the examination of the pulse, urine, excrements, and other secretions (e.g. sweat).
Book 2 [ed. Ideler (1841) I.382.20–386.38] 1 chapter	Synopsis of John's theories on pneuma.

2. AUDIENCE

The treatise was written at the request of Joseph Rhakendytes (lit. 'wearer of rags'), also known as Joseph the Philosopher (*c.*1260–*c.*1330), an intellectual and monk from the Latin-occupied island of Ithaca. In order to understand John's intentions in writing this treatise, it is worth looking briefly at Joseph's background. Joseph had spent time in Thessaloniki and on Mount Athos before arriving in Constantinople around 1308 in order to join the intellectual circles of the capital.[3] He is an intriguing figure in early-fourteenth-century Byzantine intellectual life, who lived in accordance with Christian Orthodox monastic values, as indeed his name suggests: wearing rags, renouncing possessions, living modestly, and refusing any secular office. It is not coincidental that Joseph was nominated for the post of patriarch four times, but never accepted the post.[4]

Joseph believed that the ascetic life of monks and the study of theology (*kath' hēmas*) were not sufficient to achieve the necessary spiritual elevation to a virtuous life, but that they also had to be combined with secular learning (*thyrathen paideia*).[5] This is most obvious in his ambitious project, the so-called *Synopsis Variarum Disciplinarum*, which aimed to provide contemporary students with a wide range of advanced knowledge, including works on rhetoric, logic, physics, anthropology, physiology, ethics, theology, and the four traditional subjects of the *quadrivium*, i.e. arithmetic, music, geometry, astronomy.[6] This is a compilation derived from various

[3] On Joseph, see Treu (1899b); Conticello (1995); Gielen (2011: 205–15); and Gielen (2016: lxxi–lxxiv).

[4] Theodore Metochites, *To a Friend, on the Death of the Great Philosopher and Most Pious Joseph the Younger*, 32.33–40, ed. Polemis and Kaltsogianni (2019) 664–5.

[5] See Theodore Metochites' funerary encomium for Joseph, *To a Friend, on the Death of the Great Philosopher and Most Pious Joseph the Younger*, 10.8–14, 13.1–68, ed. Polemis and Kaltsogianni (2019) 641, 644–6, in which the author refers to Joseph's decision to devote himself to the ascetic life, but also to the study of Greek philosophy, including works by authors such as Plato, Aristotle, Plotinos, Proklos. It is worth remembering that members of the clergy were sometimes characterized by conservative views on secular learning and considered that Christians should focus only on the study of the Holy Scriptures. Take, for example, the case of the Patriarch Athanasios I (1289–93, and 1303–9), on whom, see Meyendorff (1971: 59–61). On Athanasios' life, see Talbot (1975: xv–xxxi). The *Synodikon of Orthodoxy*, a liturgical document originally produced after the Triumph of Orthodoxy in 843, gradually enlarged with the inclusion of anathemas of contemporary heresiarchs, and read every year on the first Sunday of Lent in Orthodox Churches, states that the Hellenic sciences (*hellēnika mathēmata*) could be used only as tools of instruction and were not to be followed or accepted as true (*alēthesi pisteuousi)*, ed. Gouillard (1967) 59.214–8.

[6] The work is preceded in manuscripts by two dodecasyllable verses, which seem to serve as title for the entire work: '*Μέλημα καὶ φρόντισμα καὶ γλυκὺς πόνος* | *οἰκτροῦ πιναροῦ Ἰωσὴφ Ῥακενδύτου*'. See Gielen (2016: lxxiv–lxxv), who informs us that the Latin title might have been inspired by the title of Joseph's prose introduction: '*Τοῦ σοφωτάτου καὶ λογιωτάτου Ῥακενδύτου κυροῦ Ἰωσὴφ σύνοψις ἐν ἐπιτομῇ εἰς τὰ κατ' αὐτόν*'. On the manuscript tradition of the *Synopsis*, see Criscuolo (1974); and Gielen 2016 (lxxii–xcix). On the 'encyclopaedic' nature of the project

sources, including a large number of excerpts from or entire works by late Byzantine scholars such as Nikephoros Blemmydes and George Pachymeres.[7] At the beginning of his *Synopsis* Joseph echoes the Aristotelian modes of living of *bios theōrētikos* (contemplative life) and *bios politikos* (political life) as presented in the *Nicomachean Ethics*.[8] He states that he had chosen the life of contemplation at an early stage because the 'political' life did not usually involve reason as a guide and often remained attached to worldly pleasures.[9] Joseph believed that rhetoric and logic would lead to reason, while the study of natural philosophy was equally significant, since nature (*physis*) was the instrument of the creation (*organon technourgias*) of the cosmos and essential to understanding it.[10] He then described the study of the *quadrivium* (*tetras mathēmatōn*) as a ladder (*klimakos*)[11] bridging worldly and spiritual concerns, which could lead any potential student away from material concerns. The ultimate aim is assimilation with the divine (*Theou theōrias*).[12]

Interestingly, in his proem to his *On Psychic Pneuma*, John argues that philosophical contemplation resembles ladders and bridges (*klimaxi tisi kai*

and its contents, see Gielen (2013) and Gielen (2016: lxxv–lxxviii), respectively. The greater part of the *Synopsis* remains unedited. For an edition of the proem and the accompanying introductory text in iambic dodecasyllables, see Treu (1899b: 34–42). The part on rhetoric is available in Walz (1834: 478–569). Gielen (2016: 35–78) has recently provided a critical edition of the part on virtue. Judging from the manuscript tradition of Joseph's work, in which we cannot identify a constant transmission of all texts together—only three manuscripts contain all the texts—Joseph did not in the end realize his goal; see Gielen (2013: 275, and 259, n. 2), where she lists twenty-three manuscripts which contain parts of the treatise. Gielen (2016: cxxii) states that 'it is even quite likely that there never has been a definitive version, finished off completely and approved by the author himself.'

[7] See Gielen (2013: 267, 273) and (2016: lxxvi–lxxxvii), who states that Joseph's sections on logic and physics are often derived from Nikephoros Blemmydes' and George Pachymeres' works.

[8] Aristotle, *Nicomachean Ethics*, 1.5, 1095b16–19. On the contemplative life in Byzantium, see *ODB*, s.v. vita contemplativa. See also the study on this concept in early Christianity by Mason (1961).

[9] Joseph Rhakendytes, *Brief Epitome of the Most Wise and Most Erudite Joseph Rhakendytes*, ed. Treu (1899b) 34.7–35.27. See also Stiernon's (1974) entry on Joseph Rhakendytes, and Kourousis' (1984/8: 206–8, 238–9) discussion of Joseph's spiritual model.

[10] Joseph's inclination for philosophy is also praised in various places in John's work. See JZA, *On Psychic Pneuma*, 1.pr.6, 2.7.18, and 2.17.26, ed. Ideler (1841) I.313.25–8, I.369.10–12, and I.386.14–17.

[11] The ladder metaphor comes from the Neoplatonic tradition and is found more prominently in Iamblichos' (AD *c.*245–325) *Protrepticus*, 1 and 21, ed. des Places (1989) 41.17–21, and 132.7–13; and *On General Mathematical Science*, 1, ed. Festa and Klein (1891) 10.7–24. Similar references are also found in Nikomachos of Gerasa's (*fl. c.*AD 100), *Introduction to Arithmetic*, 1.3.6, ed. Hoche (1866) 7.22–8.5; in the *Commentary on Porphyry's Introduction* by Ammonios (AD *c.*435/445–517/526), ed. Busse (1891) 13.4–7, and Elias (sixth century AD), ed. Busse (1900) 28.13–15 respectively; and in David's (sixth century AD), *Introduction to Philosophy*, 19, ed. Busse (1904) 59.19. For the resurgence of interest in Neoplatonism in late Byzantium, see Meyendorff (1974: 114–15); Fryde (2000: 203, 208–10); and Bydén and Ierodiakonou (2018).

[12] Joseph Rhakendytes, *Iambic Verses*, ed. Treu (1899b) 39–42.

gephyrais), which direct the mind (*noun*) from humble things to more honourable ones (*apo tōn tapeinoterōn epi ta timiōtera*).[13] This might be seen as an allusion to Joseph's mode of life. John attempts to maintain a direct form of communication with his addressee throughout the treatise by the use of second-person singular verbs and pronouns or references to their recent meetings.[14] In fact, John starts his work by referring to the recent philosophical discussions that he had had with Joseph (*philosophois theōrēmasi synousiais*) on the psychic pneuma.[15] He then proceeds to describe the theory that he will develop throughout his treatise:

> . . . you [i.e. Joseph] also added in your account that you considered it worthwhile that I should publish a treatise for you concerning the psychic pneuma within us, on how this <psychic pneuma> can remain pure with the help of the <medical> art, and what kind of regimen is fitting for this purpose; thus, it would not be fair if we did not comply with your requests. We thus wrote this treatise for you as part of your advice, so you will be able to know easily what regimen it is necessary to follow for the health of your body and which might give you a purified mind through the psychic pneuma.[16]

John's aim is to provide all the necessary details as to how Joseph, by regulating his regimen, could keep his physical health in good condition and purify his psychic pneuma, a prerequisite for spiritual health.[17] Later on, John further clarifies his intentions by adding that the purification (*kekatharmenon*) of the psychic pneuma enables human beings to succeed in spending their lives in contemplation of realities (*bios epi theōrian tōn ontōn*).[18] When considering the involvement of the soul in bodily activities through the medium of the psychic pneuma—which, as we will see below, John describes as the vehicle and first instrument of the soul—the purified state of this pneuma, achieved through an appropriate regimen, is essential to the attainment of spiritual virtue (*aretēs psychēs*),[19] as befits Joseph's mode of life.

[13] JZA, *On Psychic Pneuma*, 1.pr.1, ed. Ideler (1841) I.313.8–12.

[14] Among the numerous examples, see, for example, JZA, *On Psychic Pneuma*, 1.pr.1, 1.20.9, 2.5.19, and 2.17.22, ed. Ideler (1841) I.312.1–15, I.348.32–349.8, I.361.11–17, and I.385.32–7.

[15] JZA, *On Psychic Pneuma*, 1.pr.1, ed. Ideler (1841) I.312.1–2. Cf. JZA, *On Psychic Pneuma*, 1. pr.3, ed. Ideler (1841) I.313.7–8. On John's relationship with Joseph, see Chapter 1, n. 203.

[16] JZA, *On Psychic Pneuma*, 1.pr.1, ed. Ideler (1841) I.312.7–15: '. . . *προσετίθης δὲ τοῖς λόγοις, ἀξιῶν βιβλίον ἐκδοθῆναι σοι περὶ τοῦ ἐν ἡμῖν ψυχικοῦ πνεύματος, ὅπερ ἂν καθαρὸν διατελοίη ἐπικουρίᾳ τέχνης, καὶ αἷς τισι κεχρῆσθαι δέον ἐπὶ τούτῳ διαίταις, οὐκ ἄν γε δίκαια δράσαιμεν, μὴ ὑπείξαντές σου ταῖς ἀξιώσεσι· καὶ ἐν ὑποθήκης μέρει τουτί σοι τὸ βιβλίον συντάξαντες, ὡς ἂν ἔχοις ἐκ τοῦ προχείρου εἰδέναι, αἷς τισί σε δέον κεχρῆσθαι διαίταις, τῷ τε σώματι τὴν ὑγίειαν, καὶ τῷ ψυχικῷ δὴ τούτῳ πνεύματι χαριζομέναις ἀκραιφνῆ τὴν διάνοιαν.*'

[17] Cf. JZA, *On Psychic Pneuma*, 2.pr.2, ed. Ideler (1841) I.350.7–15.

[18] JZA, *On Psychic Pneuma*, 1.3.2, ed. Ideler (1841) I.317.35–318.3. See also Hohlweg (1996: 519).

[19] JZA, *On Psychic Pneuma*, 2.4.26, ed. Ideler (1841) I.358.19–29. Cf. JZA, *On Psychic Pneuma*, 2.20.13 and 2.16.11, ed. Ideler (1841) I.349.23–31 and I.382.5–10. In turn, this might allude to the essential predisposition towards *theōsis* or deification, which is described by the

There are many places throughout the work, in which John provides his addressee with specialized details and takes into consideration the individual characteristics of a pious Christian monk. For example, in discussing the qualities of various foodstuffs, John refers to Joseph's special dietary requirements, including long periods of fasting, abstinence from meat, regular abstinence from drinking water, and frequency of meals.[20] Judging from the textual tradition of Joseph's *Synopsis*, it seems that the *On Psychic Pneuma* was intended to be included in it, although there is no direct mention of this in either John's work or Joseph's prologue. In fact, John's work is included in four manuscripts which contain texts of the *Synopsis*,[21] in which it appears in the form of two letters corresponding to the two books.[22] John's treatise may have served as a practical set of advice to those persons following Joseph's educative project and by extension spiritual/ethical model.[23]

Church Fathers as a process of spiritual and bodily purification. Deification is the condition in which one is as much like God and in union with God as possible, i.e. the ultimate goal of Joseph and also of every Orthodox Christian. For a brief account of deification (*theōsis*), see *ODB*, s.v. theosis. See also the study by Russell (2004); and Finlan and Kharlamov (2006). There is no explicit mention in John's text of deification. One might look at a striking reference in which John expresses his desire to be able to reach a condition in which he will be inspired (Lampe, s.v. ἐπίπνοια 1) by the Holy Spirit (*theiou d' epipneusantos pneumatos*), who in patristic literature is said to have the power to deify (see, for example, some primary sources discussed by Russell, 2004: 210–12, 222, 251–2); JZA, *On Psychic Pneuma*, 1.20.14, ed. Ideler (1841) I.349.34–6. In another case, the *theion pneuma* is mentioned in connection with the psychic *pneuma*, but their exact relationship throughout the text is not elaborated; see JZA, *On Psychic Pneuma*, 1.pr.1, ed. Ideler (1841) I.312.4–5. In Christian terms, the human soul and consequently the human pneuma are something created and not to be confused with the Holy Spirit. The Orthodox theologian Kallistos Ware (1979: 61), states that 'the created spirit of man is not to be identified with the uncreated or Holy Spirit of God, the third person of the Trinity'; on the development of the concept of Holy Spirit in early Christianity, see the recent volume by Frey and Levison (2014).

[20] JZA, *On Psychic Pneuma*, 1.15.8, 2.5.5, 2.6.28, 2.8.4, 2.10.1–3, 2.11.7, 2.11.10, and 2.17.12, ed. Ideler (1841) I.341.28–34, I.359.18–22, I.366.36–367.4, I.369.33–370.2, I.372.33–373.15, I.374.15–23, I.374.32–375.5, and I.384.22–32.

[21] Florentinus Riccardianus gr. 31 (fourteenth century); Parisinus gr. 3031 (fourteenth century); Vaticanus gr. 111 (fourteenth century); and Venetus Marcianus gr. 529 (coll. 847) (fifteenth century).

[22] In Florentinus Riccardianus gr. 31, f. 275r, Vaticanus gr. 111, f. 298v, and Venetus Marcianus gr. 529 (coll. 847), f. 405r, Book One is entitled: '*τοῦ ἀκτουαρίου κυροῦ Ἰωάννου τοῦ Ζαχαρίου ἐπιστολὴ πρὸς τὸν κῦριν Ἰωσήφ, περιέχουσα ἰατρικὰ θεωρήματα*' ('Epistle, containing medical theories, by *aktouarios kyr* John Zacharias to *kyr* Joseph'); while on ff. 290r, 315r, and 421v respectively, Book Two is entitled: '*τοῦ αὐτοῦ πρὸς αὐτόν*' ('By the same author [i.e. John] to him [i.e. Joseph]'). On this, see Gielen (2016: cxxiv–cxxv, n. 197). Interestingly, John's work is also copied in two manuscripts with a strong theological focus: Vaticanus gr. 429 (fourteenth century); and Sofiensis Centri 'Ivan Dujčev' gr. 156 (first half of the fifteenth century).

[23] Joseph's spiritual model was also appraised by many contemporary Byzantine scholars, including Theodore Metochites, Nikephoros Choumnos, Constantine Akropolites, Nikephoros Kallistou Xanthopoulos, Manuel Gabalas, Thomas Magistros, Michael Gabras, and Nikephoros Gregoras. See the study by Polemis (2007). For references to Joseph by Palaiologan scholars, see Treu (1899b: 47–63).

Ideally, John presupposes his readers to have an elementary medical background in order to be able, for example, to identify bodily mixtures.[24] Joseph himself seems to have acquired some basic medical knowledge. He used to meet John and discuss his medical inquiries with him. According to John, he was also able to perform phlebotomy.[25] However, there is no real evidence that Joseph ever practised medicine, and thus he should most probably be considered a *philiatros* ('friend of medicine' or 'amateur physician').[26]

While bearing in mind the strong connection between John's writing intentions and Joseph's request, we should also consider a wider audience consisting of physicians, who wanted to have a concise view of the theories on pneuma and how they related to an individual's regimen and the quality of human life. In fact, the details on human physiology (book one) are not covered in such detail in any part of John's *Medical Epitome*, and the same applies to the part dealing with foodstuffs and their associated capacities (book two). The presence of the work in about thirty medical codices,[27] most of them including John's other two medical works, shows that the treatise was most widely disseminated in medical circles.

3. THE SOUL AND ITS CAPACITIES

John stresses the intense interaction between medicine and philosophy in the areas of pneumatic physiology and psychology, already in his proem. He emphasizes to his reader that the theory of psychic pneuma, in which the capacities of the rational soul are reflected, constitutes a limiting factor in the medical theory (*iatrikē theōrēmatōn peras*); he then confirms that knowledge of medical theory with respect to pneuma is essential for those concerned with the intelligible cosmos (*ton noēton diakosmon politeuomenōn andrōn*), by which he most probably means contemporary intellectuals

[24] JZA, *On Psychic Pneuma*, 2.12.7, ed. Ideler (1841) I.376.16–22. See also the last chapters of the second book, *On Psychic Pneuma*, 2.13–16, ed. Ideler (1841) I.377.1–382.19, in which John gives brief details on how someone with an elementary medical background may diagnose through the examination of urine, excrements, and the pulse.

[25] JZA, *On Psychic Pneuma*, 1.20.9, ed. Ideler (1841) I.348.32–349.8. See also JZA, *On Psychic Pneuma*, 1.12.7, ed. Ideler (1841) I.333.13–19. See Chapter 4, Section 5.1, p. 132. John also asks Joseph to consult his *Medical Epitome*, a special work for *philiatroi*, if something is not clear in respect of medical matters: JZA, *On Psychic Pneuma*, 2.15.11, ed. Ideler (1841) I.380.19–21.

[26] See Pentogalos (1970), who argued that Joseph had both theoretical and practical knowledge of medicine. However, his argument is based on an overinterpretation of the available evidence, deriving mainly from a letter showing that Joseph had sent a medicine to his friend Michael Gabras, *Epistle* 293, ed. Fatouros (1973) II.453–4; cf. Hohlweg (1984: 126, n. 51). On *philiatroi*, see Chapter 4, Section 1.

[27] See Chapter 1, n. 198.

interested in the study of science and philosophy.[28] He notes, nonetheless, that before proceeding to the main topic of the book, he will give a brief introduction for those who have not the same background in philosophy as Joseph or other intellectuals, perhaps implying those who were about to start following a higher education curriculum or less highly educated people.[29] Hence, John starts his work by providing some essential philosophical knowledge in order to be able to discuss the union of soul and body through the pneuma. This part of his work does not contain any novel contributions, but it is important in order to get a first glimpse of John's intellectual context.

John distinguishes between a rational and an irrational element in the soul along Aristotelian lines; thus, man has a different kind of soul from animals, since man has a rational principle, which gives him the ability to think.[30] The next step in his account is related to how the soul may be connected to the body so one can be assisted by the art of medicine (*technēs boēthēmasin*).[31] The discussion then focuses on the capacities of the soul, where John follows Aristotelian terminology and echoes the categorization and analysis put forward by John Philoponos (AD *c.*490–*c.*570) in his commentary *On Aristotle's on the Soul*.

John refers to the soul as simple (*haplē*) as regards its substance, but complex (*poikilē*) in capacity (*tē dynamei*).[32] The first rational capacity is the intellect (*nous*), then comes discursive thinking (*dianoia*), and thirdly opinion (*doksa*).[33] John then proceeds to the non-rational capacities, i.e. imagination (*phantasia*), which he calls passive intellect (*pathētikos nous*), a term used as far back as Aristotle,[34] but which was explained and elaborated by John Philoponos,[35] and

[28] JZA, *On Psychic Pneuma*, 1.pr.3, ed. Ideler (1841) I.313.2–6; and cf. JZA, *On Psychic Pneuma*, 2.17.27, ed. Ideler (1841) I.386.21–2. The use of *noētos diakosmos* in relation to those interested in philosophy echoes Neoplatonic philosophers, such as Proklos (*c.*AD 410–85), for example, in his *Commentary on Plato's Timaeus*, ed. Diehl (1903) 308.13–14, and Damaskios (*c.*AD 462–*c.*550), for example, in his *Difficulties and Solutions of First Principles*, ed. Westerink (1991) 167.11, who used it to refer to the intelligible cosmos/order/arrangement, and is consistent with the aforementioned revival of Neoplatonic philosophy in late Byzantium.

[29] JZA, *On Psychic Pneuma*, 1.pr.6, ed. Ideler (1841) I.313.20–8. See also JZA, *On Psychic Pneuma*, 1.6.2, ed. Ideler (1841) I.321.34–5, in which he starts his account of the formation of the various kinds of pneumata right after the end of the section on philosophy, stating that this is the 'beginning and the first chapter of this treatise' (*''Επεὶ δὲ τοῦτο μὲν ὥσπερ ἀρχή τε καὶ πρῶτον τῆς ὑποθέσεως κεφάλαιον . . .*'), indicating the introductory nature of the preceding chapters.

[30] JZA, *On Psychic Pneuma*, 1.1.2, ed. Ideler (1841) I.314.17–25. Aristotle, *Nicomachean Ethics*, 1102a26–1103a3. Cf. Aristotle, *On the Soul*, 414b28ff.

[31] JZA, *On Psychic Pneuma*, 1.3.8, ed. Ideler (1841) I.318.26–35.

[32] JZA, *On Psychic Pneuma*, 1.4.1, ed. Ideler (1841) I.319.10–14. My observation on the resemblance of John's account with that of John Philoponos has also been recently noted by Kakavelaki (2018: 339–41).

[33] Cf. John Philoponos, *On Aristotle's on the Soul*, ed. Hayduck (1897) 1.10–12; and 2.21–4.

[34] Aristotle, *On the Soul*, 430a23–5. Although imagination and passive intellect are closely related in Aristotle, there is still a separation between the two. See the comments by van der Eijk (2005: 119, n. 71), and Blumenthal (1996: 159–60).

[35] John Philoponos, *On Aristotle's on the Soul*, ed. Hayduck (1897) 5.34–6.10. Cf. John Philoponos, *On Aristotle's on the Soul*, ed. Hayduck (1897) 11.5–11; and John Philoponos, *On*

finally sense perception (*aisthēsis*).[36] However, some of the soul's capacities are more divine and purer, i.e. intellect,[37] discursive thinking, and opinion, while others are more submissive and active in the body, i.e. imagination and sense perception. The soul is joined through the latter, the non-rational ones, with the psychic pneuma within the human body.[38] John is consistent in calling the psychic pneuma a vehicle/carrier (*ochēma*) of the soul, thus adopting the Neoplatonic notion of the pneumatic body (*ochēma*-pneuma).[39] This is very significant, in that John provides a tangible carrier, i.e. psychic pneuma, for the soul in the body in contrast to Galen, who was never completely confident about identifying the soul's 'substance'.[40] Finally, John's spatial subdivision of the various functions of the mind follows the localization and terminology of Posidonios of Byzantium (end of the fourth century AD), as they survive in Aetios of Amida.[41] Thus, he assigns imagination (*phantastikon*) to the anterior ventricles of the brain, reasoning (*logistikon*) to the middle ventricle, and memory (*mnēmoneutikon*) to the posterior ventricle of the brain,[42] unlike Nemesios of Emesa (late fourth century AD), who localized the so-called *dianoētikon* within the middle ventricle.[43]

the Intellect 4, ed. Verbeke (1966) 13.1–4. On this being John Philoponos' own 'new line of interpretation', see van der Eijk (2005: 2).

[36] JZA, *On Psychic Pneuma*, 1.5.1–9, ed. Ideler (1841) I.320.11–321.18.

[37] See John Philoponos, *On Aristotle's on the Soul*, ed. Hayduck (1897) 162.13–16, who argues that *nous* does not require an intermediary between itself and its objects unlike sense perception which is served by the pneuma, its organ and vehicle.

[38] JZA, *On Psychic Pneuma*, 1.4.2, ed. Ideler (1841) I.319.13–17. Cf. John Philoponos, *On Aristotle's on the Soul*, ed. Hayduck 1897, 12.14–21; and 18.34–19.3. On John Philoponos' views on the soul and his influence throughout the Byzantine era, see Bydén and Ierodiakonou (2018).

[39] JZA, *On Psychic Pneuma*, 1.5.10, ed. Ideler (1841) I.321.18–21. Cf. JZA, *On Psychic Pneuma*, 1.14.6, ed. Ideler (1841) I.340.5–7. See also Hohlweg (1996: 522–3). Cf. Kourousis (1984/8: 426–41). By identifying Plato's *ochēma* with Aristotle's pneuma, Neoplatonists, such as Porphyry, Iamblichos, and Proklos, argued that the soul acquired a pneumatic body (*ochēma*-pneuma) as it descended through the heavens, which allowed the incorporeal soul to join the body, and after death accompanied it again on its return journey. This was a significant departure from ancient Greek theories and was developed to explain how something immaterial and eternal like the soul can be joined to something material and perishable like the body. On the theory of the pneumatic body, see the specialized studies by Kissling (1922); Di Pasquale Barbanti (1998); and Zambon (2005). On the reception and development of ancient theories on pneuma in early Byzantium, see Verbeke (1945: 351–510).

[40] See nn. 51–2, below.

[41] Aetios of Amida, *Tetrabiblos*, 6.2, ed. Olivieri (1950) II.125.16–20. On the development of the concept of ventricular localization, see Manzoni (1998). Cf. Rocca (2003: 245–7); and Gäbel (2018: 327–8).

[42] JZA, *On Psychic Pneuma*, 1.20.1, ed. Ideler (1841) I.347.29–35. John also says that he is unable to locate *doxa* and *dianoia*. See also JZA, *Medical Epitome*, 1.35, ed. Ideler (1842) II.388.27–389.29.

[43] Nemesios of Emesa, *On the Nature of Man*, 13, ed. Morani (1987) 69.16–24. See van der Eijk (2008).

4. FORMATION OF PNEUMATA

4.1 Earlier theories

Before I discuss what John has to say about the formation of various kinds of pneumata, it is necessary to present a very brief background to Galenic pneumatology and, in particular, the origin and localization of the various pneumata and the development of Galenic theories in the period from Galen's death to John's day. Galen did not only assess earlier views on pneuma but always tried to test his theories by undertaking anatomical demonstrations.[44] In his opinion the production of pneuma was merely a process which took place inside the human body in several stages of elaboration.[45] The outer air enters the lungs where it receives its first elaboration, and it then proceeds to the heart and arteries in which it is fully elaborated into vital (*zōtikon*) pneuma through the action of the body's innate heat (*emphyton thermon*).[46] The vaporization (*anathymiaseōs*) of the humours in the arteries contributes further pneumatic matter to the vital pneuma.[47] The vital pneuma then enters the brain and is further elaborated in the retiform plexus (*diktyoeides plegma*) and lastly in the choroid plexuses (*chorioeidē plegmata*) in the ventricular system, which is the final repository of the psychic pneuma.[48] It is noteworthy that Galen accepts that the psychic pneuma is also nourished from the air inhaled through the nostrils directly into the brain.[49] The psychic pneuma enters the nerves, giving sensation and voluntary motion, although Galen never provided any details on exactly how this happened.[50] Furthermore, there is an overall uncertainty in Galen's theory on the role of the vital pneuma in contrast to that of the psychic pneuma.

Galen is also uncertain about the exact relation between soul and *pneuma*. Since a loss of psychic pneuma does not bring about death but only sensory

[44] On Galen's anatomical demonstrations, see von Staden (1995). For a discussion of Galenic dissections in connection with the brain's anatomy and physiology, see Rocca (2003: 50–8).

[45] On Galen's medical pneumatology, see Temkin (1951); Manzoni (2001); Rocca (1998); and Rocca (2003).

[46] Galen, *On the Function of the Parts of the Body*, 7.8, ed. Kühn (1822) III.541.15–542.1 = ed. Helmreich (1907) I.393.23–394.6.

[47] Galen, *On the Doctrines of Hippocrates and Plato*, 7.3, ed. Kühn (1823) V.608.1–609.1 = ed. de Lacy (1978–84), 444.29–446.10. Cf. Galen, *On the Use of Breathing*, 5, ed. Kühn (1822) IV.503.17–504.4 and 506.14–507.10 = ed. Furley and Wilkie (1984) 122.9–124.2 and 126.18–128.11; and Galen, *Therapeutic Method*, 12.5, ed. Kühn (1825) X.839.16–17.

[48] On this, see the discussion by Rocca (2003: 208–24), who provides a large number of relevant passages from the Galenic corpus.

[49] Galen, *On the Use of Breathing*, 5, ed. Kühn (1822) IV.504.4–6 = ed. Furley and Wilkie (1984) 124.2–4. See also Rocca (2003: 226–34).

[50] See, for example, Galen, *On the Doctrines of Hippocrates and Plato*, 7.4, ed. Kühn (1823) V.611.6–612.7 = ed. de Lacy (1978–84) 448.4–18.

and motor impairments, he is reluctant to identify it with the soul.[51] However, he generally settles for calling the psychic pneuma as the soul's first instrument (*organon*).[52] Galen follows Plato's tripartite division of the soul. The rational capacity is located in the brain, the spirited in the heart, and the desiderative in the liver.[53] He did not describe precisely how the vital and psychic pneumata act in the interests of the rational and spirited capacities. Even more problematic is the existence of the natural pneuma. Galen accepts a connection between the desiderative capacity and nutrition and pleasure,[54] but he is very reluctant to accept the existence of the natural pneuma, although he seems to admit such a possibility and that—if there were such a thing—it would be located in the liver and the veins.[55]

Galen did not make his dual system of medical pneumatology correspond to the tripartite nature of the soul. There are two surviving references to the tripartite pneumatic system in an axiomatic way, both connected with the scholastic environment of early Byzantine Alexandria.[56] In the first case, the notion of three pneumata appears in the *Commentary on Book VI of Hippocrates' Epidemics* by John of Alexandria (*c.*sixth/seventh century):

> But we should remind the more advanced student of what we have said on numerous occasions, namely that our body is composed of solids, fluids, and pneumata; that the pneumata are the psychic, natural, and vital.[57]

A significant part of the text referring to the psychic pneuma is omitted in the Greek original and the current version is derived from an addition by the editor on the basis of the Latin tradition of the text. However, it would be odd if the Greek original had indeed omitted such an important kind of pneuma.

[51] See, for example, Galen, *On the Doctrines of Hippocrates and Plato*, 7.3, ed. Kühn (1823) V.605.18–607.2 = ed. de Lacy (1978–84), 442.36–444.15.

[52] See, for example, Galen, *On the Use of Breathing*, 5, ed. Kühn (1822) IV.502.112 = ed. Furley and Wilkie (1984) 120.20–1; and *Causes of Symptoms*, 2.5, ed. Kühn (1824) VII.191.9–16; cf. Galen, *On the Doctrines of Hippocrates and Plato*, 7.7, ed. Kühn (1823) V.643.17–18 = ed. de Lacy (1978–84), 474.26–7. See also the relevant commentary by de Lacy (1978–84: 675). On the relation between pneuma and soul, see also Lewis (2017: 292–6), who discusses Praxagoras' (late fourth/early third century BC) ideas in light of Galen's views.

[53] Galen, *On the Doctrines of Hippocrates and Plato*, 7.3, ed. Kühn (1823) V.600.12–601.13 = ed. de Lacy (1978–84) 438.28–440.8.

[54] Galen, *Therapeutic Method*, 9.10, ed. Kühn (1825) X.635.10–16. On Galen's third part of the soul, see de Lacy (1988); cf. Hankinson (1991: 218–31).

[55] Galen, *Therapeutic Method*, 12.5, ed. Kühn (1825) X.839.17–840.1. On Galen and natural pneuma, see the recent study by Rocca (2012). Perhaps Galen's hesitation can be ascribed to the fact that he lacked a method to prove such a theory through anatomical demonstration.

[56] On early Byzantine Alexandrian medical tradition, see Chapter 1, n. 22.

[57] John of Alexandria, *Commentary on Book VI of Hippocrates' Epidemics*, fr. 42, ed. Duffy (1997) 102.2–6: '*ἀλλὰ δεῖ ἀναμνῆσαι τὸν τελειότερον τῶν πολλάκις ἡμῖν εἰρημένων· εἴρηται γάρ, ὅτι σύγκειται τὸ ἡμέτερον σῶμα ἐκ τῶν στερεῶν, ἐξ ὑγρῶν, ἐκ πνεύματων, καὶ πνευμάτων <ψυχικῶν>, φυσικῶν, ζωτικῶν·*'. I use Duffy's (1997: 103.1–4) English translation slightly modified.

The second mention of this threefold division of pneuma is found in the treatise *On Differences of Fevers* attributed to Stephen (*c.*sixth/seventh century) and Theophilos (seventh or ninth century):

> Thus, there is the psychic pneuma, which is located in the brain and the nerves; for this psychic pneuma is an instrument of the soul, and that is <the reason> why it is called psychic. But, there is also the vital pneuma, which is contained in the heart and the arteries and is dispersed throughout the body like a beam, and gives life, that is the innate heat. There is, however, the natural pneuma, which is produced from food and is contained in the liver.[58]

This passage, which has been overlooked by scholars working on the history of medical pneumatology,[59] provides—apart from the clear tripartite distinction—details about the localization of each pneuma.[60] The most noteworthy reference is that to the natural pneuma which originates from the liver as a product of the digestion of food. Although no similar passage is known from other Greek texts, the tripartite dogma is presented here as self-evident.[61]

The aforementioned passage shares many similarities with a chapter from the introductory medical handbook *Medical Questions* (*Masā'il fī al-Ṭibb*) by the famous Nestorian Christian physician and translator Ḥunayn ibn Isḥāq (d. 873). In addition to the reference to three pneumata and their respective places of origin in the brain, heart, and liver, Ḥunayn provides a precise correspondence between each pneuma and the three capacities of the soul, i.e. the psychic, vital, and natural, respectively.[62] The discursive form (*Mudkhal*

[58] Stephen and Theophilos, *On Differences of Fevers*, 8, ed. Sicurus (1862) 17.4–11: '*ἔστι τοίνυν ψυχικόν, ὅπερ ἐν τῷ ἐγκεφάλῳ καθίδρυται καὶ ἐν τοῖς νεύροις· τοῦτο δὲ τὸ ψυχικὸν πνεῦμα ὄργανον ὑπάρχει τῆς ψυχῆς, καὶ διὰ τοῦτο ψυχικὸν ὀνομάζεται· ἀλλὰ μὴν ἔτι καὶ ζωτικὸν πνεῦμα, ὅπερ ἐν τῇ καρδίᾳ καὶ ἐν ταῖς ἀρτηρίαις περιέχεται, ἐξαπλούμενον παρ' ὅλον τὸ σῶμα ἀκτινοειδῶς, καὶ ζωὴν χορηγοῦν, τουτέστι τὴν ἔμφυτον θερμασίαν. Ἔστι δὲ καὶ φυσικὸν πνεῦμα, ὅπερ ἐκ τῶν τροφῶν τίκτεται, καὶ ἐμπεριέχεται ἐν τῷ ἥπατι.*' Cf. Stephen and Theophilos, *On Differences of Fevers*, 2, ed. Sicurus (1862) 7.17–18, in which there is a reference to the vital, psychic, and natural [capacities] in connection with pneumata, but without any explicit reference to each kind of pneuma or any exact correspondence. This text has not been critically edited and the current edition is based on Florentinus Laurentianus gr. plut. 86.20 (fifteenth century). Several parts of the text coincide with the treatise *On Fevers* attributed to the early Byzantine scholar Palladios, ed. Ideler (1841) I.107–20. On the complicated textual transmission of the above mentioned treatises on fevers, see Garofalo (2003). On Stephen and Theophilos, see Chapter 2, n. 11 and Chapter 1, n. 28, respectively.

[59] This is mentioned neither by Temkin (1951) nor by Rocca (2012).

[60] Cf. Ps.-Galen, *Introduction, or Physician*, 13, ed. Kühn (1827) XIV.726.6–14 = ed. Petit (2009) 45.13–22.

[61] We should note that we know very little about the theories of the so-called Pneumatist sect, which was founded by Athenaeus of Attaleia in the first century BC. Perhaps this theory is based on a now lost treatise by some medical author belonging to this ancient school of medical thought. On the Pneumatist sect, see Wellmann (1895); and Kudlien (1968b).

[62] This text is available in English translation: Ḥunayn ibn Isḥāq, *Medical Questions*, 1, tr. Ghalioungui (1980: 5.22–32): 'How many are the spirits? Three: the natural spirit, the vital spirit, and the psychic spirit. The natural spirit emanates from the liver, penetrates through the veins

fī al-Ṭibb) of Ḥunayn's text was subsequently translated into Latin by Constantine of Africa (d. before 1098/1099), and became known as the *Isagoge*;[63] the text formed part of the *Articella*, an important collection of medical texts that served as a textbook in the late medieval and Renaissance West. Lastly, the tripartite pneumatology also appears in the work *Book on Fevers* (*Kitāb al-Ḥummayat*) of the Jewish philosopher and physician Isḥāq ibn Sulaymān al-Isrāʾīlī.[64]

4.2 John's theory of pneuma

I now turn to John's model for the formation of the various kinds of pneumata. He argues, like Galen, that the production of pneuma takes places within the human body. There are, however, three notable differences, which result in a significant departure from Galenic medical theories on the topic. First, John considers not only two or three but four distinct kinds of pneumata. Secondly, he says that the production of pneuma is directly connected with the process of digestion, while he says nothing about whether any kind of external air could contribute to this process.[65] Moreover, each pneuma is assigned two primary qualities (see Table 6.2), which allows John to easily correlate various

Table 6.2. Kinds of pneumata according to John's theory

Pneuma	Place of origin	Qualities
Unnamed ('gastric') pneuma	Stomach	Cold and moist
Natural pneuma	Liver	Warm and moist
Vital pneuma	Heart	Warm and dry
Psychic pneuma	Brain	Cold and dry

into the whole body, and is servant to the natural forces. The vital spirit emanates from the heart, penetrates through the arteries into the whole body, and is servant to the vital forces. The psychic spirit emanates from the brain, penetrates through the nerves into the whole body and is servant to the psychic forces.' Ghalioungui's translation is based on the unpublished edition of the text in Codex Cairensis (Library of the Faculty of Medicine, Cairo University) 625, by Galal Moussa, with occasional references to variant readings from another seven manuscripts; see Ghalioungui (1980: ix–xi).

[63] See Newton (1994: 34), who provides a discussion of the relevant passage in the *Isagoge*. The tripartite model is also found in the *Pantegni*; see Burnett (1994: 115). On medical pneumatology in the medieval Latin West, see Bono (1984).

[64] See Burnet (1994: 104). A special treatise *On the Difference between Spirit and Soul* (*Risāla fī al-Faṣl bayna al-Rūḥ wa al-Nafs*) was written by Qusṭā ibn Lūqā (c.820–c.912/913), although he refers only to two pneumata. On Qusṭā ibn Lūqā, see Wilcox (1987); on the aforementioned treatise, in particular, see Wilcox (1985).

[65] It is worth mentioning that there is no explicit discussion of the role of respired air in the process of pneumatic elaboration in John's corpus. Cf. JZA, *Medical Epitome*, 1.36, ed. Ideler (1842) II.389.30–395.9.

kinds of pneumata with the mixtures (*kraseis*) of each part of the body and of the body as a whole. John also provides a clear correspondence between the three parts of the soul and a particular organ and the relevant pneuma, although as we will see below, the system does suggest a deficiency as regards the fourth pneuma.

From the very beginning of his introductory account of the formation of pneumata, John makes an explicit connection between the production of pneumata and humours, which are the result of the digestive process.[66] He then proceeds to discuss three different cases related to the digestive process and the production of pneuma. The first case relates to foodstuffs that can produce healthy humours (*trophēs . . . euchymou*) resulting in the creation of very little or no pneuma.[67] Any pneuma thus produced makes its way either upwards or downwards. Some vapours (*atmoeidēs . . . anathymiasis*) that go to the head and have the ability to moisten its dried parts (*ta auchmōnta*) are also produced.[68] In the second case, the foodstuffs are again good (*agatha*), but the stomach suffers either from an ongoing *dyskrasia* or some lingering humours, resulting in incomplete digestion and the production of thick and foggy vapours (*atmoi pacheis te kai homichlōdeis*), which—if they become chronic—can thicken the pneuma in the body.[69] There is no explicit reference to what kind of pneuma this is, but thickening is considered a harmful condition for any pneuma. The third case deals with foodstuffs, which can produce harmful humours (*sitia . . . kakochyma*), which results in outcomes similar to those in the second case.[70] Lastly, it is clearly stated that if any organ/part of the body suffers from *dyskrasia* or is dominated by harmful humours and vapours, this results in a corresponding alteration (*alloiōsis*) to the pneuma associated with this,[71] a notion which I will discuss in the next section.

John starts by referring first to the natural (*physikon*) pneuma, showing no indication of doubting its existence or any sort of hesitation, such as is found in Galen, and thus he seems to be in line with early Byzantine medical commentators on this. The natural pneuma, in which the desiderative (*epithymētikon*) part of the soul is displayed, is born out of the best humour (*ameinōn pantōn chymos*) that has reached the liver and is warm and moist.[72] Thus the natural pneuma is seen as a product of the particular stage of the digestive

[66] JZA, *On Psychic Pneuma*, 1.6.2, ed. Ideler (1841) I.321.34–322.6.

[67] No name is given to this pneuma in the text nor is there any information as to where it goes after it has been produced. John is most probably referring to the fourth kind of pneuma, which is produced in the stomach.

[68] JZA, *On Psychic Pneuma*, 1.6.3, ed. Ideler (1841) I.322.6–18.

[69] JZA, *On Psychic Pneuma*, 1.6.4, ed. Ideler (1841) I.322.18–23.

[70] JZA, *On Psychic Pneuma*, 1.6.5, ed. Ideler (1841) I.322.23–7.

[71] JZA, *On Psychic Pneuma*, 1.6.6, ed. Ideler (1841) I.322.27–31.

[72] JZA, *On Psychic Pneuma*, 1.6.8–9, and 2.17.2, ed. Ideler (1841) I.323.2–14 and I.383.3–4. On John's theory of human digestion, see the discussion in Chapter 2, Section 2.5.

process that takes places in the liver, but there is no explicit mention of how the 'best' humour produces the natural pneuma. From John's preliminary discussion of the role of digestion, as I have shown above, we can deduce that the actual quality of foodstuffs or the potential harmful mixture in the liver can directly affect the production of the natural pneuma and the ones produced after that, since John emphatically states that the 'best' humour constitutes the substance of the creation of all pneumata (*hylē kai archē tois en hēmin ginetai pneumasin*), most probably referring to the vital and the psychic ones, too.[73]

Later on, John refers to the blood which enters the vena cava from the liver and then reaches first the right and then the left ventricle of the heart. The vital (*zōtikon*) pneuma, the instrument of life (*organon zōēs*) as it is called, is produced by the blood in the heart and is dispersed via the arteries throughout the entire body.[74] It is worth recalling that in Galen's model the vapours (*anathymiaseis*) arising from humours constitute only part of the matter of vital pneuma. Although John states on one occasion that the vital pneuma is produced after the natural pneuma,[75] which is dispersed via the veins,[76] he does not clarify whether the natural pneuma, or any quantity of it, is transformed into vital pneuma. The spirited capacity of the soul is displayed in the vital pneuma.[77] There is no detailed description of how the vital pneuma is elaborated in the brain before it is transformed into psychic pneuma, although John clearly states that it can be transformed into psychic pneuma.[78] He mentions that the psychic pneuma is produced in the ventricles and then enters the nerves. Furthermore, in his own words, John unhesitatingly acknowledges the psychic pneuma as the first instrument (*prōton organon*) of the soul.[79]

John's model recalls both Galen's and Erasistratos' (*c.*315–*c.*240 BC)[80] ideas about the refinement of pneuma inside the body. Unlike in John, Erasistratos believed all the pneuma to be derived from the external air through respiration. However, in contrast to his medical predecessors, John refers to a

[73] JZA, *On Psychic Pneuma*, 1.6.8, ed. Ideler (1841) I.323.2–3.
[74] JZA, *On Psychic Pneuma*, 1.6.16–17, and 1.16.1, ed. Ideler (1841) I.324.6–15 and I.342.2–7.
[75] JZA, *On Psychic Pneuma*, 1.6.20, ed. Ideler (1841) I.324.26–7.
[76] JZA, *On Psychic Pneuma*, 1.15.1, ed. Ideler (1841) I.340.32–4.
[77] JZA, *On Psychic Pneuma*, 2.17.3, ed Ideler (1841) I.383.9–12.
[78] JZA, *On Psychic Pneuma*, 1.6.19, ed. Ideler (1841) I.324.23–5.
[79] JZA, *On Psychic Pneuma*, 1.6.21–2, ed. Ideler (1841) I.324.30–325.4; and JZA, *Medical Epitome*, 1.33, ed. Ideler (1842) II.384.22–4. See also, JZA, *On Psychic Pneuma*, 1.6.1, ed Ideler (1841) I.321.32, in which John mentions that the psychic pneuma always (*aei*) flows in and out of the human body.
[80] On Erasistratos' theories on pneuma, see Wilson (1959); de Martini (1964: 43–4); Harris (1973: 225); von Staden (2000: 92–6); and Rocca (2003: 63–4). In particular on fineness (*leptotēta*) and thickness (*pachytēta*), see Galen's view of Erasistratos' theory in the *On the Function of the Parts of the Body*, 8.8, ed. Kühn (1822) III.540.8–11 = ed. Helmreich (1907) I.392.23–393.2.

process by which each successive kind of pneuma produced is finer and less moist than the previous one, with the psychic pneuma being the finest; it resembles the soul in terms of fineness (*leptotēti*) and is dry and cold. In terms of warmth, the pneumata that originate closer to the heart, i.e. the natural and the vital, are warmer, while the psychic pneuma is colder.[81] As we will see in the next section, John's notion of thickness/thinness of the pneuma seems to align more closely with Neoplatonic concepts on the quality of pneuma.

Meanwhile, John refers to one more pneuma which is produced in the stomach and is cold and moist. Although John does not name this pneuma and does not provide a specific chapter on its activities, as he does with the other three, he clearly refers to it in his first account of pneumatology, but only after having introduced the natural pneuma:

> But it seems that another pneuma is produced in the stomach, which is different from the others, and through this <pneuma> we partly experience sensations relating to the object of appetite . . . And this pneuma is cold and moist in contrast to those <pneumata which are produced> after it. It is the vehicle of the appetitive capacity <existing> within us <related to> the particular food <consumed> on each occasion. This [i.e. the appetitive capacity] is succeeded by the capacity found in the liver [i.e. the natural capacity], which is a stronger and much more all-embracing <capacity> and the origin of greater appetites and desires.[82]

This pneuma is related to the appetitive capacity of the soul.[83] It is a sort of local pneuma that is produced during the digestion of foodstuffs in the stomach, and there is no direct statement confirming the direction of flow of this pneuma any further from the stomach or whether it is connected directly

[81] In his conclusion John clarifies that all the pneumata are naturally warm and moist. When he calls one pneuma 'cold', this is not because it has a tendency to make something cold, but simply because it is less warm compared to other pneumata; the same applies to a pneuma that is characterized as 'dry', by which he means less moist. See JZA, *On Psychic Pneuma*, 2.17.1, ed. Ideler (1841) I.382.25–8.

[82] JZA, *On Psychic Pneuma*, 1.6.11–12, ed. Ideler (1841) I.323.20–33: '*Ὅτι δὲ κἀν τῇ γαστρὶ πνεῦμά τι ἕτερον διάφορον πρὸς ταῦτα φαίνεται γεννώμενον, καὶ διὰ τούτου τὰς κατὰ μέρος πάσχομεν αἰσθήσεις ἐπὶ τοῖς ὀρεκτοῖς . . . Καὶ τοῦτο μὲν ἤδη ψυχρόν τε καὶ ὑγρὸν τὸ πνεῦμα, τοῖς μετ' αὐτὸ προβαλλόμενον· ὄχημα δέ τι τῆς ἐν ἡμῖν τῶν κατὰ μέρος σιτίων ἑκάστοτε ὀρεκτικῆς δυνάμεως. ἐκδέχεται δὲ αὐτὴν ἡ ἐπὶ τὸ ἧπαρ, γεννικωτέρα οἷον οὖσα καὶ περιεκτικωτέρα, καὶ ἀρχὴ μειζόνων ὀρέξεων καὶ ἐπιθυμιῶν.*'

[83] Aristotle, *On the Soul*, 432b4–8, considers that the appetite (*orexis*) is found in all three parts of the soul. John Philoponos in his commentary *On Aristotle's on the Soul*, ed. Hayduck (1897) 1.11–13, 5.34–6, 18.34–5, refers to the appetitive (*orektikai*) capacities of the non-rational soul. According to Galen, *On Mixtures*, 3.1, ed. Kühn (1821) I.654.4–10 = ed. Helmreich (1904) 91.1–7, every bodily part that is nourished has four capacities, i.e. attractive (*helktikē*), retentive (*kathektikē*), alterative (*alloiōtikē*), and expulsive (*apokritikē*). In the *On Affected Parts*, 6.3, ed. Kühn (1824) VIII.400.17–18, it is specified that the attractive (*helktikē*) capacity of the stomach is also called appetitive (*orektikē*). Cf. Galen, *On the Function of the Parts of the Body*, 9.11, ed. Kühn (1822) III.727.14–16 = ed. Helmreich (1909) II.33.2–5.

with the production of the natural pneuma or any others.[84] There is no other explicit reference in the whole of John's work to this sort of 'gastric' pneuma, unlike for the other three pneumata, apart from in his conclusion where he clearly refers to four pneumata and reconfirms its existence, relevant qualities, and its connection with the appetitive capacity.[85] Furthermore, there is no evidence to suggest that John carried out any kind of anatomical dissections.[86] John's introduction of the fourth pneuma makes his theory of the correspondence between each pneuma and its two primary qualities complete. His conceptualization recalls the traditional connection between each humour and two primary qualities.[87] As we will see below, his theory will help him to introduce a detailed analysis of the role of a particular regimen in the regulation of the quality and flow of each pneuma in the human body.

[84] See also JZA, *On Psychic Pneuma*, 1.6.15, ed. Ideler (1841) I.324.4–5; and n. 67 above. Cf. JZA, *On Psychic Pneuma*, 1.6.20, ed. Ideler (1841) I.324.27–9. Also in JZA, *On Psychic Pneuma*, 1.14.8, ed. Ideler (1841) I.340.21–2, where John starts his discussion on the activities of the pneumata, he refers only to the three pneumata (natural, vital, psychic) and their place of production (liver, heart, brain) without mentioning the pneuma in the stomach. In his *On Urines*, 5.3.11, ed. Ideler (1842) II.115.30–116.4, John refers to a pneuma which is produced during the first digestion in the stomach and it can appear in the urine sample in the form of bubbles. In Ps.-Aristotle's *On Pneuma*, 483a20–2, a pneuma derived from respiration is supplied to the stomach, and in a passage in the Anonymus of London, *On Medicine*, 23.16–18, ed. Manetti (2011) 50, some kind of pneuma seems to reach the stomach, in contrast to John's case where it is clearly produced in the stomach and there is no relation to the outside air. For a discussion of the above cases, see the recent studies by Gregoric, Lewis, and Kuhar (2015: 114–17); and Lewis and Gregoric (2015: 143).

[85] JZA, *On Psychic Pneuma*, 2.17.1, ed. Ideler (1841) I.382.22–34: '*Τεττάρων οὖν διαφόρων πνευμάτων ἐξευρημένων τῷ λόγῳ, ἑνὸς μὲν τοῦ κατὰ τὴν γαστέρα φαινομένου, καὶ ψυχροῦ μὲν καὶ ὑγροῦ τούτου φαινομένου τοῦ πνεύματος . . . καὶ τούτῳ δηλονότι τῷ κατὰ τὴν γαστέρα τῆς ὀρεκτικῆς δυνάμεως ἐποχουμένης . . . ἀμέλει μᾶλλον ξηρότησι καὶ θερμότησιν αὐτὴν ὁρῶμεν τὴν δύναμιν πάσχουσαν, ἢ ταῖς ἀντικειμέναις ποιότησιν*' ('Thus, we have discovered four different pneumata in this treatise. One pneuma appears in the stomach and seems to be cold and moist . . . and it is clear that it is this <pneuma> that carries the appetitive capacity . . . We see that this capacity [i.e. appetitive] suffers more from dryness and hotness than from the opposite qualities'). This capacity is not mentioned in the relevant section of John's *Medical Epitome*, 1.5, ed. Ideler (1842) II.360.20–33.

[86] See, *On Psychic Pneuma*, 1.9.1, ed. Ideler (1841) I.328.14–25, in which John refers once to an anatomical demonstration whereby one may attest the fundamental role of the luminous (*augoeides*) pneuma in the sense of vision if one dissects the relevant nerves, the so-called canals or tubes of pneuma (*agōgoi tou pneumatos*). However, this passage most probably derives from Galen's account in his *On the Doctrines of Hippocrates and Plato*, 7.4, ed. Kühn (1823) V.612.14–613.2 = ed. de Lacy (1978–84) 448.25–9; cf. Galen, *On the Doctrines of Hippocrates and Plato*, 7.4, ed. Kühn (1823) V.614.14–18 = ed. de Lacy (1978–84) 450.18–22.

[87] The explicit connection made between humours and qualities is already present in Galen; see, for example, Galen, *On the Different Kinds of Diseases*, 12, ed. Kühn (1823) VI.875.9–11. On Galen's humoral theory, see Hankinson (2016: 30–4). On the development of the role of the humours in understanding and treating the human body in the Middle Ages, see Nutton (1993).

5. PSYCHIC PNEUMA: FUNCTION AND DYSFUNCTION

John devotes a considerable number of chapters in his work to discussing the role of the psychic pneuma in sense perception.[88] John's physiology of the sensory activity in his *On Psychic Pneuma* is often influenced by Galen,[89] although he never quotes Galen by name, as indeed he generally does for all his major sources throughout his corpus.[90] He also acknowledged the direct role of the psychic pneuma in hegemonic activity and corresponding impairments,[91] following the post-Galenic development of the localization of the functions of the mind in the brain.[92] What makes John's approach significantly different from that of his predecessors is his notion that the degree of the pneuma's fineness is directly affected by diet and other elements of a person's daily regimen. The alteration (*alloiōseis*) of psychic pneuma can cause various symptoms in the body (*sōmasi symptōmata*).[93] The psychic pneuma must be fine in order to be distributed and function properly.[94] When the psychic pneuma becomes thick (*pachyteron*), it moves more slowly. Since it is cold and dry, it functions properly in conditions of mild dryness and coldness,[95] which

[88] A discussion of sense perception, motor functions, and impairments, although in an abridged version due to the nature of the work, is found in John's *Medical Epitome*, 1.33–5, 2.6, ed. Ideler (1842) II.384.4–385.29, 442.31–443.34.

[89] See, for example, John's account of vision, *On Psychic Pneuma*, 1.8–9, ed. Ideler (1841) I.327.1–329.30. Cf. Galen, *On the Doctrines of Hippocrates and Plato*, 7.4–5, ed. Kühn (1823) V.611.6–628.15 = ed. de Lacy (1978–84) 448.4–462.19. See also n. 86, above. On Galen's theory of sight, see Boudon-Millot (2012); and Ierodiakonou (2014). See also Siegel (1970: 46–7); and Siegel (1973: 137–9).

[90] See, for example, the case of the *Medical Epitome*, discussed in Chapters 4 and 5 of this book, in which John does not refer to his sources by name. Cf. Chapter 5, n. 60.

[91] John, *On Psychic Pneuma*, 1.19.1–3, ed. Ideler (1841) I.346.19–32, mentions, for example, how the imagination is affected by the pollution of the psychic pneuma (*molynomenou pneumatos*), due to *dyskrasiai* or vapours from corrupted humours, which could lead to disturbing visions (*theamata thorybōdē*) during sleep. In his *Medical Epitome*, 1.33, ed. Ideler (1842) II.386.6–22, John also mentions impairments, such as *karos*, *lēthargos*, *kōma*, and *mōrōsis*. Interestingly, the psychic pneuma is twice called hegemonic (*hēgemonikon*) in John's treatise: JZA, *On Psychic Pneuma*, 1.6.19 and 1.16.16, ed. Ideler (1841) I.324.25 and 344.4.

[92] See nn. 41 and 43, above. See also Nemesios of Emesa, *On the Nature of Man*, 6, ed. Morani (1987) 52.2–4. Galen does not connect hegemonic activities directly with the psychic pneuma; impairments in such activities are related to an unnatural change in the mixture of the substance of the brain. See Siegel (1973: 147–53); and Julião (2018: 235–43).

[93] JZA, *On Psychic Pneuma*, 1.5.10, ed. Ideler (1841) I.321.21–4. The term 'symptom' seems to be used here in a broader sense embracing any unnatural change in the body. On this term, see Johnston (2006: 25–6). Alteration/qualitative change (*alloiōsis*) of the pneuma due to, for example, an ongoing *dyskrasia*, should not be confused with the subsequent changes (*alloiōsis*) of the pneuma to form the luminous (*augoeides*) pneuma in the eye or the airlike (*aerōdes*) pneuma in the ear; see JZA, *On Psychic Pneuma*, 1.9.2–7, ed. Ideler (1841) I.328.25–329.23.

[94] JZA, *On Psychic Pneuma*, 1.20.13, ed. Ideler (1841) I.349.23–31.

[95] Cf. Galen, *On the Use of Breathing*, 5, ed. Kühn (1822) IV.505.3–18 = ed. Furley and Wilkie (1984) 124.8–126.5, who in contrast to John's theory, states that, if the psychic pneuma is too hot, it moves better.

make the pneuma very mobile (*eukinēton*) and light (*kouphon*); an increase in wetness and warmth make it unstable (*astatein de mallon*) and its corresponding activities disappear (*teloumena . . . diarrheonta te kai aphanizomena*) accordingly.[96]

The psychic pneuma may be altered and its qualitative balance disturbed (*hēlloiōsthai kai tēs symmetrias ektetraphthai*),[97] which can be the outcome of a local *dyskrasia* during its production or its flow.[98] John also accepts that the production of foggy vapours as by-products of digestion, due to a local *dyskrasia* in the stomach or due to the existence of corrupted humours, can also affect the quality and distribution of the psychic pneuma.[99] The third reason for disturbance is related to the accumulation of a thick humour, which blocks the flow of psychic pneuma through the nerves.[100] In all cases, the pneuma will not be able to function properly and this may result in some deficiency in a sense or even be connected with medical impairments, such as apoplexy (*apoplēxiai*) and epilepsy (*epilēpsiai*).[101]

Galen rarely refers to the alteration of pneuma (*pneumatos alloiōsis*) due to harmful humours, without ascribing any particular qualities to the pneuma or providing any further details.[102] John's theory of the role of diet and other elements of one's daily regimen as factors affecting the production and quality of pneuma due to the ongoing *dyskrasiai* seems also to have been influenced by the works of some Neoplatonic authors. These authors were the first to make an explicit connection between regimen and the healthy condition of the

[96] JZA, *On Psychic Pneuma*, 1.17.4–7, ed. Ideler (1841) I.344.27–345.7.

[97] JZA, *On Psychic Pneuma*, 1.12.1–2, ed. Ideler (1841) I.332.16–30.

[98] See JZA, *On Psychic Pneuma*, 2.2.17, ed. Ideler (1841) I.353.14–18, where unusual mixtures can result in a violent disturbance of the psychic pneuma. See also n. 71, above. Furthermore, see the case of the natural pneuma, *On Psychic Pneuma*, 1.15.6 and 1.14.6, ed. Ideler (1841) I.341.23–6 and I.340.1–4.

[99] JZA, *On Psychic Pneuma*, 1.12.5 and 1.19.3, ed. Ideler (1841) I.333.3–10 and I.346.28–30; *Medical Epitome*, 1.34, ed. Ideler (1842) II.387.1–2; and n. 69, above. See Pormann (2013: 240), who informs us that, in Arabic medical commentaries, 'the idea of a vapour rising to the brain and impairing the psychic pneuma appears as early as the eleventh century.'

[100] See, for example, the case of the senses of hearing and touch respectively, JZA, *On Psychic Pneuma*, 1.13.1 and 1.13.9, ed. Ideler (1841) I.333.35–334.3 and 334.37–335.4. John agreed with Galen, who refers to cases in which the psychic pneuma cannot flow or arrives in certain areas of the brain only in small amounts because of deposits of a particular humour. See, for example, Galen, *On Affected Parts*, 3.9 and 4.2, ed. Kühn (1824) VIII.173.11–15 and 218.3–12, in the cases of epilepsy and impairment of sight respectively. See also the discussion by Rocca (1997: 235–6).

[101] JZA, *On Psychic Pneuma*, 1.13.16–18 ed. Ideler (1841) I.335.25–336.16; and JZA, *Medical Epitome*, 1.34, ed. Ideler (1842) II.386.30–387.11.

[102] Galen, *Therapeutic Method*, 12.5, ed. Kühn (1825) X.840.14–16. On the notion of alteration (*alloiōsis*), i.e. making a substance similar to the part being altered in Galen's physiology, see the brief entry by Johnston (2006: 38). See also Galen, *On the Function of the Parts of the Body*, 10.5, ed. Kühn (1822) III.783.15–16 = ed. Helmreich (1909) II.72.24, who refers to the psychic pneuma as *leptoteron* and *kouphoteron*, but he does not correlate the notion of fineness of pneuma with its qualities.

psychic pneuma. However, they never provided a detailed medical theory on the subject.

Synesios of Cyrene (AD 370–413),[103] for example, in his *On Dreams* attributed ethical connotations to a thick (*pachy*) and moist (*hygron*) psychic pneuma, which he said was connected with a *kakodaimōn* and *poinaios bios*.[104] He also accepted the use of ritual theurgy (*teletōn*)[105] and the importance of regimen (*diaitēs*)[106] for the purification of the pneuma, although he did not provide any further details on this. The closest terminological parallels to John's theory are found in the references to the thickening (*pachynthentos*) of the pneuma due to a harmful regimen (*diaitēs*) mentioned in John Philoponos' commentary *On Aristotle's on the Soul*. In this passage John Philoponos appears, in fact, to be criticizing accounts by some other philosophers, who had argued that a light (*leptoteras*) and dry (*xēroteras*) regimen (*diaitēs*) was the most appropriate for keeping the pneuma as fine as possible (*dia to mē pachynesthai to pneuma, alla leptynesthai*).[107] John Philoponos does not name his source and Robert Todd has suggested that versions of Philoponos' account may be found in the works of Porphyry (AD 234–*c.*305) and Proklos (*c.*AD 410–85), although there is no explicit reference to regimen in the

[103] There is a debate as to whether Synesios of Cyrene was born into a Christian family or whether he was later converted; see the most recent study on this by Criscuolo (2012).

[104] Synesios of Cyrene, *On Dreams*, 7.3, ed. Lamoureux in Lamoureux and Aujoulat (2004) 280.17–81.5. Cf. Synesios of Cyrene, *On Dreams*, 10.4–5, ed. Lamoureux in Lamoureux and Aujoulat (2004) 287.17–288.20. On Synesios' psychology and pneuma, see Bregman (1982: 145–54); Aujoulat in Lamoureux and Aujoulat (2004) 208–14, 249–52; and Toulouse (2016: 672–4). Although it seems that John's views on the fineness of the pneuma being achieved through an appropriate regimen are consistent with those of Synesios, I cannot see any further notable similarities between John's work and Synesios' *On Dreams*. Thus I disagree with the idea that John depended heavily on Synesios' theories, as has been proposed by Kourousis (1984/8: 466–71). In my opinion this view is merely based on Kourousis' unconvincing attempt to prove that the three anonymous philosophical Byzantine dialogues *Hermippos*, *Hermodotos*, and *Mousoklēs* were actually written by John. See also Chapter 1, nn. 95–8.

[105] Synesios of Cyrene, *On Dreams*, 6.2, ed. Lamoureux in Lamoureux and Aujoulat (2004) 278.13–22. On the purification of the soul by means of theurgy in the Neoplatonic tradition, see Shaw (1995: 45–57); and Addey (2014: 47–50). On purification of the soul in the tradition of the Chaldean oracles, see Lewy (1978: 213–26). Synesios' treatise witnessed a notable revival in Palaiologan Byzantium thanks to the commentary by Nikephoros Gregoras. Instead of the use of ritual theurgy, Gregoras, *Commentary on Synesios' on Dreams*, ed. Pietrosanti (1999) 32.14–25, suggests that the imagination (*phantasia*) could be purified through self-restraint (*sōphrosynē*), righteousness (*dikaiosynē*), vigils (*agrypnia*), and fasting (*nēsteia*) in line with the Christian mode of living. On Gregoras' reception of Synesios' text with the emphasis on the relationship between philosophy and theology in late Byzantium, see Kolovou (2012).

[106] Synesios of Cyrene, *On Dreams*, 16.1, ed. ed. Lamoureux in Lamoureux and Aujoulat (2004) 300.17–301.6. Cf. Synesios of Cyrene, *On Dreams*, 6.3, ed. Lamoureux in Lamoureux and Aujoulat (2004) 278.22–279.4. See Kissling (1922: 326–8).

[107] John Philoponos, *On Aristotle's on the Soul*, ed. Hayduck (1897) 19.22–20.4. Cf. John Philoponos, *On Aristotle's on the Soul*, ed. Hayduck (1897) 239.8–10.

passages concerned.[108] Thus, although our author was inspired by Galenic medical physiology, he seems to have combined Galen's ideas with Neoplatonic views on the role of regimen in connection with the different states of the pneuma in terms of fineness and thickness.

John recapitulates his views on the quality of various pneumata in the conclusion of his work, in which a model for the balance of various pneumata in the human body is put forward. One pneuma can predominate over others depending on the particular mixtures in the body. John states:

> Once it [i.e. the psychic pneuma] is set on the right course, advances towards what is best, and prevails over the other <pneumata> . . . we see some who abstain from <eating> too many and thick foodstuffs . . . so that the <psychic> pneuma can neither become thickened in this way nor may any other kind of pneuma, and, in particular, the natural pneuma, predominate, because of their thicker diet. For this [i.e. the natural pneuma] is the opposite of the psychic pneuma in both its qualities and capacities, and the psychic pneuma is enslaved <by the natural pneuma> and is dragged along <behind it>.[109]

The verb *epikratō* ('to prevail over or to predominate/achieve predominance'), or its cognates (*epikrateia, epikratēsasa, epikratousa*), is used only once in connection with a pneuma, but there are many references throughout the treatise in connection with the 'prevalence' or 'predominance' of a certain quality or a certain humour over others.[110] This might suggest that the 'prevalence' of a certain pneuma refers to a quantitative abundance of one over another, but this is never specified in the treatise. The main focus of the treatise and Joseph's own chief concern is on the good quality of the psychic pneuma. Nevertheless, John is eager to stress that Joseph should not neglect to take care of the other pneumata in his attempts to keep the psychic pneuma in good condition so that he might avoid the consequences connected with the lack of each pneuma's proper flow and its corresponding activities.[111] Ultimately, he emphasizes that the healthy condition of each pneuma depends on the condition of the others, and thus their 'health is restored jointly' (*synapokathistantai tais hygeiais*).[112]

[108] Todd (1984: 109 and n. 65), in which the closest parallel is identified as being in Porphyry, *The Cave of the Nymphs in the Odyssey*, 11, ed. Nauck (1886) 64.9–25 = ed. Seminar Classics 609, Buffalo (1969) 14.1–14. Cf. Lautner (2013: 390).

[109] JZA, *On Psychic Pneuma*, 2.17.10, ed. Ideler (1841) I.384.13–22: '*Ἅπαξ οὖν εὐθυπορῆσαν, ἐπὶ τἄμεινον πρόεισι καὶ τῶν λοιπῶν κατακυριεύει . . . ὁρῶμεν πλήθους τε καὶ πάχους τροφῆς ἀπέχεσθαι . . . ὡς μήτ' αὐτὸ τὸ πνεῦμα ὧδε παχύνοιτο, μήτε ταῖς ἐκ τῆς ἁδροτέρας διαίτης ἐπικρατείαις τῶν ἄλλων πνευμάτων, καὶ μάλιστα τοῦ φυσικοῦ. τοῦτο γὰρ καὶ κατ' ἀμφοτέρας τὰς δυνάμεις τε καὶ ποιότητας τῷ ψυχικῷ ἀντίκειται, καὶ δουλαγωγούμενον τὸ ψυχικὸν ἐπισύρεται πνεῦμα.*'

[110] See, for example, JZA, *On Psychic Pneuma*, 1.14.4, 1.17.8, and 2.pr.3, ed. Ideler (1841) I.339.25, I.345.9–11, and I.350.16.

[111] See, for example, JZA, *On Psychic Pneuma*, 1.16.6, ed. Ideler (1841) I.342.28–33.

[112] JZA, *On Psychic Pneuma*, 2.17.18, ed. Ideler (1841) I.385.16–20.

6. DIET AND OTHER ELEMENTS OF DAILY REGIMEN

Interestingly, John does not hesitate to call the second book of his work an account of the preservation of health (*hygieinēn pragmateian*).[113] This reference echoes Galen's treatise *On the Preservation of Health (Peri Hygieinōn)*,[114] and shows John's intention to discuss a broad spectrum of the ideal daily regimen (see Table 6.3). It indicates, moreover, his intention to make a connection between the purity (*katharotēti*) and health (*hygiainein*) of the psychic pneuma, on the one hand, and the overall health of the body, on the other.[115] As we have seen, the digestion is important both in the production of pneuma and also in ensuring that the pneuma does not lose its qualitative balance or become blocked due to the formation of *dyskrasiai*[116] and harmful humours respectively. John gives explicit advice on the best regimen to follow in order to keep each pneuma in good condition. For example, the vital pneuma, which is warm and dry, is stirred up (*diegeirousi*) by intense exercise and a diet consisting of warm and dry agents,[117] while for the psychic pneuma,

Table 6.3. Summary of contents of the daily regimen in John's *On Psychic Pneuma*

Book and reference to the edition	Contents of each thematic unit
Book 2 [ed. Ideler (1841) I.358.34–372.22] 5 chapters	Foodstuffs arranged in the following categories: a) cereals and pulses; b) vegetables and fruits; c) various kinds of meat; d) wine, water, milk, eggs, honey, various kinds of oil, vinegar, and other kinds of potions.
Book 2 [ed. Ideler (1841) I.372.23–373.15] 2 chapters	Quantity and frequency of eating.
Book 2 [ed. Ideler (1841) I.373.16–375.23] 1 chapter	Sleep, exercise, and bathing.

[113] JZA, *On Psychic Pneuma*, 2.16.12, ed. Ideler (1841) I.382.12–13. Cf. JZA, *On Psychic Pneuma*, 2.11.13, ed. Ideler (1841) I.375.17–21.

[114] Galen, *On the Preservation of Health*, ed. Kühn (1823) VI.1–452 = ed. Koch (1923) 3–198. See Wilkins (2016), who provides a fresh discussion of Galen's preventive medicine in light of the above-mentioned treatise.

[115] JZA, *On Psychic Pneuma*, 2.pr.3 and 2.16.12, ed. Ideler (1841) I.350.19–21 and I.382.17–18.

[116] In his *On Psychic Pneuma*, John does not provide a discussion on the bodily mixtures, but in his *Medical Epitome*, 1.3, ed. Ideler (1842) II.358.22–7, he clearly refers to nine different mixtures, thus following the Galenic theory on the subject. See Galen, *On Mixtures*, 1.8, ed. Kühn (1821) I.559.2–9 = ed. Helmreich (1904) 31.27–32.4. On Galen's theory, see Chapter 2, Section 1.1.

[117] JZA, *On Psychic Pneuma*, 2.17.3, ed. Ideler (1841) I.383.14–17.

which is colder and drier than the other pneumata, one should follow a moderately cold and dry diet.[118]

At the very beginning of the second book, John makes it clear that his advice will be brief, since he is not aiming to offer a therapy for every single affection.[119] According to him, digestion could be affected by various factors, including the quality and quantity of food, the harmful humours remaining in the stomach, and exercise.[120] He also gives handy advice to his reader on how to immediately diagnose the dominant quality in the stomach. For example, in the case of dryness, one may feel it on the tongue and treat it with the use of foodstuffs of the opposite quality.[121] The last part of the second book also includes details on how one can diagnose the predominance of a particular humour and the current mixture in the body through the examination of urine, excrement, the pulse, and secretions. John thus tries to provide his readers with a complete set of instructions from diagnosis to therapy.[122] The very brief and abridged nature of these instructions suggests his treatise was designed primarily for those with very little expertise on the subject of diagnosis with the aim of equipping them with the tools required for easy self-diagnosis.[123]

As I have already briefly mentioned in the context of John's example on the diagnosis of dryness, he is consistent throughout his treatise in urging his readers to treat *dyskrasia* by using the well-established ancient therapeutic approach of treatment by means of opposites (*enantia tōn enantiōn iamata*).[124] Thus every *dyskrasia* formed in the stomach should be primarily balanced with the consumption of foodstuffs of the opposite quality.[125] The order of the various foodstuffs (i.e cereals and pulses, vegetables and fruits, meat, liquids) shows many similarities with that of Galen and Paul of Aegina in *On the Capacities of Foodstuffs* and *Epitome* respectively,[126] although there are

[118] JZA, *On Psychic Pneuma*, 2.17.6, ed. Ideler (1841) I.383.23–9.

[119] JZA, *On Psychic Pneuma*, 2.3.11, ed. Ideler (1841) I.355.13–16.

[120] JZA, *On Psychic Pneuma*, 2.1.1, ed. Ideler (1841) I.350.23–8.

[121] JZA, *On Psychic Pneuma*, 2.2.3, ed. Ideler (1841) I.351.16–21.

[122] JZA, *On Psychic Pneuma*, 2.13–16, ed. Ideler (1841) I.377.1–382.19.

[123] John also makes cross references to his works *On Urines* and *Medical Epitome*, for those who prefer to consult a more detailed account on uroscopy and the examination of pulse respectively: *On Psychic Pneuma*, 2.13.8 and 2.15.9, ed. Ideler (1841) I.378.4–9 and 380.4–14.

[124] Among the various references, see JZA, *On Psychic Pneuma*, 1.13.25 and 1.16.13, ed. Ideler (1841) I.337.7–12 and 343.29–32.

[125] JZA, *On Psychic Pneuma*, 2.2.1 and 2.12.1, ed. Ideler (1841) I.351.11–12 and 375.25–7.

[126] See, for example, the first five paragraphs of the section on vegetables in *On Psychic Pneuma*, 2.6.2–7, ed. Ideler (1841) I.362.29–363.31, in which John starts by referring to *krambē* (cabbage), followed by *teutlon* (beet), *andrachnē* (purslane) and *atraphaxys* (orach), *serris* (chicory), and *thridakinē* (lettuce). In his *On the Capacities of Foodstuffs*, 2.40–6, ed. Kühn's (1823) VI.624.13–634.13 = ed. Wilkins (2013) 146.11–155.3, Galen starts by referring to *thridakinē, serreis, malachē* (mallow), *teutlon, krambē, bliton* (blite) and *atraphaxys*, and *andrachnē*. Paul of Aegina, *Epitome*, 1.74, ed. Heiberg's (1921) I.53.13–28, starts by referring to *thridakinē*, followed by *intybon* (endive), *malachē*, *teutlon*, *krambē*, and *bliton* and *atraphaxys*. Galen's

no verbatim quotations from the above authors. John follows the qualities traditionally associated with each foodstuff. For example, barley (*krithē*) is naturally cold and thus good for those who are suffering from fever and extreme warmth.[127] Some foodstuffs might have a stronger or a medicinal (*pharmakōdēs*) effect, such as radish (*raphanis*), which can be used as a cutting (*temnousa*) and thinning (*leptynousa*) agent with a direct effect on humours accumulating in the stomach.[128] John also recommends sleeping immediately after the consumption of food, since this revives (*anakainizein*) the entire body and the natural, vital, and psychic pneuma.[129]

Diet may be assisted by the use of drugs, bloodletting, exercise, or bathing according to each patient's individual characteristics. For example, in discussing an excess of blood, John simply suggests removing it by means of venesection, a commonly used method with a long tradition in the Graeco-Roman and Byzantine period.[130] If there is an excess of yellow bile in the stomach, John suggests the use of purgative drugs, such as aloe (*aloē*).[131] However, in cases of bilious excess accompanied by intense fevers, which cannot be treated by means of diet, one can use stronger drugs made, for example, from roses (*rhodōn*) and sugar (*sachar*).[132] This potion recalls recipes for sugar-based medicaments, such as juleps and syrups, that were introduced into Byzantine pharmacology from the Islamic world from the eleventh/twelfth

treatise, *On the Capacities of Foodstuffs*, is almost three hundred printed pages in Kühn's (1823) VI.453–748, edition, compared to the relevant sections in Paul of Aegina, *Epitome*, 1.73–96, ed. Heiberg (1921) I.52.11–66.26 and John, which are both around fifteen printed pages long. For a brief introduction to Galen's aforementioned work and its contents, see Wilkins (2003: ix–xxi).

[127] JZA, *On Psychic Pneuma*, 2.5.18, ed. Ideler (1841) I.361.7–11. Cf. Galen, *On the Capacities of Foodstuffs*, 1.1, ed. Kühn (1823) VI.474.3–6 = ed. Wilkins (2013) 19.11–14. On the Byzantine diet, see Dalby (2010); and Anagnostakis (2013). See also Koder (1993), who provides a useful study on the availability and use of a variety of vegetables in Byzantium.

[128] JZA, *On Psychic Pneuma*, 2.6.8, ed. Ideler (1841) I.363.22–8. There are other foodstuffs with a similar action, such as asparagus, *On Psychic Pneuma*, 2.6.14, ed. Ideler (1841) I.364.15–25. Galen wrote a special treatise *On the Thinning Diet*, 1, ed. Kalbfleisch (1923) 433.16–18, in which he clarifies that its name is derived from its effect on the thick humours of the body; see Wilkins (2002). On the use of foodstuffs as drugs, see the recent inspiring paper by Totelin (2015). See also JZA, *On Psychic Pneuma*, 1.13.28 and 1.13.33, ed. Ideler (1841) I.337.23–8 and 338.17–24, in which John suggests the use of drugs with a cutting and thinning effect (*temnōn/tmētikois, leptynōn/leptyntikois*) for those whose hearing and taste are affected as a result of an accumulation of humours.

[129] JZA, *On Psychic Pneuma*, 2.11.1, ed. Ideler (1841) I.373.17–23. See, for example, Galen, *On the Capacities of Foodstuffs*, 1.2, ed. Kühn (1823) VI.487.5–7 = ed. Wilkins (2013) 29.20–2, who refers to the beneficial role of sleep in the process of digestion.

[130] JZA, *On Psychic Pneuma*, 2.12.6, ed. Ideler (1841) I.376.14–16. See Bouras-Vallianatos (2015c: 112–21), who discusses Byzantine therapeutic approaches, including bloodletting techniques.

[131] Aloe was a well-known purgative in the ancient and medieval world; see Scarborough (1982) and Dalby (2003: 6). The use of drugs and, in particular, antidotes, in combination with a warm diet is also recommended in the case of an excess of phlegm and black bile, *On Psychic Pneuma*, 2.12.5 and 2.3.10, ed. Ideler (1841) I.376.11–14 and I.355.10–13, respectively.

[132] JZA, *On Psychic Pneuma*, 2.12.4, ed. Ideler (1841) I.376.2–11.

century onwards and gradually replaced honey-based drugs. John provides a long list of sugar-based potions in the pharmacological part of his *Medical Epitome*.[133] The references in his *On Psychic Pneuma* show John's particular interest in informing his work with new material and in line with contemporary demand. However, the most remarkable advice for the use of a drug is that of the well-known theriac of Andromachus, a compound antidote with very intense action, which he recommends if the cold quality is extremely persistent.[134]

Lastly, what makes John's account particularly interesting is that he often attempts to adapt his account to Joseph's particular needs and thus to those of his contemporaries, who followed the dietary restrictions and fasting regimen of the Orthodox monastic tradition.[135] Monks ate twice on non-fast days and only once on fast days. Meat was completely prohibited. They were expected to fast about 195 days per year, including abstaining from fish and dairy products, but not from shellfish and molluscs; on some of these days they would also abstain from oil and wine. In this context, for example, John apologizes to Joseph for paying attention to the quality of various kinds of meat.[136] Particular importance is also given to the quantity of food consumed and to dividing that food into three equal parts: the first two to be taken at midday and the third at night. This had special importance for Joseph, who—because he followed the strict rules of monastic fasting—did not always eat properly, which could produce either a state of over-warmth or over-coldness, resulting in a disturbance of the psychic pneuma.[137] In terms of exercise, John recommends speedy walking (*oxeis peripatoi*), hunting (*kynēgesiai*), wrestling (*palai*), running (*dromoi*), discus (*diskoi*), or exercise with a small ball (*to dia mikras sphairas gymnasion*)[138] for those consuming strong foodstuffs, while for Joseph, who followed a light diet, even a short walk (*brachys peripatos*) would be enough, particularly before the consumption of food in the early morning. More exercise is recommended in winter than in summer. John strongly advises avoiding exercise after meals, since it may disrupt the process of digestion and result in the accumulation of raw humours

[133] See Chapter 5, Section 5.1.

[134] JZA, *On Psychic Pneuma*, 2.17.16, ed. Ideler (1841) I.385.7–10. On theriac, see Chapter 5, n. 34.

[135] On fasting in the Orthodox tradition, see Musurillo (1956); and Louvaris (2005). On Byzantine monastic meals, see Talbot (2007). See also, Koder (1970), who provides a critical edition, German translation, and commentary on the poem on fasting by Patriarch Nicholas III Grammatikos (1084–1111) written for Protos, the head of the Athonite monastic community.

[136] JZA, *On Psychic Pneuma*, 2.6.28, ed. Ideler (1841) I.366.36–367.4.

[137] JZA, *On Psychic Pneuma*, 2.9–10, ed. Ideler (1841) I.372.24–373.15.

[138] Galen wrote a special treatise on *The Exercise with the Small Ball*, ed. Kühn (1823) V.899–910 = ed. Wenkebach (1938) 258–72, which was considered beneficial for the health of both body and soul.

(*ōmochymias thēsaurizousai*).[139] Finally, in line with his programmatic statement, in giving an account of the best way to maintain good health and thus taking into consideration a wide range of factors associated with an ideal daily regimen, John gives some brief instructions on bathing,[140] which he considers extremely beneficial, and, in particular, for Joseph, since his body is too dry due to long periods of fasting.

7. CONCLUSION

Inspired by the spiritual model of his contemporary, the monk and philosopher Joseph Rhakendytes, John wrote a special treatise on psychic pneuma, the first instrument and vehicle of the soul in the human body. In contrast to his ancient medical predecessors, such as Galen, John had no difficulty in identifying the carrier of the soul, i.e. the psychic pneuma, in the body. His endeavour was facilitated by the Neoplatonic theory of the pneumatic body (*ochēma*-pneuma). The theory of the three pneumata (i.e. psychic, vital, and natural) had been established as the main dogma in the Greek medical literature by the end of seventh century. John's addition of a fourth pneuma in the stomach allows him to ascribe two qualities to each pneuma and directly connect the production and distribution of pneuma with bodily mixtures.

John was influenced by Galen's theories on the fineness of pneuma and later Neoplatonic views, as featured in the works of Synesios of Cyrene and John Philoponos, in relation to the role of regimen. However, the systematic classification of qualitative change of the psychic pneuma as the object of treatment is John's own innovation, thus showing his ability to make original contributions to other medical fields, apart from that of uroscopy, as has been showing in examining his *On Urines*. His entire second book is a practical manual for those with little familiarity with the medical art, aimed at helping them diagnose and treat themselves easily and thus keep their bodily and spiritual health in good condition. Unlike the *Medical Epitome*, which provides its non-expert readers with details on a wide range of advice on diagnosis and therapy, here there is a particular focus on those agents that will help maintain the physiological functions of the body in good order.[141] John's efforts to classify a large number of foodstuffs and also the

[139] JZA, *On Psychic Pneuma*, 2.11.5–8, ed. Ideler (1841) I.374.6–29.

[140] JZA, *On Psychic Pneuma*, 2.11.9–10, ed. Ideler (1841) I.374.29–375.6. On the role of bathing in medicine with a strong focus on the early Byzantine period, see Zytka (2019: 117–79).

[141] In light of John's very brief treatment of foodstuffs in his *Medical Epitome*, in which he admits to using a summary from his second book *On Psychic Pneuma* (see Chapter 5, n. 42), the latter can be seen as complementary to the treatment of regimen in his *Medical Epitome*.

way he connects the role of exercise, sleep, and bathing with keeping the psychic pneuma and the health of the soul in good condition is exceptional and allows him to offer comprehensive advice on the most appropriate psychotherapeutic regimen.[142]

[142] This chapter is a revised version of Bouras-Vallianatos (2019c), which has been adapted for the purposes of the present monograph. For example, explanatory details about John's life and works have been removed, and sometimes the analysis of particular passages has been supplemented with additional discussion and/or bibliographical references.

7

Conclusion

In response to a question from an interviewer about the narrative of his novel *TransAtlantic* (published in June 2013) the novelist Colum McCann (b. 1965), astoundingly replied: 'I am trying to make sense of it now. In fact, maybe you could tell me what it means . . . that would be great. It would be nice to know what it means . . . '[1] It is impossible to be in an author's mind when s/he wrote her/his work or perfectly reconstruct their world of thought, knowledge, and expertise which would ideally offer a reliable interpretation of the work. Sometimes, as in the case of the Irish novelist cited above, even the author himself is unable to give a convincing answer about his writing intentions. Furthermore, a work acquires meaning through the response of the audience at the moment of reception. Of course, ancient and medieval treatises are not works of fiction and, in most cases, we are unable to reconstruct the original response of their medieval readers. But still the method of composing and making the texts available to an audience involves a similar intellectual process. Ancient and medieval texts present the additional challenge that their surviving version, unless an autograph is preserved, has undergone several stages of revision from scribes, readers, and modern editors. Here I have tried to provide the first critical, comprehensive assessment of John Zacharias Aktouarios' work and thought, the main findings of which are outlined below.

John was a well-educated practising physician in Constantinople and a prominent member of the early Palaiologan intelligentsia. He frequented the highest social and scholarly circles being in contact with prominent individuals, including Theodore Metochites and Alexios Apokaukos, and in close communication and correspondence with Joseph Rhakendytes, George Lakapenos, and Michael Gabras. His impact as a well-established and

[1] The interview was part of the series *Οι Κεραίες της Εποχής μας* (*The Transmitters of our Era*) broadcast on the Hellenic Radio and Television Channel 2 (*ΕΡΤ2*). It was presented by Antaios Chrysostomidis and Mikela Chartouliari and can be viewed on YouTube at https://www.youtube.com/watch?v=OxQdsdJGMBs (accessed 17 October 2018). This particular passage features in 44:08–44:37.

Innovation in Byzantine Medicine: The Writings of John Zacharias Aktouarios (c.1275–c.1330). Petros Bouras-Vallianatos, Oxford University Press (2020). © Petros Bouras-Vallianatos 2020.
DOI: 10.1093/oso/9780198850687.001.0001

successful physician had received recognition from Emperor Andronikos II, who appointed him to the office of *aktouarios*, the highest honorific title awarded to physicians in late Byzantium.

John was eager to show his admiration for the classical medical tradition in which he was well versed. And he did this by, for example, advising his readers to consult the works of the most wise (*sophōtatos*) Galen, by using Galenic models to introduce his case histories or the experience he claimed for himself in the case of pharmacology, and also by directly citing from Galen's pharmacological works in the case of the *Medical Epitome*. Although he noted omissions or substantially supplemented the views of ancient and Byzantine authors, including Hippocrates, Galen, and Theophilos, as in the case of uroscopy and pneumatology, he never chose to deploy the strong rhetoric that earlier writers such as Alexander of Tralles had used to challenge Galen or the often acerbic tone employed by Symeon Seth. Furthermore, he was remarkable in that he never introduced or cited any miraculous or popular ideas about disease or the treatment thereof. For example, he never suggested making use of amulets and incantations, although these can be found not only in *iatrosophia*, but also in works by authors such as Galen and Alexander of Tralles.[2]

John's extensive medical output makes him a unique case among middle and late Byzantine medical authors. He is distinguished by the plurality of the subjects that he addressed in detail and also for his originality and the personal contribution that he often made to the medical fields that he engaged with. The latter also makes him stand out from other Palaiologan intellectuals in that he was not only involved in the revival of the classical tradition through the creation of new and more accessible compilations of earlier authors, but he was eager to embellish ancient and earlier Byzantine material with knowledge derived from his daily contact with patients. This is most evident in his case histories. He also strove to keep up with developments taking place outside Byzantium, either in the Islamic world or in the Latin West. Beyond the strictly literary medical assessment of John's works, it is worth bearing in mind that certain improvements in the diagnosis and treatment of disease directly impacted on the everyday life of a large number of people, not only emperors, scholars, or intellectuals, but ordinary citizens, too. The same cannot be said of, for example, improvements in understanding the movements of the stars or deeper engagement with philosophical texts, which rarely had any such important practical implications.

In particular, starting from an interpretation of John's uroscopic treatise, I have shown how John brings his own point of view to bear on the subject. By marking his observations with a recurrent set of expressions, he engages his

[2] On Galen and Alexander of Tralles, see Jouanna (2011) and Bouras-Vallianatos (2016a), respectively.

reader with his conceptual world and areas of expertise. His evident authorial presence throughout the work shows John's ambition to communicate his wide knowledge of the subject to his specialist readers. His efforts to construct a detailed uroscopic theory reflect first the lack of systematization in the subject hitherto, and second the contemporary scientific debate on uroscopy. In contrast to earlier Byzantine uroscopic treatises, John did not just collect all the available data and summarize it in a long account. The author shows particular concern to structure his treatise in clear and easy-to-consult sections. This is not just a work in which John finds a place to inform readers about his original observations, it is also the long-expected, complete account of the subject. By dividing the work into three parts (on diagnosis, aetiology, and prognosis), John not only emphasizes the area of prognosis, which was often neglected in earlier uroscopic theories, but he also shows the importance of giving reasons for observations, a fundamental requirement for a professional and educated physician. His recognition of the need for precise aetiology, although mostly unnecessary in the physician's interaction with a patient, highlights the contemporary interest in scientific debate, something also illustrated in the works of early Palaiologan scholars from other disciplines such as astronomy and mathematics.

John owed his reputation as regards uroscopy to three factors. The first is that he provides his own interpretations of fundamental physiological processes, as in the case of digestion. He is the first author that we know of since Galen's times to offer a more detailed discussion of digestion, introducing a new stage. A historian of late medieval/early Renaissance medicine might look for evidence of considerable anatomical exploration as an index of a physician's innovative contribution to the subject. This seems to have been the criterion by which medical innovation was judged in the West at that period, as, for example, in the case of the celebrated professor of medicine at Bologna, Mondino de' Liuzzi (*c.*1270–1326), whose treatise on anatomy remained the standard textbook on the subject for more than two centuries.[3] At the same time, in the Islamic world, the Syro-Egyptian physician Ibn al-Nafis (d. 1288) was putting across his influential theory of pulmonary transit.[4] Although John's understanding of the digestion is not comparable in terms of impact to Ibn al-Nafis' contribution,[5] he nevertheless questioned a well-discussed function of the human body in an attempt to better understand the crucial role of the liver in this process and the consequent formation of urine; he also described previously unattested renal vessels, such as the so-called lambdoid

[3] Siraisi (1981: 66–9, 110–14); and Cunningham (1997: 42–54).

[4] On Ibn al-Nafis, see Fancy (2013). On the question of human dissection in the medieval Islamic world, see Savage-Smith (1995).

[5] See Brömer (2012)

vein. Whether this understanding was based on anatomical examination is not clear,[6] but his views on human digestion combined with the original contributions he made to pneumatology, as shown in the examination of *On Psychic Pneuma*, confirm his engagement in a process of ongoing research into human physiology.

The second factor in building his reputation was his successful attempt to encapsulate recent developments in uroscopy in the creation of his detailed, graduated urine vial. His theory on the analogies between parts of the human body and parts of the urine vial provides a significant example of parallelism between Byzantine and medieval Western medicine. Although John is aware of current theories on the subject, through the Greek translation of the uroscopic treatise ascribed to Ibn Sīnā, he is not just repeating what has been said before. He goes a step further, providing a novel and meticulous division of the urine vial, showing an eye for detail and a practical concern for the exact identification of each particular space. At the same time, traditional and well-discussed topics, such as the various colours of urine, are not simply copied from earlier treatises, but described with more clarifications, so that they can be better identified and consequently provide a more precise diagnosis and prognosis. And this leads us to the third aspect on which his reputation rests, which is John's ability to provide a stimulating presentation of his material by including stories taken from his contact with actual patients.

John gives credibility to his uroscopic theories by narrating physician–patient encounters arising out of his practical involvement with the subject. John's case histories also serve a didactic purpose for young physicians, providing advice on how to work with and react to the patients' various attitudes. More importantly, in his own way, John opens up a window onto late Byzantine medical practice, showing the particularities of treating a pregnant woman, an acquaintance, an adolescent, or a peasant. Furthermore, by showing his readers how an unfailingly successful physician could display his observations in this unique way, John was also attempting to promote himself in line with the contemporary attitude to social distinction, which was often related to an individual's literary skills.

Thanks to John's uroscopic treatise, Byzantine medicine looks much more dynamic than has been assumed till now. Although we may not have comparable examples from the field of medicine in the late Byzantine period, early

[6] In contrast to the Western medieval world, there are no reported cases of or any evidence for the practice of dissection in Palaiologan Byzantium. See Bliquez and Kazhdan (1984), and Browning (1985), who briefly reported five cases (between the eighth and twelfth century) in a variety of non-medical sources, in which Byzantine physicians are credited with undertaking human dissection. The sources have not been fully contextualized, and, at least, in the two cases dated to the twelfth century, the texts refer to the 'skill of practising dissection' (without providing any details about actual dissections) as one of the skills of a successful physician. In my opinion, this reference seems to have been employed for rhetorical effect.

Palaiologan astronomy offers a number of innovative observations. It is beside the point to judge whether Gregoras' proposal on the revision of the church calendar is more important than the introduction of John's urine vial. In a similar vein, we may point out that Gregoras' revival of the Platonic dialogue is comparable with John's decision to narrate his relationship with his patients by reviving the Galenic genre of case histories. However, it is the historian's role to emphasize that no other early Palaiologan scientific work enjoyed such a wide circulation and reception as John's *On Urines*, shaping, as it did, a particular field in a distinctive way for centuries to come in Byzantium and beyond. This is not only attested in the large-scale production of manuscripts from as early as the fourteenth century or the notable engagement with it by late Byzantine physicians and philosophers such as John Argyropoulos and his student Demetrios Angelos (*c.*1430s–early sixteenth century),[7] who copied and annotated John's work, but also in the reception of the work by Renaissance scholars in subsequent centuries.

Not surprisingly, by 1519 John's work had been published in Latin translation by Ambrogio Leone of Nola (1458/9–1525), who studied medicine in Padua. The translation is preceded by Ambrogio's letter to his son, Camillo, who has just started studying medicine, in which he equates John's treatise on urines to Galen's corpus on the pulse, emphasizing the gap in the field that John had filled in such a sophisticated way, thus substantially benefiting future physicians.[8] This becomes even more significant if we take into consideration the fact that uroscopy might also be performed by folk healers. Ambrogio's edition was widely circulated among contemporary physicians and went through two further editions and several reprints in subsequent decades.[9] John's urine vial, which must be considered his most important contribution to the history of medicine, became extremely popular, not only appearing in the work of university professors, such as the influential uroscopic treatise of the German professor of medicine at Marburg, Euricius Cordus (1484–1535) (see Figure 7.1),[10] but also showing up in sixteenth-century vernacular texts,

[7] On the manuscripts of *On Urines*, see Chapter 1, n. 184. John Argyropoulos taught medicine at the *Katholikon Mouseion* of the Kral *xenōn* shortly before the Fall of Constantinople in 1453 (see Chapter 1, n. 126) and he copied some folia from Parisinus gr. 2232, which among other works contains John's treatise; Demetrios Angelos, a student of Argyropoulos, provides marginal annotations in Parisinus gr. 2270 (fourteenth century), and partially copied Vindobonensis med. gr. 44 (first half of the fifteenth century) and Londiniensis Wellcomensis MS.MSL.52 (fifteenth century). See Mondrain (2000a: 234); and (2010).

[8] Ambrogio Leone of Nola (1519: *praefatio*). I owe this reference to Stathakopoulos (unpublished). Leone was the scribe and perhaps owner of a Greek manuscript, Dresdensis Da 5 [now in Moscow; see Appendix 5, Q=Moscquensis (ex Dresdensis Da 5)] of John's *opera omnia*. On Leone, see Spruit (2005).

[9] For a list of the Latin editions and reprints of John's *On Urines*, see Choulant (1828: 98). The second edition was by Conrad Gessner (1541) and the third by Jacques Goupyl (1548).

[10] Cordus (1543: 1, 11). On Cordus, see Dolezal (1957).

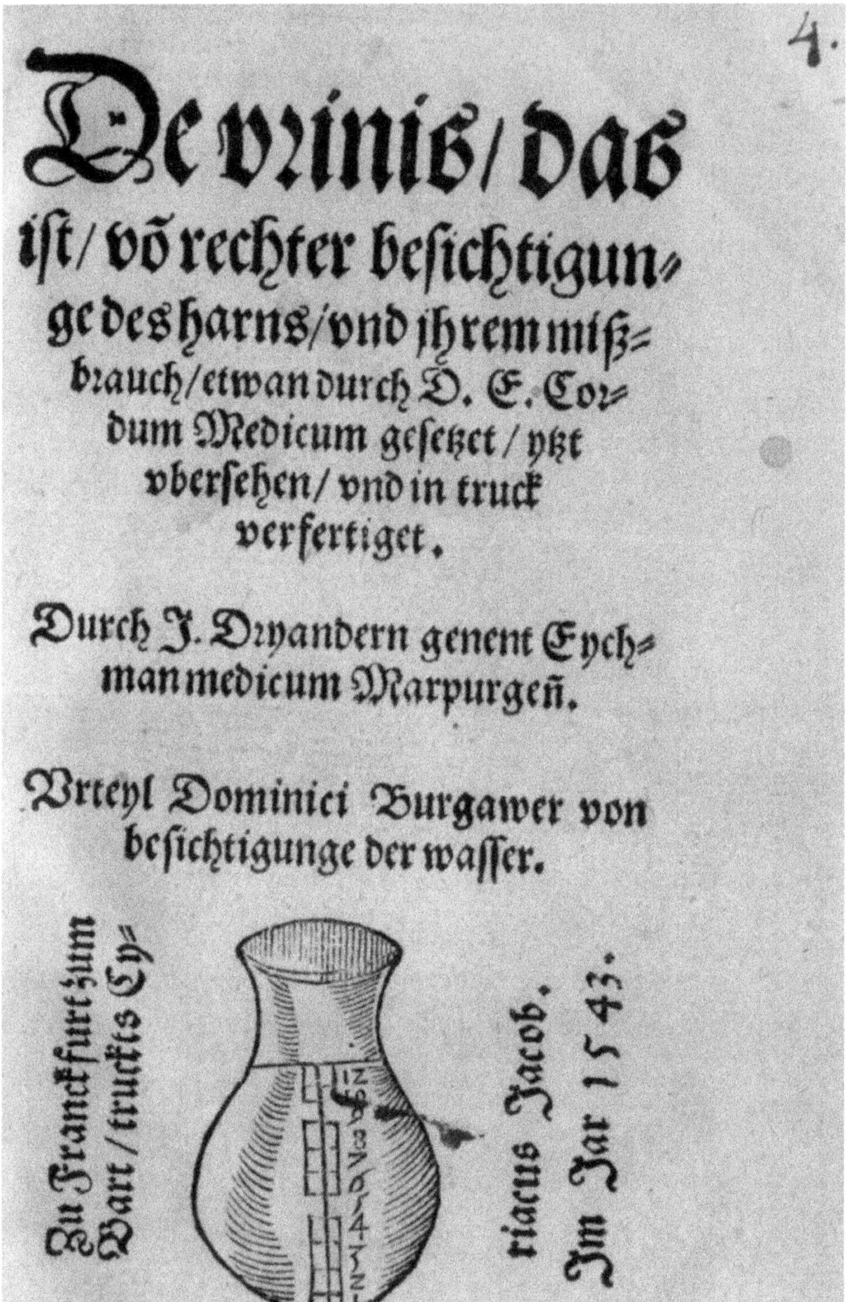
4.
De vrinis/ das
ist/ võ rechter besichtigun-
ge des harns/ vnd jhrem miß-
brauch/ etwan durch D. E. Cor-
dum Medicum gesetzet/ yetzt
vbersehen/ vnd in truck
verfertiget.

Durch J. Dryandern genent Eych-
man medicum Marpurgeñ.

Vrteyl Dominici Burgawer von
besichtigunge der wasser.

Zu Franckfurt zum
Bart/ truckts Cy-
riacus Jacob.
Im Jar 1543.

Figure 7.1. Euricius Cordus, *De Urinis*, Frankfurt, 1543, Book Cover.

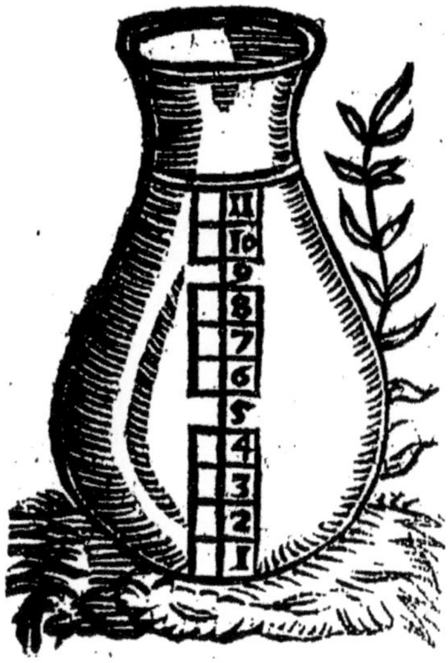

Figure 7.2. Robert Recorde, *Urinal of Physick*, London, 1548, p. 2.

such as the *Urinal of Physick* by the Welsh physician Robert Recorde (*c.*1512–58) (see Figure 7.2), which was aimed at a broad medical audience.[11] His enduring influence may be attested in the eighteenth-century urological work by the prominent Flemish anatomist and professor in Leuven, Hendrik Jozef Rega (1690–1754).[12]

In this book I have also investigated John's *Medical Epitome*, revealing his particular purpose in writing his work and its unique assemblage of material. It is not simply another Byzantine 'encyclopaedic' handbook on the subject, but was written for Alexios Apokaukos, a *philiatros* himself, and was by extension designed to appeal to other highly educated contemporaries. Through a study of John's method of composition, it was first established that John was no mere copy-paster and that the process of compiling earlier material on a specific subject was not a mechanical act for him. The first four books show him setting out to effectively and usefully reduce the size of earlier works such as Paul of Aegina's *Epitome*, which was among John's main sources. Nevertheless, when John thinks that something lacks the proper treatment for his reader, he does not hesitate to supplement the existing material with small but noticeable additions, such as in the case of differential

[11] Recorde (1547: i, viii). On Recorde, see Johnston (2008).

[12] Rega (1733: 185, 203) provides numerous references to John's work, such as the discussion of the various colours of urine and the various kinds of sediments. On Rega, see van der Corput (1905).

diagnosis, most prominently in ophthalmology. The omission of details on complicated invasive operations, which had been given, for example, by Paul of Aegina, should be understood in the light of the general scope of the work, which was intended to be read primarily by the non-expert.

John shows particular care in collecting pharmacological data, using a large variety of sources both ancient Greek and early Byzantine, as well as recently introduced Greek translations of Arabic works, thus confirming the significant transfer of Arabic pharmacological knowledge into Byzantium. Here the process of selection of sources is based on John's clinical experience (*peira*); it shows a more dynamic engagement on the part of the author and thus a more complicated synthesis of material. For example, I have managed to trace a number of connections with some late Byzantine works that have never been explored before. John makes use of Ibn al-Jazzār's *Ephodia tou Apodēmountos* and he has many recipes in common with the *Dynameron*. The addition of oriental material made John's project much more diverse and different from earlier medical manuals for *philiatroi*, such as Galen's *Therapeutics to Glaucon* or Oribasios' *For Eunapios*. This decision attests John's openness and also his eagerness to communicate with other cultures.

Furthermore, I have shown that John's *materia medica* was part of the history of late Byzantine imported spices and was not just a literary elaboration. Judging from the fact that the *Medical Epitome* had a far wider circulation than the huge and not user-friendly *Dynameron*,[13] it was John who, through his efficient amalgamation of traditional ancient Greek and Byzantine sources and foreign material, first managed to make the newly introduced knowledge of oriental *materia medica* available and accessible to the Byzantine reader. John's work fulfilled contemporary social needs to cure human diseases with new and perhaps more effective drugs, containing oriental ingredients that gradually became available in European markets from the eleventh/twelfth century onwards.

It is worth noting that among the Byzantines who had a copy of John's *Medical Epitome* in later centuries we find the scholar and later Cardinal Bishop Bessarion (1403–72) and the *archiatros* Anthony Pyropoulos, a student of John Argyropoulos. On the one hand, the luxurious parchment copy of the entire work, Venetus Marcianus gr. 298, once owned by Bessarion, shows John's work as symbolizing the outstanding Palaiologan heritage; on the other, the finest manuscript, Vindobonensis med. gr. 17 copied for Pyropoulos, unveils the working material of one of the last notable Byzantine physicians

[13] The *Medical Epitome* survives complete in twenty-six manuscripts and there are thirteen more fragmentary and excerpting manuscripts. See Appendix 5. The *Dynameron* survives almost complete in only seven manuscripts, although there are also a considerable number of excerpting manuscripts. A provisional list of witnesses is available on *Pinakes: Textes et manuscrits grecs*, at http://pinakes.irht.cnrs.fr/notices/oeuvre/2265/ (accessed 10 October 2018). See also Valiakos (2019: xiv), who lists twenty manuscripts altogether; and Touwaide (2016b: 7, 300).

practising just a few years before the Fall of Constantinople in 1453.[14] Moreover, the fifteenth-century Byzantine physician and scribe Andreiomenos also used John's pharmacological recommendations in his surviving, as yet unedited, recipe book.[15] Beyond the narrow confines of Byzantium, the French physician to King Francis I (r. 1515–47), Jean Ruelle (1474–1537), the translator of the monumental work by Dioscorides *De Materia Medica*, translated the pharmacological part of John's treatise into Latin as early as 1539,[16] fifteen years before the edition of the complete Latin translation of the *Medical Epitome* by Henry Mathys in 1554.[17]

The last work that was examined in this book is the *On Psychic Pneuma*. I have shown that John adopted the Neoplatonic theory of the pneumatic body (*ochēma*-pneuma) combined with a fundamentally Galenic understanding of the role of the psychic pneuma in consciousness, sensation, and voluntary movement, and its flow through the nerves. Unlike his predecessors, John's introduction of the fourth pneuma, produced in the stomach, allowed him to associate each of these pneumata with two qualities and thus make a direct connection with the mixtures (*kraseis*) of each part and of the body as a whole. Similar concerns as regards supplementing earlier theories on human physiology were also noted in *On Urines*, but here John's proposed model has a broader scope, beyond the practice of medicine or the theoretical understanding of the fundamental functions of the human body. In particular, his provision of a long list of foodstuffs and their qualities, as well as his advice on bathing, sleep, and exercise, makes his treatise a unique psychotherapeutic manual.

John expresses his scientific views on the role of the psychic pneuma in the body, the vehicle and first instrument of the soul, while at the same time writing a work that could serve as an essential companion for Joseph Rhakendytes and, by extension, for every other contemporary individual following

[14] On Antonios Pyropoulos' medical activity, see Kousis (1946). Moreover, the early-fifteenth-century physician Demetrios Pepagomenos is the copyist of one of the manuscripts of the *Medical Epitome*, i.e. Parisinus gr. 2256. On Pepagomenos, see Lazaris (2006: 251–7).

[15] It is preserved in Athous Iberiticus 151 (fifteenth century), ff. 228r–235v, at. f. 235r, l.13: '*κατὰ τὸν ὠκτάριον· ἡ αἰγυπτία ὠφελεῖ ἐπιληπτικοῖς*'. The titles of the recipes of Andreiomenos' recipe book were published by Kousis (1929). On Andreiomenos' connections with the circle of John Argyropoulos, see Pietrobelli (2010: 120–6). John's recipes are also found in the anonymous collections of composite drugs in Vaticanus gr. 282 (fifteenth century), f. 436v, ll. 15–19: '*πρὸς ἡμιπληξίαν τοῦ ἀκτουαρίου . . .*'; and Bononiensis 3632 (mid fifteenth century), f. 201r, ll. 1–9, f. 235r, ll. 16–18, and f. 247r, ll. 30–6: '*ἀντίδοτος ὀκταρίου . . . Ἰωάννου κυροῦ Ζαχαρίου· ὀφελὴ ὕπαρ σπλήν· καὶ νεφρούς*', '*ὀκταρίου πεσός . . .*', and '*ἡ κυρὰ τοῦ Ἀλιέος· ὀκταρίου . . .*'. '*Ὠκτάριος*' or '*Ὀκτάριος*' is found in various manuscripts instead of the usual '*ἀκτουάριος*'. On this, see Chapter 1, n. 154 and Appendix 5, *passim*.

[16] Ruelle (1539). Ruelle (1537) also made use of John's description of simple drugs in his monumental three-volume botanical work *De natura stirpium*. On this, see Hasse (2016: 157–62). On Ruelle, see Reulos and Bietenholz (1985).

[17] Mathys (1554). On Mathys, see Jacques (1897).

Joseph's mode of life. This is confirmed by the inclusion of the work in some manuscripts of Joseph's educational textbook, *Synopsis Variarum Disciplinarum*. Later on, John was appreciated as an authority on pneumatology, and his contribution was acknowledged by early modern European physicians, including the court physician to several Habsburg emperors, Julius A. von Neustein (1506–90), who published his Latin translation of *On Psychic Pneuma* in 1547.[18] This translation was included in the first edition of the Latin translation of the *Medical Epitome* in 1554 and, later, in the first complete edition of John's *opera omnia* in Latin translation in 1556.[19] Perhaps due to the fact that it was considerably briefer than *On Urines* and the *Medical Epitome*, *On Psychic Pneuma* is John's only work to have also appeared in an early printed edition in Greek by Jacques Goupyl (1525[?]–64), chair of medicine in the Collège Royal, Paris.[20] Study of the numerous annotations made by Renaissance scholars and physicians in John's manuscripts and early printed editions will further elucidate his enduring posthumous influence and reception.

[18] Von Neustein (1547). On von Neustein, see Schadelbauer (1953).

[19] Mathys (1554) and (1556). For the early printed editions and translations of John's works, see the lists by Fabricius (1724: 636–9); Choulant (1828: 97–8); and Durling (1967: 324–5).

[20] Goupyl (1557). Goupyl (1548) was also involved in the second edition of the Latin translation of John's *On Urines* (see n. 9, above) and was also the owner of the Greek manuscript Leidensis Vossianus gr. F. 32 (see Appendix 5, S=Leidensis Vossianus gr. F. 32) which contains John's entire corpus. On Goupyl, see Tétry (1985).

Appendices

APPENDIX 1

Glossary of Medical Terms

The majority of the following information is based on entries in LSJ, Leven (2005a), and the glossary in Johnston and Horsley (2011: cxii–cxxv). The reference to various illnesses/symptoms follows the relevant descriptions found in ancient and Byzantine medical texts. Modern terms in English translation, followed by the Greek term and its transliteration in parenthesis, are given for most of the entries for the convenience of the reader. However, it should be noted that in some cases such modern terms are applied retrospectively and do not correspond precisely to the Greek terms in question.

A capite ad calcem (from head to toe): This is the traditional order followed by ancient and medieval authors in listing approaches to various illnesses starting from those of the head and ending with those of the lower limbs.

Arteriotomy (ἀρτηριοτομία/artēriotomia): Opening or cutting of an artery wall.

Canthus (κανθός/kanthos): The corner of each eye where the upper and lower lids meet.

Chalazion (χαλάζιον/chalazion): A small cyst on the eyelid.

Conjuctiva (ἐπιπεφυκὼς ὑμήν/epipephykōs hymēn): The mucus, transparent membrane that covers the eyeball and the under surface of the eyelid.

Dropsy (ὕδερος/hyderos): An illness caused by the accumulation of water in parts of the body, usually resulting in swelling of the abdomen.

Ectropion (ἐκτρόπιον/ektropion): A condition in which the lower eyelid turns outwards.

Emphysema (ἐμφύσημα/emphysēma): The term could refer either to an inflation of the stomach or swelling of the eye.

Enterocele (ἐντεροκήλη/enterokēlē): A type of hernia in which the intestine erupts into the scrotum.

Erysipelas (ἐρυσίπελας/erysipelas): An acute dermatic infection characterized by redness of the skin.

Eyelid lancet (βλεφαρόξυστον/blepharoxyston): A surgical instrument used to smooth the edges of the eyelid.

Fetid polyp (ὄζαινα/ozaina): A chronic disease of the nose accompanied by a fetid discharge.

Fistula (συρίγγιον/syringion): Hard, deep, tubular ulcers in the soft tissues of the body that can reach the bones.

Gout (ποδάγρα/podagra): An illness which may appear in the upper limbs (*cheiragra*) or more commonly in the lower limbs (*podagra*) and is characterized by a red, hot swollen joint at the base of the big toe; it was thought to be caused mainly by an excess of yellow bile.

Hypochondrium (ὑποχόνδριον/hypochondrion): The soft parts of the body below the cartilage and above the navel.

Inflammation (φλεγμονή/phlegmonē): Usually characterized by redness, pain, and a throbbing sensation. In contrast to the modern understanding where it is considered a complex biological reaction of the tissues to pathogens or damaged cells, the ancient and medieval authors believed that it was caused by a wedged influx of blood.

Jaundice (ἴκτερος/ikteros): An illness characterized by the yellowish appearance of the skin as a result of the abnormal function of the liver; it was thought to be caused by an excess of yellow bile, which flowed under the skin.

Leucoma (λεύκωμα/leukōma): Listed in LSJ as 'a white spot in the eye caused by a thickening of the cornea'.

Melancholy (μελαγχολία/melancholia): A state of melancholy caused by an excess of black bile.

Midriff (φρήν/phrēn): The part of the body between the chest and the waist.

Omental hernia (ἐπιπλοκήλη/epiplokēlē): An abdominal type of hernia containing omentum, that is a layer of the peritoneum surrounding the abdominal organs.

Quartan fever (τεταρταῖος πυρετός/tetartaios pyretos): A type of fever recurring at approximately three-day intervals; it was probably connected with cases of malaria. Fever was usually considered a disease in its own right rather than a symptom as in the modern sense of the word.

Pediculosis (φθειρίασις/phtheiriasis): Infestation of the scalp and the eyebrows with lice.

Peripneumonia (περιπνευμονία/peripneumonia): Inflammation of the lungs.

Phlebotomy (φλεβοτομία/phlebotomia): Opening or cutting of a vein wall.

Pleurisy (πλευρῖτις/pleuritis): An inflammation of the pleura.

Psorophthalmia (ψωροφθαλμία/psōrophthalmia): An eye condition characterized by dryness and itchiness of the eyelid.

Pterygium (πτερύγιον/pterygion): An elevated, external, ocular mass that grows from the medical canthus of the eye onto the corneal surface.

Scirrhus (σκίρρος/skirrhos): Listed in LSJ as a 'hardened swelling or tumour, induration'.

Sclerophthalmia (σκληροφθαλμία/sklērophthalmia): Listed in LSJ as 'hardness of the eyes'.

Scrofula (χοιράς/choiras): Listed in LSJ as 'scrufulous swellings in the glands of the neck'.

Stye (κριθή/krithē): A condition characterized by an abscess or a pustule along the eyelid.

Sycosis (σύκωσις/sykōsis): An elongated, developed trachoma.

Theriac (θηριακή/thēriakē): A famous complex compound antidote against poisons with purgative action. There were various recipes for it; the most popular was the one attributed to the Greek physician Andromachus the Elder (first century AD), personal doctor to Nero.

Trachoma (τράχωμα/trachōma): A condition referring to an intense roughness on the inside of the eyelid.

Tylosis (τύλωσις/tylōsis): A chronic trachoma resembling a callus.

Ulcer (ἕλκος/helkos): The term may be used to denote a fresh or chronic wound, and also ruptured vesicles.

Xerophthalmia (ξηροφθαλμία/xērophthalmia): Listed in LSJ as 'inflammation of the eyelids, with redness and smarting'.

APPENDIX 2

Accounts of Urine Colour in Theophilos' *On Urines* and John's *On Urines*

Theophilos, *On Urines*, 6, ed. Ideler (1841) I.266.17–268.3

Περὶ χρωμάτων τῶν οὔρων.

(1) *Καιρὸς οὖν ἐξηγήσασθαι περὶ τῆς τῶν χρωμάτων διαφορᾶς, καὶ εἰπεῖν πόσαι εἰσὶ καὶ ποῖαι, καὶ μετὰ ποταπῆς συστάσεως δύνανται συμπλακῆναι ἢ πᾶσαι ἤ τινες.*

(2) *Ἐστὶ μὲν οὖν τῶν χρωμάτων πρῶτον τὸ λευκόν, καὶ τούτου πλάτος ἐν ἑαυτῷ κεκτημένου· κρύσταλλος γὰρ καὶ χιών, καὶ τίτανος, καὶ ὕδωρ ἀκραιφνές, λευκὰ μέν, οὐκ ἐν τῷ ἀκρῷ δὲ πάντα.*

(3) *Ἐνδεέστερον δὲ τούτου τοῦ χρώματος τὸ γαλακτῶδες, νοούμενον πηλίκον ἐστὶν ἐκ τῆς προσωνυμίας·*

John, *On Urines*, 1.8, ed. Ideler (1842) II.11.33–15.28

Περὶ διαφορᾶς τῶν κατὰ τὸ χῦμα χρωμάτων.

(1) *Ὁπόσα τοίνυν εἴδη χρωμάτων τοῖς οὔροις ἐμφαίνεται, καθ' ἕκαστον μὲν οὐ ῥᾴδιόν ἐστι φάναι, ταῖς πολλαῖς*[1] *τῶν χυμῶν συμπλοκαῖς τε καὶ πέψεσι πολλῶν καὶ τῶν χρωμάτων ἐπιδεικνυμένων.*

(2) *Ἔνεστί γε μὴν τῶν καιριωτέρων διορισθέντων τῷ λόγῳ, ἐκ τούτων ὡς ἀπό τινων ὡρισμένων σημείων καὶ τῶν λοιπῶν καταστοχάζεσθαι χρωμάτων, μὴ διορισθέντων τῷ λόγῳ, ὀνομάτων οἰκείων ἀπορίᾳ.*

(3) *Τῶν οὔρων τοίνυν τὰ μὲν λευκά, τὰ δ' ὠχρά, τὰ δὲ πυρρά, τὰ δὲ ξανθά, ἕτερα δὲ ἐρυθρά, τὰ δ' οἰνωπὰ κυανά τε ἐπὶ τούτοις καὶ χλωρὰ καὶ μέλαινα φαίνεται, οὐκ ἐν τούτοις τῶν πάντων ἀπαρτιζομένων χρωμάτων, ἀλλ' ἐκ τούτων καὶ*[2] *ἐμμέσων τε καὶ παραμέσων ὡς πλειόνων ἐντεῦθεν ἐπισυνηγμένων χρωμάτων.*

(4) *Τῶν οὖν λευκῶν οὔρων τὰ μὲν κρυσταλλοειδῆ, τὰ δὲ χιονοειδῆ, τὰ δὲ ὡς ἀκραιφνὲς ὕδωρ πέφυκε, καὶ ταῦτα μὲν ἐσχάτης ἂν εἴη λευκότητος.*

(5) *Ἐπεὶ δὲ τάς τε ἐπιτάσεις καὶ τὰς*[3] *ὑφέσεις ἐπιδέχεται τὰ γενικὰ τῶν χρωμάτων, τὰ δὲ δὴ ῥηθέντα ἐπιτεταμένης ἂν εἴη λευκότητος, ἐπὶ τούτοις προσθῶμεν τῷ λόγῳ καὶ ὅσα δῆτα ὑφειμένης λευκότητος πέφυκεν.*

(6) *Ἐπειδὰν τοίνυν τῆς ἄκρας λευκότητος ὑφίηται ἡ χροία, τὸ γαλακτῶδες οὕτω καλούμενον ἀπὸ τοῦ ἐοικέναι γάλακτι παρασκευάζει κρεῖττον μὲν ὂν τοῦ τε*

[1] Georgiou (2013) 418.8 reads '*ποιαῖς*'.

[2] Georgiou (2013) 419.1 reads '*καὶ τῶν*'.

[3] Georgiou (2013) 419.5 omits '*τὰς*'.

εἶτα ἀπολιπόμενον τοῦδε τὸ γλαυκόν,

ὡς κέρας διαυγές, ἢ ὡς οἱ κτηδόνες τοῦ κερατοειδοῦς χιτῶνος τοῦ ὀφθαλμοῦ· εἶτα τούτου ἀπολιπόμενον τὸ χαροπόν.

(4) Ἐστὶ δὲ τὸ χαροπὸν οἷάπερ τὰ τῶν καμήλων ἔρια τὰ ὑπόλευκα, ἢ ὡς λίθος ὀνυχίτης.

(5) Ταῦτα μὲν τὰ χρώματα λευκὰ κατὰ ποιότητα, κατὰ τὸ μᾶλλον καὶ ἧττόν ἐστιν.

(6) Εἰ δὲ βαφὴν δέξοιτό τινα χολῆς τὸ λευκὸν ὕδωρ, κατὰ μὲν πρῶτον λόγον ὕπωχρον γίνεται, ὡς ἀφέψημα χυμένης ὠμοβράστου· εἰ δὲ διαμείνῃ[6] χρόνον τινὰ ἡ ἕψησις, καταβαφὴν πλείονα ποιοῦσα, ὠχρὸν ἀποτελεῖ τὸ χρῶμα δηλοῦν περισσοτέραν χολὴν τοῦ προτέρου τὸ ὑδατῶδες ἐπιδέξασθαι.

(7) Ἀπὸ δὲ τούτου τέτακται τὸ ὑπόπυρρον, ἐοικὸς χρυσῷ τῷ ἀπὸ τῆς Κελτικῆς ἐρχομένῳ·

εἶτα τὸ πυρρόν, ὅ ἐστι κατ' ἀλήθειαν ὄβρυζος χρυσός·

εἶτα τὸ ὑπόξανθον ἐοικὸς κνίκῳ·

ὑδατώδους καὶ κρυσταλλοειδοῦς, τοῦ δ' αὖ γλαυκοῦ τόσον λειπόμενον.

(7) Αὐτὸ γὰρ ἴσως μετὰ τὸ γαλακτῶδες, ὅσον τὸ χαρωπὸν[4] ἐκπέφευγε τοῦ γλαυκοῦ τὴν λευκότητα, καὶ γλαυκὸν μὲν πέφυκεν οἷον τὸ διαυγές ἐστι κέρας, χαροπὸν δέ, ὃ καμήλων ὑπολεύκοις ἐρίοις ἔοικεν, εἶτ' οὖν ὀνυχίτῃ οὕτω πως καλουμένῳ λίθῳ.

(8) Ἀλλ' ἐπειδάν τινα βαφὴν τὰ οὖρα δέξηται τὸ πολὺ τῆς ἀπεψίας ἐκπεφευγότα, ὕπωχρα μὲν τὰ πρῶτα γίνεται, προϊόντα δὲ καὶ ὠχρά, ἀλλὰ τὰ μὲν μετρίως ζεσάσης χυμένης χυλῷ ἐῴκει, ἐκεῖνα δ' αὖ καὶ πάνυ ζεσάσης, εἰ δέ γε βούλοιο καὶ οἷον τὸ ἀπὸ τῆς ῥοιᾶς τοῦ φλοιοῦ τε καὶ περικάρπου[5] ζέσαντος ἐκείνως ὑγρὸν νόμισον.

(9) Οὐ διοίσομαι γὰρ τῶν τε χυλῶν πολλῷ ἐοικότων καὶ τοῦ τῆς ὠχρότητος ὀνόματος, μὴ διαπεφευγότος τῇ συνηθείᾳ τοὺς πλείστους.

(10) Εἴ γε μὴν καὶ τῆς οὕτω πως καλουμένης ὠχρᾶς μέτριον προσεμβάλῃς[7] χυμῷ ὀρρώδει, ὕπωχρα ποιήσεις τά[8] χρώματα· πλέον δὲ προσεμβαλὼν τῆς ὠχρᾶς,[9] καὶ ὠχρὰ τὰ χρώματα καταστήσεις ἀφ' ἑτέρων θάτερα προσονομασθέντα.[10]

(11) Ἐπειδὰν μέντοι πλείονι[11] ἐπιχρώσῃ βαφῇ[12] τὴν ὠχρότητα, τῆς πέψεως προχωρούσης, τὰ ὑπόπυρρα τῶν οὔρων, ἃ δὴ καὶ σύμμετρα ὁ λόγος οἶδε, κατασκευάζονται, μὴ πάμπαν ἀκιβδήλῳ προσεοικότα χρυσῷ.

(12) Τὸ δ' ἐπὶ τούτοις οὖρον πυρρὸν καλούμενον μᾶλλον εὐροίζῳ[13] καὶ καθαρῷ χρυσίῳ ἐῴκει.

(13) Μάθοις δ' ἂν ἴσως τοῦτο τοῖς τῶν πλουσίων παρακόψας[14] ταμείοις, εἰ μὴ παρά σοι χρυσὸς καθαρὸς καθέστηκεν.

(14) Ὑπόξανθον μετὰ ταῦτα κνίκῳ τὴν χροιὰν ἐοικός. Καὶ ἴσασιν οἱ πολλοὶ τὸ τοῦ φυτοῦ κνίκου ἄνθος, οἶμαι, ὅπερ ὡς ὑποπεπτωκός ἐστι τῇ χροιᾷ τοῦ ἄνθους τοῦ

[4] Georgiou (2013) 419.11 reads ‘χαροπὸν’.
[5] Georgiou (2013) 420.3 reads ‘περικαρπίου’.
[6] Tassinari (unpublished) reads ‘ὠμόβραστον· εἰ δὲ διαμένει’.
[7] Georgiou (2013) 420.7 reads ‘προσεπεμβάλοις’.
[8] Georgiou (2013) 420.7 omits ‘τὰ’.
[9] Georgiou (2013) 420.8 reads ‘ὤχρας’.
[10] Georgiou (2013) 420.9 reads ‘παρανομασθέντα’.
[11] Georgiou (2013) 420.9 reads ‘πλείων’.
[12] Georgiou (2013) 420.10 reads ‘βαφή’.
[13] Georgiou (2013) 420.13 reads ‘ὀβρύζῳ’.
[14] Georgiou (2013) 420.14 reads ‘παρακύψας’.

εἶτα τὸ ξανθόν, ὅπερ ἔοικε τῷ ἀληθινῷ κρόκῳ.

(8) Αὖθις δὲ τὸ ὑπέρυθρον ἀπὸ ἰχωροειδοῦς αἵματος,[20] ὡς τὸ ἐκ λευκοῦ χρώματος λαμπροῦ[21] προσελθόντος, ὅπερ καὶ οἱ βαφεῖς φλόγινον, οἱ δὲ περὶ τὸν Γαληνὸν φοινικοῦν ὀνομάζουσι.

(9) Τὸ δὲ ὑποτάξαι ἢ προτάξαι τὴν ὑπὸ πρόθεσιν ἐν τοῖς χρώμασιν οὐ πάντες ὁμοίως εἰώθασιν ὑπολαμβάνειν· ἄλλοι μὲν γὰρ προτάττουσιν, ἄλλοι δὲ ὑποτάττουσιν.

(10) Τὸ δὲ ἐρυθρόν, ὡς τὸ αἷμα τὸ καθαρὸν καὶ ἀθόλωτον· τὸ γὰρ ὑπερβάλλον τοῦδε ἢ ἐλλεῖπον οὐχ ὑγιές, ἀλλὰ νόθον.

(11) Τὸ δὲ οἰνωπόν, ἢ ὡς μελάντερος οἶνος, ἢ ὡς βαθύτερον καὶ πορφυρίζον αἷμα, καθώς ἐστιν ἡ χρόα[25] τοῦ ἥπατος.

κρόκου, ὥστε ἐκεῖθεν δεῖ συλλογίζεσθαι περὶ ὑποξάνθου χρώματος.

(15) Τό γε μὴν ἀκριβῶς ξανθὸν κατὰ μηδέν τι διενηνοχὸς φαίνεται τοῦ Κωρυκείου κρόκου, τοῦ ἐπ' ἄλλοις τόποις[15] τούτου διενεγκότος τῇ τοῦ χρώματος ἀκριβείᾳ.

(16) Ἀλλ' ἵνα μή τι πάθῃς ἀνθρώπινον πολὺ διενεγκόντα τοῦτον οἰηθεὶς τῷ χρώματι τῶν λοιπῶν τῷ ξένῳ τοῦ ὀνόματος, ἐγώ σοι τὸν ἀπὸ τοῦ Ἄθω παραθήσω κομιζόμενον καὶ τῷ ἐκείνου στοίχει χρώματι, πλὴν οὐχὶ τοῖς φαινομένοις ἔν τε κνίκῳ καὶ κρόκῳ δεῖ σε προσέχειν χρώμασιν, ἐπεὶ πολλῷ ἂν διαμάρτῃς[16] τοῦ δέοντος. ὑπερυθρὰ γὰρ καὶ ἐρυθρὰ ἤδη τὰ ἐκείνων χρώματα πέφυκεν, ἀλλὰ τοῖς ἐξ ἐκείνων ὑγρῷ λυομένων χρώμασι.

(17) Μετὰ ταῦτα τὸ ὑπέρυθρον καὶ ἐρυθρὸν τοῦ χρώματος πέφυκεν, οἷς δῆτα ἀρκέσει μὲν ἐς παράστασιν καὶ τὰ φαινόμενα, καθάπερ εἴρηται, χρώματα τοῦ τε κνίκου καὶ κρόκου. μάθοις δ' ἂν τῇ τε Ἀρμενίῳ[17] βώλῳ καὶ τῇ Λημνίᾳ σφραγίτιδι[18] τὰ ὑπέρυθρα προβάλλων.[19]

(18) Τὰ δ' ἐρυθρὰ καὶ φοινικᾶ τοῦ χρώματος τῶν ὀπωρῶν ταῖς ἐρυθρὰ προβαλλομέναις χρώματα κεράσοις δηλονότι καὶ μήλοις καί τισι παραπλησίοις, ὧν τῇ τελειότητι τῆς ἐπιφανείας καὶ τῇ πέψει καὶ τὰ χρώματα διενεγκεῖν δοκοῦσι.

(19) Τὸ οἰνωπὸν ἐπὶ τούτοις ἀπό τε[22] τῶν μελαντέρων οἴνων τοὔνομα ἐσχηκὸς καὶ οἷον πεφυκὸς τὸ χρῶμα τοῦ ἥπατος, ὥστ' ἐντεῦθεν δεῖ τὸν συνετὸν λογιζόμενον πολλάκις μὲν ἧπαρ ἑωρακότα ζῴου ἀλόγου εἰ μὴ ἀνθρώπου, πολλάκις δ' ἐπιπίοντα τοιοῦτον οἶνον, εἴτ' οὖν ἑωρακότα τὸν περὶ τοῦ οἰνωποῦ χρώματος λογίζεσθαι λόγον.

(20) Μέμνημαι γάρ[23] καὶ ἔγωγε τοιοῦτον ἐν ἀγορᾷ πολλάκις ἑωρακὼς ἀπ' ἐμπόρων κομιζόμενον οἶνον, ὃς ἐπὶ τοσούτῳ κέχρωται[24] τῷ οἰνωπῷ τοῦ χρώματος, ὥστε τοῖς μὲν ἀγγείοις, οἷς κεκόμιστο, τοῦ οἰκείου μετεδίδου

15 Georgiou (2013) 421.5 reads 'τῶν ἐπ' ἄλλους τόπους'.
16 Georgiou (2013) 421.10 reads 'διαμάρτοις'.
17 Georgiou (2013) 421.15 reads 'ἀρμενίᾳ'.
18 Georgiou (2013) 421.15 reads 'σφραγῖδι'.
19 Georgiou (2013) 422.1 reads 'παραβάλλων'.
20 Tassinari (unpublished) reads 'ὑπέρυθρον γινόμενον μὲν ἀπὸ ἰχωρόδους αἵματος'.
21 Tassinari (unpublished) reads 'λαμπρῷ'.
22 Georgiou (2013) 422.4 reads 'γε'.
23 Georgiou (2013) 422.9 reads 'γάρ τοι'.
24 Georgiou (2013) 422.11 reads 'κέχρωσται'.
25 Tassinari (unpublished) reads 'χροιά'.

	χρώματος· βραχὺς δὲ ὕδατι πολλῷ μιγνύμενος ἔτι ἐρυθρὸς τῷ χρώματι διεφαίνετο.
(12) *Τὸ δὲ κυανοῦν ὡς τὸ σεσημμένον ἐκ χολῆς ξανθῆς καὶ ὑπερωπτημένον, τῇ χροιᾷ γαρῶδες, ὡς τὰ τῶν ἰκτερικῶν οὖρα.*	(21) *Τό γε μὴν κυανοῦν τοῦ χρώματος ἐξ ἐπιταθέντος μὲν οἰνωποῦ γέγονεν ἴσως, μάλιστα δ' ἐῴκει σειραίῳ, ὃ δὴ καὶ ἕψημα ὁ λόγος οἶδε.*
(13) *Ὁ δὲ κανὼν τοῦ κυανοῦ χρώματος κατὰ τὸν Γαληνόν ἐστι τοιοῦτος· λευκὸν λαμπρῷ προσελθὸν καὶ εἰς μέλαν κατακορὲς ἐμπεσόν, κυανοῦν ἐποίησε·*	(22) *Τοῦτο δὲ πέφυκε τοιοῦτον,*[26] *ἐπειδή*[27] *τινες ἀμφιγνοήσαιεν ἂν ἔτι τοῦτο, τὸ ἀπὸ γλεύκους ἐς ἀποτρίτωσιν ἑψημένου γινόμενον. προσεπιθείης*[28] *δὲ τῇ σαφηνείᾳ τοῦ χρώματος καὶ τὸ τοῦ κάρπου τῆς κεράσου, ὃ δὴ μάλιστα πρὸς τὸ μελάντερον ἐπινένευκεν.*
τὸ δὲ φαιὸν ἐκ λευκοῦ καὶ μέλανος κραθέντων ἀλλήλοις γινόμενον, ὡς τὰ ξηρὰ ἰσχάδια.[30]	(23) *Ἐπεὶ δὲ καὶ τὸν περὶ κυανοῦ χρώματος ἱκανῶς ἔχεις λόγον, καὶ περὶ τῶν λοιπῶν νῦν μάνθανε· τὸ τοίνυν φαιὸν ἐπίδηλον οἶμαι γεγονέναι τοῖς πᾶσιν ἐξ ἀκράτου λευκοῦ καὶ μέλανος συγκραθέν.*
	(24) *Εἰ δὲ καὶ τῇ αἰσθήσει τοῦτο μαθεῖν ἐθέλεις, ψιμμίθιον ἢ λευκὴν πάνυ τίτανον ἤ τι*[29] *παραπλησίων μελανί τε καὶ πίσσῃ καὶ ἀσφάλτῳ καί τισιν ἀκράτοις μέλασιν ἑνώσας χρώμασιν ἰσοστάθμοις, τὸ φαιὸν ἂν ὧδε γνοίης χρῶμα γινόμενον.* (25) *Ἀλλὰ δὴ περὶ χλωρῶν ὧδ' εἰρηκότες πρῶτον καὶ ἐλαίωδῶν, περὶ πελιδνῶν εἶθ' οὕτως καὶ μελανῶν ἐροῦμεν.*
(14) *Τὸ δὲ χλωρόν, ὡς πράσινον κραμβίζον, καὶ ὡσεὶ*[32] *χλοή· πλάτος δὲ ἐν αὐτῷ θεωρεῖται· τὸ γὰρ ἰῶδες καὶ τὸ σμαραγδίζον καὶ τὸ ἰσατῶδες πάντα χλωρὰ κατὰ τὸ μᾶλλόν τε καὶ ἧττον. Ταῦτα δὲ ὑπὸ θερμότητος τὰ πλεῖστα*[34] *ἐγένετο.*	(26) *Τῶν τοίνυν χλωρῶν χρωμάτων τὰ μὲν κραμβίζοντά εἰσι, τὰ δ' αὖ χλοάζοντα, ἰώδη τε καὶ σμαραγδίζοντα, ὥστ' ἐξ ὧν παρωνομάσθησαν, ταῦτα δὴ*[31] *καὶ μανθάνειν τοῖς ἐκείνων χρώμασι, ταῦτα δὴ παραβάλλοντα.*
[Theophilos, *On Urines*, 17, ed. Ideler (1841) I.279.16–19: (6) *Τῆς ἀρχῆς μὲν τῶν ἐλαιωδῶν οὔρων, τὰ ἐλαιόχροα· τῆς δὲ αὐξήσεως, τὰ ἐλαιοφανῆ· τῆς δὲ ἀκμῆς, τὰ ἐλαιώδη.* (7) *Τὰ μὲν οὖν ἐλαιόχροα τὰ τὴν ἀρχὴν τῆς συντήξεως δηλοῦντα ὥσπερ ὑδατώδη φαίνεται.*]	(27) *Ἀλλὰ δὴ καὶ τῶν ἐλαιωδῶν οὕτω κοινῷ τῷ γένει καλουμένων οὔρων τὰ μὲν ἐλαιοφανῆ, τὰ δὲ ἐλαιόχροα, τὰ δ' ἐλαιώδη ὁμωνύμως τῷ κοινῷ λέγεται γένει.* (28) *Τούτων δὲ*[33] *τῶν τριῶν τοῦ μὲν πρώτου ἔτι ἀμφισβητεῖται τὸ χρῶμα, εἴθ' ὑδατῶδες ἢ ἐλαιῶδες εἴη τῇ τοῦ χρωννῦντος τοῦτο λεπτότητι· τοῦ δὲ δευτέρου ἤδη ἐπίδηλον ὡς ἤδη τὴν χροιὰν ἐπιτείναντος· ὃ δ' ἐλαιῶδες ὁ*

[26] Georgiou (2013) 423.1 omits '*τοιοῦτον*'.
[27] Georgiou (2013) 423.1 reads '*ἐπεί*'.
[28] Georgiou (2013) 423.2 reads '*προσεπιθήσεις*'.
[29] Georgiou (2013) 423.8 reads '*τι τῶν*'.
[30] Tassinari (unpublished) reads '*τὰ † ῥοῆς χάσδια †*'.
[31] Georgiou (2013) 423.14 reads '*δεῖ*'.
[32] Tassinari (unpublished) reads '*ὡς ἡ*'.
[33] Georgiou (2013) 424.2 reads '*δή*'.
[34] Tassinari (unpublished) reads '*πλείστης*'.

(15) *Τὸ δὲ πελιδνὸν βαθύτερόν ἐστι τοῦ φαιοῦ, ὡς μόλιβδος καὶ τὰ ἐπερχόμενα ἐκ τῶν πληγῶν*[41] *τῷ σώματι καὶ τὰ ἐκ θλασμάτων μελανίζοντα χρώματα. Τοῦτο δὲ ἢ ὑπὸ ψύξεως γίνεται, ἢ ὑπὸ πληγῆς.*

(16) *Ἀπὸ δὲ τούτου τὸ μέλαν, ἐνδεικνύμενον ποτὲ μὲν ψύξιν, ποτὲ δὲ θερμότητα· εἰ μὲν γὰρ ἐκ χλωροῦ προηγησαμένου, θερμότητα· εἰ δ' ἐκ πελιδνοῦ, ψύξιν.*

(17) *Ἐστὶ δὲ ἐπέκεινα πάντων τῶν χρωμάτων· καὶ τοῦτο πλάτος ἱκανὸν ἔχει κατὰ μᾶλλον καὶ ἧττον· πολλὰ γὰρ μέλανα ἄλλα ἄλλων κατακορῆ καὶ ἀνόμοια.*

λόγος ὥρισε, τῇ τοῦ ἐλαίου μάλιστα προσέοικε χροιᾷ, πλὴν οὐχὶ τῶν παχέων τούτων καὶ τῷ χρώματι ἐπιτεταμένων, ἀλλὰ τῶν μάλιστα λεπτῶν. ἐκεῖνα γὰρ τοῖς ὑπὸ τὸ χλωρὸν ἁρμόζει μᾶλλον εἴδεσιν.

(29) *Ἐπεὶ δ' ἱκανῶς καὶ τὸν περὶ χλωρῶν καὶ ἐλαιωδῶν οὔρων ἐν διαφοραῖς ἐξεθέμεθα λόγον, ἑξῆς ἐπὶ τῶν πελιδνῶν τῷ λόγῳ ἴωμεν καὶ μελάνων φαινομένων οὔρων.*

(30) *Τὸ τοίνυν πελιδνὸν τοῦ χρώματος μολιβδόχρουν μὲν ἂν εἴπῃ*[35] *τις σαφηνίζων τὸν λόγον, ὥστε ἐκεῖθεν δεῖ καὶ περὶ τούτων*[36] *στοχάζεσθαι.*

(31) *Τοσούτῳ*[37] *δὲ προσνένευκε τῷ μέλανι χρώματι, ὅσον, οἶμαι, λέλειπται τοῦ φαιοῦ, ὥστε καὶ εἰ διπλασίῳ λόγον ἕξει, τὰ μέλανα πρὸς τὰ λευκὰ χρώματα, τῇ συνθήκῃ, ἂν*[38] *πελιδνὰ ἐντεῦθεν ὀφθείη χρωματα, καὶ πελιδνὰ τοιαῦτ' ἂν εἴη.*

(32) *Μέλανα δὲ οὐδεὶς ἂν ἀγνοήσῃ*[39] *χρώματα πᾶσιν ἔκδηλα γεγονότα. προσήκει τοίνυν ἐντεῦθεν τῷ περὶ τὰ τοιαῦτα σπουδαίῳ ἐπινοῆσαι μὲν τὰ ῥηθέντα χρώματα καὶ τοῖς*[40] *πλαξὶν ἐγγράψαι τῆς διανοίας, οὐκ ὀλίγων ἐπ' αὐτοῖς ῥηθησομένων διαγνώσεων τε καὶ προγνώσεων.*

(33) *Προσεπινοῆσαι δὲ τῷ λόγῳ δεῖ καὶ ἃ τῶν χρωμάτων μὴ διώρισται τῷ ἐξαπορῆσαι οἰκείων ὀνομάτων, ἤτοι ἐξυδαρωθέντα ἢ ἐπιταθέντα ἀπὸ τῶν ὁρισθέντων τούτων χρωμάτων, ὥστε ἂν εἴ τις ἀκριβῶς ταῦτα γνοίη, ῥᾳδίως καὶ τὰ διαπεπτωκότα τῶν ὡρισμένων τούτων χρωμάτων δι' οἱονδήτινα*[42] *καταγνοίη λόγον.*

(34) *Οὐκοῦν οὐκ ἐπὶ πλέον προσανέχειν τῷ περὶ διαφορᾶς χρωμάτων προσήκει λόγῳ, ἱκανῶς ἐνταῦθα πρὸς συνετοὺς τῶν πάντων διωρισμένων.*

(35) *Τοῖς γὰρ δή τοι μέρος παιδιᾶς τὰ τῇ τέχνῃ τιθεμένοις σπουδαῖα, οὐδ' ἂν πάντα τις συνελών, πολλάκις φαίη τὰ ἐνδεχόμενα*

[35] Georgiou (2013) 424.11 reads '*εἴποι*'.
[36] Georgiou (2013) 424.12 reads '*τούτου*'.
[37] Georgiou (2013) 424.13 reads '*τοσοῦτο*'.
[38] Georgiou (2013) 424.15 reads '*ἀκριβῶς ἂν*'.
[39] Georgiou (2013) 425.1 reads '*ἄν, οἶμαι ἀγνοήσειε*'.
[40] Georgiou (2013) 425.4 reads '*ταῖς*'.
[41] Tassinari (unpublished) reads '*τὰ ἐκ τῶν ἐπερχομένων πληγῶν*'.
[42] Georgiou (2013) 425.9 reads '*οἷον δή τινα*'.

(18) Καὶ περὶ μὲν τῶν χρωμάτων ἱκανὴ ἡ διδασκαλία, συλλεχθεῖσα ἀπὸ τῶν διδαχῶν τῶν παλαιοτέρων σοφῶν τε καὶ ἰατρῶν.

(19) Τούτων τῶν χρωμάτων, οἷα δύνανται συμπλακῆναι μετὰ παχείας συστάσεως, ἢ μετὰ λεπτῆς, καὶ τίνα ἐξ αὐτῶν σημαινόμενα εἴτε ἐν ὑγιαίνουσι σώμασιν εἴτε ἐν νοσοῦσι, προϊὼν ὁ λόγος διδάξει.

συνίστασθαι χρώματα, πρὸς ἀποχρῶσαν τούτοις διδασκαλίαν ἀρκέσειε. καὶ ὁ μὲν περὶ διαφορᾶς χρωμάτων οὔρων λόγος ᾧδέ πη κείσθω. ἐνταῦθα δὲ προσήκει φάναι καὶ περὶ διαφορᾶς τῶν ἐπὶ τῷ χύματι συνισταμένων συστάσεων.

APPENDIX 3

John's Diagram of the Urine Vial in his *On Urines*

The diagram appears in twenty-three out of forty-one surviving manuscripts of the work or parts of it. There are basically two types of diagram. In the first (no. 1; see, for example, Figure App.3.1) sub-areas nos 5 and 9 (these are the two sub-areas that are in between the three main areas) are wider than the other bands, with some minor variations from one manuscript to another. In the second (no. 2) each sub-area is followed by the next one without any extra space in between some of them. The latter appears only in two manuscripts, Florentinus Laurentianus gr. plut. 74.13 (see Figure App.3.2) and Cracoviensis (ex Berolinensis gr. fol. 7).[1] I have adopted diagram no. 2, which corresponds more closely with John's description, who states that the vial consists of eleven sub-areas each of them having the width of a finger.[2] Ambrogio Leone of Nola's (see Figure App.3.3) and Julius Ludwig Ideler's (see Figure App.3.4) editions have adopted no. 2, but both depict a vial with a round bottom, which is not found in any surviving manuscript.[3] Stavroula Georgiou prints diagram no. 1 following Parisinus gr. 2270, f. 246r.[4] In most of the manuscripts, the diagram is accompanied by the Greek numbers of the eleven sub-areas on the left and three Greek numbers on the right indicating the main areas. The names of the main areas, i.e. '*νεφέλη*', '*ἐναιώρημα*', and '*ὑπόστασις*' are also found in the vast majority of the manuscripts. I have adopted both the numbering (Arabic numbers are given in parenthesis for the convenience of the modern reader) and the labelling of the various areas as in most of the manuscripts that retain the diagram (see Chapter 2, Section 2.7).

[1] The Florence manuscript presents only ten sub-areas, compared to the Cracow one, which correctly shows eleven subdivisions.

[2] JZA, *On Urines*, 1.13.9, ed. Ideler (1842) II.20.36–21.1.

[3] Ideler (1842: II.22); Leo of Nola (1519: f. 13r). There are three manuscripts (Parisinus gr. 2153, Parisinus gr. 2256, Varsoviensis Zamoyscianus 155 Cim.) in which the outer shape of the vial is indicated, but the bottom is flat.

[4] Georgiou (2013: 437, 582).

Manuscript[5]	Urine vial diagram no. 1	Urine vial diagram no. 2	No urine vial diagram
Venetus Marcianus V. 13 (coll. 1221), f. 36r, AD 1376[6]	✓		
Parisinus gr. 2270, f. 246r, 14th c.[7]	✓		
Parisinus gr. 2304, f. 14v, 14th c.[8]	✓		
Parisinus Coislinianus 334, 14th c.[9]			✓
Varsoviensis Zamoyscianus 155 Cim., p. 398, 14th c.[10]	✓		
Vaticanus gr. 299, f. 29r, 14th c.[11]	✓		
Venetus Marcianus gr. 296 (coll. 632), f. 21v, 14th c.[12]	✓		
Venetus Marcianus gr. 510 (coll. 769), 14th c.[13]			✓
Florentinus Laurentianus gr. plut. 75.11, f. 9r, AD 1411/12[14]	✓		
Parisinus gr. 2305, f. 12v, AD 1418[15]	✓		
Scorialensis Φ.III.12, f. 22r, AD 1432[16]	✓		
Oxoniensis Bodleianus Auct. T.4.3 (Misc. 241), f. 17v, 15th c. (first half)[17]	✓		
Vindobonensis med. gr. 26, 15th c. (first half)[18]			✓
Vindobonensis med. gr. 44, f. 149v, 15th c. (first half)[19]	✓		
Parisinus gr. 2260, 15th c. (second quarter)[20]			✓
Berolinensis Phillippicus gr. 1582, f. 11v, 15th c.[21]	✓		
Cantabrigiensis, Trinity College O.8.11, 15th c.[22]			✓
Florentinus Laurentianus gr. plut. 74.13, f. 108v, 15th c.[23]		✓	
Florentinus Laurentianus gr. plut. 75.9, 15th c.[24]			✓
Florentinus Laurentianus gr. plut. 75.16, f. 14r, 15th c.[25]	✓		
Londoniensis Wellcomensis MS.MSL.52, f. 54r, 15th c.[26]	✓		
Mediolanensis Ambrosianus gr. 707 (R 20 sup.), 15th c.[27]			✓

[5] I give the reference to the latest catalogue, including any recent study which has provided a more precise, revised dating. If a manuscript consists of two or more parts dated to different centuries, I give the date of the part in which John's urine vial is depicted.

[6] Mioni (1972: 273–6). Autopsy, February 2012.

[7] Omont (1888: II.227, III.397); Mondrain (2003: 375–6). Autopsy, October 2012.

[8] Omont (1888: II.233); Mondrain (2003: 381–2). Autopsy, September 2012.

[9] Devreesse (1945: 317–18). Autopsy, October 2012.

[10] Turyn (1928: 508–11); Aland (1956: 22–3); Kaliszuk and Szyller (2012: 61). I read this manuscript on microfilm.

[11] Mercati and Franchi de' Cavalieri (1923: 425–30). Autopsy, February 2012.

[12] Mioni (1981: 423–4). Autopsy, February 2012.

[13] Mioni (1985: 365–7). Autopsy, February 2012.

[14] Bandini (1770: III.158–9). Autopsy, February 2012.

[15] Omont (1888: II.233). Autopsy, October 2012.

[16] De Andrés (1965: 64–6) refers to AD 1433. Autopsy, October 2018. On the date of this manuscript, see the description in Appendix 5, E=Scorialensis Φ.III.12.

[17] Coxe (1853: 788–9); *RGK* I 106, II 140, III 175. Autopsy, January 2013.

[18] Hunger (1969: II.72–4). Autopsy, March 2012.

[19] Hunger (1969: II.95–6). Autopsy, March 2012.

[20] Omont (1888: II.225–6); Cronier (2006: 56–64). Autopsy, October 2012.

[21] Studemund and Cohn (1890: 78). Autopsy, June 2012.

[22] James (1902: 398). Autopsy, March 2014.

[23] Bandini (1770: III.102–15). Autopsy, February 2012.

[24] Bandini (1770: III.155–6). Autopsy, February 2012.

[25] Bandini (1770: III.164–5). Autopsy, February 2012.

[26] Bouras-Vallianatos (2015b: 286–92). Autopsy, March 2014.

[27] Martini and Bassi (1906: 818–19). Autopsy, February 2012.

Mutinensis a.T.8.20, 15th c.[28]			✓
Oxoniensis Bodleianus Thomae Roe 15, f. 112v, 15th c.[29]	✓		
Parisinus gr. 2153, f. 463r, 15th c.[30]	✓		
Parisinus gr. 2232, 15th c.[31]			✓
Parisinus gr. 2256, f. 154v, 15th c.[32]	✓		
Parisinus gr. 2306, f. 9v, 15th c.[33]	✓		
Parisinus gr. 2308, f. 60r, 15th c.[34]	✓		
Vaticanus gr. 2182, 15th c.[35]			
Londiniensis Wellcomensis MS.MSL.60, f. 186r, 15th c. (second half)[36]			
Cantabrigiensis, Gonville and Caius College 76/43, 15th and 16th c.[37]			✓
Londiniensis Arundelianus 537, 15th and 16th c.[38]			✓
Mosquensis (ex. Dresdensis Da 5), *c.*AD 1519[39]			
Leidensis Vossianus gr. F. 32, *c.*AD 1548[40]			✓
Berolinensis Phillippicus gr. 1531, 16th c.[41]			✓
Cracoviensis (ex Berolinensis gr. fol. 7), f. 6r, 16th c.[42]		✓	
Mediolanensis Ambrosianus gr. 190 (C 89 sup.), f. 10r, 16th c.[43]	✓		
Monacensis gr. 362, 16th c.[44]			✓
Parisinus gr. 2307, f. 11v, 16th c.[45]	✓		
Londiniensis Wellcomensis MS.MSL.124, 17th c.[46]			✓
Edition			
Leo of Nola (1519) f. 13r		✓	
Ideler (1842) II, p. 22		✓	
Georgiou (2013) p. 437	✓		

[28] Puntoni (1896: 474, no. 141); *RGK* I 18, II 25, III 31; *RGK* I 183, II 242, III 302. I read this manuscript on microfilm.

[29] Coxe (1853: 468–9). Autopsy, January 2013.

[30] Omont (1888: II.205, III.396). Autopsy, September 2012.

[31] Omont (1888: II.218). Autopsy, October 2012.

[32] Omont (1888: II.224–5). Autopsy, October 2012.

[33] Omont (1888: II.233). Autopsy, October 2012.

[34] Omont (1888: II.234). Autopsy, October 2012.

[35] Lilla (1985: 75–9). This manuscript contains an excerpt from books five and six (ff. 81r–96v). Autopsy, February 2012.

[36] Bouras-Vallianatos (2015b: 292–302). Autopsy, March 2014. This manuscript contains a list of contents of John's *On Urines* (ff. 185v–187v) only. There is a diagram in which the urine vial is divided into the three main areas, i.e. '*νεφέλη*', '*ἐναιώρημα*', and '*ὑπόστασις*', without any subdivisions.

[37] James (1907: 73–5). Autopsy, March 2014.

[38] McKendrick (1999: 19). Autopsy, November 2011.

[39] Schnorr von Carolsfeld (1882: 283–4) von Gebhardt (1898: 537–8). The manuscript is now in the Russian State Archive of Ancient Acts in Moscow (Российский Государственный Архив Древних Актов, РГАДА). It has not been possible to access this manuscript. See also Appendix 5, Q=Mosquensis (ex Dresdensis Da 5).

[40] De Meyier (1955: 34–7). Autopsy, October 2012.

[41] Studemund and Cohn (1890: 51–2). Autopsy, June 2012.

[42] De Boor (1897: 125). The manuscript is now in Biblioteka Jagiellońska, Krakow. I read this manuscript on microfilm.

[43] Martini and Bassi (1906: 205); Georgiou (2013: 274–6). Autopsy, February 2012.

[44] Hardt (1810: 50–6). Autopsy, March 2012.

[45] Omont (1888: II.233–4). Autopsy, October 2012.

[46] Bouras-Vallianatos (2015b: 311–13). Autopsy, March 2014.

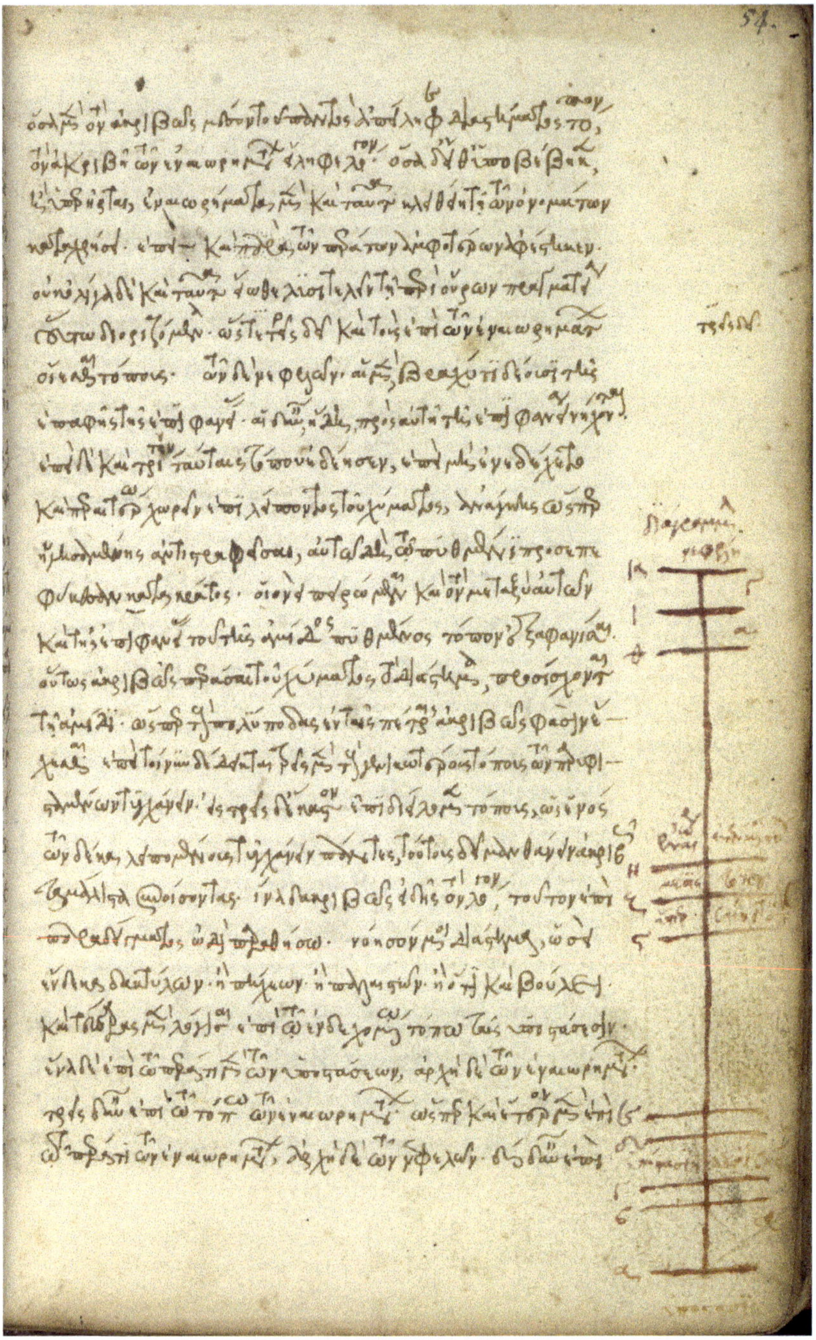

App. 3.1. Diagram of the urine vial in John's *On Urines*. Londiniensis Wellcomensis MS.MSL.52 (fifteenth century), f. 54r.

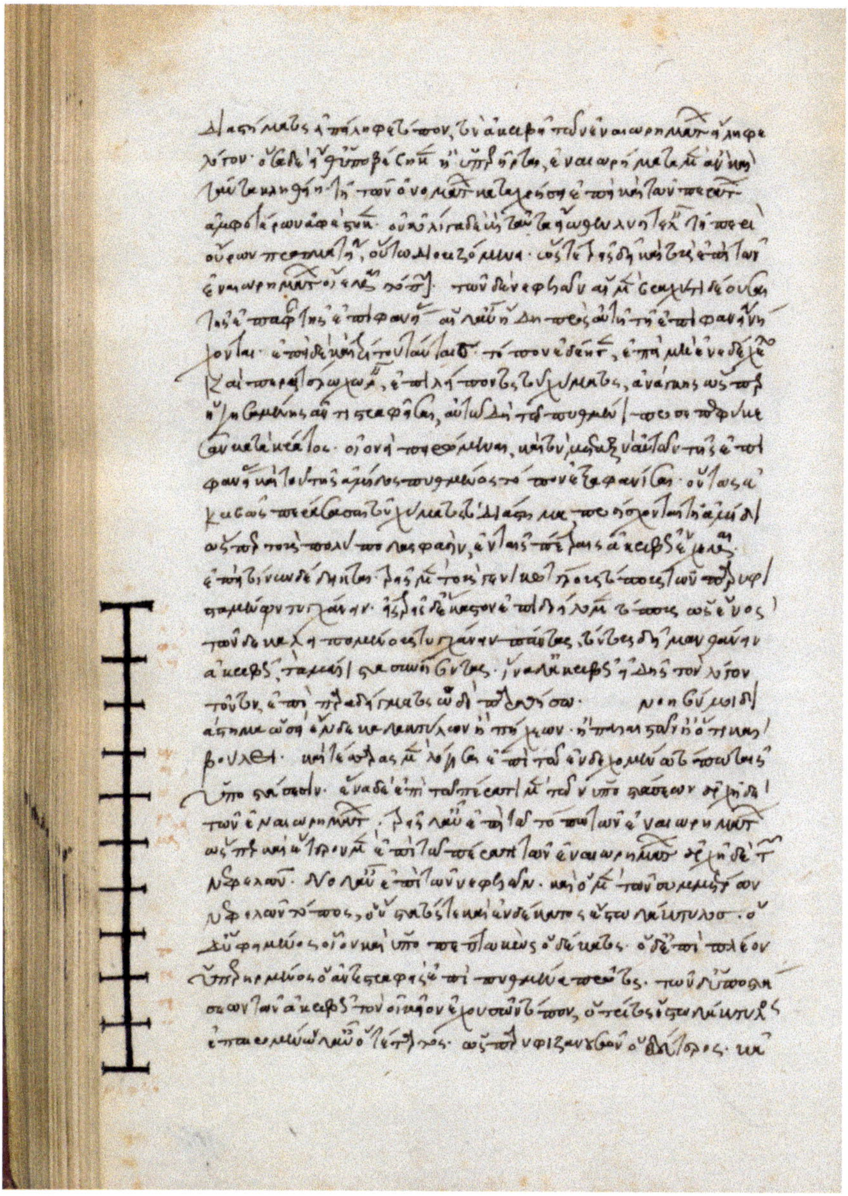

App. 3.2. Diagram of the urine vial in John's *On Urines*. Florentinus Laurentianus gr. plut. 74.13 (fifteenth century), f. 108v.

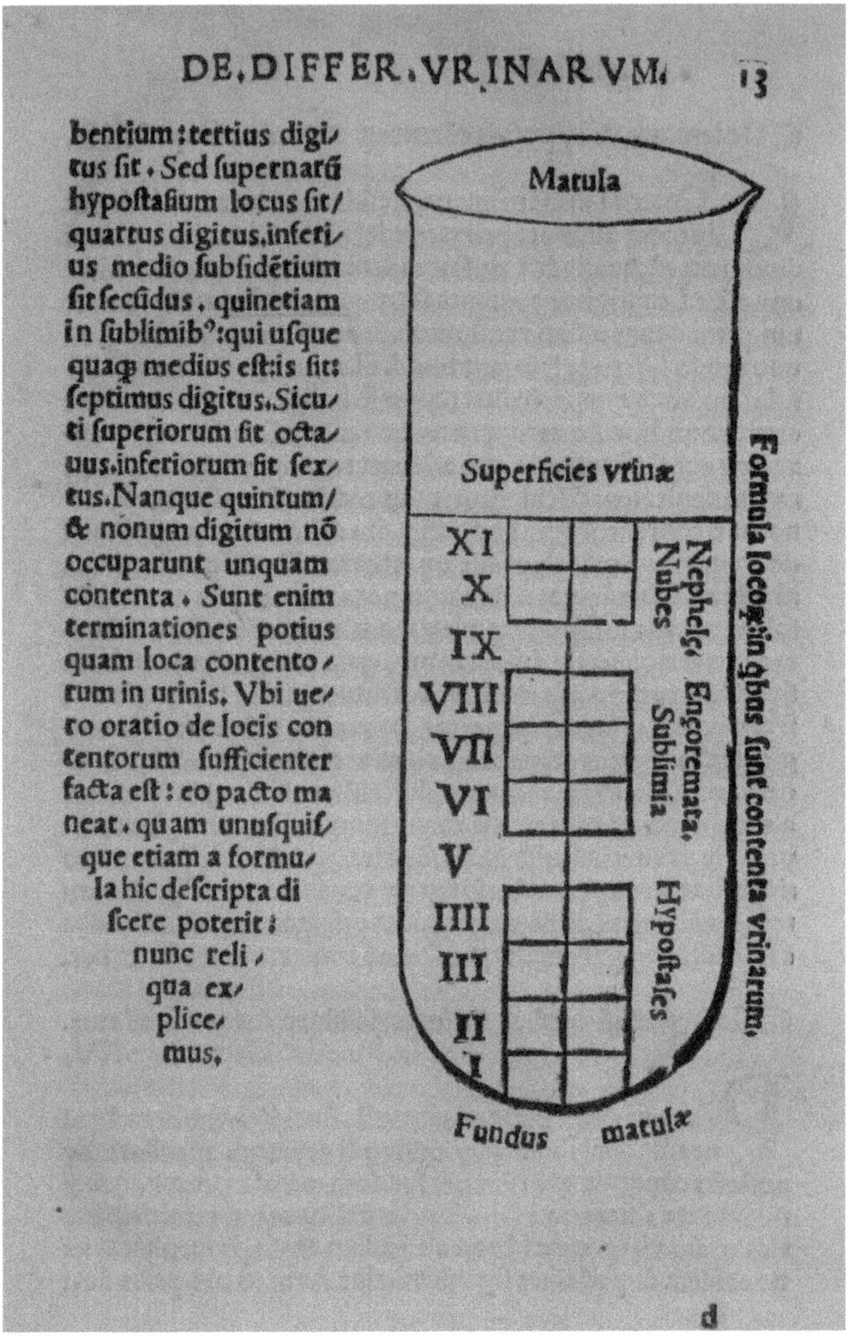
DE. DIFFER. VRINARVM. 13

bentium: tertius digi-
tus ſit. Sed ſupernarũ
hypoſtaſium locus ſit,
quartus digitus. inferi-
us medio ſubſidẽtium
ſit ſecũdus, quinetiam
in ſublimib⁹: qui uſque
quaq; medius eſt: is ſit:
ſeptimus digitus. Sicu-
ti ſuperiorum ſit octa-
uus. inferiorum ſit ſex-
tus. Nanque quintum,
& nonum digitum nõ
occuparunt unquam
contenta. Sunt enim
terminationes potius
quam loca contento-
rum in urinis. Vbi ue-
ro oratio de locis con
tentorum ſufficienter
facta eſt: eo pacto ma
neat. quam unuſquiſ-
que etiam a formu-
la hic deſcripta di
ſcere poterit:
nunc reli-
qua ex-
plice-
mus.

App. 3.3. Diagram of the urine vial in John's *On Urines*. First Latin edition. A. Leone of Nola (tr.), *De urinis libri*, Venice, 1519, f. 13r.

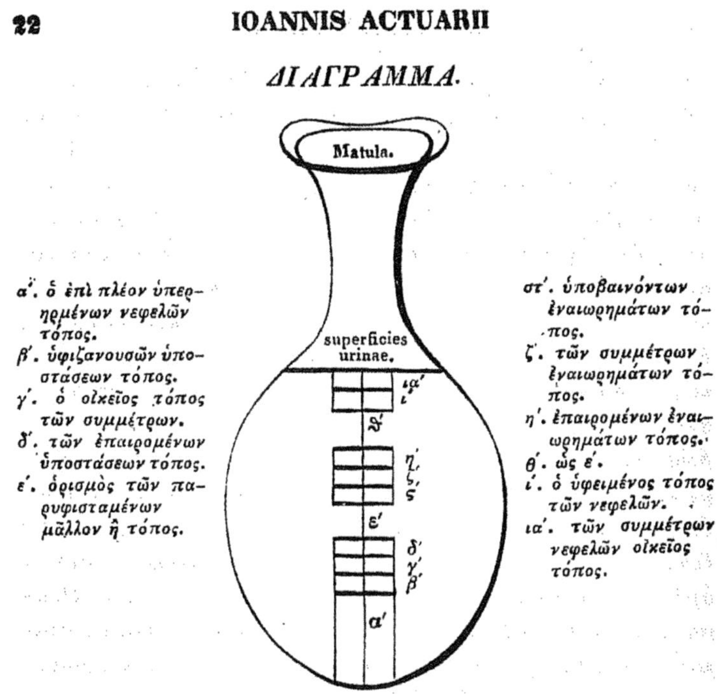

App. 3.4. Diagram of the urine vial in John's *On Urines*. First Greek edition. J. L. Ideler (ed.), *Physici et medici Graeci minores*, Berlin, 1842, vol. 2, p. 22.

APPENDIX 4

Treatment of Eye Affections and Scirrhus in John's *Medical Epitome*, Book Four

In the transcription I provide below, I have kept the same spelling and punctuation as in the codex, apart from the fact that I have supplied the iota subscript.

JZA, *Medical Epitome*, 4, Vindobonensis med. gr. 17, f. 102v, l. 6–f. 103v, l. 17:

Τράχωμα δὲ καὶ σύκωσις καὶ τύλος τὰ αὐτὰ τῷ γένει τυγχάνοντα, διαφέροντα δ' ἀλλήλων τῷ χρόνῳ καὶ τῇ δυνάμει· κολλουρίοις θεραπεύεται τῷ τε δι' οἴνου καὶ τῷ διὰ τῶν δύο λίθων καὶ τῷ αἵματι (here I follow E: *αἱματίτῃ*) *πλυθέντι· καθ' ὑπερβολὴν γὰρ ὑποσμήχει τὸ βλέφαρον· καὶ τὸ ἁρμάτιον δὲ μετ' ὀλίγου τοῦ κυκναρίου καὶ τὸ διὰ κρόκου πρὸς τούτοις, καὶ ταῖς ψωροφθαλμίαις ἁρμόζει ταῖς χωρὶς ἑλκώσεως, ἐκστρεφομένου τοῦ βλεφάρου ἐπιχριόμενα· εἰ δὲ μικρὸς ὢν ὁ τύλος μὴ εἴκει, ἐκστρέψαντες τὸ βλέφαρον ξέσωμεν διὰ κεσσήρεως* (E: *κισσήρεως*) *ἢ σηπίας ὀστράκου· ἢ φύλλων συκῆς· τὸ δὲ χαλάζιον ἀμμωνιακὸν ὄξει λειώσας ἅμα χαλβάνῃ, χρίε· δεῖ γὰρ ὧδε τῶν μαλακτικῶν καὶ διαφορητικῶν μετὰ τοῦ λεπτομεροῦς· τὴν δ' οὕτω καλουμένην κριθήν, μυίας τὴν κεφαλὴν ἀποβαλόντες καὶ τῷ λοιπῷ ταύτης σώματι παρατρίβοντες, τὸ πάθος θεραπεύομεν· ἔνιοι δὲ καὶ κριθῶν ἀποβρέγματι καταντλοῦντες βοηθοῦσι· κριθαῖς κριθὰς ἐκκρούοντες· φθειριάσεως δ' ἐνοχλούσης, πρῶτον μὲν δεῖ τὰς φθείρας ἐκκαθᾶραι· εἶτα θαλάσσῃ ἀποκλύσαι χλιαρᾷ· κἄπειθ' οὕτως* (E: *οὕτω*) *προσάπτεσθαι τοῦ ταρσοῦ τῷ φαρμάκῳ· δυοῖν μὲν μετέχοντος στυπτηρίας σχιστῆς· ἑνὸς δὲ σταφίδος ἀγρίας, λείων ἀκριβῶς . . . περὶ δὲ πτερυγίων τοσοῦτον ἔνεστιν εἰπεῖν ὡς τὰ μὲν μεγάλα καὶ χρόνια, χειρουργίᾳ ἰᾶται· τὰ δὲ νεώτερα, τὰ σμηκτικὰ τῶν βοηθημάτων, ὁποῖον ὁ χαλκὸς ὁ κεκαυμένος· καὶ τὸ χάλκανθον ἅμα χολῇ χοιρείᾳ· καὶ ἡ χολὴ τῆς αἰγὸς ἅμα μέλιτι·*

JZA, *Medical Epitome*, Book 4, Vindobonensis med. gr. 17, f. 110r, ll. 16–23:

Περὶ σκίρρου: ὁ δὲ ἀκριβὴς σκίρρος, ἀνίατος· ἤδη ὢν ἀναίσθητος, καὶ μὴ φαρμάκοις εἴκων· ὁ δ' ἕτερος, οὐκ εὐίατος, μετρίαν ἔχων αἴσθησιν· διαφορητικοῖς οὖν ἅμα καὶ μαλακτικοῖς οὗτοι θεραπεύονται· ὁποῖα οἵ τε μυελοὶ καὶ τὰ στέατα καὶ μᾶλλον τῶν ἀγρίων ζῴων· ἔτι τε ἀμμωνιακόν· καὶ βδέλλιον· καὶ στύραξ· καὶ ταῦτα μέν, ἐν τοῖς κατὰ πᾶν τὸ σῶμα σκίρροις ἐπιτίθεται· ἐπὶ δὲ τῶν τενόντων καὶ συνδέσμων πεπονθότων, προπυρωθέντα πυρίτιν (E: *πυρίτην*) *ἢ μυλίτιν* (E: *μυλίτην*) *λίθον, δεῖ σβεννύειν ὄξει δριμυτάτῳ· καὶ τὸν ἀναφερόμενον ἀτμὸν δέχεσθαι τῷ πεπονθότι μορίῳ· καὶ μετὰ τοῦτο πάλιν, μαλακτικὸν ἐπιτιθέναι φάρμακον· ἀμοιβηδὸν* (E: *ἀμοιβαδὸν*) *ταῦτα ποιοῦντα μέχρι τελείας λύσεως·*

APPENDIX 5

The Manuscripts of the *Medical Epitome*

Georgios Costomiris (1849–1902), a Greek ophthalmologist and scholar active in Paris, was the first person to attempt to record the large number of manuscripts of John's corpus, providing a detailed list of contents for some of them.[1] Hermann Diels (1848–1922) catalogued the majority of the codices in the second volume of his monumental *Die Handschriften der antiken Ärzte* published in 1906.[2] More recently, Stavroula Georgiou provided the first extensive study of the manuscripts of John's *On Urines* in her doctoral thesis.[3]

The textual tradition of John's *Medical Epitome* is one of the richest in Byzantine medical literature. We are aware of twenty-six manuscripts preserving the entire text (although sometimes some chapters of either books five or six are missing), dating from the fourteenth to the eighteenth century, with only two of them dating to before 1400. Furthermore, there are thirteen fragmentary and excerpting[4] manuscripts.[5] It is noteworthy that none of these manuscripts is significantly older than the complete copies. In addition, there are two sixteenth-century printed Latin translations of the work or parts of it. For the Greek text there is only a partial edition by Julius Ludwig Ideler of books one and two. As we shall see below, the lack of a full edition is not simply a matter of chance, since the textual tradition is complicated for books three, four, five, and six.

In this Appendix, I provide a description of the contents of all surviving manuscripts and Latin editions. The manuscripts are given in chronological order. For each manuscript, I give the reference to the latest catalogue, including any recent study which has provided a more precise, revised dating. The transcriptions follow the original spelling and punctuation of the relevant codex, apart from the iota subscript which I have supplied. Sometimes, where they are known, details of provenance are

[1] Costomiris (1897: 414–45).

[2] Diels (1906: II.108–11) and (1908: 69). See also Touwaide (2016: 38, 48, 59, 143, 174, 187, 288, 294, 297–9, 314, 345, 347, 359); and *Pinakes: Textes et manuscrits grecs*, at http://pinakes.irht.cnrs.fr/notices/auteur/1529/ (accessed 17 August 2018).

[3] Georgiou (2013: 175–307).

[4] Since the text is very long and encompasses various topics, several books or particular excerpts, especially from the last two books on pharmacology, were often transmitted independently.

[5] At an advanced stage in the completion of the final manuscript of this book I became aware of an uncatalogued codex (MS II.4237) in the Bibliothèque royale de Belgique (Brussels), which contains some excerpts from John's works, but I was not able to consult it. I would like to thank Lucien Reynhout from the Bibliothèque royale for his help in identifying this manuscript. One cannot exclude the possibility that some very small, unidentified excerpts, including a few chapters from the *Medical Epitome*, may also survive in other poorly catalogued manuscripts. According to De Andrés (1968: 114), there was one more codex preserving an excerpt from John's *Medical Epitome*, books four and five, i.e. Scorialensis Δ.IV.13, ff. 142r–175v or 176r, which is now missing.

also provided and, in particular, in cases of owners or places with a distinct medical interest or association. The presentation of contents is synoptic as regards works of other authors and John's other works.[6] For the *Medical Epitome*, I always give the full title of the work as found in each manuscript and a detailed list of contents followed by reference to Ideler's edition for books one and two and to Henry Mathys' Latin edition for books three to six.[7] In most cases my conclusions on the contents of the text have been substantiated through autopsy. My objective has been to select the most appropriate witnesses to use as sources for my examination of the *Medical Epitome* throughout this book pending the appearance of the *editio princeps*, on which I am currently working, based on all available witnesses.

As is clear from Table App.5.1, in which I present an overview of the contents of John's *Medical Epitome* in the complete copies, we can mainly divide the witnesses into four large groups depending on the order of books. As I have already demonstrated in Chapter 5, a significant confusion has been caused in the textual tradition due to the twofold arrangement of the recipes in book six. In particular, the first part of book six ($\Sigma T\alpha$) is arranged in an *a capite ad calcem* order, while the second part of book six ($\Sigma T\beta$) is arranged according to the various kinds of drugs, as in book five. As a result, the second part of book six is copied immediately after book five (Group II), or the first part of book six is copied between books three and four (Group III); the arrangement of Group III is also reflected in Jean Ruelle's (1539) Latin edition of the last two books (see Section 2.3, below). Unfortunately, the oldest witnesses, i.e. **R** and **C** (Group IV), present numerous inconsistencies in the structure of books five and six, causing disarray in various chapters in the last two books and occasional omissions. However, there are seven manuscripts (Group I) which give the contents in the correct order, also followed, in most cases, by Mathys (1556) in his Latin edition of the entire work. My transcriptions are based on **V** and any important variant readings attested in **E** are indicated within parenthesis. **E** and **V** have been selected because they are the earliest manuscripts of Group I, both securely dated to the first half of the fifteenth century. Finally, I have checked all the relevant passages in **Pd** (Group I, fifteenth century), which does not provide any further, notable variant readings.

1. List of manuscripts

1.1 Complete manuscripts

R=Vaticanus Reginensis gr. 181	AD 1364
C=Parisinus Coislinianus 334	14th c.
F=Florentinus Laurentianus gr. plut. 75.11	AD 1411/12
P=Parisinus gr. 2305	AD 1418
E=Scorialensis Φ.III.12	AD 1432
V=Vindobonensis med. gr. 17	15th c. (first half)
Va=Vindobonensis med. gr. 26	15th c. (first half)

[6] I provide a transcription of the titles of John's other works, i.e. *On Urines* and *On Psychic Pneuma*, only when they give important details about John's appellations.

[7] The order of recipes in books five and six can vary a good deal in some manuscripts, including several omissions. In these cases, the reference to Mathys' (1556) edition is approximate and is indicated by '~'.

B=Berolinensis Phillippicus gr. 1582	15th c.
G=Florentinus Laurentianus gr. plut. 75.9	15th c.
H=Florentinus Laurentianus gr. plut. 75.16	15th c.
W=Londiniensis Wellcomensis MS.MSL.52	15th c.
A=Mediolanensis Ambrosianus gr. 707	15th c.
O=Oxoniensis Bodleianus Thomae Roe 15	15th c.
Pa=Parisinus gr. 2153	15th c.
Pb=Parisinus gr. 2256	15th c.
Pc=Parisinus gr. 2304	15th c.
Pd=Parisinus gr. 2306	15th c.
M=Venetus Marcianus gr. 298	AD 1465
D=Padovanus C.M. 644	15th c. (second half)
Q=Mosquensis (ex Dresdensis Da 5)	AD 1519
S=Leidensis Vossianus gr. F. 32	*c.*AD 1548
N=Monacensis gr. 69	AD 1551
X=Bruxellensis 11337–41 (Omont 46)	16th c.
Pe=Parisinus gr. 2307	16th c.
Pf={Parisinus gr. 2233/Berolinensis Phillippicus gr. 1528}	16th c.
Li=Lipsiensis gr. 60	AD 1786/7

1.2 Excerpting and fragmentary manuscripts

Z=Varsoviensis Zamoyscianus 155 Cim.	14th c.
I=Athous Iberiticus 151	15th c.
Ea=Scorialensis Υ.III.14	15th c.
Vt=Vaticanus gr. 2182	15th c.
L=Londiniensis Arundelianus 537	16th c.
Aa=Mediolanensis Ambrosianus gr. 598	16th c.
Ab=Mediolanensis Ambrosianus gr. 779	16th c.
Oa=Oxoniensis Bodleianus Laudianus gr. 62	16th c.
Pg=Parisinus gr. 2235	16th c.
Vp=Vaticanus Palatinus gr. 370	16th c.
Vb=Vindobonensis med. gr. 11	16th c.
Wa=Londiniensis Wellcomensis MS.MSL.112	AD 1732–63
Cr=Cracoviensis (ex Berolinensis gr. fol. 39)	19th c.

1.3 List of Latin editions

Rue=J. **Ruelle**	Paris (1539)
Math=C. H. **Mathys**	Paris (1556)

1.4 Greek edition

Idel=J. L. **Ideler**	Berlin (1842)

1.5 List of Books of the Medical Epitome *with reference to the relevant edition*

A=Book 1, inc. *Ἐπειδή σοι*, des. *τὴν σπουδὴν τρέψωμεν*. {Ideler (1842) II.353–417}

B=Book 2, inc. *Οὐ κατ᾽ ἐκείνους τῶν φίλων*, des. *λέγειν τὰ δέοντα*. {Ideler (1842) II.418–63}

Bα[8]=First part of Book 2, inc. *Οὐ κατ' ἐκείνους τῶν φίλων*, des. *μεθόδων ἐφάψασθαι*. {Ideler (1842) II.418–440.15}

Bβ=Second part of Book 2, inc. *Περὶ διαγνώσεως τῶν κατὰ τὸ δέρμα παθῶν*, des. *λέγειν τὰ δέοντα*. {Ideler (1842) II. 440.16–463}

Γ=Book 3, inc. *Ἐπειδὴ πᾶσα διδασκαλία*, des. *πᾶν τοῦ λόγου μέτρον συμπεραντέον*. {Mathys (1556) II.153–213}

Δ=Book 4, inc. *Ἡ μὲν παροιμία φησί*, des. *ἐνταῦθά πη συγκαταπαύειν*. {Mathys (1556) II.213–316}

E=Book 5, inc. *Ἤδη σοι καὶ τὸν ἐπὶ τοῖς τέσσαρσι βιβλίοις*, des. *ὑποσχέσεως ἄρτιον*. {Mathys (1556) II.317–432}

*E*p=It stands for a substantial part or a selection of various excerpts of *E*.

ΣT=Book 6, inc. *Ἐδόκει μοι διὰ βραχέων*, des. *δοκῶμεν ἐκπεπονηκότες τὴν βίβλον*. {Mathys (1556) II.433–563}

ΣTα[9]=First part of Book 6, inc. *Ἐδόκει μοι διὰ βραχέων*, des. *ἄρτιος ὁ λόγος τελοίη*. {Mathys (1556) II.433–526}

*ΣTα*Gal=It stands for a substantial part of *ΣTα*, inc. *Ἐγὼ φησὶν ὁ Γαληνός· καὶ τὰ τῶν κεράμων ὄστρακα*. {Mathys (1556) II.452ff}

ΣTβ=Second part of Book 6, inc. *Ἡ διὰ χαλκίτεως ἔμπλαστρος*, des. *δοκῶμεν ἐκπεπονηκότες τὴν βίβλον*. {Mathys (1556) II.526–63}

*ΣTβ*p=It stands for a substantial part or a selection of various excerpts of *ΣTβ*.

2. Description of manuscripts

2.1 Complete manuscripts

R=Vaticanus Reginensis gr. 181

Vatican City, Biblioteca Apostolica Vaticana (autopsy, February 2012).

Stevenson (1888: 121–3).

AD 1364, paper, 215 × 150 mm, ff. xiv+325; at least two main unidentified scribes; several folia in poor condition.

Text: [ir–xiiir] Table of contents: *Πίναξ τοῦ πρώτου λόγου τοῦ περὶ κράσεων καὶ φυσικῶν δυνάμεων καὶ παθῶν τῶν ὀργανικῶν*, inc. *Περὶ τοῦ ποῖα χρή*, des. *τοῦ Φίλωνος*. [xiiir–v] Magic spells. [xivv] Later hand: *Ἀκτουαρίου πρὸς τὸν προκαθήμενον τοῦ βασιλικοῦ κοιτῶνος ἰατρικὰ βιβλία ἕξ ὧν ἐμνημόνευσεν ἐν τῷ δευτέρῳ λόγῳ τῶν περὶ ἐνεργειῶν καὶ παθῶν τοῦ ψυχικοῦ πνεύματος καὶ τῆς κατ' αὐτὸ διαίτης*. [1r–45v] **Book 1 *Medical Epitome***, title: *Περὶ κράσεων καὶ φυσικῶν δυνάμεων· καὶ παθῶν τῶν ὀργανικῶν καὶ καιρίων μορίων· καὶ σφυγμῶν· καὶ οὔρων καὶ τῶν ἄλλων· ὅσα δι' ἐκκρίσεων φαίνεται· καὶ τῆς ἀπὸ τούτων διαγνώσεως*. {Ideler (1842) II.353–417}. [45v–79r] **Book 2 *Medical Epitome*** {Ideler (1842) II.418–63}. [79r–109r] **Book 3 *Medical Epitome*** {Mathys (1556) II.153–213}. [109r–159r] **Book 4 *Medical Epitome*** {Mathys (1556) II.213–316}. [159v–187r] **Excerpt from Book 6 *Medical Epitome***, inc. *Ἐγὼ φησὶν ὁ Γαληνός· καὶ τὰ τῶν κεράμων ὄστρακα*, des. *διὸ καὶ ταχέως ἑλκοῦνται μὴ θεραπευόμενοι ὡς προσήκει*. {~Mathys (1556) II.452–98}. [187r–200v] **Excerpt from**

[8] Book two was not originally divided by the author into two distinct parts. For referencing purposes, I call the two parts 'first' and 'second', following the form in which they appear in **Pa**.

[9] For referencing purposes, I call the two parts of book six 'first' and 'second', following the form in which they appear in a large number of manuscripts.

App. 5.1. Contents of complete manuscripts and early printed editions of the *Medical Epitome* according to book order

Group		I	II	III	IV
Book Order		*Α, Β, Γ, Δ, Ε, ΣΤ*	*Α, Β, Γ, Δ, Ε, ΣΤβ, ΣΤα*	*Α, Β, Γ, ΣΤα, Δ, Ε, ΣΤβ*	*Α, Β, Γ, Δ, ΣΤα*Gal, *Ep*, *ΣΤβ*p, *Ep*
COMPLETE MANUSCRIPTS	R				✓
	C				✓
	F		✓		
	P			✓	
	E	✓			
	V	✓			
	Va			✓	
	B	✓			
	G			✓	
	H			✓	
	W			✓ (minus *ΣΤβ*)	
	A			✓	
	O	✓			
	Pa			✓ (order: *Α, Βα, Γ, Ββ, ΣΤα, Δ, Ε, ΣΤβ*)	
	Pb			✓	
	Pc			✓ (minus *ΣΤβ*)	
	Pd	✓			
	M		✓		
	D			✓	
	Q		✓[?]		
	S				~
	N		✓		
	X		✓		
	Pe	✓			
	Pf	✓			
	Li		✓		
LATIN EDITIONS	Rue			✓ (order: *Ε, ΣΤβ*; minus *Α, Β, Γ, ΣΤα, Δ*)	
	Math	✓			

Book 5 *Medical Epitome*, inc. ~~*Διατοῦτο*~~ *καὶ χρονίου ὀφθαλμίας*, des. *καὶ πρὸ τῶν καθαρσίων συμπέττοντα μὲν τοῦς χυμούς*. {~Mathys (1556) II.413–16, 392–413, 388–92}. [200v–222v] **Excerpt from Book 6 *Medical Epitome***, inc. *Ἀποφράττον δὲ τοὺς πόρους· ἐπεὶ δύναμις ἐστιν αὔτη· χαμαιπιτύος*, des. *ἐκπεπονηκότες τὴν βίβλον ταύτην*. {~Mathys (1556) II.532–63}. [223r–266r] **Excerpt from Book 5 *Medical Epitome***, *Ἐπεὶ τοῖς ῥηθεῖσι τέταρσι βιβλίοις ἐπιτίθεμεν λόγον*, des. *σὺν αὐτοῖς ἐλέβορος λευκὸς καθαίρει αἷμα καὶ χολήν*. {~Mathys (1556) II.317–88}. [266v–271r] Aetios of Amida, *Tetrabiblios*, Book 3.175–83. [271r–281v] Anonymous treatises on urines. [281v, 283r] Excerpt from Ps.-Hippocrates' *Epistle to King Ptolemy on the Constitution of Man*. [282r] Short drug glossary. [282v, 283v] Opuscules on measurements. [284r] Tachygraphic abbreviations. [284v] Anonymous recipe. [285r–295r] Ps.-Galen, *On Urines*. [295r–324v] Anonymous treatise on the pulse. [324r] Scribal colophon: *Τέλος τῶν φυσικῶν λογιδίων τοῦ ἰατρὸς βίβλου· ἐν μηνὶ Ἀπριλλίῳ...ἔτους ͵ϛωοβʹ· ᾧ ἡ δόξα καὶ τὸ κράτος ἀμήν.*

C=Parisinus Coislinianus 334

Paris, Bibliothèque nationale de France (autopsy, October 2012).

Devreesse (1945: 317–18).

14th c., paper, 223 × 145 mm, ff. 355; several unidentified scribes; several folia in poor condition.

Text: [1r–8v] Table of contents (first folia in very poor condition): inc. (first semi-readable line) *Περὶ τῆς κατὰ μέγεθ[ος τῶν σφυγμῶν διαφορᾶς]*, des. *περὶ τῶν βασιλικοδήκτων*. [8v] Short treatise on unlucky days. [10r–18r] Ps.-Galen, *On Urines*. [19r–47v] **Book 1 *Medical Epitome***, title: *Περὶ κράσεων· καὶ φυσικῶν δυνάμεων· καὶ παθῶν τῶν ὀργανικῶν καὶ καιρίων μορίων· καὶ σφυγμῶν· καὶ οὔρων καὶ τῶν ἄλλων· ὅσα δι' ἐκρίσεων φαίνεται· καὶ τῆς ἀπὸ τούτων διαγνώσεως*. {Ideler (1842) II.353–417}. [47v–72v] **Book 2 *Medical Epitome*** {Ideler (1842) II.418–63}. [72v–95v] **Book 3 *Medical Epitome*** {Mathys (1556) II.153–213}. [95v–133r] **Book 4 *Medical Epitome*** {Mathys (1556) II.213–316}. [133r–154r] **Excerpt from Book 6 *Medical Epitome***, inc. *[Ἐ]γὼ φησὶν ὁ Γαληνός, καὶ τὰ τῶν κεράμων ὄστρακα*, des. *διὸ καὶ ταχέως ἑλκοῦνται μὴ θεραπευόμενοι ὡς προσήκει*. {~Mathys (1556) II.452–98}. [154r–165v] **Excerpt from Book 5 *Medical Epitome***, inc. *Διατοῦτο καὶ χρονίου ὀφθαλμίας*, des. *καθὼς ἑξῆς ἐροῦμεν παρὰ πάντων· ἵν' οὖν*. {~Mathys (1556) II.413–16, 392–413, 388–92}. [166r] **Short excerpt from Book 4 *Medical Epitome*** {Mathys (1556) II.315–316}. [166r–180v] **Excerpt from Book 5 *Medical Epitome***, inc. *Βιβλίοις ἐπιτίθεμεν λόγον· ὃς πέμπτος τῆς ὅλης πραγματείας ἐστί*, des. *καὶ ἀκίνδυνον ἔσται πρὸς τούς*. {~Mathys (1556) II.317–53}. [181r–193v] **Excerpt from Book 6 *Medical Epitome***, inc. *Οὐγγ. ϛʹ· τὰ τηκτὰ κατὰ τῶν ξηρῶν· ἐὰν δὲ ἀνωδυνότερον εἶναι*, des. *δοκῶμεν ἐκπεπονηκότες τὴν βίβλον*. {~Mathys (1556) II.536–63}. [195r–198v] Aetios of Amida, *Tetrabiblos*, Book 3.175–83. [198v–214v] Anonymous collection of therapeutic recommendations. [215r–281v] ***On Urines***, title: *[Τ]οῦ σοφωτάτου καὶ λογιωτάτου πανσεβάστου σεβαστοῦ τοῦ ἀκτου[αρίου...]*. [282r–289v, 310r–345v] Excerpts from Aetios of Amida's *Tetrabiblos*, Book 16. [290r–309v] **Various excerpts from Books 5 & 6 *Medical Epitome***, inc. *Δι' οὐρητικὸν πρὸς ἴκτερον*, des. *στόμαχου· σμύρνης δραχμὰς βʹ· πεπέρ[εως]*. [346r–355v] Excerpt from [Ibn Sīnā's], *On Urines*.

F=Florentinus Laurentianus gr. 75.11

Florence, Biblioteca Medicea Laurenziana (autopsy, February 2012).

Bandini (1770: III.158–9).

AD 1411/12, paper, 283 × 205 mm, ff. iv+287+iii; one scribe (ff. 1r–287v): Stephen (*RGK* I 366, II 503, III 584), who later became Metropolitan of Media, active in the monastery of St John the Baptist at Petra in Constantinople in the early fifteenth century (see also Parisinus gr. 2304, described below).[10]

Text: [1r–82r] ***On Urines***. [82r–116v] ***On Psychic Peuma***. [116v–144r] **Book 1 *Medical Epitome***, title: *Τοῦ αὐτοῦ βιβλίον ἰατρικὸν περιέχον πᾶσαν τέχνην ἐν ἐπιτόμῳ.* {Ideler (1842) II.353–417}. [144r–163v] **Book 2 *Medical Epitome*** {Ideler (1842) II.418–63}. [163v–181r] **Book 3 *Medical Epitome*** {Mathys (1556) II.153–213}. [181r–213v] **Book 4 *Medical Epitome*** {Mathys (1556) II.213–316}. [213v–247v] **Book 5 *Medical Epitome*** {Mathys (1556) II.317–432}. [247v–259r] **Second part of Book 6 *Medical Epitome*** {Mathys (1556) II.526–63}. [259r–286r] **First part of Book 6 *Medical Epitome*** {Mathys (1556) II.433–526}. [286r] Opuscule on measurements. [286r–287v] Paul of Aegina, *Epitome*, Book 7.25. [287v] Scribal colophon: *Ἡ παροῦσα βίβλος ἐγράφη παρ' ἐμοῦ τοῦ ἐν ἱερομονάχοις ἐλαχίστου Στεφάνου· καὶ οἱ ἀναγινώσκοντες εὔχεσθε ὑπὲρ ἐμοῦ διὰ τὸν Κύριον· ἐν ἔτει ͵ϛϡκ΄· (ἰνδικτιῶνος) ε΄.*

P=Parisinus gr. 2305

Paris, Bibliothèque nationale de France (autopsy, October 2012).

Omont (1888: II.233).

AD 1418, paper, 205 × 145 mm, ff. iii+401; one main scribe (ff. 1r–19r, 22r–399v): Manuel Iagaris (*RGK* II 345); various later hands (19v–21v, 400r–401v).

Text: [1r–120v] ***On Urines***. [120v] Scribal endnote: *Τέλος σὺν Θεῷ ἁγίῳ τὸ περὶ οὔρων: δόξα σοι ἁγία τριᾶς· δόξα σοι τῷ δείξαντι ἀρχὴν καὶ τέλος οὔρων· Θεοῦ τὸ δῶρον καὶ Μανουὴλ ὁ πόνος· ἅγιος· ἅγιος· ἅγιος.* [121r–158r] ***On Psychic Pneuma***. [158r–200v] **Book 1 *Medical Epitome***, title: *Τοῦ αὐτοῦ βιβλίον ἰατρικὸν καὶ περιέχον πᾶσαν τέχνην ἐν ἐπιτόμῳ.* {Ideler (1842) II.353–417}. [200v–227r] **Book 2 *Medical Epitome*** {Ideler (1842) II.418–63}. [227r–251r] **Book 3 *Medical Epitome*** {Mathys (1556) II.153–213}. [251r–288r] **First part of Book 6 *Medical Epitome*** {Mathys (1556) II.433–526}. [288v–331v] **Book 4 *Medical Epitome*** {Mathys (1556) II.213–316}. [332r–384r] **Book 5 *Medical Epitome*** {Mathys (1556) II.317–432}. [384r–399r] **Second part of Book 6 *Medical Epitome*** {Mathys (1556) II.526–63}. [399r] Scribal endnote: *Τῷ δὲ Θεῷ ἡμῶν εἴη δόξα εἰς τοὺς αἰώνας ἀμήν· δόξα σοι τῷ δείξαντι ἀρχὴν καὶ τέλος· Θεοῦ τὸ δῶρον καὶ Μανουὴλ ὁ πόνος.* [399v] Scribal colophon: *Ἐτελειώθη ἡ παροῦσα βίβλος ἐν ἔτει ͵ϛϡκϛ΄ μηνὶ Φεβρουαρίῳ κϛ΄ (ἰνδικτιῶνος) ια΄· γραφεῖσα διὰ χειρὸς Μανουὴλ Ἰάγαρι Δουκὸς τοῦ Τυρί· καὶ οἱ ἀναγιγνώσκωντες αὐτὴν εὔχεσθαί με διὰ τὸν Κύριον: ἵνα εὕρω ἔλεος ἐν τῇ ἡμέρᾳ τῆς κρίσεως.* [399v] Anonymous recipe. [400r–402v] Excerpt from Isidore of Kiev's *On the Council of Florence*.

E=Scorialensis Φ.III.12

San Lorenzo de El Escorial, Real Biblioteca del Monasterio (autopsy, October 2018).

De Andrés (1965: 64–6).

AD 1432,[11] paper, 208 × 144 mm, ff. iv+463; one main unidentified scribe (ff. 1r–472v).

[10] Kakoulidi (1968: 26–9). On Stephen of Media, see Cataldu Palau (2008).

[11] De Andrés (1965: 64) refers to 'An. 1433', but, according to the scribal colophon, the manuscript was completed in October, thus it should be 1432, as we must subtract the figure

Text: [1r–v] **Excerpt from Book 5 *Medical Epitome***, inc. *Ξανθῆς χολῆς εἰς κενώσεως προκειμένης*, des. *χυλὸν ὑποκυστίδος σάχαρ*. {~Mathys (1556) II.391–3}. [2r–4v] Various anonymous recipes and notes on the pulse. [5r–8v] [Ibn Sīnā], *On Urines*. [8v] Ps.-Galen, *On Urines*. [9r–v] Excerpts from [Hippocrates'] *Prognostic*. [10r–11v] Various medical diagrams. [12r–128v] ***On Urines***, title: *Τοῦ σοφωτάτου καὶ λογιωτάτου πανσεβάστου σεβαστοῦ ἀκτουαρίου κυροῦ Ἰωάννου τοῦ Ζαχαρίου· τάδε ἔνεισιν ἐν τῷ περὶ διαφορᾶς οὔρων λόγῳ*. [129r–v] Anonymous excerpts on sweats and various recipes. [130r–174r] ***On Psychic Pneuma***. [174r–v] Opuscule on measurements and various anonymous recipes. [174v–211r] **Book 1 *Medical Epitome***, title: *Παρακοιμωμένῳ τῷ Ἀποκαύχῳ· τῷ καὶ ὕστερον χρηματίσαντι μεγάλῳ Δουκί· τοῦ σοφωτάτου ἀκτουαρίου κυροῦ Ἰωάννου*. (175r) title: *Τοῦ σοφωτάτου ἰατροῦ ἀκτουαρίου κυροῦ Ἰωάννου τοῦ Ζαχαρίου, θεραπευτικῆς μεθόδου, βιβλίον πρῶτον*. {Ideler (1842) II.353–417}. [211r–237r] **Book 2 *Medical Epitome*** {Ideler (1842) II.418–63}. [237r–260v] **Book 3 *Medical Epitome*** {Mathys (1556) II.153–213}. [261r–305r] **Book 4 *Medical Epitome*** {Mathys (1556) II.213–316}. [305r–352v] **Book 5 *Medical Epitome*** {Mathys (1556) II.317–432}. [352v–393r] **First part of Book 6 *Medical Epitome*** {Mathys (1556) II.433–526}. [393v] Short treatise on calendars. [394r] Table of lunar phases and months. [394v–395r] Opuscules on astrology. [395v] Anonymous recipes. [396r–419v] **Second part of Book 6 *Medical Epitome*** {Mathys (1556) II.526–63}. [419v] Scribal endnote: *Ἐτελειώθη κατὰ μῆνα Ὀκτωβρίου· τῆς νῦν τρεχούσης (ἰνδικτιῶνος) ια´ τοῦ ͵ϛϡμα´ ἔτους*. [420r–v] Various excerpts on fevers. [421r–443r] Excerpts from Paul of Aegina, *Epitome*, Book 2.1–60. [443v–457r] [Hippocrates], *Aphorisms*. [457r–461r] [Hippocrates], *Prognostic*. [461r–466v] [Hippocrates], *On Winds*. [467r–469v] Paul of Aegina, *Epitome*, Book 7.25. [469v] Opuscule on measurements. [470r–472v] Various anonymous recipes.

V=Vindobonensis med. gr. 17

Vienna, Österreichische Nationalbibliothek (autopsy, March 2012).

Hunger (1969: II.62–3).

first half of the 15th c., paper, 260/270 × 210 mm, ff. i+243; one scribe (ff. 1r–242v): Simon Makrodoukas (*Σίμων ὁ Μακροδούκας*).[12] The manuscript was commissioned for the fifteenth-century physician *archiatros* Anthony Pyropoulos.

Text: [1r–31v] **Book 1 *Medical Epitome***, title: *Πυροπούλου νέου ἀρχιητροῦ, ἰατρικῆς βιβλία ι´*. {Ideler (1842) II.353–417}. [32r–54v] **Book 2 *Medical Epitome*** {Ideler (1842) II.418–63}. [55r–76r] **Book 3 *Medical Epitome*** {Mathys (1556) II.153–213}. [76r–112v] **Book 4 *Medical Epitome*** {Mathys (1556) II.213–316}. [112v–167r] **Book 5 *Medical Epitome*** {Mathys (1556) II.317–432}. [167r–242v] **Book 6 *Medical Epitome*** {Mathys (1556) II.433–563}.

Va=Vindobonensis med. gr. 26

5509 (used when calculating dates falling between 1 September and 31 December), from 6941 (͵ϛϡμα´), not 5508, which is used when calculating dates falling between 1 January and 31 August.

[12] According to Lambeck and Kollár (1780: VI.263), although the actual note was probably lost during a later rebound of the codex. See Hunger (1969: II.63).

Vienna, Österreichische Nationalbibliothek (autopsy, March 2012).

Hunger (1969: II.72–4).

first half of the 15th c., paper, 222/225 × 145/148 mm, ff. i+ii(parchment)+446 (445–446, parchment)+i; one main scribe (ff. 1r–412v, 416r–443v).[13] According to the note in f. 444v the manuscript may have belonged to the Pantokrator monastery in Constantinople.

Text: [1r–118r] ***On Urines***. [118v] Scribal endnote: *Τέλος σὺν Θεῷ ἁγίῳ ἀμήν· ὥσπερ ξένοι χαίρουσιν ἰδεῖν πατρίδα καὶ οἱ θαλαττεύοντες ἰδεῖν λιμένα, οὕτω καὶ οἱ βιβλογράφοντες ἰδεῖν βιβλίου τέλος*. [120r–173r] ***On Psychic Pneuma***. [173r–215r] **Book 1 *Medical Epitome***, title: *Τοῦ αὐτοῦ βιβλίον ἰατρικὸν περιέχον πᾶσαν τέχνην ἐν ἐπιτόμῳ*. {Ideler (1842) II.353–417}. [215r–244r] **Book 2 *Medical Epitome*** {Ideler (1842) II.418–63}. [244r–267v] **Book 3 *Medical Epitome*** {Mathys (1556) II.153–213}. [268r–303r] **First part of Book 6 *Medical Epitome*** {Mathys (1556) II.433–526}. [303r–305v] Paul of Aegina, *Epitome*, Book 7.25. [305v] Scribal endnote: *Τέλος συν Θεῷ ἁγίῳ ἀμήν· διπλοῦν τὸν ἁπλοῦν ἡ κυήσασα λόγον, ῥῶσιν διπλὴν δίδου τῷ γεγραφότι*. [307r–350r] **Book 4 *Medical Epitome*** {Mathys (1556) II.213–316}. [350r–396v] **Book 5 *Medical Epitome*** {Mathys (1556) II.317–432}. [397r–412r] **Second part of Book 6 *Medical Epitome*** {Mathys (1556) II.526–63}. [412v] Scribal endnote: *Τῷ Θεῷ ἡμῶν εἴη δόξας εἰς τοὺς αἰῶνας ἀμήν· τέλος ἁπάσης τῆς πραγματείας, τοῦ σοφωτάτου ὀκταρίου· διπλοῦν τὸν ἁπλοῦν ἡ κυήσασα λόγον, ῥῶσιν διπλὴν δίδου τῷ γεγραφότι* (*μοὶ τῷ κεκτημένῳ*, *superscriptum*). [413v] Anonymous recipes. [415r] Anonymous recipes. [416r–443v] Excerpts from Theophanes Chrysobalantes' *Synopsis*. [444r–v, 445v–446r] Anonymous recipes by various late hands. [445r] Cryptographic abbreviations. [444v] Mark of ownership: *Τουτο το βηβηβλιο ηνε του Παντοκρατορα εχι φηλα…και οπου το παρη να εχι τον αφορεσμον τον παρη*.

B=Berolinensis Phillippicus gr. 1582

Berlin, Staatsbibliothek (autopsy, June 2012).

Studemund and Cohn (1890: 78).

15th c., paper, 218 × 314 mm, ff. ii+391+iii; one main scribe (ff. 1r–154v, 159r–387r): Demetrios Vranas.[14]

Text: [1r–110v] ***On Urines***. [111r–154v] ***On Psychic Pneuma***. [155v–156r, 157v–158r] Various anonymous recipes. [159r–195v] **Book 1 *Medical Epitome***, title: *Τοῦ σοφωτάτου ἀκτουαρίου κυροῦ Ἰωάννου τοῦ Ζαχαρίου· περὶ διαγνώσεως παθῶν*. {Ideler (1842) II.353–417}. [195v–221v] **Book 2 *Medical Epitome*** {Ideler (1842) II.418–63}. [221v–245v] **Book 3 *Medical Epitome*** {Mathys (1556) II.153–213}. [245v–285v] **Book 4 *Medical Epitome*** {Mathys (1556) II.213–316}. [286r–334r] **Book 5 *Medical Epitome*** {Mathys (1556) II.317–432}. [334r–387r] **Book 6 *Medical Epitome*** {Mathys (1556) II.433–563}. [387r] Scribal colophon followed by a monokondylion: *Ὡς ταῖς ἐλάφοις καύματος ὥρα πέλει / πηγὴ ποθεινὴ ἄκος οὖσα τοῦ θέρους / οὕτω πέφυκε καὶ γραφεῦσιν*

[13] The scribal notes on ff. 305v and 412v are in part identical with the one produced by the copyist Demetrios Vranas in Berolinensis Phillippicus gr. 1582. Cf. Vassis (2005: 149).

[14] The surname of the scribe derives from the reading of the *monokondylion* in f. 387r by Georgiou (2013: 182): '*Δημήτριος ὁ Βρανᾶς*'. Studemund and Cohn (1890: 78) previously suggested the erroneous reading '*Δημήτριος ὁ Γράψας*'. The scribal colophon on f. 387r is in part identical with those ones found in Vindobonensis med. gr. 26.

ἡδύτης / τὸ τέρμα βίβλου, τοῖσδε τῶν πονουμένων· / διπλοῦν τὸν ἁπλοῦν ἡ κυήσασα λόγον, διπλῆν ῥῶσιν δίδου μοι τῷ γεγραφότι. [388v–389v] Ps.-Galenic treatise on the pulse. [390r] Notes on mathematics. [391r] Various anonymous recipes. [391v] Long invocation to the Ecumenical Patriarch.

G=Florentinus Laurentianus gr. 75.9

Florence, Biblioteca Medicea Laurenziana (autopsy, February 2012).

Bandini (1770: III.155–6).

15th c., paper, 208 × 138 mm, ff. v+468+vi; two main unidentified scribes: A (ff. 1r–112v, 220r–427v, 468v) and B (ff. 117r–219v, 428r–468r).

Text: [1r–4r] Anonymous recipes. [5r–112v] ***On Urines***, title: *Τοῦ σοφωτάτου καὶ λογιωτάτου πανσεβάστου σεβαστοῦ τοῦ ἀκτουαρίου κυροῦ Ἰωάννου τοῦ Ζαχαρίου· τάδε ἔνεστιν, ἐν τῷ περὶ διαφορᾶς οὔρων λόγῳ.* [117r–174r] ***On Psychic Peuma.*** [174r–219v] Galen, *Therapeutics to Glaucon.* [219v] Scribal endnote: *Δόξα τῷ Θεῷ τῷ δόντι πέρας· ἔληξεν ἀρχήν, δάκτυλοι τρεῖς καὶ γόνυ.* [220r–222v] Incomplete table of contents of the ***Medical Epitome.*** [226v] Medical notes in aphoristic form. [228r–263v] **Book 1 *Medical Epitome*,** no title {Ideler (1842) II.353–417}. [263v–288v] **Book 2 *Medical Epitome*** {Ideler (1842) II.418–63}. [288v–312v] **Book 3 *Medical Epitome*** {Mathys (1556) II.153–213}. [312v–346v] **First part of Book 6 *Medical Epitome*** {Mathys (1556) II.433–526}. [346v–386v] **Book 4 *Medical Epitome*** {Mathys (1556) II.213–316}. [386v–427v] **Book 5 *Medical Epitome*** {Mathys (1556) II.317–432}. [428r–465r] **Second part of Book 6 *Medical Epitome*** {Mathys (1556) II.526–63}. [465v, 468v] Opuscules on measurements. [465v–468r] Paul of Aegina, *Epitome*, Book 7.25.

H= Florentinus Laurentianus gr. 75.16

Florence, Biblioteca Medicea Laurenziana (autopsy, February 2012).

Bandini (1770: III. 164–5).

15th c., paper, 206 × 137 mm, ff. i+403+ii; at least three main unidentified scribes.

Text: [1r–2v] Incomplete table of contents of John's works, title: *Πίναξ ἀκριβής, τῆς παρούσης πικτίδος, τοῦ σοφωτάτου καὶ λογιωτάτου ἀκτουαρίου κυροῦ Ἰωάννου του Ζαχαρίου.* [3r] Various anonymous recipes. [4r–104r] ***On Urines***, title: *Τοῦ σοφωτάτου καὶ λογιωτάτου πανσεβάστου σεβαστοῦ τοῦ ἀκτουαρίου κυροῦ Ἰωάννου τοῦ Ζαχαρίου· ταδ' ἔνεστιν, τῷ περὶ διαφορας οὔρων λόγῳ.* [106r–149v] ***On Psychic Pneuma.*** [149v–192r] Galen, *Therapeutics to Glaucon.* [194r–223r] **Book 1 *Medical Epitome*,** title: *Τῷ παρακοιμωμένῳ τῷ Ἀποκαύχῳ, τῷ καὶ ὕστερον χρηματίσαντι μεγάλῳ δουκί· τοῦ σοφωτάτου ἀκτουαρίου κυροῦ Ἰωάννου· περὶ διαγνώσεως παθῶν· λόγος αʹ.* {Ideler (1842) II.353–417}. [223v–244r] **Book 2 *Medical Epitome*** {Ideler (1842) II.418–63}. [244r–263v] **Book 3 *Medical Epitome*** {Mathys (1556) II.153–213}. [263v–292r] **First part of Book 6 *Medical Epitome*** {Mathys (1556) II.433–526}. [292r–323r] **Book 4 *Medical Epitome*** {Mathys (1556) II.213–316}. [323r–353v] **Book 5 *Medical Epitome*** {Mathys (1556) II.317–432}. [355r–386v] **Second part of Book 6 *Medical Epitome*** {Mathys (1556) II.526–63}. [386v] Opuscule on measurements. [386v–389r] Paul of Aegina, *Epitome*, Book 7.25. [393r–400r, 401r–403v] Various anonymous recipes.

W=Londiniensis Wellcomensis MS.MSL.52

London, Wellcome Library (autopsy, March 2014).

Bouras-Vallianatos (2015b: 286–92).

15th c., paper, 215 × 145 mm, ff. v+202+i and i+210+i. Provenance: Manuel Kantakouzenos Gerakes—Stavronikita Monastery, Mount Athos—brought to England in 1749 by the English physician Anthony Askew (1722–74).

Note: This MS consists of two volumes bound separately but foliated continuously. Volume 52B comprises two distinct parts, 52B1 and 52B2. 52A and 52B1 are the work of the same scribe and were originally bound together. These are described below under I, while 52B2 (ff. 333r–403v) is described under II.

I.

Shortly before AD 1463 (from the note on f. 332v); one main scribe (ff. 1r–332v) attributed by Brigitte Mondrain to Demetrios Angelos.[15]

Text: [vr] Mark of ownership: *Καὶ τόδε σὺν τῆς ἅλης μονῆς τοῦ Σταυρονικήτα· τοῦ μεγάλου Νικολάου τῆς ἐν τῷ Ἁγίῳ Ὄρει.* [vv] *τοῦ σοφωτάτου· καὶ λογιωτάτου· καὶ ἄκρου· ἰατροῦ· πανσεβάστου· σεβαστοῦ κυροῦ Ἰωάννου Ζαχαρίου τοῦ ἀκτουαρίου.* [1r–43v] ***On Psychic Pneuma***. [44r–143v] ***On Urines***, title: *Τοῦ σοφωτάτου καὶ λογιωτάτου πανσεβάστου σεβαστοῦ τοῦ ἀκτουαρίου κυροῦ Ἰωάννου τοῦ Ζαχαρίου· λόγος α*[ος]. [145r–178r] **Book 1 *Medical Epitome***, title: *Περὶ διαγνώσεως καὶ αἰτιῶν κατὰ μέρος παθῶν· λόγος α΄· τοῦ αὐτοῦ σοφωτάτου ἰατροῦ ἀκτουαρίου κυροῦ Ἰωάννου τοῦ Ζαχαρίου· θεραπευτικῆς μεθόδου, βιβλίον, πρῶτον.* Title added: *Πρὸς τὸν παρακοιμώμενον τὸν Ἀπόκαυχον τῷ καὶ ὕστερον χρηματίσαντι μεγάλῳ δουκί.* {Ideler (1842) II.353–417}. [178r–202v] **Book 2 *Medical Epitome*** {Ideler (1842) II.418–63}. [203r–224r] **Book 3 *Medical Epitome*** {Mathys (1556) II.153–213}. [224r–257v] **First part of Book 6 *Medical Epitome*** {Mathys (1556) II.433–526}. [257v–295v] **Book 4 *Medical Epitome*** {Mathys (1556) II.213–316}. [296r–332v] **Book 5 *Medical Epitome*** {Mathys (1556) II.317–432}. [332v] Historical note: *Κατὰ τὴν κς΄ τοῦ Μαρτίου μηνὸς*, des. *νυκτὸς ὥρᾳ δ΄ τοῦ ͵ς϶οβ΄ ἰν(δικτιῶνος) ια΄.*

II.

*c.*1445; one main hand (ff. 333r–403v): similar to those of (according to Georgi Parpulov) Constantine Triboles (*RGK* II 318) and (according to Rudolf Stefec) Mark (*RGK* III 437).

Original order of leaves: 333–379, 388–395, 380–387, 396–403.

Text: [333r–v] Theophilos and Stephen, *On Differences of Fevers*, chapter on sweats. [333v–341r] Anonymous, *On the Pulse*, in the form of questions and answers. [341r–345v] Paul of Aegina, *Epitome*, excerpt on the pulse. [345v–346r] Brief anonymous text on the pulse. [346r–v] Aetios of Amida, *Tetrabiblos*, excerpt on the pulse. [346v–354r] Excrerpt from Galen's *On the Pulse for Beginners*. [354v–361v] Theophilos, *On Excrements*. [361v–363r] Ps.-Hippocrates, *Sayings about Life and Death*. [363r] Mark of ownership: *Ἰησοῦ Χριστὲ β[οή]θει τῷ σῷ δούλῳ [—]δικω τῷ Ἀρδυρομ*ᵀ ᵀ [?] [the following three lines of text are completely blotted out]. [363v] Anonymous recipes. [364r–366v] Excerpt from Ps.-Galen's *On Procurable*

[15] Mondrain (2000a: 236–7, 250); (2003: 366); and (2010: 295, 299, 301, 305).

Remedies. [366v–403v] Anonymus of Paris, *On Acute and Chronic Diseases*. [404r] Mark of ownership: *Μανουῆλ Καντακουζινὸς ο Γεράκης*.

A=Mediolanensis Ambrosianus gr. 707 (R 20 sup.)

Milan, Biblioteca Ambrosiana (autopsy, February 2012).

Martini and Bassi (1906: 818–19).

15th c., paper, 219 × 141 mm, ff. i+539+ii; at least three main unidentified scribes.

Text: [4r–18r] Table of contents of John Zacharias Aktouarios' works. [20r–185v] ***On Urines***. [186r–251r] ***On Psychic Pneuma***. [251r–323v] **Books 1 & 2 *Medical Epitome***, title: *Τοῦ αὐτοῦ βιβλίον ἰατρικόν, περιέχον πᾶσαν τέχνην ἐν ἐπιτόμῳ*. {Ideler (1842) II.353–463}. [324r–354r] **Book 3 *Medical Epitome*** {Mathys (1556) II.153–213}. [354r–400r] **First part of Book 6 *Medical Epitome*** {Mathys (1556) II.433–526}. [400v–455v] **Book 4 *Medical Epitome*** {Mathys (1556) II.213–316}. [456r–513v] **Book 5 *Medical Epitome*** {Mathys (1556) II.317–432}. [514r–532r] **Second part of Book 6 *Medical Epitome*** {Mathys (1556) II.526–63}. [532v] Opuscule on measurements. [533r–534r] Merkourios, *On the Pulse*. [534v–535v]. [Ibn Sīnā], *On the Pulse*. [536r–539r] Paul of Aegina, *Epitome*, Book 7.25.

O=Oxoniensis Bodleianus Thomae Roe 15

Oxford, Bodleian Library (autopsy, January 2013).

Coxe (1853: 468–9).

15th c., paper, 284 × 214 mm, ff. viii+404+ii; at least three main unidentified scribes. According to the note in f. 404r the manuscript belonged to the Patriarch Metrophanes III (1565–72, 1579–80) and the monastery of Holy Trinity on the island of Halki in the Sea of Marmara.

Text: [1r–42v] Meletios, *On the Constitution of Man*. [42r–68r] Manuel Moschopoulos, *Sholia on the Works of Hesiod*. [68r–73v] *Letters to Brutus*. [74r–84r] [Ibn Sīnā], *On Urines*. [86r–89v] Excerpt from Theophilos' *On Urines*. [89v–90v] Ps.-Galen, *On Urines*. [90v–97v] Theophilos, *On Urines*. [98r–101r] Theophilos, *On Excrements*. [101r–102v] Anonymous text *On Urine Vials*. [102v–103r] Ps.-Galen, *On Urine Vials*. [103r–104r] Brief astrological text on the connections between plants and stars. [104v] Opuscule on the examination of blood. [105r–181v] ***On Urines***. [184r–210v] ***On Psychic Pneuma***. [215r–217r] Incomplete table of contents of John's ***Medical Epitome***. [218r–251v] **Book 1 *Medical Epitome***, title: *Ἀρχὴ τοῦ πρώτου λόγου τῆς θεραπευτικῆς ὀκταρίου τοῦ Ζαχαρίου, τοῦ ἐν τῇ πασῶν τεχνῶν ἐπιφανεστάτῃ ἰατρικῇ περιβοήτου καὶ θαυμαστοτάτου*. {Ideler (1842) II.353–417}. [251v–274r] **Book 2 *Medical Epitome*** {Ideler (1842) II.418–63}. [274v–295v] **Book 3 *Medical Epitome*** {Mathys (1556) II.153–213}. [295v–325r] **Book 4 *Medical Epitome*** {Mathys (1556) II.213–316}. [325r–354r] **Book 5 *Medical Epitome*** {Mathys (1556) II.317–432}. [354v–389v] **Book 6 *Medical Epitome*** {Mathys (1556) II.433–563}. [389v] Opuscule on measurements. [390r–404r] **Excerpt from Book 6 *Medical Epitome***, title: *Οὗτος ὁ λόγος ἐγράφη δίς, διότι ἔναι οὗτος πλεῖστος· ἔναι γοῦν τοῦ ὀκταρίου*, inc. *Ἡ διὰ δυοῖν ἀριστολοχίαιν*, des. *ἐκπεπονηκότες τὴν βίβλον*. {~Mathys (1556) II.532–63}. [404r] Mark of ownership: *Ἡ βίβλος αὔτη πεφυκε τῆς παντουργου τριἄδος τῆς ἐν τινήσο Χάλκης τε μονης τῆς τοῦ ἐσόπτρου καὶ...τῆς βουληθη ποτὲ ταύτην ἀποστερίσε καὶ χορισμένος ἔσετε τριἄδος τῆς γίας ἐν τῷ αιῶνι τοῦτο γε καὶ τῷ αιλευσομένῳ· οἱ πατέρες μέμνησθε τοῦ Μητροφάνους*.

Pa=Parisinus gr. 2153

Paris, Bibliothèque nationale de France (autopsy, September 2012).

Omont (1888: II.205, III.396).

15th c., paper, 284 × 214 mm, ff. iii+517+iii; several unidentified scribes. The manuscript once came to the possession of Demetrios Angelos.[16]

Text: [1r–12v] Ps.-Galen, *Introduction, or the Physician*. [13r–27v] Galen, *On the Different Kinds of Fever*. [29r–36v] Ps.-Galen, *On Medical Definitions*. [37r–46v] Galen, *Art of Medicine*. [47r–78v] Galen, *On the Different Kinds of the Pulse*. [81v–106r] Galen, *On Diagnosis by the Pulse*. [106r–130r] Galen, *On the Causes of the Pulse*. [130v–169r] Galen, *On Prognosis by the Pulse*. [170r–173v] [Ibn Sīnā], *On Urines*. [173v–174v] Anonymous treatises on urines. [174v–175r] [Hippocrates], *Aphorisms*, brief excerpt. [176r–187r] Galen, *Therapeutics to Glaucon*. [188r–216v] Galen, *On Crises*. [217r–v] Anonymous recipes. [218r–284r] Soranus, *Diseases of Women*. [290r–312v] **Book 1 *Medical Epitome***, title: *Βιβλίον ἰατρικὸν περιέχων πᾶσαν τέχνην ἐν ἐπιτόμῳ*. {Ideler (1842) II.353–417}. [312v–320r] **First part of Book 2 *Medical Epitome*** {Ideler (1842) II.418–440.15}. [320r–330v] **Book 3 *Medical Epitome*** {Mathys (1556) II.153–213}. [331r–338r] **Second part of Book 2 *Medical Epitome*** {Ideler, II (1842) 440.15–463}. [339r–358r] **First part of Book 6 *Medical Epitome*** {Mathys (1556) II.433–526}. [358v–379v] **Book 4 *Medical Epitome*** {Mathys (1556) II.213–316}. [379v–405r] **Book 5 *Medical Epitome*** {Mathys (1556) II.317–432}. [405r–413r] **Second part of Book 6 *Medical Epitome*** {Mathys (1556) II.526–63}. [413v–424v] Anonymous collection of recipes. [424v–425v] Paul of Aegina, *Epitome*, Book 7.25. [426r] Opuscule on purgative drugs. [426r–426v] Opuscule on the nature of the human body. [426v–427v] Anonymus, *On Offspring*. [427v–434r] Anonymous collection of recipes. [435r–457v] ***On Psychic Pneuma***. [458r–517v] ***On Urines***.

Pb=Parisinus gr. 2256

Paris, Bibliothèque nationale de France (autopsy, October 2012).

Omont (1888: II.224–5); Lebègue (1924: 164–76).

15th c., paper, 215 × 139 mm, ff. i(parchment)+i+627+xi+i(parchment); two main scribes: Demetrios Pepagomenos (*RGK* II 133) (ff. 2r–142r, 382v–625v) and unidentified (ff. 144v–382r). The manuscript once belonged to one of the main scribes, the early-fifteenth-century physician Demetrios Pepagomenos (see f. 8v).

Text: [1r] Brief recipe. [2r–5v] Table of contents of the codex, title: *Ἐνταῦθ' ὅρα μοι τῆς παρούσης πυκτίδος, σύνοψιν χειρὸς τῆς ἐμῆς ταχυτάτην ἰητρικῆς τ' ἄριστον ξυλλογὴν ξένε· Δημητρίου θέσει τε Πεπαγωμένου*. [6v–8r] Drawings of the human body. [8v] Acrostic poem (*Α–Ω*): *Ἅπας ὁρῶν μοι τήνδε τὴν βίβλον νόει /...ἤκουσε τὸ πρίν, Δημήτριος τὴν κλῆσιν / θέσει δὲ Πεπαγωμένον τοῦτον νόει /...τοίνυν ὁ τήνδε τὴν βίβλον κεκτημένος /...ὡς ἂν τύχω χάριν τι τῆς δέλτου μνήμης*. [9r–23r] [Hippocrates], *Aphorisms*. [23r–33r] [Hippocrates], *Prognostic*. [34r–142r] Excerpt from Aetios of Amida's *Tetrabiblos*, Books 1–2. [144v–237v] ***On Urines***, (144v, *infra*): *Τοῦ σοφωτάτου καὶ λογιωτάτου βασιλικοῦ ἰατροῦ, κυροῦ Ζαχαρίου, τοῦ ἀκτουαρίου*. [240r–279v] ***On Psychic Pneuma***. [280r–311v] **Book 1 *Medical Epitome***, title: *Τοῦ αὐτοῦ βιβλίον ἰατρικὸν περιέχον πᾶσαν τέχνην ἐν ἐπιτόμῳ*. (280r) title: *Τοῦ αὐτοῦ κυροῦ Ἰωάννου τοῦ ἀκτουαρίου θεραπευτικῆς μεθόδου*. {Ideler (1842) II.353–417}. [311v–336v] **Book 2**

[16] Mondrain (2010: 301–19).

Medical Epitome {Ideler (1842) II.418–63}. [336v–360v] **Book 3** ***Medical Epitome*** {Mathys (1556) II.153–213}. [360v–393v] **First part of Book 6** ***Medical Epitome*** {Mathys (1556) II.433–526}. [394r–433r] **Book 4** ***Medical Epitome*** {Mathys (1556) II.213–316}. [434r–473r] **Book 5** ***Medical Epitome*** {Mathys (1556) II.317–432}. [473r–484v] **Second part of Book 6** ***Medical Epitome*** {Mathys (1556) II.526–63}. [484v] Opuscule on measurements. [488v–505v] Anonymous collection of recipes. [505v–508r] Paul of Aegina, *Epitome*, Book 7.25. [508r] Opuscule on purgative drugs. [508r–509r] Opuscule on the nature of the human body. [509r–510v] Anonymus, *On Offspring*. [510v–520r] Anonymous collection of recipes. [529r–535v] [Ibn Sīnā], *On Urines*. [535v–538v] Ps.-Galen, *On Urines*. [540r–544v] Neophytos Prodromenos, *Glossary of Plant Names*. [546r–562r] Ps.-Galen, *Glossary of Plant Names*. [562r–565r] *Glossary of Plant Names* attributed to Aetios of Amida. [565v–579r] Anonymous treatise on birds. [580r–592v] Hermes Trismegistos, *On Plants*. [593v–594r] Ps.-Pythagoras, *Epistle to Telauges*. [595r–596r] Opuscule on birds. [600r–625v] Michael Attaleiates, *Ponēma Nomikon*. [626v] Anonymous recipes.

Pc=Parisinus gr. 2304

Paris, Bibliothèque nationale de France (autopsy, September 2012).

Omont (1888: II.233); Mondrain (2003: 381–2).

14th c. (ff. 1–190) and 15th c. (ff. 192–361), paper, 217 × 143 mm, ff. ii+x+361; three main scribes: unidentified hand A (ff. 1r–190v); Stephen (*RGK* I 366, II 503, III 584) (ff. 191–352v), who later became Metropolitan of Media, active in the monastery of St John the Baptist at Petra in Constantinople in the early fifteenth century (see also Florentinus Laurentianus gr. plut. 75.11, described above); unidentified hand B (ff. 359v–361v). The manuscript once came into the possession of Demetrios Angelos.[17]

Text: [a*r*–j*v*] Anonymous treatise on urines. [k*r*–*v*] List of contents of John's works. [1r–113v] ***On Urines***, title: *Τοῦ σοφωτάτου καὶ λογιωτάτου πανσεβάστου σεβαστοῦ τοῦ ἀκτουαρίου κυροῦ Ἰωάννου τοῦ Ζαχαρίου*. [114r–155v] **On Psychic Pneuma**. [155v–190v] Galen, *Therapeutics to Glaucon*. [191r–220r] **Book 1** ***Medical Epitome***, title: *Τῷ παρακοιμωμένῳ τῷ Ἀποκαύχῳ τῷ καὶ ὕστερον χρηματίσαντι μεγάλῳ δουκί· τοῦ σοφωτάτου ἀκτουαρίου κυροῦ Ἰωάννου, περὶ διαγνώσεως παθῶν, λόγος α'*. {Ideler (1842) II.353–417}. [220r–241r] **Book 2** ***Medical Epitome*** {Ideler (1842) II.418–63}. [241r–260r] **Book 3** ***Medical Epitome*** {Mathys (1556) II.153–213}. [260r–289r] **First part of Book 6** ***Medical Epitome*** {Mathys (1556) II.433–526}. [289r–320v] **Book 4** ***Medical Epitome*** {Mathys (1556) II.213–316}. [320v–352r] **Book 5** ***Medical Epitome*** {Mathys (1556) II.317–432}. [359v–361v] Anonymous brief medical treatise.

Pd=Parisinus gr. 2306

Paris, Bibliothèque nationale de France (autopsy, October 2012).

Omont (1888: II.233).

15th c., paper, 208 × 134 mm, ff. iii+369+iii; one main scribe (ff. 1r–367r): Athanasios (*RGK* II 11, III 11), active in Constantinople in the fifteenth century. The manuscript once came to the possession of Anthony Eparchos (1491–1571).[18]

Text: [1r–83r] ***On Urines***. [83r–113r] **Book 1** ***Medical Epitome***, title: *Τοῦ σοφωτάτου καὶ λογιωτάτου κυροῦ Ἰωάννου Ζαχαρίου τοῦ ἀκτουαρίου, βιβλίον ἰατρικόν· περιέχον ἐν ἐπιτόμῳ τὴν πᾶσαν τέχνην τῆς ἰατρικῆς, ἐν λόγοις ς'· γραφὲν πρὸς τὸν*

[17] Mondrain (2010: 301, 305, 320).

[18] Mondrain (2000b: 157); and Stefec (2012: 256–7).

Ἀπόκαυκον τὸν τοῦ βασιλικοῦ κοιτῶνος προϊστάμενον, καὶ εἰς πρεσβείαν τηνικαῦτα σταλέντα. {Ideler (1842) II.353–417}. [113r–133v] **Book 2 *Medical Epitome*** {Ideler (1842) II.418–63}. [134r–152r] **Book 3 *Medical Epitome*** {Mathys (1556) II.153–213}. [152r–185r] **Book 4 *Medical Epitome*** {Mathys (1556) II.213–316}. [185v–232r] **Book 5 *Medical Epitome*** {Mathys (1556) II.317–432}. [232r–287v] **Book 6 *Medical Epitome*** {Mathys (1556) II.433–563}. [287v–288v] Selected recipes from **Book 5, *Medical Epitome*.** [289r–325r] ***On Psychic Pneuma*.** [329r–338r] Theophilos, *On Urines*. [338r–343r] Theophilos, *On Excrements*. [345r–359r] Ps.-Galen, *Introduction, or the Physician*. [360r–367r] Galen, *Art of Medicine*. [368–369r] Anonymous recipes in Greek and Latin.

M=Venetus Marcianus gr. 298 (coll. 583)

Venice, Biblioteca nazionale Marciana (autopsy, February 2012).

Mioni (1981: 426–7).

AD 1465, parchment, 320 × 225 mm, ff. 200; one hand (ff. 1r–200v): similar to that of John Plousiadinos (*RGK* I 176, II 234, III 294) according to Ciro Giacomelli;[19] ff. 185–200 in very poor condition. The manuscript was commissioned by the cardinal Bessarion (1403–72).

Text: [1r–33v] ***On Psychic Pneuma*.** [33v–58v] **Book 1 *Medical Epitome*,** title: *Τοῦ αὐτοῦ βιβλίον ἰατρικὸν περιέχον πᾶσαν τέχνην ἐν ἐπιτόμῳ.* (34r) title: *Τοῦ σοφωτάτου ἀκτουαρίου κυροῦ Ἰωάννου, θεραπευτικῆς μεθόδου βιβλίον πρῶτον τῷ παρακοιμωμένῳ τῷ Ἀποκαύκῳ, τῷ καὶ ὕστερον χρηματίσαντι μεγάλῳ δουκί.* {Ideler (1842) II.353–417}. [58v–76v] **Book 2 *Medical Epitome*** {Ideler (1842) II.418–63}. [76v–93r] **Book 3 *Medical Epitome*** {Mathys (1556) II.153–213}. [93r–123v] **Book 4 *Medical Epitome*** {Mathys (1556) II.213–316}. [123v–158r] **Book 5 *Medical Epitome*** {Mathys (1556) II.317–432}. [158r–169v] **Second part of Book 6 *Medical Epitome*** {Mathys (1556) II.526–63}. [170r, *supra*] Scribal note: *Οὔτε εὗρον εἰς τὸ ἀντιβόλαιον κἀγώ. Ὁ παρὼν λόγος τρίτος ἐστίν· ἔλαθε δέ, διὰ τοῦτο ἐγράφη περὶ τὸ τέλος τοῦ βιβλίου.* [170r–198v] **First part of Book 6 *Medical Epitome*** {Mathys (1556) II.433–526}. [199r–200v] Paul of Aegina, *Epitome*, Book 7.25. [200v] Fragmentary mark of onwership:...*γράφη...ων προστάξει, τοῦ κυρίου μου [Βησσαρίωνος] καρδινάλεως [τῆς] ἁγιωτάτης τοῦ Θεοῦ ἐκκλη[σίας]...καὶ [πατριάρχου]...Κωνσταν[τινουπόλεως]...ἰνδικτιῶνος· ιγʹ.*

D=Padovanus C.M. 644

Padua, Biblioteca civica (microfilm access)

Mioni (1965: 237–8); Giacomelli (2018).[20]

Second half of the 15th c., paper, 238 × 170 mm, ff. iii+216+ii; one main unidentified scribe (ff. 1r–216v).

Text: [1r–36v] ***On Psychic Pneuma*.** [37r–67v] **Book 1 *Medical Epitome*,** title: *Τοῦ αὐτοῦ βιβλίον ἰατρικὸν περιέχον πᾶσαν τέχνην ἐν ἐπιτόμῳ.* {Ideler (1842) II.353–417}. [68r–86v] **Book 2 *Medical Epitome*** {Ideler (1842) II.418–63}. [86v–104v] **Book 3 *Medical Epitome*** {Mathys (1556) II.153–213}. [105r–134r] **First part of Book 6 *Medical Epitome*** {Mathys (1556) II.433–526}. [134v–167v] **Book 4 *Medical Epitome*** {Mathys (1556) II.213–316}. [169r–203v] **Book 5 *Medical Epitome*** {Mathys (1556) II.317–432}. [203v–216r] **Second part of Book 6 *Medical Epitome*** {Mathys (1556) II.526–63}.

[19] Giacomelli (2018: 114, n. 75).

[20] This manuscript was first described by Teza (1903).

Q=Mosquensis (ex Dresdensis Da 5)

Moscow, Russian State Archive of Ancient Acts (Российский Государственный Архив Древних Актов, РГАДА). It has not been possible to consult this manuscript and the description is based on the nineteenth-century catalogues.

Schnorr von Carolsfeld (1882: 283–4); von Gebhardt (1898: 537–8).

AD 1519 (scribal notes on ff. 178r, 242r), paper, 350 × 235 mm, ff. 254[?]. According to the existing catalogues, the manuscript was copied by Ambrogio Leone of Nola (scribal notes on ff. 178r, 242r), translator of John's *On Urines* into Latin, which was first published in 1519, thus coinciding with the date of the codex. So perhaps it contains the Greek copy of *On Urines* on which Leo based his Latin translation. Mosquensis is most probably a direct copy of Venetus Marcianus gr. 298.[21] The manuscript once belonged to Christian Frederick Matthaei (1744–1811), who is known for having brought many manuscripts from the Moscow Synodal (Patriarchal) Library which were ultimately purchased by the Dresden Library. However, it cannot be securely confirmed whether this particular manuscript (no. 11 in Matthaei's collection) was originally in Moscow. The manuscript is known to have been brought to the Soviet Union in 1947.[22]

Text: [2r–?] ***On Psychic Pneuma*** and ***Medical Epitome***, title: *Περὶ ἐνεργειῶν τοῦ ψυχικοῦ πνεύματος καὶ τῆς λοιπῆς ἰατρικῆς πραγματείας λόγοι θʹ*. [176v] Opuscule on measurements. [176v–?] Paul of Aegina, *Epitome*, Book 7.25. [182r–?] ***On Urines***. [243r–?] Anonymous treatise on phlebotomy. [247r–?] Anonymous treatise on the pulse. [249r–?] Excerpt on urines attributed to Oribasios.

S=Leidensis Vossianus gr. F. 32

Leiden, Universiteitsbibliotheek (autopsy, October 2012).

De Meyier (1955: 34–7).

*c.*AD 1548, paper, 310 × 215 mm (1–156, 213–262, 311–395), 295 × 200 mm (157–212, 263–310), ff. iii+395+iii; seven main scribes: A (ff. 1r, 46r, 66r–67r, 67v–68r, 123r–124r, 251r–261v), B (ff. 2r–45v, 48r–66v), C (ff. 69r–122r, 157r–212v, 263r–376v), D (ff. 127r–156v, 213r–218v), E (ff. 219r–221v, 223v–225r), F (ff. 222r–223r, 225r–249r), and G (ff. 377r–395v). According to the scribal colophon in f. 156r, scribe D is Franciscus Vagenus. The manuscript once belonged to Jacques Goupyl (f. 2r).

Text: [1r] Incomplete list of contents of ***On Urines***. [2r] Mark of ownership: *Κτῆμα Ἰακώβου τοῦ Γουπύλου*. [2r–66v] ***On Urines***. [66v–68r] Excerpt from Theophilos' *On Urines*. [68r] Opuscule on urines. [68v] Brief text of theological/pharmacological content. [69r–122r, 123r] ***On Psychic Pneuma***. [123v] Brief text on *materia medica* synonyms. [124r] Brief text on the anatomy of brain. [127r–156r] **Book 1 *Medical Epitome***, title: *Παρακοιμωμένῳ τῷ Ἀποκαύχῳ τῷ καὶ ὕστερον χρηματίσαντι μεγάλῳ δουκὶ τοῦ σοφοτάτου ἀκτουαρίου κυροῦ Ἰωάννου περὶ διαγνώσεως παθῶν λόγος πρῶτος*. {Ideler (1842) II.353–417}. [156v] Scribal endnote: *Μετέγραψε ὁ Φραγκίσκος Βαγῆνος νορμανὸς τῇ πατρίδι τοῦτο τὸ σύνταγμα ἐν τῇ Λευκετίᾳ ἔτει χιλιοστῷ ͵φμηʹ*. [157r–185v] **Book 2 *Medical Epitome*** {Ideler (1842) II.418–63}. [186r–212v] **Book 3 *Medical***

[21] On this, see the description of the modern partial copy of Mosquensis, which was produced in 1786/7 (Li=Lipsiensis gr. 60, below).

[22] Schnorr von Carolsfeld (1882: iv). I would like to thank Kerstin Schellbach (Librarian, Sächsische Landesbibliothek—Staats- und Universitätsbibliothek Dresden) for her assistance in tracing the provenance of this codex.

Epitome {Mathys (1556) II.153–213}. [213r–218v] **Excerpt from Book 6** ***Medical Epitome***, inc. *Ἐδόκει μοι διὰ βραχέων*, des. *διαττόμενα λεπτῷ κοσκίνῳ*. {~Mathys (1556) II.433–52}. [219r–247r] **Excerpt from Book 6** ***Medical Epitome***, inc. *Ἐγώ φησιν ὁ Γαληνός, καὶ τὰ τῶν κεράμων ὄστρακα*, des. *μὴ θεραπευόμενοι ὡς προσήκει*. {~Mathys (1556) II.452–98}. [247r–249r] **Excerpt from Book 5** ***Medical Epitome***, inc. *Διὰ τοῦτο καὶ χρονίου ὀφθαλμίας*, des. *ἤδη ἱκανῶς σοι ἐκτεθειμένον*. {~Mathys (1556) II.413–15}. [251r–261v] **Excerpt from Book 6** ***Medical Epitome***, inc. *Διὰ τοῦτο καὶ ξηραντικωτέρων*, des. *ἄρτιος ὁ λόγος τελείῃ*. {~Mathys (1556) II.498–526}. [263r–310v] **Book 4** ***Medical Epitome*** {Mathys (1556) II.213–316}. [311r–360r, 377r–395v] **Book 5** ***Medical Epitome*** {Mathys (1556) II.317–432}. [360r–365v] Excerpt from Aetios of Amida's *Tetrabiblos*, Book 3.175–83. [365v–376v] Anonymous treatise on urines.

N=Monacensis gr. 69

Munich, Bayerische Staatsbibliothek (autopsy, March 2012).

Pradel (2013: 120–2).

AD 1551, paper, 340 × 235 mm, ff. i+300+i; one scribe (ff. IIv, 1r–300v): Kornelios Mourmouris (*RGK* III 354e). This is most probably a direct copy of Venetus Marcianus gr. 298 (see notes on ff. IIv, 255v; and cf. note in Venetus Marcianus gr. 298, f. 170r).

Text: [IIv] Scribal notes: *Σημειῶσαι, ὅτι τὸ τρίτον βιβλίον τῆς παρούσης βίβλου, διὰ λάθος τοῦ πρωτοτύπου ἤ ἀντιβολαίου, μετετέθη ἐν τῷ τέλει τῆς βίβλου· ἡ παροῦσα βίβλος διὰ χειρὸς ἐμοῦ Κουρελλίου Μουρμούρεως υἱοῦ Ἀνδρέου· τοῦ ἐκ τῆς Ναυπλιέων πόλεως, Ἐνετίησι διατρίβοντος μετεγράφη: ἔτους ἀπὸ τῆς τοῦ Σωτῆρος γεννήσεως, ͵αφνα΄ μουνιχιῶνος εἰκάδι*. [1r–46r] ***On Psychic Pneuma***. [46r–84r] **Book 1** ***Medical Epitome***, title: *Τοῦ αὐτοῦ βιβλίον ἰατρικὸν περιέχον~~τος~~ πᾶσαν τέχνην ἐν ἐπιτόμῳ*. (47r) title: *Τοῦ σοφωτάτου ἀκτουαρίου κυροῦ Ἰωάννου, θεραπευτικῆς μεθόδου βιβλίον πρῶτον· τῷ παρακοιμωμένῳ. τῷ Ἀποκαύκῳ, τῷ καὶ ὕστερον χρηματίσαντι μεγάλῳ δουκί.* {Ideler (1842) II.353–417}. [84r–113r] **Book 2** ***Medical Epitome*** {Ideler (1842) II.418–63}. [113r–139r] **Book 3** ***Medical Epitome*** {Mathys (1556) II.153–213}. [139r–188v] **Book 4** ***Medical Epitome*** {Mathys (1556) II.213–316}. [188v–238r] **Book 5** ***Medical Epitome*** {Mathys (1556) II.317–432}. [238r–255r] **Second part of Book 6** ***Medical Epitome*** {Mathys (1556) II.526–63}. [255v–298r] **First part of Book 6** ***Medical Epitome*** {Mathys (1556) II.433–526}. [255v] Scribal note: *Οὕτως εὗρον εἰς τὸ ἀντιβόλαιον κἀγῶ· ὁ παρὼν λόγος τρίτος ἐστίν· ἔλαθε δὲ διατοῦτο ἐγράφη περὶ τὸ τέλος τοῦ βιβλίου*. [298r] Opuscule on measurements. [298r–300v] Paul of Aegina, *Epitome*, Book 7.25. [300v] Scribal colophon: *Τῷ Θεῷ δόξα, τῷ δόντι τέλος*.

X=Bruxellensis 11337–41 (Omont 46)

Brussels, Bibliothèque royale de Belgique (autopsy, October 2012).

Omont (1885: 18); Calcoen (1975: III.54–5).

16th c., parchment (ff. 1–277) and paper (ff. 278–328), 208 × 140 mm, ff. 328.

Note: This MS consists of two distinct parts, described below separately as I. and II.

I.

16th c.; one main unidentified scribe (ff. 2r–277v).

Text: [2r–49r] ***On Psychic Pneuma***. [49v–88r] **Book 1** ***Medical Epitome***, title: *Τοῦ σοφωτάτου ἀκτουαρίου κυροῦ Ἰωάννου· περὶ διαγνώσεως παθῶν, λόγος α΄.* {Ideler (1842) II.353–417}. [88r–115r] **Book 2** ***Medical Epitome*** {Ideler (1842) II.418–63}.

[116r–139v] **Book 3** ***Medical Epitome*** {Mathys (1556) II.153–213}. [140r–179v] **Book 4** ***Medical Epitome*** {Mathys (1556) II.213–316}. [180r–225r]: **Book 5** ***Medical Epitome*** {Mathys (1556) II.317–432}. [225r–240r] **Second part of Book 6** ***Medical Epitome*** {Mathys (1556) II.526–63}. [242r–277v] **First part of Book 6** ***Medical Epitome*** {Mathys (1556) II.433–526}.

II.

16th c.; one main unidentified scribe different from that of part I. (ff. 278r–327v).
Text: [278r–327v] Symeon Seth, *Treatise on the Capacities of Foodstuffs*.

Pe=Parisinus gr. 2307

Paris, Bibliothèque nationale de France (autopsy, October 2012).
Omont (1888: II.233–4).
16th c., paper, 213 × 162 mm, ff. i+622+ii+ii; two main scribes: George Moschos (*RGK* I 67, II 88, III 111) (ff. 1r–565r) and unidentified (ff. 569r–622v).
Text: [1r–122v] ***On Urines***. [122v–168r] **Book 1** ***Medical Epitome***, title: *Τοῦ σοφωτάτου καὶ λογιωτάτου κυροῦ Ἰωάννου Ζαχαρίου τοῦ ἀκτουαρίου βιβλίον ἰατρικόν· περιέχον ἐν ἐπιτόμῳ τὴν πᾶσαν τέχνην τῆς ἰατρικῆς ἐν λόγοις ϛʹ· γραφὲν πρὸς τὸν Ἀπόκαυκον τὸν τοῦ βασιλικοῦ κοιτῶνος προϊστάμενον, καὶ εἰς πρεσβείαν τηνικαῦτα σταλέντα*. {Ideler (1842) II.353–417}. [168r–201r] **Book 2** ***Medical Epitome*** {Ideler (1842) II.418–63}. [201r–230r] **Book 3** ***Medical Epitome*** {Mathys (1556) II.153–213}. [230r–284r] **Book 4** ***Medical Epitome*** {Mathys (1556) II.213–316}. [284r–362v] **Book 5** ***Medical Epitome*** {Mathys (1556) II.317–432}. [362v–451v] **Book 6** ***Medical Epitome*** {Mathys (1556) II.433–563}. [452r–453v] Selected recipes from **Book 5,** ***Medical Epitome***. [453v–508v] ***On Psychic Pneuma***. [508v–523v] Theophilos, *On Urines*. [523v–531r] Theophilos, *On Excrements*. [531v–553v] Ps.-Galen, *Introduction, or the Physician*. [554r–565r] Galen, *Art of Medicine*. [569r–592r] [Ibn Sīnā], *On Urines*, long version. [593r–598v] [Ibn Sīnā], *On Urines*, abridged version. [599r–600r] Merkourios, *On the Pulse*. [600r–601r] [Ibn Sīnā], *On the Pulse*. [601r–622v] Anonymous collection of recipes.

Pf=Parisinus gr. 2233/

Paris, Bibliothèque nationale de France (autopsy, October 2012).
Omont (1888: II.218).
16th c., paper, 340 × 250 mm, ff. iv+182+ii; one main unidentified scribe identical with the one in Phillippicus gr. 1528. The manuscript is fragmentary and its remaining part is Berolinensis Phillippicus gr. 1528, described below.
Text: [1r–33r] **Book 1** ***Medical Epitome***, title: *Περὶ διαγνώσεως παθῶν λόγος πρῶτος*. {Ideler (1842) II.353–417}. [33v–57r] **Book 2** ***Medical Epitome*** {Ideler (1842) II.418–63}. [57v–80r] **Book 3** ***Medical Epitome*** {Mathys (1556) II.153–213}. [80r–121r] **Book 4** ***Medical Epitome*** {Mathys (1556) II.213–316}. [121v–181r] **Book 5** ***Medical Epitome*** {Mathys (1556) II.317–432}. [181v–182v] Table of contents, **Book 6** ***Medical Epitome***.

/Berolinensis Phillippicus gr. 1528

Berlin, Staatsbibliothek (autopsy, June 2012)
Studemund and Cohn (1890: 50–1).

16th c., paper, 340 × 250 mm, ff. ii+76+iii; one main unidentified scribe identical with the one in Parisinus gr 2233. The manuscript is fragmentary and its remaining part is Parisinus gr. 2233, described above.

Text: [1r–74r] **Book 6 *Medical Epitome*** {Mathys (1556) II.433–563}. [74v–76r] Selected recipes from **Book 5, *Medical Epitome.***

Li=Lipsiensis gr. 60

Leipzig, Universitätsbibliothek (autopsy, July 2012).

Gardthausen (1898: 75).[23]

AD 1786/7, paper, unbound, 210 × 175 mm, ff. 210 (paginated 1–420), one scribe: most probably Christian Frederick Matthaei (1744–1811), who was once the possessor of Mosquensis (ex Dresdensis Da 5). This manuscript is a modern copy of one of the medieval manuscripts containing both the *Medical Epitome* and the *On Urines*. The modern transcriber copied two scribal colophons of the original manuscript on pp. 298 and 304 indicating Ambrogio Leone of Nola as the scribe of the original manuscript, while the date of completion is given as 1519. Both the name of this scribe and the same date are likewise copied twice in Mosquensis (ex Dresdensis Da 5, ff. 178r and 242r, see above). Furthermore, both manuscripts have the same sequence of contents. In contrast, however, to Mosquensis (ex Dresdensis Da 5), the modern copy does not include *On Psychic Pneuma* at the beginning. Thus Lipsiensis gr. 60 is a partial apograph of Mosquensis (ex Dresdensis Da 5), which in turn is most probably a direct copy of Venetus Marcianus gr. 298 (see the scribal note on p. 298; and cf. note in Venetus Marcianus gr. 298, f. 170r).

Text: [1] Scribal note in the outer margin: d. 12. Jul. 1786. [1–31] **Book 1 *Medical Epitome***, title: *Τοῦ αὐτοῦ σοφωτάτου ἀκτουαρίου Ἰωάννου ἰατρικῆς μεθόδου περι-εχούσης πᾶσαν τέχνην ἐν ἐπιτόμῳ· βιβλίον πρῶτον περὶ τῶν τῶν καθόλου διαγνώσεων.* {Ideler (1842) II.353–417}. [31–96] **Book 2 *Medical Epitome*** {Ideler (1842) II.418–63}. [97–128] **Book 3 *Medical Epitome*** {Mathys (1556) II.153–213}. [129–80] **Book 4 *Medical Epitome*** {Mathys (1556) II.213–316}. [181–239] **Book 5 *Medical Epitome*** {Mathys (1556) II.317–432}. [239–56] **Second part of Book 6 *Medical Epitome*** {Mathys (1556) II.526–63}. [256–98] **First part of Book 6 *Medical Epitome*** {Mathys (1556) II.433–526}. [298] Scribal endnote (copied from the original): *Τέλος τοῦ ενάτου καὶ ὑστάτου βιβλίου τῆς ὅλης ιατρικῆς πραγματείας κατὰ τὸν σοφώτατον ακτουάριον. Ἰστέον δὲ ὅτι ἐν τῷ ἀντιβολαίῳ εὕρικα οὕτω γραφέν· ὁ παρὼν λόγος τρίτος ἐστίν· ἔλαθε δε, διὰ τοῦτο ἐγράφη περὶ το τέλος τοῦ βιβλίου, ἀλλὰ καγὼ Ἀμβρόσιος Λέων γράφων ταῦτα ἐποίησα τούτον λόγον ἕνατον ἕνεκα δέουσης πραγματείας· ἔγραφον δε Ἐνετίησι θ' ποσειδεῶνος ͵αφιθ'.* [299] Opuscule on measurements. [299–304] Paul of Aegina, *Epitome*, Book 7.25. [304] Scribal endnote (copied from the original): *Τῷ θεῷ δόξα καὶ χάρις τῷ δόντι τέλος· ἔγραψε ὁ Ἀμβρόσιος ὁ Λέων Νωλανεὺς ὁ τοῦ Μαρινοῦ Ἐνετίησι δεκάτῃ ἱσταμένου ποσειδεῶνος ͵αφιθ'*...[305–420] ***On Urines***. [420] Scribal colophon (copied from the original): *Ἔγραφε ὁ Ἀμβρόσιος ὁ Λέων ὁ Νωλανευς Ἐνετίησι ͵αφίθ' Ν' τοῦ φθίνοντος γαμηλιῶνος*...[420] Scribal note: d. Mai 16, 87.

[23] See also the entry by Friederike Berger on *Manuscripta-Mediaevalia*, at http://www.manuscripta-mediaevalia.de/?xdbdtdn!%22obj%2031587764%22&dmode=doc#|4 (accessed 17 August 2018).

2.2 Excerpting and fragmentary manuscripts

Z=Varsoviensis Zamoyscianus 155 Cim.

Warsaw, Biblioteka Narodowa (microfilm access).

Turyn (1928: 508–11); Aland (1956: 22–3); Kaliszuk and Szyller (2012: 61).

14th c., paper, 225 × 145 mm., ff. ix+372(paginated 1–744)+viii; one main unidentified scribe (pp. 1–744).

Text: [1–84] ***On Psychic Pneuma***. [85–168] **Book 1 *Medical Epitome***, title: *Τοῦ αὐτοῦ ἀκτουαρίου, τῷ προκαθημένῳ του βασιλικοῦ κοιτῶνος κυροῦ, περὶ διαγνώσεως καὶ αἰτίας τῶν τε καθ' ὅλον καὶ τῶν κατὰ μέρος τοῦ σώματος παθῶν, καὶ τῆς τούτων θεραπείας· περὶ διαγνώσεως καὶ αἰτίας*. {Ideler (1842) II.353–417}. [168–226] **Book 2 *Medical Epitome*** {Ideler (1842) II.418–63}. [226–280] **Book 3 *Medical Epitome*** {Mathys (1556) II.153–213}. [280–376] **Book 4 *Medical Epitome*** {Mathys (1556) II.213–316}. [376] Scribal note: *Ζήτει καὶ τοὺς ἑξῆς περὶ συνθέσεως φαρμάκων λόγους*. [377–614] ***On Urines***, title: *Τοῦ σοφωτάτου καὶ λογιωτάτου πανσεβάστου σεβαστοῦ τοῦ ἀκτουαρίου κυροῦ Ἰωάννου τοῦ Ζαχαρίου, περὶ οὔρων*. [614–615] Paul of Aegina, *Epitome*, Book 2.12. [615–618] **Excerpt from Book 5 *Medical Epitome***, title: *Ἐκ τῶν τοῦ ἀκτουαρίου· ζουλάπια τοῖς καθαρθησομένοις διδόμενα πρὸ τῶν καθαρσίων φαρμάκων*, inc. *Ξανθῆς χολῆς προκειμένης εἰς κένωσιν*, des. *μετὰ τοῦ μὴ ἀδικεῖν τὸν στόμαχον*. {~Mathys (1556) II.394–409}. [619–706] Galen, *Therapeutics to Glaucon*. [706–714] Galen, *On Mixtures*. [715–731] Paul of Aegina, *Epitome*, Book 2.11. [732–734] Anonymous short text *On the Taste of Foodstuffs*. [734–743] Excerpt from [Hippocrates'] *On Regimen*.

I=Athous Iberiticus 151 (Lambros 4271)

Mount Athos, Library of Iviron Monastery (autopsy, November 2012).

Lambros (1900: II.34–5).

15th c., paper, 220 × 145 mm, ff. i+236+i; several unidentified scribes; the last folia (228r–235v) contain an autograph collection of recipes by the fifteenth-century medical author Andreiomenos.[24] The codex consists of various medical treatises by well-known authors such as Theophanes Chrysobalantes and Galen; there are also numerous collections of anonymous recipes. I give the list of contents related to John's work only. There is a note on f. 18v confirming that the manuscript was once found in the infirmary of the monastery of Iviron.[25]

Text: [176r–182v] **Excerpt from Book 5 *Medical Epitome***, title: *Ἀρχὴ σὺν Θεῷ διαφόρων ζουλαπίων, σύνθεσις Γαληνοῦ*, inc. *Ζουλάπιον εἰς βῆχα*, des. *Τροχίσκος ἕτερος ὁ διὰ σπερμάτων...οσκιάμου οὐγγ. ς'*. {~Mathys (1556) II.329–40}. [184r–198r] **Excerpt from Book 5 *Medical Epitome***, title: *Ἀρχὴν σὺν Θεῷ λόγου πέμπτου περὶ συνθέσεως φαρμάκων ὠκταρίου*, inc. *Ἐπὶ τοῖς προεκτεθεῖσι βιβλίοις ἐπιτίθεμεν λόγον*, des. *Ἀντίδοτος ἡ τοῦ Φίλο*[s.l.-*ω*]*νος...μέλιτος τὸ ἀρκοῦν*. {~Mathys (1556) II.317–29, 342–59}. [200r–202v] **Excerpt from Book 6 *Medical Epitome***, title: *Περὶ συνθέσεως ἐλαίων*, inc. *Τὸν περὶ συνθέσεως τῶν ἐλαίων*, des. *εἰ βουληθεῖς σκεβάσαι ἄν*. {~Mathys

[24] Pietrobelli (2010: 121–6).

[25] Athous Iberiticus 151, f. 18v, ll. 8–9: '*Η παροῦσα βίβλος πέλει μονῆς τῆς τῶν Ἰβίρων· ἤγουν ἰατρονσόφει· ἀφιεροθεν δὲ παρ' ἐμοῦ Σάβα ἱεροδιακόνου εἰς το νοσοκομίον εἰς ἰατρεῖα τῶν ἐκεῖσε νοσούντων·*'. I would like to thank Father Theologos, librarian of the Iviron Monastery, for his hospitality and for allowing access to the codex.

(1556) II.545–53}. [202v–211r] **Excerpt from Book 5 *Medical Epitome***, inc. *Τοῖς ὑποχρονίου ὀφθαλμίας ἐνοχλουμένοις*, des. *ἀποφράττοντα δὲ τοὺς πόρους*. {~Mathys (1556) II.413–16, 392–411, 388–92}. [211r–217r] Various **excerpts from Books 5 & 6 *Medical Epitome***, inc. *Ἡ μαστιχηρὰ πρὸς πλῆξιν*, des. *τὸν φάρυγγα βέλτιον δὴ λειόσαντα ἀναπλάτειν καταπότια σὺν μέλιτι ἐφθῷ*.

Ea=Scorialensis Y.III.14

San Lorenzo de El Escorial, Real Biblioteca del Monasterio (autopsy, September 2018).

De Andrés (1965: 161–4).

AD 1323 (ff. 188–241), 1486 (ff. 22–148, 156–187), 15th c. (ff. 1–21, 149–155), paper, 212 × 149 mm, ff. vii+242; five main scribes, including Nikephoros the Hieromonk (*RGK* II 420) (ff. 22r–148v, 156r–187r) and George the monk and physician (*PLP* 244) (ff. 188r–241v). The codex consists of a collection of excerpts from authors such as Galen, Paul of Aegina, and Theophilos, and Arabic works in Greek translation by, for example, Ibn al-Jazzār. I give the list of contents related to John's work only.

Text: [6v–17v] **Excerpt from Book 1 *Medical Epitome***, title: *Ἐκ τῶν ἀκτουαρίου περὶ σφυγμῶν· καὶ τῆς ἐξ αὐτῶν διαγνώσεως*, inc. *Τῆς θέρμης ἐπιδιδουμένης*...(7r) *καὶ γοῦν μή τινος ἔξωθεν ἢ ἔσωθεν ἐνοχλοῦντος*, des. *ἀλλοκότοις χυμοῖς ἠθροισμένοις περὶ τὸν στόμαχον*. {~Ideler (1842) II.362–388.25}.

Vt=Vaticanus gr. 2182

Vatican City, Biblioteca Apostolica Vaticana (autopsy, February 2012).

Lilla (1985: 75–9).

15th c., paper, 291 × 207 mm, ff. ii+194+ii; three main scribes: unidentified hand A (ff. 1r–47v), Athanasios (*RGK* II 11, III 11) (ff. 48r–80v), unidentified hand B (ff. 81r–192v).

Text: [1r–47v] Excerpts from the *Ephodia tou Apodēmountos*. [48r–57v] Excerpt from Galen's *Therapeutics to Glaucon*. [58r–80v] Dioscorides *De Materia Medica*, Books 2–4. [81r–88v] **Excerpt from Book 5 *On Urines***. [89r–96v] **Excerpt from Book 6 *On Urines***. [97r–126v] **Book 1 *Medical Epitome***, title: *Τοῦ αὐτοῦ περὶ διαγνώσεως παθῶν ἑκάστου τῶν ὀργανικῶν μορίων*. {Ideler (1842) II.353–417}. [126v–139v] **Book 2 *Medical Epitome*** {Ideler (1842) II.418–63}. [139v–159r] **Book 3 *Medical Epitome***, title: *Τοῦ σοφωτάτου ὀκταρίου κυροῦ Ἰωάννου θεραπευτικῆς μεθόδου βιβλίον πρῶτον*. {Mathys (1556) II.153–213}. [159r–192v] **Excerpt from Book 4 *Medical Epitome***, inc. *Ἡ μὲν παροιμία φησὶ χελώνης κρέα*, des. *διάφορα ὑπαγορεύῃ πάθη*. {Mathys (1556) II.213–311}.

L=Londiniensis Arundelianus 537

London, British Library (autopsy, November 2011).

McKendrick (1999: 19).

15th (ff. 24–194) and 16th c. (ff. 1–23, 195–238), paper, 200 × 150 mm, ff. iii+238 +iv; two main unidentified scribes: A (ff. 24r–194v) and B (ff. 1r–23v, 195r–238v).

Text: [1r–114r] ***On Urines***. [114r–156r] Galen, *Therapeutics to Glaucon*. [156r–196v] ***On Psychic Peuma***. [196v–238v] **Excerpt from Book 1 *Medical Epitome***, title: *Τοῦ αὐτοῦ βιβλίον ἰατρικόν, περιέχον πᾶσαν τέχνην ἐν ἐπιτόμῳ*, inc. [*Ἐ*]*πειδή σοι τὴν ὑπὲρ τοῦ γένους ἡμῶν στελλομένῳ πρεσβείαν*, des. *ἐντεῦθεν οὖν ἀποσιτίαι τε καὶ ἄλγη*. {Ideler (1842) II.353–405.28}.

Aa=Mediolanensis Ambrosianus gr. 598 (O123 Sup.)

Milan, Biblioteca Ambrosiana (autopsy, February 2012).

Martini and Bassi (1906: 689–94).

Note: This MS consists of two distinct parts, I and II; I provide a description of part I, which contains John's excerpt.

I. 16th c., paper, 221 × 161 mm, ff. 10, one unidentified scribe (ff. 1r–9r).

Text: [1r–5v] **Excerpt from Book 5 *Medical Epitome*,** title: *Τοῦ σοφωτάτου καὶ λογιωτάτου τοῦ κυροῦ Ἰωάννου ἀκτουαρίου τοῦ Ζαχαρίου, λόγος ε´ τῆς περὶ συνθέσεως φαρμάκων τῶν ἐντὸς τοῦ σώματος*, inc. *Ἤδη σοι καὶ τὸν ἐπὶ τοῖς τέσσαρσι βιβλίοις ἐπιτίθεμεν λόγον*, des. *μήλων καὶ ῥοῶν ζωμός, ἀνὰ οὐγγ. γ´.* {~Mathys (1556) II.317–32}. [5v–9r] Excerpt from Eustathios Makrembolites' *Aenigmata*.

Ab=Mediolanensis Ambrosianus gr. 779 (&147 Sup.)

Milan, Biblioteca Ambrosiana (autopsy, February 2012).

Martini and Bassi (1906: 875).

16th c., paper, 226 × 161 mm, ff. i+7+ii; two unidentified scribes: A (ff. 1r–3v) and B (ff. 5v–7r).

Text: [1r–3v] Michael Psellos, *On the Properties of Stones*. [5r] Excerpt from Theophanes Chrysobalantes' *Synopsis*. [5v–7r] **Excerpt from Book 1 *Medical Epitome*,** title: *Τῷ παρακοιμωμένῳ τῷ καὶ ὕστερον χρηματίσαντι μεγάλῳ δουκί· βιβλίον περιέχον πᾶσαν τέχνην ἰατρικὴν ἐν ἐπιτόμῳ· παρὰ τοῦ σοφωτάτου κυροῦ Ἰωάννου ἀκτουαρίου*, inc. *Ἐπειδή σοι εἰς τὴν ὑπὲρ τοῦ γένους ἡμῶν στελλομένῳ πρεσβείαν*, des. *καὶ τῆς ὑποθέσεως σὺν Θεῷ ἅψασθαι.* {Ideler (1842) II.353–354.33}.

Oa=Oxoniensis Bodleianus Laudianus gr. 62

Oxford, Bodleian Library (autopsy, January 2013).

Coxe (1853: 542).

16th c., paper, 340 × 235 mm, ff. i+110+i; one scribe: John Nathanael (*RGK* I 173, II 231, III 285) (ff. 1r–109v).

Text: [1r–39v] **Book 4 *Medical Epitome*,** title: *Τοῦ σοφωτάτου καὶ λογιωτάτου ὠκταρίου θεραπευτικῆς μεθόδου βιβλίον τέταρτον, τῶν κατὰ μέρος παθῶν.* {Mathys (1556) II.213–316}. [39v–95r] **Book 5 *Medical Epitome*** {Mathys (1556) II.317–432}. [95r–109v] **Second part of Book 6 *Medical Epitome*** {Mathys (1556) II.526–63}.

Pg=Parisinus gr. 2235

Paris, Bibliothèque nationale de France (autopsy, September 2012).

Omont (1888: II.219).

16th c., paper, 240 × 174 mm, ff. iii+205+iv; one main unidentified hand (ff. 2r–205r).

Text: [2r–64r] **Book 5 *Medical Epitome*,** title: *Πίναξ τοῦ ε´ βιβλίου περὶ συνθέσεων φαρμάκων.* (7r) Title: *Λόγος ε´ περὶ συνθέσεως φαρμάκων*, inc. *Ἐπὴ τοῖς ῥηθέσι τέταρσι βιβλίοις*, des. *ἐλέβορος λευκὸς καθαίρει αἷμα καὶ χολήν.* {~Mathys (1556) II.317–429}. [64v–71r] Excerpt from Aetios of Amida's *Tetrabiblos*, Book 3.175–83. [71r–85r] Anonymous text on urines. [88r–94v] Table of contents of **Book 6 *Medical Epitome*.** [96r–135r] **Excerpt from Book 6 *Medical Epitome*,** title: *Θεραπείας διαφόρων νοσημάτων τοῦ δ^ου^ βιβλίου*, inc. *[Ἐ]γὼ φησὶν ὁ Γαληνός· καὶ τὰ τῶν κεράμων ὄστρακα*, des. *διὸ καὶ ταχέως ἑλκοῦνται μὴ θεραπευόμενοι ὡς προσήκει.* {~Mathys (1556) II.452–98}. [135r–157r] **Excerpt from Book 5 *Medical Epitome*,** inc. *Διὰ τοῦτο καὶ χρονίου ὀφθαλμίας ἐνοχλουμένοις*, des. *ἀποφράττον δὲ τοὺς πόρους.* {~Mathys (1556) II.413–16, 392–413, 388–92}. [157r–190v] **Excerpt from Book 6 *Medical Epitome*,** inc.

Ἐπεὶ δύναμίς ἐστιν αὕτη χαμαιπίτυος, des. *ἐκπεπονηκότες τὴν βίβλον ταύτην· τέλος τοῦ δ' βιβλίου*. {~Mathys (1556) II.530–63}. [192r–205r] Excerpt from Symeon Seth's *Treatise on the Capacities of Foodstuffs*.

Vp=Vaticanus Palatinus gr. 370

Vatican City, Biblioteca Apostolica Vaticana (autopsy, February 2012).

Stevenson (1885: 238–9).

16th c., paper, 300 × 210 mm, ff. i+256+i; one main unidentified scribe (ff. 1r–255v).

Text: [1r–59r] Nemesios, *On the Nature of Man*. [59r–71r] Proklos, *Elements of Physics*. [71r–150v] Aristotle, *Physics*. [151r–188v] **Book 4 *Medical Epitome***, title: *Τοῦ σοφωτάτου καὶ λογιωτάτου ὠκταρίου θεραπευτικῆς μεθόδου βιβλίον τέταρτον· τῶν κατὰ μέρος παθῶν*. {Mathys (1556) II.213–316}. [189r–242r] **Book 5 *Medical Epitome*** {Mathys (1556) II.317–432}. [242v–255v] **Second part of Book 6 *Medical Epitome*** {Mathys (1556) II.526–63}.

Vb=Vindobonensis med. gr. 11

Vienna, Österreichische Nationalbibliothek (autopsy, March 2012).

Hunger (1969: II.52–3).

16th c., paper, 307/310 × 205/210 mm, ff. i+61; two unidentified scribes: A (ff. 1r–55v) and B (ff. 56r–60v); according to Hunger, hand B is also found in Vindobonensis phil. gr. 14, 15, and 16. Marginal annotations by Arnout van Eyndhouts (*c.*1510–*c.*1574) (*RGK* I 28, II 39, III 48).[26]

Text: [1r–48v] **Book 4 *Medical Epitome***, title: *Ἰατρικὴ μέθοδος*. {Mathys (1556) II.213–316}. [49r–55v] **Excerpt from Book 5 *Medical Epitome***, inc. [*Ἤ*]*δη σοὶ καὶ τὸν ἐπὶ τοῖς τέταρσιν βιβλίοις ἐπιτίθεμεν λόγον*, des. *μήλων καὶ ῥοῶν ζωμὸς ἀνὰ οὐγγ. γ'· [ἕ]τερον ἐφεκτικόν*. {~Mathys (1556) II.317–32}. [56r–58r] Diocles, *Epistle to King Antigonus*. [58v] Excerpt on the pulse. [59r–60r] Excerpt on lecanomancy.

Wa=Londiniensis Wellcomensis MS.MSL.112

London, Wellcome Library (autopsy, January 2014).

Bouras-Vallianatos (2015*b*: 307–8).

AD 1732–63, paper, 320 × 195 mm, ff. v+217+vii, one unidentified scribe (ff. 1r–217r). This MS was copied directly from Wellcomensis MS.MSL.52 (203r–332v). The manuscript was most probably commissioned by the English physician Anthony Askew.

Text: [1v–32v] **Book 3 *Medical Epitome***, title: *Περὶ θεραπευτικῶν μεθόδων βιβλίον πρῶτον*. {Mathys (1556) II.153–213}. [32v–78v] **First part of Book 6 *Medical Epitome*** {Mathys (1556) II.433–526}. [79v–139v] **Book 4 *Medical Epitome*** {Mathys (1556) II.213–316}. [140v–217v] **Book 5 *Medical Epitome*** {Mathys (1556) II.317–432}.

Cr=Cracoviensis (ex Berolinensis gr. fol. 39)

Krakow, Biblioteka Jagiellońska (microfilm access).

De Boor (1897: 142–4).

19th c., paper, large folder containing forty-two items of working notes, most probably, by Karl Weigel (1769–1845). Items 27 and 29 contain parts of John's *Medical Epitome* copied most probably from Mosquensis (ex Dresdensis Da 5, described above).

[26] Stefec (2014: 177).

Text: [Item 27] **Book 1, Chapter 56, *Medical Epitome***, title: *Περὶ τῶν κατὰ τὴν μήτραν παθῶν*, inc. *Γυναῖκες δὲ πλεονεκτοῦσι τοῖς ἀπὸ τῆς μήτρας πάθεσι*. {~Ideler (1842) II.412.24–16.4}; scribal note: L. II cp. 24 aus dem Codex Dresdensis. [Item 29] **Books 1 and 2 *Medical Epitome***, title: *Παρακοιμωμένῳ τῷ Ἀποκαύχῳ τῷ καὶ ὕστερον χρηματίσαντι μεγάλῳ δουκὶ τοῦ σοφωτάτου ἀκτουαρίου κυροῦ Ἰωάννου περὶ διαγνώσεως παθῶν*. {~Ideler (1842) II.353–463}.

2.3 List of contents of the Latin editions of the Medical Epitome.[27]

Ruelle (1539) ff. 1r–192v	**Mathys** (1556) II, pp. 1–563
	(**Book 1**) p. 1, title: Actuarii Zachariae Medicus, sive Methodi Medendi, Liber primus, inc. Quoniam ad Hyperboreos Scythas.
	(**Book 2**) 90, title: Actuarii Zachariae Methodi Medendi, Liber 2, inc. Quoniam, cum felicibus.
	(**Book 3**) 153, title: Actuarii Zachariae Methodi Medendi, Liber tertius, inc. Cum omnis doctrina.
	(**Book 4**) 213, title: Actuarii Zachariae De affectibus qui singulis partibus incidunt, medendi ratione, Liber quartus, inc. Testudinis caro.
(**Book 5**) f. 1r, title: Actuarii Zachariae De medicamentorum compositione liber, inc. Postquam editis antea quautor voluminibus.	(**Book 5**) 317, title: Actuarii Zachariae Methodi Medendi, Liber quintus. De medicamentorum compositorum formis, inc. Absolutis quatuor libris.
2r, title: Sumendorum medicamentorum formae.	
2v, title: Admovendorum medicaminum formae.	
3r, title: De potionibus febricitantium.	319, title: De potionibus febricitantium.
5r, title: De potionibus medicamentariis.	
7v, title: Obstructionis curatio.	
9r, title: Antidotorum usus et compositio varia.	326, title: De antidotis et iis quae intus assumuntur.
9v, title: Pastillorum compositio et usus.	
10r, title: Catapotiorum componendi ratio.	
10v, title: Pulveres.	
10v, title: Medicamentorum formae, quae quatenus durent.	
12r, title: De zulapiis et serapiis.	329, title: De serapiis et zulapiis.
18v, title: De pastillis.	335, title: De pastillis.

[27] The contents of individual chapters in Ruelle's edition do not always correspond closely with the contents of the same chapter in Mathys. Furthermore, separate recipes from different chapters are sometimes put together in Ruelle's edition.

30r, title: De antidotis.	342, title: De antidotis.
81v, title: De liquoribus medicatis.	376, title: De liquoribus medicatis.
91v, title: De purgantibus medicamentis.	379, title: De purgantibus medicamentis
92v, title: De simplicibus medicamentis purgantibus.	
100r, title: De purgantibus medicamentis compositis.	394, title: De purgantibus medicamentis compositis.
101r, title: De flava bile repurganda.	
101v, title: De pituitae purgatione.	
102v, title: Deiectio atrae bilis.	
103r, title: De coniunctis humoribus purgandis praecepta.	
122v, title: Medicamenta quae vel appositu vel iniectione purgat.	409, title: Medicamenta quae vel apposita, vel iniecta purgant.
124r, title: Unguenti alvum resoluentis compositio.	
126r, title: De balanis seu glandibus et clysteribus.	412, title: De glandibus medicamentis quae naribus induntur.
127v, title: De errhinis et gargarizatu.[28]	
129v, title: Apophlegmatismi.	416, title: De medicamentis exitialibus.
131r, title: De eliciendo vomitu.	
133v, title: De myrobalanorum generibus.	
135v, title: Ratio miscendorum medicamentorum.	
***ΣTα* is missing**	**(Book 6)** 433, title: Actuarii Zachariae Methodi Medendi, Liber sextus, inc. Videor mihi qui omnium.
	435, title: Ad capitis affectus qui oculis deprehenduntur.
	458, title: De capitis internis vitiis.
	464, title: De aurium affectibus et parotidibus.
	474, title: De nasi vitiis.
	479, title: De affectionibus oculorum.
	498, title: De faciei vitiis.
	506, title: De oris affectibus.
	521, title: De ulceribus communibus toti corpori.
Book 6 (***ΣTβ***) 137v, title: De emplastris et linimentis.[29]	526, title: De emplastris malagmatis et linimentis.
166r, title: De pessis.	544, title: De pessis.[30]
174r, title: De compositorum oleorum viribus et ratione.	545, title: De unguentorum et oleorum compositorum viribus ac ratione.
184r, title: De morsibus venenatorum et rabidorum.	553, title: De venenatis.

[28] From this point onwards many recipes are omitted and the order of the remaining recipes is often rearranged.

[29] Several recipes are missing from the beginning of the chapter on plasters.

[30] Some recipes are missing.

APPENDIX 6

Chapter Titles of John's *Medical Epitome*, Books Three and Four, and List of Recipes of Books Five and Six

This appendix gives a list of chapter titles of the unedited books (i.e. three, four, five, and six) of the *Medical Epitome* as they appear in Vindobonensis med. gr. 17. There is a considerable variation in the titles in surviving manuscripts, especially for the recipes in the last two books. Furthermore, sometimes one title covers more than one recipe or a group of them. The chapter titles appear in the form of marginal annotations in Vindobonensis med. gr. 17. There are two hands involved in this process. The first (in red; e.g. f. 88r) is identical with that of the main scribe of the codex, i.e. Simon Makrodoukas (see also Appendix 5, Vindobonensis med. gr. 17), and the second (in brick red; e.g. f. 121v) is an unidentified hand. In the transcription I provide below, I have kept the same spelling and punctuation as in the codex, apart from the fact that I have supplied the iota subscript.[1] Where a spelling is clearly erroneous, I have indicated the correct, or most probably correct, spelling of the term in parenthesis preceded by *sc.* (i.e. scilicet), for example, *ῥυέντα* (*sc. ῥυέντος*). Lastly, one can also find a list of the chapter titles in John's *Medical Epitome* books three to six in Georgios Costomiris' article,[2] in which he transcribed the lists of contents introducing each book (a practice found in some manuscripts) as they appear in Parisinus gr.2307 (see also Appendix 5, Parisinus gr. 2307). In this case, the list, in particular, for books five and six, is sometimes more synoptic.

JZA, *Medical Epitome*, 3, Vindobonensis med. gr. 17, ff. 55r–76r:

(1) *Περὶ φλεβοτομίας*:
(2) *Περὶ τομῆς ἀρτηρίας*:
(3) *Περὶ χρήσεως βδελλῶν*:
(4) *Περὶ σικύας*:
(5) *Περὶ βαλάνων καὶ κλυσμάτων*:
(6) *Περὶ ἐρρίνων*:
(7) *Περὶ χρήσεως καθαρτικῶν φαρμάκων*:
(8) *Περὶ τῶν μετρίως καθαιρόντων φαρμάκων*:
(9) *Περὶ τῶν ὀξέως καθαιρόντων*:
(10) *Περὶ ὑγιεινῆς διαίτης*:
(11) *Περὶ χρήσεως βαλανείων καὶ ὕπνων καὶ γυμνασίων*:
(12) *Περὶ γυμνασίων*:
(13) *Περὶ διαίτης τροφῶν*:

[1] Chapter numbers are not in the manuscript. The numbers in parenthesis preceding each chapter title have been added for convenience in referencing.

[2] Costomiris (1897: 417–22).

(14) *Περὶ διαίτης ἐμέτου ὑπὸ πολυτροφίας:*
(15) *Περὶ διαίτης τῶν βαρυνομένων ἢ δακνομένων τὸν στόμαχον:*
(16) *Περὶ διαίτης τῶν βαρυνομένων τὰ σπλάγχνα ἢ τὴν κεφαλήν ἢ τοὺς πόδας ὑπὸ πληρώσεως:*
(17) *Περὶ διαίτης τῶν κατεσκληκότων ὑπό τε κόπου λύπης τε καὶ φρενίτιδος· κενώσεως τε τυχὸν καὶ ἀγρυπνίας· ἀσιτίας τε καὶ καταχρήσεως γυμνασίων:*
(18) *Περὶ διαίτης πυρετῶν:*
(19) *Περὶ διαίτης συνεχῶν πυρετῶν:*
(20) *Περὶ τῶν διαλειπόντων πυρετῶν· καὶ πρῶτον περὶ τριταίου:*
(21) *Περὶ ἀφημερινοῦ:*

JZA, *Medical Epitome*, 4, Vindobonensis med. gr. 17, *Medical Epitome*, ff. 76r–112v:

(1) *Περὶ θεραπείας ὀδύνης κεφαλῆς:*
(2) *Περὶ φρενίτιδος:*
(3) *Περὶ τῶν τῆς καρδίας παθῶν:*
(4) *Περὶ τῶν παθῶν τοῦ πνεύμονος:*
(5) *Περὶ δυσπνοίας ὑπὸ καταρροῆς ἀπὸ κεφαλῆς:*
(6) *Περὶ πλευρίτιδος:*
(7) *Περὶ θεραπείας πτύσεως αἵματος:*
(8) *Θεραπεία ἐμέτου:*
(9) *Περὶ ἐμουμένου αἵματος:*
(10) *Περὶ ἐπισχέσεως γαστρός:*
(11) *Περὶ ὀδύνης κώλου:*
(12) *Περὶ θεραπείας ἰσχιάδος:*
(13) *Θεραπεία τῶν διὰ γαστρὸς ὑπιόντων:*
(14) *Περὶ θεραπείας εἰς ῥυέντα* (sc. *ῥυέντος*) *χυμοῦ εἰς τὰ ἔντερα:*
(15) *Περὶ τεινεσμοῦ:*
(16) *Περὶ ῥευματισμοῦ κατὰ τῶν αἱμορροΐδων:*
(17) *Θεραπεία σύριγγος ἤτοι διατρήσεως:*
(18) *Περὶ ἡπατικῆς δυσεντερίας:*
(19) *Θεραπεῖαι τῶν τε τοῦ ἥπατος καὶ τοῦ σπληνός καὶ τῶν ἀπὸ τούτων τῷ λοιπῷ σώματι συμβαινόντων παθῶν· καὶ πρῶτον, θεραπεία θέρμης καὶ ψύξεως αὐτῶν:*
(20) *Θεραπεία φλεγμονῆς καὶ καταψύξεως ἥπατος καὶ σπληνός:*
(21) *Θεραπεία σκιρρωθέντος ἥπατος καὶ σπληνός· καὶ τῆς διὰ τοῦτο ὑδερικῆς διαθέσεως:*
(22) *Θεραπεία τῆς τε διὰ ψυχρότητος καὶ πλημμύρης τοιούτων χυμῶν καχεξίας· καὶ τῆς διὰ ταῦτα τε καὶ ἕτερα τινα αἴτια ὑδερικῆς διαθέσεως:*
(23) *Περὶ θεραπείας ἰκτέρου:*
(24) *Περὶ θεραπείας διαβήτου:*
(25) *Περὶ θεραπείας τῶν κατὰ τὰ οὐρητικὰ ἀγγεῖα παθῶν:*
(26) *Περὶ θεραπείας λιθιάσεως:*
(27) *Περὶ θεραπείας πριαπισμοῦ:*
(28) *Περὶ παρέσεως καυλοῦ:*
(29) *Περὶ γονορροίας:*
(30) *Περὶ ὑδροκύλης* (sc. *-ήλης*)*· στεατοκύλης* (sc. *-ήλης*)*· ἐντεροκύλης* (sc. *-ήλης*) *καὶ ἐπιπλοκύλης* (sc. *-ήλης*)*:*
(31) *Περὶ θεραπείας τῶν κατὰ τὴν μήτραν παθῶν:*
(32) *Περὶ ῥεουσῶν τριχῶν:*

(33) *Περὶ θεραπείας τῶν κατὰ τὰ ὦτα παθῶν:*
(34) *Περὶ θεραπείας τῶν κατὰ τοὺς ὀφθαλμοὺς παθῶν:*
(35) *Περὶ τῶν κατὰ τὴν ῥίνα παθῶν:*
(36) *Περὶ τῆς ἀπὸ ῥινὸς αἱμορραγίας:*
(37) *Περὶ τῆς κατὰ τὸ πρόσωπον μελανίας:*
(38) *Περὶ θεραπείας τῶν ἐντὸς τοῦ στόματος παθῶν:*
(39) *Θεραπεία περὶ ὀδύνης ὀδόντων:*
(40) *Θεραπεία περὶ τοῦ κατὰ στόμα γινομένου βατράχου:*
(41) *Θεραπεία πρὸς ἄφθας καὶ ἐξανθήματα:*
(42) *Περὶ κατάρρου:*
(43) *Περὶ κυνάγχης:*
(44) *Περὶ ἐλέφαντος:*
(45) *Θεραπεία λεύκης:*
(46) *Θεραπεία περὶ ἀλφῶν:*
(47) *Περὶ φλεγμονῆς:*
(48) *Περὶ γαγραίνης* (*sc. γαγγραίνης*) *καὶ σφακέλου:*
(49) *Περὶ ἕρπητος:*
(50) *Περὶ καρκίνου:*
(51) *Περὶ σκίρρου:*
(52) *Περὶ στεατωμάτων καὶ μελικηρίδων:*
(53) *Περὶ συκαμίνου:*
(54) *Περὶ δρακοντίων:*
(55) *Περὶ ἕλκους:*

JZA, *Medical Epitome*, 5, Vindobonensis med. gr. 17, *Medical Epitome*, ff. 112v–167r:

(1) *Εἰς πυρεκτικούς:*
(2) *Περὶ ἰοζουλαπίου:*
(3) *Νουφαροζούλαπον:*
(4) *Περὶ ὀξοσαχάριτος:*
(5) *Ὀξοσάχαρ τὸ διὰ τῶν ῥιζῶν:*
(6) *Ἕτερον ὀξοσάχαρ τὸ διὰ τῶν κυδωνίων:*
(7) *Ῥοδοζούλαπον:*
(8) *Σανταλοζούλαπον:*
(9) *Μηλοζούλαπον:*
(10) *Δαμασκηνοζούλαπον:*
(11) *Ζιζιφοζούλαπον:*
(12) *Ἀγουριδοζούλαπον:*
(13) *Σέρεως ἢ κιχωρίου ῥίζαν:*
(14) *Περὶ μετοχετεύσεως ῥευμάτων:*
(15) *Περὶ δυσκρασίας ἥπατος:*
(16) *Περὶ δυσεντερίας:*
(17) *Περὶ ἀναγωγῆς αἵματος:*
(18) *Περὶ ψυχρότητος στομάχου καὶ γαστρός:*
(19) *Περὶ τροχίσκων:*
(20) *Περὶ κοκκίων:*
(21) *Περὶ ὀξοσαχάριτος:*
(22) *Εἰς σπληνικούς· ἡπατικούς· καὶ στομαχικούς:*
(23) *Σεράπιον τὸ δι' ἀψινθίου:*

(24) *Περὶ ζουλαπίων*:
(25) *Βηχικόν*:
(26) *Ἕτερον βηχικόν*:
(27) *Ἕτερον ζουλάπιον εἰς θέρμην τοῦ ἥπατος*:
(28) *Ἕτερον ψυχρότερον τοῦ ῥηθέντος*:
(29) *Ἕτερον καταστέλλον τὰς ἀκρίτους καὶ ἀμέτρους ὁρμὰς τῆς χολῆς*:
(30) *Ἕτερον ἐφεκτικὸν τῶν ἀμέτρων δριμέων ῥευμάτων τῆς γαστρός*:
(31) *Ἕτερον εἰς αἵματα ὑπιόντα*:
(32) *Εἰς ψύγματα* (sc. *ψήγματα*[?]) *τὰ ἐν τοῖς οὔροις φαινόμενα*:
(33) *Εἰς αἷμα καὶ πῦον ἀπό τε τῶν νεφρῶν καὶ τῆς κύστεως φερόμενον*:
(34) *Ἕτερον εἰς βῆχα ἀπὸ λεπτοῦ ῥεύματος· ἀπὸ τῆς κεφαλῆς φερόμενον καὶ εἰς θέρμην τοῦ σώματος*:
(35) *Ἕτερον εἰς παλμοὺς καρδίας· καὶ ἀναισθησίας*:
(36) *Εἰς ἐποχὴν ἐμμήνων*:
(37) *Εἰς ἐμφράξεις τὲ καὶ ὄγκους τῶν σπλάχνων καὶ πλανήτας πυρετούς*:
(38) *Περὶ τροχίσκων*:
(39) *Ὁ διὰ τοῦ σποδίου*:
(40) *Ὁ διὰ ῥόδων*:
(41) *Ὁ διὰ σαντάλων*:
(42) *Ὁ δι᾽ ὀξυακάνθης*:
(43) *Ὁ διὰ τῆς μαστίχης*:
(44) *Εἰς θερμότητα καὶ ξηρότητα τοῦ στήθους*:
(45) *Εἰς κοιλιακὸν τὸν ἀπὸ λειεντερίας*:
(46) *Ἕτερος ἅπαξ ποθεὶς βοηθῶν*:
(47) *Εἰς τὸ καταστεῖλαι αἷμα*:
(48) *Ἕτερος εἰς τὸ πάθος τοῦ εἰλεοῦ*:
(49) *Ἕτερος εἰς ἴκτερον*:
(50) *Ἕτερος εἰς οἰδήματα τοῦ σπληνός*:
(51) *Ὁ διὰ τῆς μήκωνος ὀπός*:
(52) *Ἕτερος εἰς πληγὰς τῶν νεφρῶν καὶ τοῦ ἥπατος*:
(53) *Εἰς τοὺς οὐροῦντας ἢ πτύοντας αἷμα*:
(54) *Σκευασίας τοῦ κυφαίου τροχίσκου*:
(55) *Εἰς διαβήτην*:
(56) *Εἰς στραγγουρίαν*:
(57) *Εἰς πλῆθος οὔρου*:
(58) *Πρὸς χαυνότητα τῆς κύστεως*:
(59) *Εἰς ἠπατικοὺς στομαχικούς*:
(60) *Εἰς τοὺς συνεχῶς καταρροϊζομένους*:
(61) *Ὁ διὰ κοραλλίου*:
(62) *Ἑτέρα σκευασία τοῦ αὐτοῦ*:
(63) *Ὁ διὰ φυσαλίδων*:
(64) *Ὁ τοῦ Ἀμαζόνος* (sc. *τῶν Ἀμαζόνων*):
(65) *Ὁ τοῦ ἀνικήτου*:
(66) *Πρὸς τοὺς ἔχοντας ἕλκη κατὰ κύστιν ἢ νεφρούς*:
(67) *Ὁ τοῦ Νεαπολίτου*:
(68) *Ὁ Φιλίππου*:
(69) *Ἕτερος ἡ σφραγίς*:
(70) *Ἕτερος ὁ ἀστὴρ ἀνώδυνος*:

(71) *Περὶ ἀντιδότων*:
(72) *Σκευασία τοῦ ἡδυχρόου*:
(73) *Σκευασία τῆς θηριακῆς*:
(74) *Σκιλλητικοὶ ἄρτοι*:
(75) *Ἀρτίσκοι θηριακοί*:
(76) *Ἡ ἑκατοντάειδος Γαληνοῦ*:
(77) *Ἀντίδοτος τοῦ Ἔσδρα*:
(78) *Ἡ διὰ παιωνίας*:
(79) *Ἡ τοῦ Φίλωνος*:
(80) *Ἡ διὰ πρασίου*:
(81) *Ἡ δι᾽ ὀρόβου*:
(82) *Ἡ διὰ ἀνακαρδίων*:
(83) *Ἡ διὰ μόσχου*:
(84) *Ἡ διὰ καλαμίνθης*:
(85) *Ἡ Διοσπολίτου*:
(86) *Ἡ δι᾽ ἑρμοδακτύλου*:
(87) *Ἡ Αἰγυπτία*:
(88) *Ἡ Μιθριδάτου*:
(89) *Ἡ διὰ σκίγγου*:
(90) *Τὸ διὰ καρκίνων*:
(91) *Πρὸς παντὸς ἑρπετοῦ πληγήν*:
(92) *Ἐπίθεμα ἐχεόδηκτον*:
(93) *Ἡ ζωπύρειος*:
(94) *Ἡ λυσιπόνιος*:
(95) *Ἡ Ἱπποκράτους*:
(96) *Ἀντίδοτος κωλική*:
(97) *Ἑτέρα κωλική*:
(98) *Ἑτέρα εἰς ψυχρὰν νόσον*:
(99) *Ἀντίδοτος εἰς δυσουρίαν*:
(100) *Τροχίσκος*:
(101) *Πρὸς τοὺς οὐροῦντας αἷμα ἀπὸ κύστεως*:
(102) *Ἕτερος τροχίσκος*:
(103) *Ἀντίδοτος νεφριτικοῖς*:
(104) *Ἀντίδοτος ἰσχιαδικοῖς*:
(105) *Ἀντίδοτος*:
(106) *Ἡ διὰ λιθοσπέρμου*:
(107) *Πόμα ὑδρωπικόν*:
(108) *Ἡ διὰ κοραλλίου*:
(109) *Ἡ Πρόκλου*:
(110) *Ἑτέρα ποδαγρική*:
(111) *Ἀντίδοτος ὑστερική*:
(112) *Ἀντίδοτος εἰς κοιλιακούς*:
(113) *Ἡ διὰ χαμαιμήλου*:
(114) *Ἑτέρα πρὸς ποδαγρικοὺς καὶ ἀρθριτικούς*:
(115) *Ἡ πανάκεια*:
(116) *Ἡ ἀσύγκριτος*:
(117) *Ἡ χρυσῆ*:
(118) *Ἡ διὰ κομεροῦ* (*sc. καμερῶν*[?]):

(119) *Ἡ διὰ κυμίνου:*
(120) *Ἡ διὰ κιτρίου:*
(121) *Ἡ διὰ λαχᾶ* (*sc. λαχᾶν*):
(122) *Ἡ διὰ μήλων:*
(123) *Ἡ διάροδος:*
(124) *Ἡ δι' ἀνθῶν:*
(125) *Ἡ διὰ σατυρίου:*
(126) *Ἡ διὰ πενιδίων:*
(127) *Ἡ διὰ λιβάνου:*
(128) *Ἡ διὰ τραγακάνθης:*
(129) *Ἡ διὰ κόστου:*
(130) *Ἡ διὰ ἴρεως:*
(131) *Ἡ διὰ κωδιῶν:*
(132) *Ἡ διὰ μαργάρων:*
(133) *Ἡ διὰ ἄμπαρος:*
(134) *Ἡ διὰ μόσχου:*
(135) *Ἡ διάροδος ἢ διὰ τῶν λαχῶν:*
(136) *Ἡ δι' ἀρωμάτων βασιλική:*
(137) *Εἴλιγμα πρὸς ἐπάνοδον ὑγρότητος:*
(138) *Ἕτερον πρὸς θλιβομένους:*
(139) *Ἕτερον διὰ μαργαριτῶν:*
(140) *Εἰς ἐπιληπτικούς:*
(141) *Εἰς ἐμπυϊκοὺς καὶ φθισικούς:*
(142) *Ἀντίδοτος εἰς ῥευματισμὸν στομάχου:*
(143) *Εἰς ἀφημερινούς:*
(144) *Ἕτερον:*
(145) *Πρὸς τεταρταίους καὶ ἀρθριτικούς:*
(146) *Ἕτερον πρὸς πᾶσαν περίοδον:*
(147) *Ἕτερον ἄγον ἱδρῶτα:*
(148) *Πρὸς ἡλκωμένην ἀρτηρίαν:*
(149) *Ἡ διὰ τῆς πτέρεως Ἀνδρομάχου:*
(150) *Καταπότιον:*
(151) *Ἐκλεικτὸν δυσπνοϊκοῖς:*
(152) *Ἄλλο:*
(153) *Ἄλλο:*
(154) *Ἕτερον:*
(155) *Ἕτερον:*
(156) *Ἡ διὰ τῶν ὀπωρῶν:*
(157) *Πρὸς ἀνατροπὰς στομάχου:*
(158) *Ἄλλο:*
(159) *Ὠριγενίας πρὸς στομάχου ἀνατροπάς:*
(160) *Ἄδιψον καταπότιον:*
(161) *Ἡπατικὴ Ἀνδρομάχου:*
(162) *Πότιμα πρὸς ἡπατικούς:*
(163) *Ἡ διὰ κωδίας:*
(164) *Ὀξόμελι:*
(165) *Ἄλλως:*
(166) *Ἡ διὰ μελικράτου:*

(167) *Ἡ διὰ μώρων* (sc. *μόρων*) *ἢ βαττίνων* (sc. *βατίνων*):
(168) *Κονδύτης*:
(169) *Οἶνος σκιλλιτικός* (sc. *σκιλλητικός*):
(170) *Τὸ διὰ τοῦ χυλοῦ τοῦ κυδωνίου*:
(171) *Κυδωνοζούλαπον*:
(172) *Ῥοδίτης οἶνος*:
(173) *Ὁ μυρτίτης*:
(174) *Μυρσινίτης*:
(175) *Κεδρίτης*:
(176) *Πισσίτης*:
(177) *Ἀψινθίτης*:
(178) *Στιχαδίτης* (sc. *Στοιχαδίτης*):
(179) *Θυμίτης*:
(180) *Ἀρωματίτης*:
(181) *Οἶνος πρὸς κατάρρους ὠμότητας*:
(182) *Ἐλελυσφακίτης* (sc. *Ἐλελισφακίτης*):
(183) *Μανδραγορίτης*:
(184) *Ὀξόμελι*:
(185) *Ὀξάλμη*:
(186) *Θυμοξάλμη*:
(187) *Ὄξος σκιλιτικόν* (sc. *σκιλλητικόν*):
(188) *Οἶνος μελιτίτης*:
(189) *Θαλασσόμελι*:
(190) *Περὶ καθαιρόντων φαρμάκων*:
(191) *Ἀλόη*:
(192) *Σκαμωνία* (sc. *Σκαμμωνία*):
(193) *Πέπλιον*:
(194) *Ἐλέβορος*:
(195) *Ἐπίθυμον*:
(196) *Πολυπόδιον*:
(197) *Γλήχων*:
(198) *Ἀρμένειον* (sc. *Ἀρμένιον*) *ὃ* (sc. *ᾧ*) *οἱ ζωγράφοι χρῶνται*:
(199) *Κενταύριον*:
(200) *Κολοκυνθίς*:
(201) *Τιθύμαλος* (sc. *Τιθύμαλλος*):
(202) *Ἐλατήριον*:
(203) *Κνίδειος κόκκος*:
(204) *Ἀγαρικόν*:
(205) *Κνίκου σπέρμα*:
(206) *Λαθυρίς*:
(207) *Ἀριστολοχίας τῆς κληματίδος ὁ καρπός*:
(208) *Λινόζωστης* (sc. *Λινόζωστις*):
(209) *Σικύου τοῦ ἀγρίου τῆς ῥίζης ὁ φλοιός*:
(210) *Στύραξ*:
(211) *Θῦμος*:
(212) *Κυκλάμινος*:
(213) *Σκόροδον*:
(214) *Λεπὶς χαλκοῦ*:

(215) *Εὐφόρβιον*:
(216) *Χαμαιλέα* (sc. *Χαμελαία*):
(217) *Ἐλέβορος λευκός*:
(218) *Σησαμοειδές*:
(219) *Τοῦ ἡμέρου σικίου* (sc. *σικύου*) *ἡ ῥίζα*:
(220) *Σταφὶς ἀγρία*:
(221) *Θαψία*:
(222) *Σπάρτος*:
(223) *Βολβός*:
(224) *Ἱππόφαιστον*:
(225) *Ἀκτὴ καὶ χαμαιακτή*:
(226) *Ἄλυπον*:
(227) *Κληματίς*:
(228) *Σένε*:
(229) *Περὶ μάννα καὶ κασίας*:
(230) *Ζουλάπιον εἰς κένωσιν χολῆς ξανθῆς ζεούσης τε καὶ ἐκκαιούσης τὸν ἄνθρωπον*:
(231) *Εἰς ἧττον ζεούσης τε καὶ καιούσης*:
(232) *Εἰς φλέγματος*:
(233) *Εἰς μελαγχολικοῦ χυμοῦ*:
(234) *Κατασκευὴ κοκκίων· τῶν δι᾽ εὐφορβίου· εἰς ὑδρωπικούς*:
(235) *Ἕτερον κενοῦν κίτρινον ὕδωρ*:
(236) *Ἕτερον καθαρτικὸν ξανθῆς χολῆς καὶ μελαίνης*:
(237) *Ὀξοσάχαρ· εἰς ὀξεῖς πυρετούς*:
(238) *Τὸ διὰ καπνίου εἰς ἔμφραξιν τοῦ ἥπατος*:
(239) *Ἕτερον εἰς ἔμφραξιν τοῦ ἥπατος*:
(240) *Ἕτερον ἀφέψημα λύον τὴν γαστέρα· καθαρτικὸν χυμῶν παντοίων*:
(241) *Σύνθεσις διδομένη ἐν ἔαρι καὶ μετοπώρῳ εἰς τοὺς ὀξεῖς πυρετούς*:
(242) *Κοκκία τὰ διὰ τοῦ σαγαπηνοῦ· εἰς ἀρθριτικούς*:
(243) *Κοκκία ὠφέλημα* (sc. *ὠφέλιμα*) *εἰς ποδαλγίαν*:
(244) *Ἕτερον εἰς ποδαλγίαν τὸ βασιλικόν*:
(245) *Ζουλάπιον καθαῖρον χολὴν ξανθὴν καὶ μέλαιναν*:
(246) *Ἕτερον καθαῖρον τὸν στόμαχον ἀπὸ χολῆς ξανθῆς*:
(247) *Ἡ μικρὰ τρύφυλλος* (sc. *τρίφυλλος*):
(248) *Ἡ ἱερὰ πικρὰ τοῦ Γαληνοῦ*:
(249) *Τὰ διὰ τῆς κολοκυνθίδος καταπότια*:
(250) *Ῥοδόμελι καθαρτικόν*:
(251) *Ἀντίδοτος ἡ τοῦ Συγγέλου*:
(252) *Ἡ τῶν πενταειδῶν κοκκίων σκευασία*:
(253) *Ὀξομέλιτος καθαρτικοῦ σκευασίας*:
(254) *Ἡ ἱερὰ τοῦ Γαληνοῦ πρὸς τὰ μέγιστα καὶ χείριστα τῶν παθῶν*:
(255) *Ἱερὰ Ῥούφου*:
(256) *Ἱερὰ Λογαδίου*:
(257) *Ἱερὰ τοῦ Μεμφίτου*:
(258) *Ἡ διὰ δαμασκήνων*:
(259) *Κόκκοι στομαχικοί*:
(260) *Καταπότια τὰ διὰ τοῦ ἀρμενικοῦ λίθου*:
(261) *Οἶνος καθαρτικός*:
(262) *Οἰνόμελι ἐκκοπροτικόν* (sc. *ἐκκοπρωτικόν*):

(263) *Ἀψινθάτου σκευασία:*
(264) *Δροσάτον χολῆς ξανθῆς ἀγωγόν:*
(265) *Φοῦσκα μαλακτικὴ κοιλίας:*
(266) *Ζωμὸς μαλακτικός:*
(267) *Ἐλαῖαι καθαρτικαί:*
(268) *Τὸ διὰ τῶν κυδωνίων μήλων:*
(269) *Καθαρτικὸν διὰ κυδωνίων μήλων:*
(270) *Καθαρτικὸν τὸ διὰ κίτρου:*
(271) *Καθαρτικὸν διὰ μαλάθρου:*
(272) *Πάστιλλος καθαρτικὸς χολῆς:*
(273) *Ἁλάτιον ὑπακτικόν:*
(274) *Ἕτερον καθαῖρον ἀκινδύνως:*
(275) *Ὑδραγωγὸν καθαρτικόν:*
(276) *Ἕτερον καθαρτικὸν ἄλυπον:*
(277) *Ἐπομφάλιον καθαρτικόν:*
(278) *Ἔμπλαστρος καθαρτικὴ ἡ καλουμένη χεζανάγκη:*
(279) *Ἕτερον ἐπαγγελόμενον διὰ ῥινὸς αἷμα:*
(280) *Σύνθεσις ἀλείματος* (*sc. ἀλείμματος*) *καθαρτικοῦ:*
(281) *Ἐπίθεμα κατὰ τοῦ ὀμφαλοῦ τιθέμενον καὶ καθαῖρον τὸν σπλῆνα:*
(282) *Ἐπίθεμα αἱμαγωγὸν ὥς τε ὑπομνῆσαι αἱμορροΐδας:*
(283) *Ἑτέρα ἀλοιφὴ ἀλειφομένη ὑπὸ τῶν πελμάτων τῶν ποδῶν· καὶ ἐκβάλλει τὸ ὠμὸν φλέγμα:*
(284) *Περὶ κλυσμάτων καὶ βαλάνων:*
(285) *Σύνθεσις βαλάνου:*
(286) *Ὀξόμελι κωλικοῖς ἐνιέμενον:*
(287) *Καθαρτικὸν ἔρρινον Ἀσκληπιάδου:*
(288) *Ἕτερον ἄπονον ἀλύπως καθαῖρον:*
(289) *Ἕτερον πταρμικὸν καθαῖρον τὴν κεφαλήν:*
(290) *Ἕτερον:*
(291) *Ἕτερον χρονίως κεφαλαλγοῦσι:*
(292) *Ἕτερον:*
(293) *Ἕτερον:*
(294) *Ἄλλο:*
(295) *Ἕτερον:*
(296) *Ἕτερον ἔρρινον ἀποφλεγματίζων* (*sc. -ον*):
(297) *Ἀποφλεγματισμοί:*
(298) *Ἀποφλεγματισμὸς διὰ μασήματος:*
(299) *Ἕτερον:*
(300) *Ἄλλο:*
(301) *Ἕτερον:*
(302) *Ἕτερος:*
(303) *Ἕτερος:*
(304) *Περὶ ζῴων φθαρτικῶν:*
(305) *Περὶ κανθαρίδων:*
(306) *Περὶ πιτυοκάμπης:*
(307) *Περὶ βουπρήστεως:*
(308) *Περὶ σαλαμάνδρας:*
(309) *Περὶ λαγωοῦ θαλασσίου:*

(310) *Περὶ φρύνου:*
(311) *Περὶ βδελλῶν:*
(312) *Περὶ ὑοσκύαμου:*[3]

JZA, *Medical Epitome*, 6, Vindobonensis med. gr. 17, *Medical Epitome*, ff. 167r–242v:

(1) *Πρὸς τοὺς παρ' ἡλικίας φαλακρωμένους:*
(2) *Ἕτερον:*
(3) *Πρὸς τὸ μὴ ἀπορρεῖν τὰς ἐν τῇ κεφαλῇ τρίχας:*
(4) *Εἰς τὸ γεννῆσαι τρίχας:*
(5) *Πρὸς ῥῦσιν τριχῶν:*
(6) *Ἕτερον:*
(7) *Ἕτερον:*
(8) *Μελαῖνον πώγονα* (*sc. πώγωνα*):
(9) *Πυρὰς* (*sc. Πυρρὰς*) *ποιῆσαι τρίχας:*
(10) *Ψίλωθρον τριχῶν:*
(11) *Ἄλλο:*
(12) *Ἕτερον:*
(13) *Ἕτερον:*
(14) *Περὶ ἀχώρων τῶν ἐν τῇ κεφαλῇ:*
(15) *Ἕτερον:*
(16) *Ἕτερον:*
(17) *Ἕτερον:*
(18) *Πρὸς τοὺς προσφάτους ἀχῶρας:*
(19) *Μηλίνη Λευκίου ἀναξηραντική:*
(20) *Σμῆγμα πρὸς ἀχῶρας:*
(21) *Ἕτερον:*
(22) *Πρὸς ψυδράκια:*
(23) *Ἕτερον:*
(24) *Ἕτερον:*
(25) *Πρὸς πυορροοῦντα καὶ χρονίας διαθέσεως:*
(26) *Πρὸς ἤχους ὤτων:*
(27) *Εἰς παρωτίδας:*
(28) *Περὶ πολυπόδων:*
(29) *Εἰς ὀζένας* (*sc. ὀζαίνας*) *καὶ πολύποδας:*
(30) *Χειρουργία πρὸς πολύποδας:*
(31) *Πρὸς τὰ ἐν μυκτῆρσιν ἕλκη:*
(32) *Εἰς αἱμορραγίαν ῥινός:*
(33) *Περὶ τῶν ἐν ὀφθαλμοῖς παθῶν:*
(34) *Προφυλακτικὸν ὑγιαίνουσιν ὀφθαλμοῖς:*
(35) *Εἰς βεβρωμένους κανθούς:*

[3] The codex also includes the chapters on the remaining vegetal and mineral poisons, although it lacks chapter titles. For example, the relevant list in Parisinus gr. 2306 (**Pd**), f. 186v, ll. 11–15, reads as follows: '*περὶ κορίου· περὶ ψιλλίου· περὶ ὀποῦ μήκωνος· περὶ ἀγρίου βολβοῦ· περὶ σμίλακος ἤγουν τάξου· περὶ τοξικοῦ· περὶ ἰξίου· περὶ μυκήτων· περὶ ταυρείου αἵματος· περὶ ψυχροῦ ὕδατος· περὶ ψιμμιθίου· περὶ γύψου· περὶ λιθαργύρου· περὶ ὑδραργύρου· περὶ τιτάνου καὶ ἀρσενικοῦ·*'.

(36) *Εἰς ξηροφθαλμίαν*:
(37) *Ἄλλο*:
(38) *Εἰς ψωριῶντα βλέφαρα*:
(39) *Πρὸς μιλφώσεις*:
(40) *Καλλιβλέφαρον*:
(41) *Εἰς κνησμώδεις κανθούς*:
(42) *Πρὸς τραχώματα*:
(43) *Ὀξυδερκική*:
(44) *Φαίδρου τὸ ῥινίον*:
(45) *Ὀξυδερκές*:
(46) *Ὀξυδερκική*:
(47) *Εἰς ὑποχύσεις*:
(48) *Ὑγρὰ ἡ βασιλίς*:
(49) *Εἰς γλαυκοφθάλμους*:
(50) *Ἀνακόλλημα τριχῶν*:
(51) *Εἰς κριθάς*:
(52) *Ἄλλο*:
(53) *Εἰς αἰγύλωπας* (sc. *αἰγίλωπας*):
(54) *Ἄλλο*:
(55) *Καταπλάσματα ὀφθαλμιώντων*:
(56) *Εἰς περιωδυνίας*:
(57) *Ἐπίχριστον παραχρῆμα ἐπέχει τὸ ῥεῦμα*:
(58) *Ῥευμάτων ἐφεκτικόν*:
(59) *Ἄλλο*:
(60) *Ἥρωνος*:
(61) *Διάσμυρνον*:
(62) *Πρὸς πᾶσαν φλεγμονήν*:
(63) *Τὸ φαιόν*:
(64) *Τὸ νεκτάριον*:
(65) *Μονοήμερον*:
(66) *Τὸ τοῦ Νεαπολίτου*:
(67) *Φαιὸν τὸ ὀλυμπιακόν*:
(68) *Τὸ σκυλάκιον*:
(69) *Μαλάθρινον* (sc. *Μαλαβάθρινον*) *Γαληνοῦ*:
(70) *Φιλαδέλφιον*:
(71) *Λευκὸν τὸ τρυφερόν*:
(72) *Τὸ διὰ λιβάνου*:
(73) *Ἀνώδυνον*:
(74) *Πρὸς μεγίστας περιωδυνίας*:
(75) *Ἔρινον* (sc. *Ἔρρινον*) *Γαληνοῦ*:
(76) *Ὑγείδιον*:
(77) *Ἀνίκητος ἀστήρ*:
(78) *Λιβιανὸν ἐπιγραφόμενον*:
(79) *Τὸ διὰ τοῦ ἐλαφίου* (sc. *ἐλαφείου*) *κέρατος*:
(80) *Χλωρὸν Ζωΐλου ὀφθαλμικόν*:
(81) *Τὸ ψιττάκιον*:
(82) *Τὸ διὰ χαλβάνης*:
(83) *Διάροδον Νείλου*:

(84) *Ἕτερον*:
(85) *Ἕτερον*:
(86) *Τὸ διὰ τῶν λευκοΐων*:
(87) *Δήλινον* (*sc. Μήλινον*) *τρυφερόν*:
(88) *Τὸ Ζωΐλου, πρὸς παλαιὰς ὀφθαλμίας*:
(89) *Ἀσκληπιάδου*:
(90) *Ἀντιγόνου*:
(91) *Διάσμυρνον*:
(92) *Ὁ Λυγγεύς*:
(93) *Εἰς τετυλωμένας διαθέσεις*:
(94) *Ἁρμάτια ἐπιγραφόμενον σμηκτικόν*:
(95) *Ἰνδικὸν βασιλικόν*:
(96) *Ψωρικόν*:
(97) *Κολλύριον μέλαν ὀξυδερκικόν*:
(98) *Πρὸς πολὺ καὶ παλαιὸν καὶ λεπτὸν ἄκρως ποιεῖ*:
(99) *Παρακόλλημα πρὸς ῥεῦμα*:
(100) *Πρὸς δὲ τὰς ἀπὸ πληγῆς αἱματώδεις ὑποχύσεις*:
(101) *Εἰς ψωροφθαλμίαν καὶ ξηροφθαλμίας* (*sc. ξηροφθαλμίαν*):
(102) *Πρὸς φυομένας τρίχας ἐπὶ τῶν βλεφάρων*:
(103) *Πρὸς σταφυλώματα*:
(104) *Εἰς ἀμαύρωσιν δὲ πᾶσαν ἢ ἀρχομένην ὑπόχυσιν*:
(105) *Ἐπὶ νυκταλωπιώντων*:
(106) *Περὶ αἰγίλωπος*:
(107) *Εἰς τοὺς ἐπὶ τῶν γενείων προσφάτους λειχῆνας*:
(108) *Τροχίσκος λειχηνικός*:
(109) *Ἄλλο*:
(110) *Ὑγρὰ πρὸς λειχήνων* (*sc. λειχῆνας*) *διαθέσεις*:
(111) *Περίχριστος ἑφθὴ πρὸς λειχῆνας*:
(112) *Ἔμπλαστρος λειχινική* (*sc. λειχηνική*):
(113) *Ἕτερον*:
(114) *Ἐκδορίου λειχήνων*:
(115) *Ἑτέρα ποιοῦσα καὶ πρὸς ἀλωπεκίαν*:
(116) *Πρὸς πυρίκαυτα*:
(117) *Πρὸς τὰ ἐπὶ τοῦ γενείου ἐξανθήματα*:
(118) *Περὶ ὀδόντων*:
(119) *Πρὸς σειομένους ὀδόντας*:
(120) *Εἰς βεβρωμένους ὀδόντας*:
(121) *Ἕτερον ἀνώδυνον*:
(122) *Προφυλακτικὰ ὀδόντων*:
(123) *Πρὸς σειομένους ὀδόντας*:
(124) *Πρὸς ἡλκωμένα οὖλα*:
(125) *Μύλην ἀπόνως ἆραι*:
(126) *Πρὸς βεβρωμένους*:
(127) *Ἕτερον*:
(128) *Ἦρα* (*sc. Ἥρα*) *στοματική*:
(129) *Ἕτερον*:
(130) *Πρὸς ἐσχάρας καὶ οὖλα δυσώδη*:
(131) *Πρὸς ἄνθας* (*sc. ἄφθας*):

(132) *Περὶ ἐπινυκτίδων*:
(133) *Περὶ κατακαυμάτων ἀφ' ὕδατος θερμοῦ*:
(134) *Περὶ ἀνθράκων*:
(135) *Περὶ καρκίνων*:
(136) *Ἀρχιγένους*:
(137) *Ἡ διὰ χαλκίτεως ἔμπλαστρος τοῦ Γαληνοῦ*:
(138) *Τὸ δι' ὑδρελαίου*:
(139) *Τὸ δι' ὀξελαίου*:
(140) *Ἦρα* (sc. *Ἥρα*) *λευκή*:
(141) *Χρυσίζουσα*:
(142) *Μήλινον*:
(143) *Ἄλλη*:
(144) *Ἡ κιρρὰ τοῦ Ἁλιέως*:
(145) *Ἡ Μοσχίονος* (sc. *Μοσχίωνος*):
(146) *Ἡ διὰ καδμίας* (sc. *καδμείας*) *ἀπουλωτική* (sc. *ἐπουλωτική*):
(147) *Ἡ Παμφύλειος* (sc. *Παμφίλειος*):
(148) *Ἡ μέλαινα*:
(149) *Ἡ Πυθίωνος*:
(150) *Ἡ κεφαλικὴ Ἥρα*:
(151) *Τροχίσκος τριμίγματος*:
(152) *Μέλαινα ἔμπλαστρος*:
(153) *Πρὸς τὰ Χειρώνεια*:
(154) *Ἡ διὰ λαδάνου*:
(155) *Ἀνδρομάχου*:
(156) *Ἀνδρέου*:
(157) *Ἡ διὰ καλάμων*:
(158) *Μελάχλωρος κεφαλή* (sc. *κεφαλική*):
(159) *Ἄμοιρος* (sc. *Ἄκηρος*) *Γαληνοῦ*:
(160) *Ἄλλη τοῦ αὐτοῦ*:
(161) *Ἡ διὰ δυοῖν ἀριστολοχίαιν*:
(162) *Ἡ δυσραχίτης* (sc. *δυσραχῖτις*):
(163) *Ἡ τοῦ χαλκίτεως*:
(164) *Χλωρὰ ἡ Ἀλκιμίωνος ἢ Νικομάχου*:
(165) *Ἡ διὰ βοτανῶν*:
(166) *Χλωρὰ ἡ διὰ σκίλλης*:
(167) *Διαπνευστική*:
(168) *Διαφορητική*:
(169) *Ἡ Κιφισιφῶντος* (sc. *Κτησιφῶντος*):
(170) *Ἄλλη ἐπισπαστική*:
(171) *Ἄλλη πῦον διαφοροῦσα*:
(172) *Ἑτέρα ἐπισπαστική*:
(173) *Ἡ διὰ ἰξοῦ*:
(174) *Κενωτικὴ πύων*:
(175) *Ἑτέρα*:
(176) *Ἡ δι' ἀσβέστου*:
(177) *Ἡ διάσμυρνος*:
(178) *Τὸ διὰ σπερμάτων*:
(179) *Τὸ διὰ πηγάνου*:

(180) *Τὸ διὰ καππάρεως*:
(181) *Πρὸς ῥευματισμὸν στομάχου καὶ ἐντέρων*:
(182) *Πρὸς ὑδρωπικούς*:
(183) *Τὸ διὰ μέλιτος*:
(184) *Φάρμακον ἐπιτετευγμένον*:
(185) *Εἰς κοπώδεις διαθέσεις*:
(186) *Εἰς ὀπισθοτονικούς*:
(187) *Τὸ Βάσσου*:
(188) *Διὰ καστορίου*:
(189) *Τὸ διὰ τῶν ἁλῶν*:
(190) *Τὸ διὰ φρύνων*:
(191) *Τὸ Νεαπολίτου*:
(192) *Τὸ τοῦ Ἁλιέως*:
(193) *Φαυλίνου* (sc. *Φλαβίου*) *Κλήμεντος*:
(194) *Ἄκοπον*:
(195) *Προς ἰσχιάδα χρονίαν*:
(196) *Χλωράκοπον*:
(197) *Ἡ χρυσῆ καὶ τὸ πολυάρχιον*:
(198) *Ἡ χρυσῆ*:
(199) *Τὸ εὐῶδες*:
(200) *Τὸ κοπτόν*:
(201) *Τὸ μάλαγμα*:
(202) *Τὸ μέγα*:
(203) *Τὸ μικρόν*:
(204) *Τὸ διὰ σπερμάτων*:
(205) *Τὸ δι᾽ οἰνάνθης*:
(206) *Τὸ τοῦ Ἀμιθάωνος* (sc. *Ἀμυθάωνος*):
(207) *Ἡ παναληθής*:
(208) *Ἡ τῆς ἁπλουστέρου* (sc. *ἁπλουστέρας*) *βαρβάρου σύμμιξις*:
(209) *Ἡ πηγανερά*:
(210) *Τὸ διὰ βουτύρου*:
(211) *Ἡ δι᾽ ἰτεῶν*:
(212) *Ἡ διὰ χυλοῦ*:
(213) *Ἡ τοῦ Μνασίου* (sc. *Μνασέ(/αί)ου*) *μαλακτική*:
(214) *Ἡ δι᾽ ἁλῶν*:
(215) *Ἡ διὰ μέλιτος*:
(216) *Ἡ διὰ ψυχῶν* (sc. *ψιχῶν*):
(217) *Ἡ δι᾽ ὄχρας* (sc. *ὤχρας*):
(218) *Ἡ μαστιχηρά*:
(219) *Τὸ ξανθὸν ἄλειμμα*:
(220) *Ἡ τετραφάρμακος*:
(221) *Τὸ διὰ ψιμιθίου* (sc. *ψιμυθίου*):
(222) *Τὸ πράσινον*:
(223) *Ἡ Αἰγυπτία Ἀνδρομάχου*:
(224) *Τὸ μυρσινάτον*:
(225) *Τὸ δι᾽ ὀστρέου*:
(226) *Τὸ δι᾽ ἀγχούσης*:
(227) *Τὸ διὰ σάντιγος* (sc. *σάνδυκος*):

(228) *Τὸ διὰ θείου*:
(229) *Τὸ νευροχαλαστικόν*:
(230) *Ἡ Τυρεία* (*sc. Τυρία*):
(231) *Ἡ πεντάθετος*:
(232) *Τὸ δι᾽ ἀλθαίας*:
(233) *Τὸ διὰ καστορίου*:
(234) *Ἡ τοῦ Μαχερίωνος* (*sc. Μαχαιρίωνος*):
(235) *Ἡ τοῦ Πριμμίωνος* (*sc. Πριμίωνος*):
(236) *Ἡ δι᾽ εὐφορβίου*:
(237) *Τὸ ξανθὸν ἔμπλαστρον*:
(238) *Ἡ τοῦ Ἀζανίτου*:
(239) *Τὸ ψωράλειμμα*:
(240) *Το δι᾽ ἄμβραν* (*sc. ἄμπαρος*):
(241) *Τὸ διὰ χάρτου*:
(242) *Πρὸς τὰς ἐντὸς αἱμορραγίας*:
(243) *Κοραλλίου ὁ τροχίσκος κατωτερικός*:
(244) *Ψωρικὸν ἐπὶ ἀρχομένης ἐλεφαντιάσεως*:
(245) *Μάλαγμα τὸ μοναχικόν*:
(246) *Ὁ δι᾽ ἀλικακάβων*:
(247) *Ἰαρείου* (*sc. Ἀρείου*) *πρὸς ψώραν*:
(248) *Πρὸς ῥαγάδας*:
(249) *Ἡ ἀρετή*:
(250) *Τὸ Μοῦσα* (*sc. Μούσα*):
(251) *Τροχίσκος ὁ Βιθυνός*:
(252) *Ἄδηκτον*:
(253) *Τροχίσκος ὁ λεπτὸς δυσεντερικός*:
(254) *Εἰς αἱμορροΐδας*:
(255) *Πρὸς ὑστερικὰς πνίγας*:
(256) *Ἕτερος*:
(257) *Περὶ πεσσῶν*:
(258) *Περὶ ὑδρωπιώσης μήτρας*:
(259) *Εἰς φλεγμονὴν μήτρας*:
(260) *Ἕτερον*:
(261) *Ἕτερον ὁ χρυσοῦς*:
(262) *Ἕτερον ἐπὶ πυρρωδεστέρας* (*sc. πυρωδεστέρας*) *φλεγμονῆς*:
(263) *Πρὸς σκληρίας*:
(264) *Ἄλλο*:
(265) *Ἕτερον*:
(266) *Πρὸς ῥαγάδας*:
(267) *Πρὸς κεχρονισμένους* (*sc. κεχρονισμένας*) *μυρμηκίας*:
(268) *Περὶ συνθέσεως ἐλαίων*:
(269) *Ναρδίνου σκευασία*:
(270) *Γλεύκινον*:
(271) *Κύπρινον*:
(272) *Σικυόνιον*:
(273) *Ῥόδινον*:
(274) *Ἀνήθινον*:
(275) *Χαμαιμήλινον*:

(276) *Κρίνινον*:
(277) *Πηγάνινον*:
(278) *Ἰέλαιον*:
(279) *Μυρσίνινον*:
(280) *Μήλινον*:
(281) *Ἴρινον*:
(282) *Μαστίχινον*:
(283) *Δάφνινον*:
(284) *Ὀμφάκινον*:
(285) *Ἀμυγδάλινον*:
(286) *Ῥαφάνινον*:
(287) *Μελάνθινον*:
(288) *Σινήπινον*:
(289) *Ἕτερον μήλινον*:
(290) *Σαμψύχινον*:
(291) *Περὶ ἰοβόλων*:
(292) *Περὶ λυσσῶντος κυνός*:
(293) *Περὶ σφηκῶν*:
(294) *Περὶ σκολοπένδρας*:
(295) *Περὶ τρυγόνος*:
(296) *Μυγαλῆς*:
(297) *Περὶ ἐχίδνης*:
(298) *Περὶ δρυΐνου*:
(299) *Περὶ αἱμόρρου*:
(300) *Περὶ ὕδρου*:
(301) *Περὶ κέγχρου*:
(302) *Περὶ κεράστου*:
(303) *Περὶ ἀσπίδος*:
(304) *Περὶ βασιλίσκου*:

Bibliography

Dictionaries and Encyclopaedias

(*DNP*). Cancik, H., Schneider, H., and M. Landfester. (eds.). 1996–2003. *Der neue Pauly: Enzyklopädie der Antike*. 19 vols. Stuttgart: J. B. Metzler.

(*GMG*). Holton, D., Horrocks, G., Janssen, M., Lendari, T., Manolessou, I., and N. Toufexis. 2019. *The Cambridge Grammar of Medieval and Early Modern Greek*. 4 vols. Cambridge: Cambridge University Press.

(Kriaras). Kriaras, E. (ed.). 1968–2014. *Λεξικὸ τῆς Μεσαιωνικῆς Ἑλληνικῆς Δημώδους Γραμματείας, 1100–1669*. 19 vols. Thessaloniki: Kentro Ellēnikēs Glōssas.

(Lampe). Lampe, G. W. H. 1961. *A Patristic Greek Lexicon*. Oxford: Clarendon Press.

(*LexLat*). Cervenka-Ehrenstrasser, I. and J. Diethart. 1995–2000. *Lexikon der lateinischen Lehnwörter in den griechischsprachigen dokumentarischen Texten Ägyptens*. 2 vols. Vienna: Hollinek/Österreichische Nationalbibliothek.

(LSJ). Liddell, H. G., Scott, R., and H. S. Jones. (eds.). 1996. *A Greek-English Lexicon*. [9th edn. 1940; with a revised supplement edited by P. G. W. Glare] Oxford: Clarendon Press.

(*OCD*). Hornblower, S., Spawforth, A., and E. Eidinow. (eds.). 2012. *The Oxford Classical Dictionary*. [4th edn.] Oxford: Oxford University Press.

(*ODB*). Kazhdan, A. (ed.). 1991. *The Oxford Dictionary of Byzantium*. 3 vols. Oxford: Oxford University Press.

(*PBW*). Jeffreys, M. et al. (eds.). 2016. *Prosopography of the Byzantine World*, 1025–1150, available at http://pbw2016.kdl.kcl.ac.uk (accessed 20 September 2018).

(*PLP*). Trapp, E., Walther, R. and H.-V. Beyer. (eds.). 1976–91. *Prosopographisches Lexikon der Palaiologenzeit*. 11 vols. Vienna: Verlag der Österreichischen Akademie der Wissenschaften.

(*PmBZ*). Winkelmanns, F. et al. (eds.). 1998–2013. *Prosopographie der mittelbyzantinischen Zeit*. 14 vols. Berlin: De Gruyter.

(*RGK*). Hunger, H. et al. (eds.). 1981–97. *Repertorium der griechischen Kopisten 800–1600*. 3 vols in 9 pts. Vienna: Verlag der Österreichischen Akademie der Wissenschaften. [Cited with volume no. followed by catalogue no., e.g. *RGK* II 120]

Primary Sources

Unpublished

Andreiomenos. *Recipe Book*. Athous Iberiticus 151, ff. 228r–235v.

Chariton. *Recipe Book*. Parisinus gr. 2240, ff. 1r–39v.

George-Gregory Chioniades. *Antidotes from Persia*. Venetus Marcianus gr. V.8 (coll. 1334), ff. 138r–156r.

George Oinaiotes. *Epistles* nos. 43, 168, 171, 174. Florentinus Laurentianus San Marco 356, ff. 65v–67v, 275r–276v, 279r–291r; Matritensis gr. 4796, ff. 26v–27r, 105r–106r, 107r–112r; Monacensis gr. 198, ff. 355v–356r, 405r–v, 407v–409r. Unpublished critical edition by G. Fatouros, S. Kourousis, and D. R. Reinsch.

Ibn al-Jazzār. *Ephodia tou Apodēmountos* (Greek translation of *Zād al-Musāfir wa-Qūt al-Ḥāḍir*). Vaticanus gr. 300, ff. 11r–267r.

John Zacharias Aktouarios. (JZA). *Medical Epitome*. Vindobonensis med. gr. 17, ff. 1r–242v.

[Nicholas Myrepsos]. *Dynameron*. Parisinus gr. 2243, ff. 2v–624v.

Published (editions and translations)

Adams, F. 1844–7. *Paulus Aegineta*. 3 vols. London: Syndenham Society of London.

Alexanderson, B. 1967. *Περὶ κρίσεων: Überlieferung und Text*. Gothenburg: Acta Universitatis Gothoburgensis.

[Anonymus]. 1525. *Here Begynneth the Seynge of Uryns* [...] *Man to Knowe*. London: J. Rastell for Richard Banckes.

al-ʿĀṣī, Ḥ. 1992. *Minhāj al-Dukkān*. Beirut: Dār al-Manāhil.

Bazou, A. 2011. *Γαληνοῦ Ὅτι ταῖς τοῦ Σώματος Κράσεσιν αἱ τῆς Ψυχῆς Δυνάμεις Ἕπονται*. Athens: Akadēmia Athēnōn.

Beck, L. 2005. *De materia medica*. Hildesheim: Olms-Weidmann.

Bekker, I. et al. 1829–55. *Nicephori Gregorae Byzantina historia*. 3 vols. Bonn: Weber.

Bell, A. T. et al. 1997. *Ioannis Alexandrini in Hippocratis De natura pueri commentarium*. Berlin: Akademie Verlag. [C.M.G., XI.1.4: 130–74]

Bennett, D. 2003. *Xenonika: Medical Texts Associated with Xenones in the Late Byzantine Period*. University of London: PhD thesis, available at https://ethos.bl.uk/OrderDetails.do?uin=uk.bl.ethos.404391 (accessed 17 August 2018).

Bernard, J. S. 1749. *Synesius de Febribus: quem nunc primum ex codice ms. Bibliothecæ Lugduno Batavæ edidit, vertit, notisque inlustravit Jo. Steph. Bernard. Accedit Viatici Constantino Africano interprete lib. VII. Pars*. Amsterdam: G. de Groot.

Bezdeki, St. 1924. 'Epistolae XC', *Ephemeris Dacoromana* II: 239–377.

Bos, G. 1997. *Ibn al-Jazzār on Sexual Diseases and their Treatment: A Critical Edition of Zād al-Musāfir wa-Qūt al-Ḥāḍir*. London: Kegan Paul International.

Bos, G. 2000. *Ibn Al-Jazzār on Fevers: A Critical Edition of Zād al-Musāfir wa-Qūt al-Ḥāḍir = Provisions for the Traveller and the Nourishment for the Sedentary. Bk. 7, chs. 1–6*. London: Kegan Paul International.

Bos, G. 2015. *Ibn al-Jazzār's Zād al-Musāfir wa-Qūt al-Ḥāḍir, Provisions for the Traveller and Nourishment for the Sedentary, Book 7 (7–30)*. Leiden: Brill.

Boudon-Millot, V. 2007a. *Galien: Introduction générale; Sur l'ordre de ses propres livres; Sur ses propres livres; Que l'excellent médecin est aussi philosophe*. Paris: Les Belles Lettres.

Boudon-Millot, V., Jouanna, J., and A. Pietrobelli. 2010. *Galien: Ne pas se chagriner*. Paris: Les Belles Lettres.

Busse, A. 1891. *Ammonius in Porphyrii Isagogen sive quinque voces*. Berlin: Reimer.

Busse, A. 1900. *Eliae in Porphyrii Isagogen et Aristotelis Categorias commentaria*. Berlin: Reimer.

Busse, A. 1904. *Davidis Prolegomena et in Porphyrii Isagogen commentarium*. Berlin: Reimer.

Bussemaker, U. C. 1845. '*ΣΤΕΦΑΝΟΥ ΠΕΡΙ ΟΥΡΩΝ*. Traité d'Etienne sur les urines, publié pour le première fois d'après un manuscrit de la Bibliothèque royale', *Revue de Philologie* 1: 415–38, 545–60.

Capone Ciollaro, M. 2003. *Demetrio Pepagomeno: Prontuario medico*. Naples: Bibliopolis.

Casson, L. 1989. *The Periplus Maris Erythraei*. Princeton: Princeton University Press.
Cordus, E. 1543. *De urinis, das ist, von rechter Besichtigungen des Harns, und ihrem Mißbrauch* [ed. by J. Dryander]. Frankfurt: Jacob.
Cramer, J. A. 1836. *Anecdota graeca e codicibus manuscriptis bibliothecarum Oxoniensium*, vol. 3. Oxford: Oxford University Press.
Criscuolo, U. 1972. 'Un discorso e una monodia inediti di Michele Italico', *Atti dell'Accademia delle Scienze di Torino, II, Cl. di Scienze mor., stor. e filol.* 106: 593–634.
Daremberg, C. and C. É. Ruelle. 1879. *Oeuvres de Rufus d'Éphèse*. Paris: Imprimé par l'autorisation du gouvernement à l'Imprimerie Nationale.
Deichgräber, K. 1965. *Die griechische Empirikerschule: Sammlung der Fragmente und Darstellung der Lehre*. Berlin: Widemannsche Verlagsbuchhandlung.
Delatte, A. 1927–39. *Anecdota Atheniensia*. 2 vols. Liège: Faculté de philosophie et lettres.
Delehaye, H. 1921. 'Deux typica byzantins de l'époque des Paléologues', *Mémoires de l'Académie royale de Belgique, Classe de Lettres, 2é série* 8: 1–213.
Diehl, E. 1903. *Procli Diadochi in Platonis Timaeum commentaria*, vol. 1. Leipzig: Teubner.
Diels, H. 1915. *Galeni in Hippocratis Prorrheticum I commentaria III*. Leipzig and Berlin: Teubner. [C.M.G., V.9.2]
Dorini, U. and T. Bertelè. 1956. *Il Libro dei Conti di Giacomo Badoer*. Rome: Istituto poligrafico dello stato.
Downey, G. 1957. 'Nikolaos Mesarites: Description of the Church of the Holy Apostles at Constantinople', *Transactions of the American Philosophical Society* 47: 855–924.
Drexl, F. 1925. *Achmetis Oneirocriticon*. Leipzig: Teubner.
Dübner, L. 1907. *Kosmas und Damian. Texte und Einleitung*. Leipzig and Berlin: Teubner.
Duffy, J. M. 1983. *Stephani Philosophi In Hippocratis Prognosticum*. Berlin: Akademie Verlag. [C.M.G., XI.1.2]
Duffy, J. M. 1992. *Michaelis Pselli philosophica minora*. Leipzig: Teubner.
Duffy, J. M. 1997. *Ioannis Alexandrini In Hippocratis Epidemiarum librum VI commentarii fragmenta*. Berlin: Akademie Verlag. [C.M.G., XI.1.4]
Eideneier, H. 1991. *Ptochoprodromus: Einführung, kritische Ausgabe, deutsche Übersetzung, Glossar*. Cologne: Romiosini.
Eijk, P. J. van der. 2005. *On Aristotle on the Soul 1.1–2*. London: Duckworth.
Elter, A. F. 1898. *Io. Katrarii Hermodotus et Musocles dialogi*. Bonn: Ex Caroli Georgi Typographeo Academico.
Ermerins, F. Z. 1840. *Anecdota medica Graeca e codicibus MSS. expromsit*. Leiden: S. et J. Luchtmans.
Ernout, A. 1949. *Pline l'Ancien. Histoire naturelle. Livre XII*. Paris: Les Belles Lettres.
Evans, A. 1936. *Francesco Balducci Pegolotti: La pratica della mercatura*. Cambridge MA: The Medieval Academy of America.
Failler, A. and V. Laurent. 1984. *Georges Pachymérès. Relations historiques*. 2 vols. Paris: Les Belles Lettres.
Fatouros, G. 1973. *Die Briefe des Michael Gabras, ca. 1290 – nach 1350*. 2 vols. Vienna: Verlag der Österreichischen Akademie der Wissenschaften.
Festa, N. and U. Klein. 1891. *Iamblichi de Communi mathematica scientia liber*. Leipzig: Teubner.

Fischer, J. F. 1774. *Ἀκτουαρίου Περὶ Ἐνεργειῶν και Παθῶν τοῦ Ψυχικοῦ Πνεύματος καὶ τῆς κατ' αὐτὸ Διαίτης Λόγοι B*. Leipzig: Sumtu J. F. Langenhemii.

Fuchs, L. 1549. *Nicolai Myrepsi Medicamentorum opus*. Basel: I. Opori.

Furley, D. and J. Wilkie. 1984. *Galen on Respiration and the Arteries*. Princeton: Princeton University Press.

Garofalo, I. 2000. *Anatomicarum administrationum libri qui supersunt novem, earundem interpretatio arabica Hunaino Isaaci filio ascripta; tomus alter libros V–IX continens*. Naples: Instituto Universitario Orientale.

Garofalo, I. 2005. *Galien: Les os pour les débutants; L'anatomie des muscles*. Paris: Les Belles Lettres.

Gautier, P. 1972. *Michel Italikos. Lettres et discours*. Paris: Institut français d'études byzantines.

Gautier, P. 1974. 'Le typikon du Christ Sauveur Pantocrator', *Revue des Études Byzantines* 32: 1–145.

Georgiou, S. 2013. *Edition critique, traduction et commentaire critique du livre 1 "De Urinis" de Jean Zacharias Actouarios*. Paris, École Pratique des Hautes Études: PhD thesis.

Gessner, C. 1541. *Compendium ex Actuarii Zachariae libris de differentiis urinarum iudiciis & praevidentiis. Universalis doctrina Claudii Galeni de compositione pharmacorum secundum locos affectos. Sylvula Galeni experimentorum et aliorum aliquot*. Zurich: Apud C. Froschouerum.

Ghalioungui, P. 1980. *Questions on Medicine for Scholars by Ḥunayn ibn Isḥāq*. Cairo: A R E Al-Ahram Center for Scientific Translations.

Giros, C., Kravari, V., and M. Zivojinovic. 1998. *Actes de Chilandar. I: Des Origines a 1319*. Paris: P. Lethielleux.

Gouillard, J. 1967. 'Le Synodikon de l'orthodoxie', *Travaux et mémoires* 2: 45–107.

Goupyl, J. 1548. *Actuarii Joannis Zachariae filii medici praestantissimi, Libri VII de urinis; Ambrosio Leone Nolano interprete, ad. graecorum exemplarium fidem a Iacobo Goupylo recogniti. Aristotelis Stagiritae Lib. de coloribus Antonii Thylesii Cosentini de eadem re liber*. Paris: Apud Iacobum Gazellum, sub insigni scuti Coloniensis.

Goupyl, J. 1557. *Ἀκτουαρίου Περὶ ἐνεργειῶν καὶ παθῶν τοῦ ψυχικοῦ πνεύματος, καὶ τῆς κατ' αὐτὸ διαίτης, λόγοι β. Actuarii de actionibus & affectibus spiritus animalis, eiusque victu libri II*. Paris: Apud Martinum Juvenum.

Gysseling, M. and A. C. F. Koch. 1950. *Diplomata Belgica ante annum millesimum centesimum scripta*. 2 vols. Brussels: Belgisch Inter-Universitair Centrum voor Neerlandistiek.

Hayduck, M. 1897. *Ioannis Philoponi in Aristotelis de Anima libros commentaria*. Berlin: Reimer.

Heiberg, J. L. 1921–4. *Paulus Aegineta*. 2 vols. Leipzig: Teubner. [C.M.G., IX.1–2]

Heisenberg, A. 1903. *Georgii Acropolitae opera*. Leipzig: Teubner.

Helmreich, G. 1893. *Claudii Galeni Pergameni Scripta minora*, vol. 3. Leipzig: Teubner.

Helmreich, G. 1904. *Galeni De temperamentis*. Leipzig: Teubner.

Helmreich, G. 1907–9. *Galeni De usu partium libri xvii*. 2 vols. Leipzig: Teubner.

Helmreich, G. 1923. *Galeni De bonis malisque sucis*. Leipzig; Berlin: Teubner. [C.M.G., V.4.2: 387–429]

Hoche, R. 1866. *Nicomachi Geraseni Pythagorei Introductionis arithmeticae libri ii.* Leipzig: Teubner.

Ibn Sīnā. 1593. *Al-Qānūn fī al-Ṭibb.* 1 vol. in 2. Rome: In Typographia Medicea.

Ideler, J. L. 1841–2. *Physici et medici Graeci minores.* 2 vols. Berlin: G. Reimeri.

Irigoin, J. 1993. *Bacchylide. Dithyrambes, épinicies, fragments.* Paris: Les Belles Lettres.

Jahier, H. and A. Noureddine. 1956. *Avicenne: Poème de la médecine.* Paris: Les Belles Lettres.

Johnston, I. 2016. *On the Constitution of the Art of Medicine. The Art of Medicine; A Method of Medicine to Glaucon.* Cambridge MA: Harvard University Press.

Jones, W. H. S. 1931. *Hippocrates, with an English Translation*, vol. 4. Cambridge MA: Harvard University Press.

Jouanna, J. 2000. *Hippocrate: Épidémies V et VII.* Paris: Les Belles Lettres.

Jouanna, J. 2013. *Hippocrate: Pronostic.* Paris: Les Belles Lettres.

Jouanna, J. 2016. *Hippocrate: Épidémies I et III.* Paris: Les Belles Lettres.

Kalbfleisch, K. 1923. *Galeni de Victu attenuante.* Leipzig: Teubner. [C.M.G., V.4.2: 430–51]

Karpozilos, A. and G. Fatouros. 2017. *The Letters of Theodoros Hyrtakenos.* Athens: Ekdoseis Kanakēs.

Kliegel, P. 1972. *Die Harnverse des Gilles de Gorbeil.* Rheinische Friedrich-Wilhelms-Universität Bonn: PhD thesis.

Koch, K. 1923. *De sanitate tuenda.* Leipzig; Berlin: Teubner. [C.M.G., V.4.2: 3–198]

Koder, J. 1970. 'Das Fastengedicht des Patriachen Nikolaos III Grammatikos', *Jahrbuch der Österreichischen Byzantinistik* 19: 203–41.

Kotzia, P. and P. Sotiroudis. 2010. '*Γαληνού Περί Αλυπίας*', *Ἑλληνικά* 60: 63–150.

Kousis, A. P. 1909. *Ραζῆ Λόγος Περὶ Λοιμικῆς.* Athens: Vasilikon Typographeion N. Chiōtē kai K. Rousea.

Kousis, A. P. 1929. '*Τὸ ἀνέκδοτον ἔτι ἰατρικὸν ἔργον τοῦ Ἀνδρειωμένου*', *Ἐπετηρὶς Ἑταιρείας Βυζαντινῶν Σπουδῶν* 6: 383–6.

Kousis, A. P. 1939a. '*Χαρίτωνος Περὶ Τροχίσκων*', in *Τεσσαρακονταετηρὶς Θεοφίλου Βορέα*. vol. 1. Athens: Pyrsos, 109–15.

Kousis, A. P. 1939b. 'Quelques considerations sur les traductions en grec des oeuvres médicales orientales et principalement sur les deux manuscrits de la traduction d'un traité persan par Constantin Melitiniotis', *Πρακτικὰ Ἀκαδημίας Ἀθηνῶν* 14: 205–20.

Kousis, A. P. 1944a. 'The Apotherapeutic of Theophilos according the Laurentian Codex, plut. 75.19', *Πρακτικὰ Ἀκαδημίας Ἀθηνῶν* 19: 35–45.

Kousis, A. P. 1944b. 'Les oeuvres médicales de Nicéphoros Blémmydès selon les manuscrits existants', *Πρακτικὰ Ἀκαδημίας Ἀθηνῶν* 19: 56–75.

Kroll, G. and P. Viereck. 1895. *Anonymi Christiani Hermippus De astrologia dialogus.* Leipzig: Teubner.

Kühn, C. G. 1821–33. *Claudii Galeni opera omnia.* 20 vols. in 22. Leipzig: Knobloch.

Kurtz, E. and F. Drexl. 1936–41. *Michaelis Pselli Scripta minora.* 2 vols. Milan: Società editrice "Vita e pensiero".

Kyriakidis, S. 1961. *Eustazio di Tessalonica. La espugnazione di Tessalonica.* Palermo: Istituto Siciliano di studi bizantini e neoellenici.

Lacy, P. de. 1978–84. *Galen on the Doctrines of Hippocrates and Plato.* 3 vols. Berlin: Akademie Verlag. [C.M.G., V 4.1.2]

Lamagna, M. 1999. 'Un anonimo de Urinis laurenziano', in A. Garzya and J. Jouanna (eds.), *I testi medici greci: tradizione e ecdotica*. Naples: D'Auria, 305–14.

Lamagna, M. 2017. *Giovanni Attuario. L'eccellente trattato sulle urine di Avicenna*. Cuenca: Ediciones de la Universidad de Castilla-La Mancha.

Lambros, S. P. 1880. *Μιχαὴλ Ἀκομινάτου τοῦ Χωνιάτου τα Σωζόμενα*, vol. 2. Athens: Parnassos.

Lamoureux, J. and N. Aujoulat. 2004. *Synésios de Cyrène: Opuscules I*. Paris: Les Belles Lettres.

Langkavel, B. A. 1868. *Simeonis Sethi Syntagma de alimentorum facultatibus*. Leipzig: Teubner.

Legrand, P.-E. 1932–68. *Hérodote. Histoires*. 9 vols. Paris: Les Belles Lettres.

Leone, P. A. 1972. *Ioannes Tzetzes Epistulae*. Leipzig: Teubner.

Leone, P. A. 1982. *Nicephori Gregorae Epistulae*, vol. 2. Matino: Tipografia di Matino.

Leone, P. A. 1991. *Maximi Monachi Planudis Epistulae*. Amsterdam: Hakkert.

Leone of Nola, A. 1519. *Hoc in volumine digesti sunt De urinis libri septem de graeco sermone in latinum conversi*. Venice: Bernardinus Vitalis.

Lindstam, S. 1910. *Georgii Lacapeni Epistulae X priores cum epimerismis editae*. Uppsala: E. Berling.

Lindstam, S. 1924. *Georgii Lacapeni et Andronici Zaridae epistulae XXII cum epimerismis*. Gothenburg: Typis descripsit Elanders Boktryckeri Aktiebolag.

Littré, É. 1839–61. *Oeuvres complètes d'Hippocrate: traduction nouvelle avec le texte grec en regard, collationné sur les manuscrits et toutes les éditions; accompagnée d'une introduction, de commentaires médicaux, de variantes et de notes philologiques; suivie d'une table générale des matières*. 10 vols. Paris: J.–B. Baillière.

Manetti, D. 2011. *Anonymus Londinensis: De medicina*. Berlin: De Gruyter.

(Mathys, 1554) Mathisius, C. H. and I. A. Tridentinus. 1554. *Actuarii Ioannis filii Zachariae, Methodi medendi libri sex, quibus omnia*. Venice: [Apud Gualterum Scottum].

(Mathys, 1556) Mathisius, C. H., Leone Nolanus, A., and I. A. Tridentinus. 1556. *Actuarii Ioannis filii Zachariae Opera. De actionibus et spiritus animalis affectibus eiusque: nutritione Lib. II. De Urinis Lib. VII. Methodi Medendi Lib. VI. Rerum ac verborum memorabilium Index*. 2 vols. Paris: Guil. Morelium, in Greacis typographum Regium.

Mohler, L. 1927. *Kardinal Bessarion als Theologe Humanist und Staatsmann. Funde und Forschungen*, vol. 2. Paderborn: Ferdinand Schöningh.

Morani, M. 1987. *Nemesii Emeseni De natura hominis*. Leipzig: Teubner.

Moraux, P. 1985. 'Anecdota Graeca minora VI: Pseudo-Galen, De signis ex urinis', *Zeitschrift für Papyrologie und Epigraphik* 60: 63–74.

Munitiz, J. 1988. *Nikephoros Blemmydes. A Partial Account*. Leuven: Spicilegium Sacrum Lovaniense.

Nauck, A. 1886. *Porphyrii philosophi Platonici opuscula selecta*. Leipzig: Teubner.

Neustein, J. A. von. 1547. *Actuarii Zachariae De victus ratione in spiritu animali libri duo: Iulio Alexandrino Tridentino interprete. De puerorum educatione liber versibus*. Venice: Apud Petrum de Nicolinis de Sabio.

Nutton, V. 2014. '*Avoiding Distress*', in P. Singer (ed.), *Galen: Psychological Writings*. Cambridge: Cambridge University Press, 43–106.

Oder, E. and K. Hoppe. 1924. *Corpus Hippiatricorum Graecorum*, vol. 1. Leipzig: Teubner.

Olivieri, A. 1935–50. *Aetii Amideni Libri medicinales*. 2 vols. Leipzig: Teubner. [C.M.G., VIII.1–2].

Papadopoulos, I. 1927. '*Γρηγορίου Χιονιάδου τοῦ Ἀστρονόμου: Ἐπιστολαί*', *Ἐπιστημονικὴ Ἐπετηρὶς τῆς Φιλοσοφικῆς Σχολῆς Πανεπιστημίου Θεσσαλονίκης* 1: 151–204.

Papazoglou, G. K. 2014. *Τυπικόν Ισαακίου Αλεξίου Κομνηνού Της Μονής Θεοτόκου της Κοσμοσώτειρας*. Thessaloniki: Ekdoseis Zētē.

Perrin, B. 1919. *Plutarch Lives, VII, Demosthenes and Cicero. Alexander and Caesar (Loeb Classical Library, vol. VII)*. Cambridge MA: Harvard University Press.

Petit, C. 2009. *Galien: Le médecin, introduction*. Paris: Les Belles Lettres.

Pietrosanti, P. 1999. *Nicephori Gregorae explicatio in librum Synesii "De insomniis"*. Bari: Levante.

Pino Campos, L. M. 2019. *Sobre las causas en los pulsos de Galeno*. Madrid: Ediciones Clásicas.

Places, E. S. J. des. 1989. *Jamblique: Protreptique*. Paris: Les Belles Lettres.

Polemis, I. 2002. *Θεόδωρος Μετοχίτης. Ἠθικὸς ἢ Περὶ Παιδείας*. [2nd edn.] Athens: Ekdoseis Kanakēs.

Polemis, I. 2014. *Michael Psellus: Orationes funebres*. Berlin: De Gruyter.

Polemis, I. and E. Kaltsogianni. 2019. *Theodorus Metochites: Orationes*. Berlin: De Gruyter.

Puschmann, T. 1878–9. *Alexander von Tralles: Original-Text und Übersetzung nebst einer einleitenden Abhandlung. Ein Beitrag zur Geschichte der Medicin*. 2 vols. Vienna: W. Braumüller.

Raeder, H. 1926. *Synopsis ad Eustathium. Libri ad Eunapium*. Leipzig; Berlin: Teubner. [C.M.G., VI.3]

Raeder, H. 1928–33. *Oribasii Collectionum medicarum reliquiae*. 2 vols in 4 pts. Leipzig; Berlin: Teubner. [C.M.G., VI.1.1–2.2]

Rallis, G. A. and M. Potlis. 1852–9. *Σύνταγμα τῶν* [. . .] *καὶ τῶν ἱερῶν οἰκουμενικῶν καὶ τοπικῶν συνόδων*. 6 vols. Athens.

Recorde, R. 1548. *The Urinal of Physick*. London: Reynolde Wolfe.

Rega, H. J. 1733. *De Urinis tractatus duo. Prior quaestio quodlibetica alter de urinis ut signo*. Leuven: Martini van Overbeke.

Reinsch, R. and A. Kambylis. 2001. *Annae Comnenae Alexias*. Berlin: De Gruyter.

Renzi, S. 1854. *Collectio Salernitana*, vol. 3. Naples: Tipografia del Filiatre-Sebezio.

Ricettario Fiorentino. 1499. *Ricettario Fiorentino*. Florence: Compagnia del Drago.

Romano, R. 1991. *Costantino Acropolita, Epistole*. Naples: D'Auria.

Rossetti, D. G. 1904. *The New Life*. New York: Thomas Y. Crowell & Co.

Ruelle, J. 1537. *De natura stirpium libri tres*. Basel: In Officina Frobeniana [per Hieronymum Frobenium et Nicolaum Episcopium.

Ruelle, J. 1539. *Actuarius de medicamentorum compositione*. Paris: Per Conradum Neobarium ad D. Hilarium.

Scalon, C. 1995. *Produzione e fruizione del libro nel basso Medioevo: Il caso Friuli*. Padua: Antenore.

Schopen, L. 1828–32. *Ioannis Cantacuzeni eximperatoris historiarum libri iv*. 3 vols. Bonn: Weber.

Seminar Classics 609, Buffalo. 1969. *Porphyrius: The Cave of the Nymphs in the Odyssey*. Buffalo: Seminar Classics 609, State University of New York at Buffalo.

Sicurus, D. 1862. *Theophili et Stephani Atheniensis De febrium differentia ex Hippocrate et Galeno*. Florence: Bencini.

Singer, P. 1997. *Galen. Selected Works*. Oxford: Oxford University Press.

Singer, P. (ed.). 2014. *Galen: Psychological Writings*. Cambridge: Cambridge University Press.

Suwaysī, M. et al. 1999. *Zād al-Musāfir wa-Qūt al-Ḥāḍir*. 2 vols. Tunis: al-Majmaʿ al-Tūnisī lil-ʿUlūm wa-al-Ādāb wa-al-Funūn, Bayt al-Ḥikmah.

Stefec, R. 2013. 'Weitere Briefe des Michael Gabras', *Byzantinoslavica* 71: 313–23.

Tassinari, P. (unpublished). *Theophilos: On Urines*.

Thomson, M. H. 1955. *Textes grecs inédits relatifs aux plantes*. Paris: Les Belles Lettres.

Treu, M. 1899a. *Theodori Pediasimi eiusque amicorum quae exstant*. Potsdam: P. Brandt.

Trot, B. 1515. *Omnia opera Ysaac* [. . .]. Lyon: Johannis de Platea, 156r–203. [repr. in Fontana, E. 1966. *Il libro delle urine di Isacco l'Ebreo tradotto dall'arabo in latino da Constantino Africano*. Pisa: Giardini, 143–239].

Valiakos, I. 2019. *Das Dynameron des Nikolaos Myrepsos*. Heidelberg: Proprylaeum.

Verbeke, G. 1966. *Commentaire sur le 'de Anima' d'Aristote*. Louvain: Publications universitaires.

Vranousi, E. L. 1980. *Βυζαντινὰ Ἔγγραφα τῆς Μονῆς Πάτμου*, vol. Α΄: *Αὐτοκρατορικά*. Athens: Ethniko Idryma Ereunōn.

Walz, C. 1934. *Rhetores Graeci*, vol. 3. Stuttgart: Cotta.

Wellmann, M. 1907–14. *Pedanii Dioscuridis Anazarbei De materia medica libri quinque*. 3 vols. Berlin: Weidmann.

Wenkebach, E. 1938. 'Galenos von Pergamon: Allgemeine Ertüchtigung durch Ballspiel Eine sporthygienische Schrift aus dem zweiten Jahrhundert n. Chr.', *Archiv für die Geschichte der Medizin* 31: 254–97.

Westerink, L. G. 1991. *Damascius: Traité des premiers principes*, vol. 3. Paris: Les Belles Lettres.

Westerink, L. G. 1992. *Michaelis Pselli Poemata*. Leipzig: Teubner.

Wilkins, J. 2013. *Galien: Sur les facultés des aliments*. Paris: Les Belles Lettres.

Zaccagnini, G. 1927. *Chartularium Studii Bononiensis*, vol. 8: *Memoriali del Comune bolognese. anno 1268*. Bologna: Presso l'Istituto per la storia dell'Università di Bologna.

Zipser, B. 2009. *John the Physician's Therapeutics: A Medical Handbook in Vernacular Greek*. Leiden: Brill.

Secondary Sources

Abou-Aly, A. M. A. 1992. *The Medical Writings of Rufus of Ephesus*. University College London: PhD thesis, available at http://discovery.ucl.ac.uk/1317541/1/246073.pdf (accessed 17 August 2018).

Addey, C. 2014. *Divination and Theurgy in Neoplatonism: Oracles of the Gods*. Farnham: Ashgate.

Agrimi, J. C. 1994. *Les consilia médicaux*. Turnhout: Brepols.

Ahrweiler, H. 1966. 'Le Sébaste, chef de groupes ethniques', in P. Wirth (ed.), *Polychronion: Festschrift Franz Dölger zum 75. Geburtstag*. Heidelberg: Carl Winter Universitätsverlag, 34–8.

Ahrweiler, H. 1996. 'Le récit du voyage d'Oinaiôtès de Constantinople à Ganos (Texte du lettre d'Oinaiôtès, établi par G. Fatouros)', in W. Seibt (ed.), *Geschichte und Kultur der Palaiologenzeit*. Vienna: Verlag der Österreichischen Akademie der Wissenschaften, 9–27.

Aland, K. 1956. *Die Handschriftenbestände der polnischen Bibliotheken: insbesondere an griechischen und lateinischen Handschriften von Autoren und Werken der klassischen bis zum Ende der patristischen Zeit; ein vorläufiger Bericht auf Grund einer Studienreise im November/Dezember 1955*. Berlin: Akademie-Verlag.

Álvarez-Millán, C. 1999. 'Graeco-Roman Case Histories and their Influence on Medieval Islamic Clinical Accounts', *Social History of Medicine* 12: 19–43.

Álvarez-Millán, C. 2000. 'Practice versus Theory: TenthCentury Case Histories from the Islamic Middle East', *Social History of Medicine* 13: 293–306.

Álvarez-Millán, C. 2010. 'The Case History in Medieval Islamic Medical Literature: *Tajārib* and *Mujarrabāt* as Source', *Medical History* 54: 195–214.

Álvarez-Millán, C. 2015. 'Disease in Tenth-Century Iran and Irak according to al-Rāzī's Casebook', *Suhayl. Journal for the History of the Exact and Natural Sciences in Islamic Civilisation* 14: 49–88.

Alwis, A. 2012. 'Men in Pain: Masculinity, Medicine and the *Miracles* of St Artemios', *Byzantine and Modern Greek Studies* 36: 1–19.

Amar, Z. and E. Lev. 2017. *Arabian Drugs in Early Medieval Mediterranean Medicine*. Edinburgh: Edinburgh University Press.

Amar, Z., Lev, E., and Y. Serri. 2014. 'On Ibn Juljul and the Meaning and Importance of the List of Medicinal Substances not Mentioned by Dioscorides', *Journal of the Royal Asiatic Society* 24: 529–55.

Anagnostakis, I. (ed.). 2013. *Flavours and Delights: Tastes and Pleasures of Ancient and Byzantine Cuisine*. Athens: Armos.

Andorlini, I. 2007. 'Teaching Medicine in Late Antiquity: Methods, Texts and Contexts', in P. Lendinara, L. Lazzari, and M.-A. D'Aronico (eds.), *Form and Content of Instruction in Anglo-Saxon England in the Light of Contemporary Manuscript Evidence*. Turnhout: Brepols, 401–14.

André, J. 1981. *L'alimentation et la cuisine* à *Rome*. Paris: Les Belles Lettres.

André, J. and J. Filliozat. 1986. *L'Inde vue de Rome*. Paris: Les Belles Lettres.

Andrés, G. de. 1965. *Catálogo de los códices griegos de la Real Biblioteca de El Escorial*, vol. 2. Madrid: [Real biblioteca de el Escorial].

Andrés, G. de. 1968. *Catálogo de los códices griegos desaparecidos de la Real Biblioteca de El Escorial*. El Escorial: [Real biblioteca de el Escorial].

Angeletti, L. R. et al. 2009. *Il 'De Urinis' di Teofilo Protospatario*. Rome: Casa Editrice Università La Sapienza.

Angeletti, L. R. and B. Cavarra. 1994. 'Critical and Historical Approach to Theophilus' *De Urinis*', *American Journal of Nephrology* 14: 282–9.

Angeletti, L. R. and B. Cavarra. 1997. 'The *Peri ouron* Treatise of Stephanus of Athens: Byzantine Uroscopy of the 6th-7th Centuries AD', *American Journal of Nephrology* 17: 228–32.

Angeletti, L. R. and V. Gazzaniga. 1999. 'Theophilus' *Auctoritas*: The Role of *De urinis* in the Medical Curriculum of the 12th-13th Centuries', *American Journal of Nephorology* 19: 165–71.

Angelov, D. 2007. *Imperial Ideology and Political Thought in Byzantium, 1204–1330.* Cambridge: Cambridge University Press.

Antonaras, A. C. 2010. 'Early Christian and Byzantine Glass Vessels: Froms and Uses', in F. Daim and J. Drauschke (eds.), *Byzanz: das Römerreich im Mittelalter*, vol. 1: *Welt der Ideen, Welt der Dinge.* Mainz: Römisch-Germanisches Zentralmuseum, 383–430.

Asper, M. 2007. *Griechische Wissenschaftstexte: Formen, Funktionen, Differenzierungsgeschichten.* Stuttgart: F. Steiner Verlag.

Balander, C. 1993. 'Production et usages du miel dans l'antiquité Gréco–Romaine,' in M.-C. Amouretti and G. Comet (eds.), *Des hommes et des plantes.* Aix-en-Provence: Université de Provence, Service des publications, 93–125.

Bandini, A. 1764–70. *Catalogus codicum manuscriptorum Bibliotheae Mediceae Laurentianae, varia continens opera Graecorum partum.* 3 vols. Florence: Typis Caesareis.

Barclay, C. R. 1996. 'Autobiographical Remembering: Narrative Constraints on Objectified Selves', in D. C. Rubin (ed.), *Remembering Our Past: Studies in Autobiographical Memory.* Cambridge: Cambridge University Press, 94–125.

Beck, H.-G. 1952. *Theodoros Metochites: Die Krise des byzantinischen Weltbildes im 14. Jahrhundert.* Munich: Beck.

Bennett, D. 2017. *Medicine and Pharmacy in Byzantine Hospitals.* Abingdon: Routledge.

Bénou, L. 1998. *Le codex B du Monastère Saint-Jean-Prodrome (Serrès). A XIIIe–XVe siècles.* Paris: Association Pierre Belon.

Bernabò, M. (ed.). 2010. *La collezione di testi chirurgici di Niceta: Firenze, Biblioteca medicea laurenziana, Plut. 74.7.* Rome: Edizioni di storia e letteratura.

Beyer, H.-V. 1971. 'Nikephoros Gregoras als Theologe und sein erstes Auftreten gegen die Hesychasten', *Jahrbuch der Österreichischen Byzantinistik* 20: 171–88.

Beyer, H.-V. 1978. 'Eine Chronologie der Lebensgeschichte des Nikephoros Gregoras', *Jahrbuch der Österreichischen Byzantinistik* 27: 127–55.

Bianconi, D. 2004. 'Le traduzioni in greco di testi latini', in G. Cavallo (ed.), *Lo spazio letterario del Medioevo, 3. Le culture circostanti,* vol. 1: *La cultura bizantina.* Rome: Salerno, 519–68.

Bianconi, D. 2006. 'Qualcosa di nuovo su Giovanni Catrario', *Medioevo Greco* 6: 69–91.

Biran, M. 2015. 'The Mongol Empire and Inter-Civilizational Exchange', in B. Z. Kedar and M. E. Wiesner-Hanks (eds.), *Expanding Webs of Exchange and Conflict, 500CE–1500CE.* Cambridge: Cambridge University Press, 534–58.

Birchler-Argyros, U. B. 1988. 'Die Quellen zum Kral-Spital in Konstantinopel', *Gesneros* 45: 419–44.

Bliquez, L. J. 1984. 'Two Lists of Greek Surgical Instruments and the State of Surgery in Byzantine Times', *Dumbarton Oaks Papers* 38: 187–204.

Bliquez, L. J. 1999. 'The Surgical Instrumentarium of Leon Iatrosophistes', *Medicina nei Secoli* 11: 291–322.

Bliquez, L. J. 2015. *The Tools of Asclepius. Surgical Instruments in Greek and Roman Times.* Leiden: Brill.

Bliquez, L. J., and A. Kazhdan. 1984. 'Four Testimonia to Human Dissection in Byzantine Times', *Bulletin of the History of Medicine* 58: 554–7.

Bloch, I. 1902. 'Byzantinische Medizin', in M. Neuburger and J. Pagel (eds.), *Handbuch der Geschichte der Medizin*, vol. 1. Jena: G. Fischer: 492–588.

Blumenthal, H. 1996. *Aristotle and Neoplatonism in Late Antiquity: Interpretations of the* De Anima. London: Duckworth.

Böhm, K., Köhler, C. O., and R. Thome. 1978. *Historie der Krankengeschichte*. Stuttgart: Schattatauer.

Bono, J. 1984. 'Medical Spirits and the Medieval Language of Life', *Traditio* 40: 91–130.

Boor, C. de. 1897. *Verzeichniss der griechischen Handschriften der Königlichen Bibliothek zu Berlin 2*). Berlin: A. Asher.

Bos, G. 1993. 'Ibn Al-Jazzār on Women's Diseases and their Treatment', *Medical History* 37: 296–312.

Bosch, U. V. 1965. *Kaiser Andronikos III. Palaiologos. Versuch einer Darstellung der byzantinischen Geschichte in den Jahren 1321–1341*. Amsterdam: Hakkert.

Boudon-Millot, V. 2007b. 'Biographie', in *eadem*, *Galien: Introduction générale; Sur l'ordre de ses propres livres; Sur ses propres livres; Que l'excellent médecin est aussi philosophe*. Paris: Les Belles Lettres, vii–xc.

Boudon-Millot, V. 2010. 'Aux origines de la thériaque: la recette d'Andromaque', *Revue d'Histoire de la Pharmacie* 58: 261–70.

Boudon-Millot, V. 2012. 'Vision and Vision disorders: Galen's Physiology of Sight', in M. Horstmanshoff, H. King, and C. Zittel (eds.), *Blood, Sweat and Tears – The Changing Concepts of Physiology from Antiquity into Early Modern Europe*. Leiden: Brill, 551–67.

Boudon-Millot, V. 2016. 'Stéphanos d'Athènes', in R. Goulet (ed.), *Dictionnaire des philosophes antiques*, vol. 6. Paris: Centre National de la Recherche Scientifique, 579–88.

Bouras-Vallianatos, P. 2014. 'Clinical Experience in Late Antiquity: Alexander of Tralles and the Therapy of Epilepsy', *Medical History* 58: 337–53.

Bouras-Vallianatos, P. (with contributions by S. Xenophontos). 2015a. 'Galen's Reception in Byzantium: Symeon Seth and his Refutation of Galenic Theories on Human Physiology', *Greek, Roman, and Byzantine Studies* 55: 431–69.

Bouras-Vallianatos, P. (with contributions by G. Parpulov). 2015b. 'Greek Manuscripts at the Wellcome Library in London: A Descriptive Catalogue', *Medical History* 59: 275–326.

Bouras-Vallianatos, P. 2015c. 'Contextualizing the Art of Healing by Byzantine Physicians', in B. Pitarakis (ed.), *Life Is Short, Art Long: The Art of Healing in Byzantium*. Istanbul: Pera Museum Publication, 104–22. [Extended version in Modern Greek: 2016. '*Η Ιατρική Τέχνη στο Βυζάντιο*', *ΝΕΥΣΙΣ* 24: 189–223.]

Bouras-Vallianatos, P. 2015d. 'A New Witness to Michael Psellos' Poem *On Medicine* (*De Medicina*)', *Jahrbuch der Österreichischen Byzantinistik* 65: 9–12.

Bouras-Vallianatos, P. 2016a. 'Modelled on Archigenes *theiotatos*: Alexander of Tralles and his Use of Natural Remedies (*physika*)', *Mnemosyne* 69: 382–96.

Bouras-Vallianatos, P. 2016b. 'Medizinisches Schrifttum', in F. Daim (ed.), *Byzanz. Historisch-kulturwissenschaftliches Handbuch* [Der Neue Pauly. Supplemente 11]. Stuttgart, J. B. Metzler, 1025–31.

Bouras-Vallianatos, P. 2016c. 'Case Histories in Late Byzantium: Reading the Patient in John Zacharias Aktouarios' *On Urines*', in G. Petridou and C. Thumiger (eds), *Approaches to the Patient in the Ancient World*. Leiden: Brill, 390–409.

Bouras-Vallianatos, P. 2018a. 'Enrichment of the Medical Vocabulary in the Greek-Speaking Medieval Communities of Southern Italy: The Lexica of Plant Names', in B. Pitarakis and G. Tanman (eds.), *Life Is Short, Art Long: The Art of Healing in Byzantium. New Perspectives*. Istanbul: Istanbul Research Institute, 155–84.

Bouras-Vallianatos, P. 2018b. 'Reading Galen in Byzantium: The Fate of *Therapeutics to Glaucon*', in P. Bouras-Vallianatos and S. Xenophontos (eds.), *Greek Medical Literature and Its Readers: From Hippocrates to Islam and Byzantium*. New York: Routledge, 180–229.

Bouras-Vallianatos, P. 2019a. 'Galen in Late Antique Medical Handbooks', in P. - Bouras–Vallianatos and B. Zipser (eds.), *Brill's Companion to the Reception of Galen*. Leiden: Brill, 38–61.

Bouras-Vallianatos, P. 2019b. 'Galen in Byzantine Medical Litertarue', in P. Bouras–Vallianatos and B. Zipser (eds.), *Brill's Companion to the Reception of Galen*. Leiden: Brill, 86–110.

Bouras-Vallianatos, P. 2019c. 'Theories on Pneuma in the Work of the Late Byzantine Physician John Zacharias Aktouarios', in S. Coughlin, D. Leith, and O. Lewis (eds.), *The Concept of Pneuma after Aristotle*. Berlin: Edition Topoi.

Bouras-Vallianatos, P. (forthcoming). 'Cross-Cultural Transfer of Medical Knowledge in the Medieval Mediterranean: The Introduction and Dissemination of Sugar-Based Potions from the Islamic World to Byzantium'.

Bouras-Vallianatos, P. and B. Zipser. (eds.). 2019. *Brill's Companion to the Reception of Galen*. Leiden: Brill.

Brain, P. 1986. *Galen on Bloodletting: A Study of the Origins, Development and Validitly of His Opinions, with a Translation of the Three Works*. Cambridge: Cambridge University Press.

Brams, J. 2006. 'Traductions et traducteurs latins dans l'empire de Nicée et sous les Paléologues', in M. Cacouros and M.-H. Congourdeau (eds.), *Philosophie et Sciences à Byzance de 1204 à 1453*. Leuven: Peeters, 101–12.

Brams, J. and W. Vanhamel (eds.). 1989. *Guillaume de Moerbeke: recueil d'études à l'occasion du 700e anniversaire de sa mort (1286)*. Leuven: Leuven University Press.

Bravos, S. 1974. *Das Werk des Aetios v. Amida und seine medizinischen und nichtmedizinischen Quellen*. Universität Hamburg: PhD thesis.

Bregman, J. 1982. *Syensius of Cyrene, Philospher-Bishop*. Berkeley: University of California Press.

Brewer, W. F. 1996. 'What Is Recollective Memory?', in D. C. Rubin (ed.), *Remembering our Past: Studies in Autobiographical Memory*. Cambridge: Cambridge University Press, 19–66.

Brody, H. 2003. *Stories of Sickness*. Oxford: Oxford University Press.

Brömer, R. 2012. 'The Nature of the Soul and the Passage of Blood through the Lungs. Galen, Ibn al-Nafīs, Servetus, İtaki 'Aṭṭār', in M. Horstmanshoff, H. King, and C. Zittel (eds.), *Blood, Sweat and Tears – The Changing Concepts of Physiology from Antiquity into Early Modern Europe*. Leiden: Brill, 339–62.

Brown, P. G. 2012. 'The Great Calculation According to the Indians, of Maximus Planudes – The Digits of the System', *Loci*, available at http://www.maa.org/publications/periodicals/convergence/the-great-calculation-according-to-the-indians-of-maximus-planudes-the-digits-of-the-system-i (accessed 23 October 2018).

Browning, R. 1978. 'The Language of Byzantine Literature', in S. Vryonis, jr (ed.), *The Past in Medieval and Modern Greek Culture*. Malibu: Undena Publications, 103–33.

Browning, R. 1985. 'A Further Testimony to Human Dissection in the Byzantine World', *Bulletin of the History of Medicine* 59: 518–20.

Buchwald, W. et al. (eds.). 1982. *Tusculum-Lexikon: grieschischer und lateinischer Autoren des Altertums und des Mittelalters*. Munich: Artemis.

Bühler, W. 1990/3. 'Johannes Zacharias, de urinis, ed. J. L. Ideler', *Museum Criticum* 25–8: 409–15.

Burnett, C. 1994. 'The Chapter on the Spirits in the Pantegni of Constantine the African', in C. Burnett and D. Jacquart (eds.), *Constantine the African and 'Alī Ibn Al-'Abbās Al-Magūsī. The* Pantegni *and Related Texts*. Leiden: Brill, 99–120.

Bussemaker, U. C. 1847. 'Über Magnus von Emesa und des-sen Buch vom Harne', *Janus* 2: 273–97.

Bydén, B. and K. Ierodiakonou. 2018. 'Byzantine Philosophy', available at http://plato.stanford.edu/entries/byzantine-philosophy/ (accessed 15 October 2018).

Cacouros, M. 2006. 'La philosophie et les sciences du Trivium et du Quadrivium à Byzance de 1204 à 1453 entre tradition et Innovation: les textes et l'enseignement, le cas de l'école du Prodrome (Pétra)', in M. Cacouros and M.-H. Congourdeau (eds.), *Philosophie et Sciences à Byzance de 1204 à 1453*. Leuven: Peeters, 1–51.

Calà, I. 2012a. *Per l'edizione del primo dei Libri medicinales di Aezio Amideno*. Università di Bologna: PhD thesis.

Calà, I. 2012b. 'Il medico Andreas nei *Libri medicinales* di Aezio Amideno', *Galenos* 6: 53–64.

Calà, I. 2016. 'Terapie tra magia e religione. La gravidanza e il parto nei testi medici della Tarda Antichità', in M. T. Santamaría Hernández (ed.), *Traducción y transmisión doctrinal de la Medicina grecolatina desde la Antigüedad hasta el Mundo Moderno: nuevas aportaciones sobre autores y textos*. Cuenca: Ediciones de la Universidad de Castilla-La Mancha, 11–24.

Calcoen, R. 1975. *Inventaire des manuscrits scientifiques de la Bibliothèque royale Albert Ier*, vol. 3. Brussels: Centre National d'Histoire des Sciences.

Caldwell, L. 2018. 'Roman Medical Sects: The Asclepiadeans, the Methodists, and the Pneumatists', in P. T. Keyser with J. Scarborough (eds.), *The Oxford Handbook of Science and Medicine in the Classical World*. Oxford: Oxford University Press, 637–54.

Canart, P. 1978. 'Le livre grec en Italie méridionale sous les règnes normand et souabe: aspects matériels et sociaux', *Scrittura e Civiltà* 2: 103–62.

Cange, C. du. 1688. *Glossarium ad scriptores mediae et infimae Graecitatis*. 2 vols. Lyon: Anisson; Posuel; Rigaud.

Cataldi Palau, A. 2008. 'I colleghi di Giorgio Baiophoros: Stefano di Medea, Giorgio Crisococca, Leone Atrapes', in B. Atsalos and N. Tsironi (eds.), *Actes du VIe Colloque International de Paléographie Grecque*. Athens: Ellēnikē Etaireia Vivliodesias, 191–224.

Charon, R. 2006. *Narrative Medicine: Honoring the Stories of Illness*. Oxford: Oxford University Press.

Cheynet, J.-C. 2003. 'Les sceaux byzantins de Londres', in J.-C. Cheynet and C. Sode (eds.), *Studies in Byzantine Sigillography*, vol. 8. Munich: K. G. Saur, 85–100.

Chipman, L. 2007. 'Islamic Pharmacy in the Mamlūk and Mongol Realms: Theory and Practice', *Asian Medicine* 3: 265–78.

Chipman, L. 2010. *The World of Pharmacy and Pharmacists in Mamlūk Cairo*. Leiden: Brill.

Chipman, L. 2019. 'The Reception of Galenic Pharmacology in the Arabic Tradition', in P. Bouras-Vallianatos and B. Zipser (eds.), *Brill's Companion to the Reception of Galen*. Leiden: Brill, 304–16.

Choulant, L. 1828. *Handbuch der Bücherkunde für die aeltere Medicin*. Leipzig: L. Voss.

Chrysochoou, S. 2014. 'Maximos Planoudes and the 'Diagram' of Ptolemy', in T. G. Kolias and K. G. Pitsakis (eds.), *Aureus: Volume Dedicated to Professor Evangelos K. Chrysos*. Athens: Ethniko Idryma Ereunōn, 113–29.

Cirenei, F. 1961. *La fisiologia di Galeno*. Genoa: Sampierdarena.

Class, M. 2014. 'Introduction. Medical Case Histories as Genre: New Approaches', *Literature and Medicine* 32: vii–xvi.

Cocchi, A. 1754. *Graecorum chirurgici libri Soranianus de fracturarum signis Oribasii duo de fractis et de luxatis e collectione Nicetae ab antiquissimo et optimo codice florentino descripti atque editi*. Florence: ex Typographio Imperiali.

Colapinto, L. 1993. 'The "Nuovo Receptario" of Florence', *Medicina nei Secoli* 5: 39–50.

Collins, K. E. and M. Sussman. 1999. 'Isaac Israeli and his *Book of Urine*', *Scottish Medical Journal* 44: 86–8.

Congourdeau, M.-H. 1996. 'Le traducteur grec du traité de Rhazès sur la variole', in A. Garzya and J. Jouanna (eds.), *Storia e ecdotica dei testi medici greci*. Naples: D'Auria, 99–111.

Congourdeau, M.–H. 2012. 'La médecine byzantine à la croisée de l'Orient et de l'Occident', in A. Speer and P. Steinkrüger (eds.), *Knotenpunkt Byzanz: Wissensformen und kulturelle Wechselbeziehungen*. Berlin: De Gruyter, 223–31.

Constantinides, C. N. 1982. *Higher Education in Byzantium in the Thirteenth and Early Fourteenth Centuries, 1204–ca.1310*. Nicosia: Cyprus Research Centre.

Conticello, V. 1995. 'Pseudo-Cyril's 'De SS. Trinitate'. A Compilation of Joseph the Philosopher', *Orientalia Christiana Periodica* 61: 117–29.

Corput, E. van der. 1905. 'Réga (Henri-Joseph)', *Biographie nationale de Belgique*, vol. 18. Brussels: Bruylant-Christophe & Cie, 842–52.

Costomiris, G. A. 1891. 'Études sur les écrits inédits des anciens médecins grecs', *Revue des Études Grecques* 4: 97–110.

Costomiris, G. A. 1897. 'Études sur les écrits inédits des anciens médecins grecs. Cinquième série, XIIe–XIVe siècles: Jean Tzetzès, Nicolas Myrepsus, Jean Actuarius', *Revue des Études Grecques* 10: 405–45.

Coxe, H. O. 1853. *Catalogi codicum manuscriptorum bibliothecae Bodleianae pars prima, recensionem codicum Graecorum continens*. Oxford: e Typographeo Academico.

Craik, E. M. 2015. *The 'Hippocratic' Corpus: Content and Context*. Abingdon: Routledge.

Criscuolo, R. 1974. 'Note sull' Enciclopedia del filosofo Giuseppe', *Byzantion* 44: 255–81.

Criscuolo, U. 2012. 'Sinesio di Cirene fra neoplatonismo e teologia patristica', in L. M. Hoffmann and H. Seng (eds.), *Synesios von Kyrene: Politik – Literatur – Philosophie*. Turnhout: Brepols, 164–82.

Cronier, M. 2006. 'Quelques aspects de l'histoire du texte du *De materia medica* de Dioscoride', in A. Roselli (ed.), *Ecdotica e ricezione dei testi medici greci*. Naples: D'Auria, 43–65.

Cronier, M., Guardasole, A., Madgelaine, C. and A. Pietrobelli. 2015. 'Galien en procès à Byzance: L'*Antirrhétique* de Syméon Seth', *Galenos* 9: 71–121.

Csepregi, I. 2002. 'The Miracles of Saints Cosmas and Damian: Characteristics of Dream Healing', *Annual of medieval studies at the CEU* 8: 89–123.

Cunningham, A. 1992. 'Transforming Plague: The Laboratory and the Identity of Infectious Disease', in A. Cunningham and P. Williams (eds.), *The Laboratory Revolution in Medicine*. Cambridge: Cambridge University Press, 209–44.

Cunningham, A. 1997. *The Anatomical Renaissance: The Resurrection of the Anatomical Projects of the Ancients*. Aldershot: Scolar Press.

Dalby, A. 2003. *Food in the Ancient World from A–Z*. London: Routledge.

Dalby, A. 2010. *Tastes in Byzantium: The Cuisine of a Legendary Empire*. London: I. B. Tauris.

Dampasis, I. N. 1967. '*Ἰωάννης ὁ Ἀκτουάριος*', *Ἰατρικὰ Χρονικά* 7: 947–61.

Danielewicz, J. 2001. 'Metatext and its Functions in Greek Lyric Poetry', in S. J. Harrison (ed.), *Texts, Ideas, and the Classics*. Oxford: Oxford University Press, 46–61.

Daremberg, Ch. 1853. *Notices et extraits des manuscrits médicaux grecs, latins et français des principales bibliothèques de l'Europe*. Paris: J.-B. Baillière.

Daskas, B. 2016. 'Nikolaos Mesarites, Description of the Church of the Holy Apostles at Constantinople. New Critical Perspectives', *Parekbolai* 6: 79–102.

Debru, A. 1996. 'Les démonstrations médicales à Rome au temps de Galien', in P. J. van der Eijk, H. F. J. Horstmanschoff and P. H. Schrijvers (eds.), *Ancient Medicine in Its Socio-Cultural Context*, vol. 1. Amsterdam: Rodopi, 69–81.

Debru, A. 2008. 'Physiology', in R. J. Hankinson (ed.), *The Cambridge Companion to Galen*. Cambridge: Cambridge University Press, 263–82.

Deichgräber, K. 1971. *Die Epidemien und das Corpus Hippocraticum*. Berlin: Verlag der Akademie der Wissenschaften.

Deichgräber, K. 1982. *Die Patienten des Hippokrates: historisch-prosopographische Beiträge zu den Epidemien des Corpus Hippokraticum*. Mainz: Akademie der Wissenschaften und der Literatur und Wiesbaden.

DelVecchio Good, M.-J. 1995. *American Medicine: The Quest for Competence*. Berkeley: University of California Press.

Demand, N. 1998. 'Women and Slaves as Hippocratic Patients', in S. R. Joshel and S. Murnaghan (eds.), *Women and Slaves in Greco-Roman Culture: Differential Equations*. London: Routledge, 69–84.

Desnos, E. 1914. 'Histoire de l'urologie', in E. Desnos and A. Pousson (eds.), *Encyclopédie française d'urologie*. Paris: O. Doin, I: 1–294.

Devreesse, R. 1945. *Le fonds Coislin*. Paris: Imprimerie Nationale.

Diamandopoulos, A. 1995. *Μουσική Ουροσκοπία*. Patra: Achaikes Ekdoseis.

Diamandopoulos, A. 1997. 'Uroscopy in Byzantium', *American Journal of Nephrology* 17: 222–7.

Diamandopoulos, A. 2000. *Ιστορία της Ελληνικής Νεφρολογίας*. Athens: Papazēsēs.

Diamandopoulos, A. 2001. 'Joannes Zacharias Actuarius. A Witness of Late Byzantine Uroscopy, Closely Linked with Thessaloniki', *Nephrology Dialysis Transplantation* 16 [Suppl. 6]: 2–3.

Diamandopoulos, A. and P. Goudas. 2009. 'Juxtaposition of Actuarius' versus Galen's ideas on Renal Physiology: The Impact of 12 Centuries', *Journal of Nephrology* 22 [Suppl. 14]: 21–32.

Diels, H. 1905–6. *Die Handschriften der antiken Ärzte*. 2 vols. Berlin. [*Abhandlungen der Königlich-Preussischen Akademie der Wissenschaften* 1905, *Phil.-Hist. Kl.* 3 and 1906, *Phil.-Hist. Kl.* 1].

Diels, H. 1908. *Bericht über den Stand des interakademischen Corpus medicorum antiquorum und Erster Nachtrag zu den in den Abhandlungen 1905 und 1906 veröffentlichten Katalogen: Die Handschriften der antiken Ärzte, I. und II. Teil.* [*Abhandlungen der Königlich-Preussischen Akademie der Wissenschaften* 1907, *Phil.-Hist. Kl.* 2].

Diepgen, P. 1949–55. *Geschichte der Medizin: die historische Entwicklung der Heilkunde und des ärztlichen Lebens.* 2 vols. Berlin: De Gruyter.

Dietrich, A. 2012. 'Halīladj', in P. J. Bearman et al. (eds.), *Encyclopedia of Islam.* [2nd edn.] Leiden: Brill, available at http://dx.doi.org/10.1163/1573-3912_islam_SIM_8591 (accessed 21 October 2018).

Dimitriadis, K. 1971. *Byzantinische Uroskopie.* Rheinische Friedrich-Wilhelms-Universität Bonn: PhD thesis.

Dolezal, H. 1957. 'Cordus, 1)', in *Neue deutsche Biographie*, vol. 3. Berlin: Duncker & Humblot, 358–9.

Doyen-Higuet, A. M. 2006. *L'Épitomé de la Collection d'hippiatrie grecque*, vol. 1. Louvain-la-Neuve: Université catholique de Louvain, Institut orientaliste.

Draycott, J. 2016. 'Literary and Documentary Evidence for Lay Medical Practice in the Roman Republic and Empire', in G. Petridou and C. Thumiger (eds.), *Approaches to the Patient in the Ancient World.* Leiden: Brill, 432–50.

Durak, K. 2018. 'From the Indian Ocean to the Markets of Constantinople: Ambergris in the Byzantine World', in B. Pitarakis and G. Tanman (eds.), *Life Is Short, Art Long: The Art of Healing in Byzantium. New Perspectives.* Istanbul: Istanbul Research Institute, 201–25.

Durling, R. J. 1967. *A Catalogue of Sixteenth Century Printed Books in the National Library of Medicine.* Bethesda MD: National Library of Medicine.

Efthymiadis, S. 2014. 'Collections of Miracles (Fifth–Fifteenth Centuries)', in S. Efthymiadis (ed.), *The Ashgate Research Companion to Byzantine Hagiography*, vol. II: *Genres and Contexts.* Farnham: Ashgate, 104–42.

Eftychiades, A. 1983. *Εἰσαγωγὴ εἰς τὴν Βυζαντινὴν Θεραπευτικήν.* Athens: Parisianos.

Eichholz, D. E. 1959. 'Galen and his Environment', *Greece and Rome* 51: 60–71.

Eijk, P. van der. 1997a. 'Towards a Rhetoric of Ancient Scientific Discourse: Some Formal Charecteristics of Greek Medical and Philosophical Texts (Hippocratic Corpus, Aristotle)', in E. J. Bukker (ed.), *Grammar as Interpretation: Greek Literature in Its Linguistic Contexts.* Leiden, Brill, 77–129.

Eijk, P. van der. 1997b. 'Galen's Use of the Concept of "Qualified Experience" in his Dietetic and Pharmacological Works', in A. Debru (ed.), *Galen on Pharmacology.* Leiden: Brill, 35–57.

Eijk, P. van der. 1999. 'Antiquarianism and Criticism: Forms and Functions of Medical Doxography in Methodism (Soranus, Caelius Aurelianus)', in P. J. van der Eijk (ed.), *Ancient Histories of Medicine. Essay in Medical Doxography and Historiography in Classical Antiquity.* Leiden: Brill, 397–452.

Eijk, P. van der. 2008. 'The Art of Medicine: Nemesius of Emesa and Early Brain Mapping', *The Lancet* 371(9637): 440–1.

Eijk, P. van der. 2010. 'Principles and Practices of Compilation and Abbreviation in the Medical "Encyclopaedias" of Late Antiquity', in M. Horster and C. Reitz (eds.), *Condensing Text – Condensed Texts.* Stuttgart: Steiner, 519–54.

Eijk, P. van der. 2015. 'Galen on the Assessment of Bodily Mixtures', in B. Holmes and K.-D. Fischer (eds.), *The Frontiers of Ancient Science: Essays in Honor of Heinrich von Staden*. Berlin: De Gruyter, 675–98.

Eijk, P. van der, Geller, M., Lehmhaus, L., Martelli, M., and C. Salazar. 2015. 'Canons, Authorities and Medical Practice in the Greek Medical Encyclopaedias of Late Antiquity and in the Talmud', in E. Cancik-Kirschbaum and A. Traninger (eds.), *Wissen in Bewegung: Institution – Iteration – Transfer*. Wiesbaden: Harrassowitz, 195–221.

Epstein, J. 1995. *Altered Conditions: Disease, Medicine, and Storytelling*. New York: Routledge.

Fabricius, C. 1972. *Galens Exzerpte aus älteren Pharmakologen*. Berlin: De Gruyter.

Fabricius, J. A. 1724. *Bibliothecae Grecae*, vol. 12. Hamburg: Apud Christian Liebezeit & Theodor Christoph Felginer.

Fancy, N. A. G. 2013. *Science and Religion in Mamluk Egypt: Ibn al-Nafīs, Pulmonary Transit and Bodily Resurrection*. London: Routledge.

Featherstone, J. M. 2011. 'Theodore Metochites's *Semeioseis gnomikai* – Personal encyclopedism', in P. van Deun and C. Macé (eds.), *Encyclopedic Trends in Byzantium?*. Leuven: Peeters.

Fellmann, I. 1986. *Das Aqrābāḏīn al-Qalānisī*. Beirut: Kommission bei F. Steiner Verlag Wiesbaden.

Finlan, S. and V. Kharlamov. 2006. *Theōsis: Deification in Christian Theology*. Eugene OR: Pickwick Publications.

Fischer, E. A. 2004. 'Planoudes' Technique and Competence as a Translator of Ovid's *Metamorphoses*', *Byzantinoslavica* 62: 143–60.

Fischer, K.-D. 1987. '"Universorum ferramentorum nomina": Fruhmittelalterliche Listen chirurgischer Instrumente und ihr griechisches Vorbild', *Mittellateinisches Jahrbuch* 22: 28–44.

Flemming, R. 2007. 'Women, writing and medicine in the classical world', *Classical Quarterly* 57: 257–79.

Fontana, E. 1966. *Il libro delle urine di Isacco l'Ebreo tradotto dall'arabo in latino da Constantino Africano*. Pisa: Giardini.

Formisano, M. 2001. *Tecnica e scrittura: le letterature tecnico-scientifiche nello spazio letterario tardolatino*. Rome: Carocci.

Foust, C. M. 1994. 'Mysteries of Rhubarb: Chinese Medicinal Rhubarb through the Ages', *Pharmacy in History* 36: 155–9.

Frank, A. W. 1995. *The Wounded Storyteller: Body, Illness, and Ethics*. Chicago: University of Chicago Press.

Freind, J. 1744. *The History of Physick*. [4th edn.] London.

Frey, J. and J. Levison. 2014. *The Holy Spirit, Inspiration, and the Cultures of Antiquity: Multidisciplinary Perspectives*. Berlin: De Gruyter.

Fryde, E. B. 2000. *The Early Palaeologan Renaissance (1261–c.1360)*. Leiden: Brill.

Fuchs, F. 1926. *Die höheren Schulen von Konstantinopel im Mittelalter*. Leipzig: Teubner.

Gäbel, R. 2018. 'Mental Illnesses in the Medical Compilations of Late Antiquity: The Case of Aëtius of Amida', in C. Thumiger and P. Singer (eds.), *Mental Illness in Ancient Medicine: From Celsus to Paul of Aegina*. Leiden: Brill, 315–40.

Gabrieli, G. 1905. 'Il <<Zād al Musāfir>> di Ibn al Gazzār in un ms. Greco Corsiniano', *Rendiconti della Reale Accademie dei Lincei, Classe di scienze morali, storiche e filologiche* 14: 29–50.

Gaide, F. and F. Biville. (ed.) 2003. *Manus Medica.* Paris: Publications de l'Université de Provence.

García Ballester, L. 1995. 'Elementos para la construción de las historias clínicas en Galeno', *Dynamis* 15: 47–65.

García Bueno, C. 2017. *El copista griego Jacobo Diasorino (s. XVI): estudio paleográfico y codicológico de sus manuscritos.* Universidad Complutense de Madrid: PhD thesis, available at https://eprints.ucm.es/45368/1/T39363.pdf (accessed 17 August 2018).

García-Sánchez, E. 1998. 'Les techniques de distillation de l'eau de roses à al–Andalus', in R. Gyselen and F. Auballe-Sallenave (eds.), *Parfums d'Orient.* Bures-sur-Yvette: Groupe pour l'etude de la civilisation du Moyen-Orient, 125–40.

Gardthausen, V. E. 1898. *Katalog der griechischen Handschriften der Universitäts-Bibliothek zu Leipzig.* Leipzig: Harrassowitz.

Garofalo, I. 2003. 'Note sulla tradizione alessandrina del *De Differentiis Febrium* di Galeno', in A. Garzya and J. Jouanna (eds.), *Trasmissione e ecdotica dei testi medici greci.* Naples: D'Auria, 149–64.

Garofalo, I. 2019. 'Galen's legacy in Alexandrian texts written in Greek, Latin, and Arabic', in P. Bouras-Vallianatos and B. Zipser (eds.), *Brill's Companion to the Reception of Galen.* Leiden: Brill, 62–85.

Garzya, A. 1984. 'Problèmes relatifs à l'édition des livres IX–XVI du *Tétrabiblon* d'Aétios d'Amida', *Revue des Études Anciennes* 86: 245–57.

Gaul, N. 2007. 'The Twitching Shroud: Collective Construction of *Paideia* in the Circle of Thomas Magistros', *Segno e Testo* 5: 263–340.

Gaul, N. 2011. *Thomas Magistros und die späbyzantinische Sophistik: Studien zum Humanismus urbaner Eliten der frühen Palaiologenzeit.* Wiesbaden: Harrassowitz.

Gaul, N. 2016. 'All The Emperor's Men (And His Nephews): Paideia and Networking Strategies at the Court of Andronikos II Palaiologos, 1290–1320', *Dumbarton Oaks Papers* 70: 153–78.

Gaul, N. 2018. 'Performative Reading in the Late Byzantine *Theatron*', in T. Shawcross and I. Toth (eds.), *Reading in the Byzantine Empire and Beyond.* Cambridge: Cambridge University Press, 215–33.

Geanakoplos, D. J. 1959. *Emperor Michael Palaeologus and the West, 1258–1282: A Study in Byzantine-Latin Relations.* Cambridge MA: Harvard University Press.

Gebhardt, O. von. 1898. 'Christian Friedrich Matthaei und seine Sammlung griechischer Handschriften', *Centralblatt für Bibliothekswesen* 15.12: 537–66.

Geroulanos, S. 2007. 'Surgery in Byzantium', in M. Grünbart, E. Kislinger, A. Muthesius, and D. Stathakopoulos (eds.), *Material Culture and Well-Being in Byzantium (400–1453).* Vienna: Verlag der Österreichischen Akademie der Wissenschaften, 129–34.

Giacomelli, C. 2018. 'Su di un codice greco di Giovanni Zaccaria Attuario nella Biblioteca civica di Padova (C.M. 644)', *Revue d'Histoire des Textes* 13: 93–127.

Gielen, E. 2011. 'Joseph the Philosopher, an Outstanding Outsider: Philosophy and Rhetoric at the Court of Andronikos II', in G. Nathan and L. Garland (eds.),

Basileia: Essays on Imperium and Culture. Brisbane: Australian Association for Byzantine Studies, 205–15.

Gielen, E. 2013. '*Ad Maiorem Dei Gloriam*. Joseph Rhakendytès' Synopsis of Byzantine Learning', in J. König and G. Woolf (eds.), *Encyclopaedism from Antiquity to the Renaissance*. Cambridge: Cambridge University Press, 260–76.

Gielen, E. 2016. *Nicephori Blemmydae de virtute et ascesi. Iosephi Racendytae de virtute*. Turnhout: Brepols.

Gielen, E. 2018. 'Physician versus Physician: Comparing the Audience of *On the Constitution of Man* by Meletios and *Epitome on the Nature of Men* by Leo the Physician', in P. Bouras-Vallianatos and S. Xenophontos (eds.), *Greek Medical Literature and Its Readers: From Hippocrates to Islam and Byzantium*. New York: Routledge, 153–79.

Gill, C. 2010. *Naturalistic Psychology in Galen and Stoicism*. Oxford: Oxford University Press.

Gleason, M. W. 2009. 'Shock and Awe: The Perfomance Dimension of Galen's Anatomy Demonstrations', in C. Gill, T. Whitmarsh, and J. Wilkins (eds.), *Galen and the World of Knowledge*. Cambridge: Cambridge University Press, 85–114.

Glick, T. F. 2005. 'Translation Movements', in T. F. Glick, S. J. Livesey, and F. Wallis (eds.), *Medieval Science, Technology, and Medicine: An Encyclopedia*. London: Routledge, 482–6.

Glycofrydi-Leontsini, A. 2003. 'Demetrius Cydones as a Translator of Latin Texts', in C. Dendrinos et al. (eds.), *Porphyrogenita: Essays on the History and Literature of Byzantium and the Latin East in Honour of Julian Chrysostomides*. Aldershot: Ashgate, 175–85.

Goffman, E. 1959. *The Presentation of Self in Everyday Life*. Garden City NY: Doubleday.

Golitsis, P. 2008. 'Georges Pachymère comme didascale: essai pour une reconstitution de sa carrière et de son enseignement philosophique', *Jahrbuch de Österreichischen Byzantinistik* 58: 53–68.

Good, B. 1994. *Medicine, Rationality, and Experience*. Cambridge: Cambridge University Press.

Gossen, H. 1916. 'Johannes Aktuarios', in G. Wissowa (ed.), *Realencyclopädie der classischen Altertumswissenschaft*, vol. 9. Stuttgart: J. B. Metzler: 1799–800.

Gourevitch, D. 2001. *I giovani pazienti di Galeno: per una patocenosi dell'impero romano*. Rome: Laterza.

Gregoric, P., Lewis, O., and M. Kuhar. 2015. 'The Substance of *De Spiritu*', *Early Science and Medicine* 20: 101–24.

Grimm-Stadelmann, I. 2008. *Θεοφίλου περὶ τῆς τοῦ ἀνθρώπου κατασκευῆς. Theophilos. Der Aufbau des Menschen. Kritische Edition des Textes mit Einleitung, Übersetzung und Kommentar*. Ludwig-Maximilians-Universität München: PhD thesis, available at https://edoc.ub.uni-muenchen.de/9393/1/Grimm_Stadelmann_Isabel.pdf (accessed 17 August 2018).

Grumel, V. 1949. 'La profession médicale à Byzance à l'époque des Comnènes', *Revue des Études Byzantines* 7: 42–6.

Guardasole, A. 2004a. 'L'héritage de Galien dans l'oeuvre d'Alexandre de Tralles', in J. Jouanna and J. Leclant (eds.), *Colloque La médecine grecque antique, Cahiers de la Villa «Kérylos»*. Paris: Académie des Inscriptions et Belles Lettres, 211–26.

Guardasole, A. 2004b. 'Alexandre de Tralles et les remédes naturels', in F. Collard and E. Samama (eds.), *Mires, physiciens, barbiers et charlatans: les marges de la medicine de l' Antiquité au XVIe siècle*. Langres: D. Gueniot, 81–99.

Guardasole, A. 2015. 'Les traités de pharmacologie de Galien et les extraits des médecins antérieurs: un témoignage important sur la formation du langage scientifique spécialisé', in S. Morlet (ed.), *Lire en extraits: lecture et production des textes de l'Antiquité à la fin du Moyen Âge*. Paris: PUPS, 73–90.

Gutas, D. 2012. 'Arabic into Byzantine Greek: Introducing a Survey of the Translations', in A. Speer and P. Steinkrüger (eds.), *Knotenpunkt Byzanz: Wissensformen und kulturelle Wechselbeziehungen*. Berlin: De Gruyter, 246–64.

Gutas, D., Kaldellis, A., and B. Long. 2017. 'Intellectual Exchanges with the Arab World', in A. Kaldellis and N. Siniossoglou (eds.), *The Cambridge Intellectual History of Byzantium*. Cambridge: Cambridge University Press, 79–98.

Haeser, H. 1875–82. *Lehrbuch der Geschichte der Medizin und der epidemischen Krankheiten*. 3 vols. Jena: Hermann Dufft.

Hagedorn, U. and D. Hagedorn. 2004. 'Thessalos über die Amateurärzte', in H. Harrauer and R. Pintaudi (eds.), *Gedenkschrift Ulrike Horak*. Florence: Gonnelli, 5–8.

Hankinson, R. J. 1991. 'Galen's Anatomy of the Soul', *Phronesis* 36: 197–233.

Hankinson, R. J. 2016. 'Humours and Humoral Theory', in M. Jackson (ed.), *The Routledge History of Disease*. Abingdon: Routledge, 21–37.

Hanson, A. E. 1989. 'Diseases of Women in the *Epidemics*', in G. Baader and R. Winau (eds.), *Die Hippokratischen Epidemien: Theorie–Praxis–Tradition*. Stuttgart: Steiner, 38–53.

Hanson, J. 2010. 'The Rise and Fall of the Macedonian Renaissance', in L. James (ed.), *A Companion to Byzantium*. Hoboken: John Wiley, 341–50.

Hardt, I. 1810. *Catalogus codicum manuscriptorum graecorum Bibliothecae Regiae Bavaricae*, vol. 4. Munich: Typis I. E. Seidelii Solisbacensis.

Hardwick, L. 2003. *Reception Studies*. Oxford: Oxford University Press.

Hardy, F. G. and L. M. V. Totelin. 2016. *Ancient Botany*. London: Routledge.

Harig, G. 1967. 'Von den arabischen Quellen des Symeon Seth', *Medizinhistorisches Journal* 2: 248–68.

Harig, G. 1971. 'Zum Problem "Krankenhaus" in der Antike', *Klio* 53: 179–96.

Harris, C. R. S. 1973. *The Heart and the Vascular System in Ancient Greek Medicine, from Alcmaeon to Galen*. Oxford: Clarendon Press.

al-Hassan, A. Y. and D. R. Hill. 1992. *Islamic Technology: An Illustrated History*. Cambridge: Cambridge University Press.

Hasse, D. N. 2016. *Success and Suppression: Arabic Sciences and Philosophy in the Renaissance*. Cambridge MA: Harvard University Press.

Hecker, J. F. C. 1829. *Geschichte der neueren Heilkunde*. Berlin: Enslin.

Helmreich, G. 1913. *Handschriftliche Studien zu Symeon Seth*. Ansbach: Brügel.

Hinterberger, M. 2001. 'Studien zu Theodoros Metochites', *Jahrbuch der Österreichischen Byzantinistik* 51: 285–319.

Hirschberg, J. 1887. 'Die Augenheilkunde bei den Griechen', *Albrecht von Graefe's Archiv für Ophthalmologie* 33: 47–78.

Hohlweg, A. 1983. 'Johannes Aktuarios. Leben, Bildung und Ausbildung. *De Methodo Medendi*', *Byzantinische Zeitschrift* 76: 302–21.

Hohlweg, A. 1984. 'John Actuarius' *De Methodo Medendi* – On the New Edition', *Dumbarton Oaks Papers* 38: 121–33.

Hohlweg, A. 1988. 'Medizinischer "Enzyklopädismus" und das *ΠΟΝΗΜΑ ΙΑΤΡΙ-ΚΟΝ* des Michael Psellos', *Byzantinische Zeitschrift* 81: 39–49.

Hohlweg, A. 1989. 'La formazione culturale e professionale del medico a Bisanzio', *Koinonia* 13: 165–88.

Hohlweg, A. 1991. 'Terminologie in byzantinischen medizinischen Texten und Lexikographie', in W. Hörandner and E. Trapp (eds.), *Lexicographica Byzantina*. Vienna: Verlag der Österreichischen Akademie der Wissenschaften, 129–35.

Hohlweg, A. 1995. 'Drei anonyme Texte suchen einen Autor', *Βυζαντιακά* 15: 13–45.

Hohlweg, A. 1996a. 'Astronomie und Geschichtsbetrachtung bei Nikephoros Gregoras', in W. Seibt (ed.), *Geschichte und Kultur der Palaiologenzeit*. Vienna: Verlag der Österreichischen Akademie der Wissenschaften, 51–63.

Hohlweg, A. 1996b. 'Seelenlehre und Psychiatrie bei dem Aktouarios Johannes Zacharias', in P. Pellegrin and R. Wittern (eds.), *Hippokratische Medizin und antike Philosophie*. Hildesheim: Olms-Weidmann, 513–30.

Hohlweg, A. 1997. '*Στάγματα* I', in U. Criscuolo and R. Maisano (eds.), *Synodia: studia humanitatis Antonio Garzya septuagenario ab amicis atque discipulis dicata*. Naples: D'Auria, 423–9.

Holmes, C. 2010. 'Byzantine Political Culture and Compilation Literature in the Tenth and Eleventh Centuries: Some Preliminary Inquiries', *Dumbarton Oaks Papers* 64: 55–80.

Holton, D. and I. Manolessou. 2010. 'Medieval and Early Modern Greek', in E. J. Bakker (ed.), *A Companion to the Ancient Greek Language*. Oxford: Wiley-Blackwell, 539–63.

Hörandner, W. 2012. 'The Byzantine Didactic Poem – A Neglected Literary Genre? A Survey with Special Reference to the Eleventh Century', in F. Bernard and K. Demoen (eds.), *Poetry and its Contexts in Eleventh-century Byzantium*. Farnham: Ashgate, 55–67.

Horden, P. 2005. 'How Medicalised were Byzantine Hospitals', *Medicina e Storia* 10: 45–74.

Horrocks, G. 2010. *Greek: A History of the Language and its Speakers*. [2nd edn.] Malden MA: Wiley-Blackwell.

Horstmanshoff, H. F. J. 1990. 'The Ancient Physician: Craftsman or Scientist?', *Journal of the History of Medicine and Allied Sciences* 45: 176–97.

Horstmanshoff, H. F. J. 1995. 'Galen and his Patients', in P. J. van der Eijk, H. F. J. Horstmanschoff, and P. H. Schrijvers (eds.), *Ancient Medicine in Its Socio-Cultural Context*, vol. 1. Amsterdam: Rodopi, 83–99.

Hult, K. 2002. *Theodore Metochites on Ancient Authors and Philosophy: Semeioseis Gnomikai 1–26 & 71, A Critical Edition with Introduction, Translation, Notes, and Indexes*. Gothenburg: Acta Universitatis Gothoburgensis.

Hummel, C. 1999. *Das Kind und seine Krankheiten in der griechischen Medizin: von Aretaios bis Johannes Aktuarios (1. bis 14. Jahrhundert)*. Frankfurt am Main: Peter Lang.

Hunger, H. 1961–94. *Katalog der griechischen Handschriften der Österreichischen Nationalbibliothek*. 4 vols. Vienna: G. Prachner Verlag.

Hunger, H. 1978. *Die hochsprachliche profane Literatur der Byzantiner*. 2 vols. Munich: Beck.

Hunter, K. M. 1991. *Doctors' stories: The Narrative Structure of Medical Knowledge*. Princeton: Princeton University Press.

Ieraci Bio, A. M. 1982. 'Testi medici di uso strumentale', *Jahrbuch der Österreichischen Byzantinistik* 32: 33–43.

Ieraci Bio, A. M. 1989. 'La trasmissione della letteratura medica Greca nell'Italia meridionale fra X e XV secolo', in A. Garzya (ed.), *Contributi alla cultura greca nell'Italia meridionale*. Naples: Bibliopolis, 133–255.

Ieraci Bio, A. M. 1991. 'Sulla concezione del medico pepaideuménos in Galeno e nel Tardoantico', in J. A. Lopez Férez (ed.), *Galeno: obra, pensamiento e influencia*. Madrid: Universidad Nacional de Educación a Distancia, 133–51.

Ieraci Bio, A. M. 1996. *Paolo di Nicea. Manuale medico*. Naples: Bibliopolis.

Ieraci Bio, A. M. 2003. '*Disiecta membra* della scuola iatrosofistica alessandrina', in I. Garofalo and A. Roselli (eds.), *Galenismo e medicina tardoantica: fonti greche, latine e arabe*. Naples: Annali dell'Istituto Universitario Orientale di Napoli, 9–51.

Ieraci Bio, A. M. 2006. 'La medicina greca dello Stretto (Filippo Xeros ed Eufemio Siculo)', in F. Burgarella and A. M. Ieraci Bio (eds.), *La cultura scientifica e tecnica nell'Italia meridionale Bizantina*. Soveria Mannelli: Rubbettino.

Ieraci Bio, A. M. 2007. 'Testi ginecologi tra Oriente ed Occidente. 1. *Metrodora* ed il *Dynameron* di Nicola Mirepso. 2. Una testimonianza italo-greca su una *Quaestio medicalis* salernitana', in D. Jacquart and A. Paravicini-Bagliani (eds.), *La Scuola Medica Salernitana. Gli autori e i testi*. Firenze: SISMEL, 283–314.

Ieraci Bio, A. M. 2010. 'Giovanni Argiropulo e un inedito commento anonimo a Galeno (*ars. med.* 1, 1a–b7) nel Vat. gr. 285', in V. Boudon-Millot, A. Garzya, J. Jouanna, and A. Roselli (eds.), *Storia della tradizione e edizione dei medici greci*. Naples: D'Auria, 271–90.

Ieraci Bio, A. M. 2013. 'Giovanni Argiropulo e la medicina, tra l'Italia e Constantinopoli', in A. Rigo, A. Babuin, and M. Trizio (eds.), *Vie per Bisanzio*. Bari: Edizioni di Pagina, 788–803.

Ieraci Bio, A. M. 2014. 'Nuovi apporti sull'ippocratismo a Bisanzi', in J. Jouanna and M. Zink (eds.), *Hippocrate et les hippocratismes: Médecine, religion, société*. Paris: Académie des Inscriptions et Belles Lettres, 401–20.

Ieraci Bio, A. M. 2017. 'La sistematizzazione della farmacologia a Bisanzio: il *Dynameron* di Nicola Mirepso e le fonti 'occidentali'', in L. Lehmhaus and M. Martelli (eds.), *Collecting Recipes: Byzantine and Jewish Pharmacology in Dialogue*. Berlin: De Gruyter, 301–14.

Ierodiakonou, K. 2014. 'On Galen's Theory of Vision', in P. Adamson, R. Hansberger, and J. Wilberding (eds.), *Philosophical Themes in Galen*. London: Institute of Classical Studies, 235–47.

Irigoin, J. 1959. 'Pour une étude des centres de copie bizantins (suite)', *Scriptorium* 13: 177–209.

Iskandar, A. 1976. 'An Attempted Reconstruction of the Late Alexandrian Medical Curriculum', *Medical History* 20: 235–58.

Jackson, R. P. J. 1993. 'Roman Medicine: The Practitioners and their Practices', *Aufstieg und Niedergang der römischen Welt* II. 37.1: 80–101.

Jackson, R. P. J. 2003. 'The Domus 'del chirurgo' at Rimini: An Interim Account of the Medical Assemblage', *Journal of Roman Archaeology* 16: 312–21.

Jacoby, D. 1995. 'Les Italiens en Egypte aux XIIe et XIIIe siecles: du comptoir a la colonie?', in M. Balard and A. Duceller (eds.), *Coloniser au Moyen Âge. Méthodes d'expansion et techniques de domination en Méditerranée du 11e au 16e siècle*. Paris: A. Colin, 76–88.

Jacoby, D. 1998. 'The Trade of Crusader Acre in the Levantine Context: An Overview', *Archivio Storico del Sannio*, n.s., 3: 103–20.

Jacoby, D. 2008. 'Marino Sanudo Torsello on Trade Routes, Commodities, and Taxation', in M. Losacco, C. Maltezou, and P. Schreiner (eds.), *Philanagnostes. Studi in onore di Marino Zorzi*. Venice: Instituto Ellenico di Studi Zizantini e Postbizantini di Venezia, 185–97.

Jacoby, D. 2016. 'Constantinople as Commercial Transit Center, Tenth to Mid-Fifteenth Century', in P. Magdalino, N. Necipoğlu, and I. Jevtić (eds.), *Trade in Byzantium*. Istanbul: Koç Üniversitesi, Anadolu Medeniyetleri Araştirma Merkezi, 193–210.

Jacques, V. 1897. 'Mathys (Henri *ou* Corneille-Henri)', in *Biographie nationale de Belgique*, vol. 14. Brussels: Bruylant-Christophe & Cie, 69–71.

James, M. R. 1902. *The Western Manuscripts in the Library of Trinity College Cambridge. A Descriptive Catalogue*, vol. 3. Cambridge: Cambridge University Press.

James, M. R. 1907. *A Descriptive Catalogue of the Manuscripts in the Library of Gonville and Caius College*, vol. 1. Cambridge: Cambridge University Press.

Janin, R. 1969. *La géographie ecclésiastique de l'Empire byzantin, Première partie: Le siege de Constantinople et le patriarcat oecuménique*, vol. 3. *Les églises et les monastères*. [2nd edn.] Paris: Institut français d'études byzantines.

Jeffreys, M. 2017. 'Summaries of the Letters of Michael Psellos', in M. Jeffreys and M. D. Lauxtermann (eds.), *The Letters of Psellos: Cultural Networks and Historical Realities*. Oxford: Oxford University Press, 143–445.

Johnson, W. 2010. *Readers and Reading Culture in the High Roman Empire: A Study of Elite Communities*. Oxford: Oxford University Press.

Johnson-Eilola, J. and S. Selber. 2007. 'Plagiarism, Originality, Assemblage', *Computers and Composition* 24: 375–403.

Johnston, I. 2006. *Galen: On Diseases and Symptoms*. Cambridge: Cambridge University Press.

Johnston, I. 2018. 'Galen and His System of Medicine', in P. T Keyser with J. Scarborough (eds.), *The Oxford Handbook of Science and Medicine in the Classical World*. Oxford: Oxford University Press, 765–87.

Johnston, I. and G. H. R. Horsley. 2011. *Galen Method of Medicine, Books 1–4*. Cambridge MA: Harvard University Press.

Johnston, S. 2008. 'Robert Recorde', in *Oxford Dictionary of National Biography*. Oxford: Oxford University Press, available at https://doi.org/10.1093/ref:odnb/23241 (accessed 17 Octover 2018).

Jordanova, L. J. 2006. *History in Practice*. [2nd edn.] London: Hodder Arnold.

Jori, A. 2009. 'Medizinische Bildung für Laien: Der Beitrag Plutarchs', *Sudhoffs Archiv* 93: 67–82.

Jouanna, J. 1999. *Hippocrates*. Baltimore: Johns Hopkins University Press. [Originally published in French: 1992. *Hippocrate*. Paris: Librairie Arthème Fayard.]

Jouanna, J. 2006. 'La postérité du traité hippocratique la *Nature de l'homme*: la théorie des quatre humeurs', in C. W. Müller, C. Brockmann, and C. W. Brunschön (eds.), *Ärzte und ihre Interpreten. Medizinische Fachtexte der Antike als Forschungsgegenstand der klassischen Philologie: Fachkonferenz zu Ehren von Diethard Nickel.* Munich: Saur, 117–41.

Jouanna, J. 2011. 'Médecine rationnelle et magie: le statut des amulettes et des incantations chez Galien', *Revue des Études Grecques* 124: 47–77.

Julião, R. 2018. 'Galen on Memory, Forgetting and Memory Loss', in C. Thumiger and P. Singer (eds.), *Mental Illness in Ancient Medicine: From Celsus to Paul of Aegina.* Leiden: Brill, 222–44.

Kakavelaki, A. 2012. *Η Έννοια του Πνεύματος κατά την Αρχαία και τη Βυζαντινή Περίοδο.* University of Athens: PhD thesis, available at https://www.didaktorika.gr/eadd/handle/10442/33268 (accessed 17 August 2018).

Kakavelaki, A. 2016. '*Η Θεωρία της Τριμερούς Διάκρισης του Πνεύματος στην Αρχαία Ελληνική Ιατρική: Ανασύσταση της Θεωρίας Αυτής Μέσω Βυζαντινών Κειμένων και Παρουσίαση της Σχετικής Θεωρίας του Βυζαντινού Ιατρού Ιωάννη Ζαχαρία Ακτουάριου*', *ΝΕΥΣΙΣ* 24: 225–41.

Kakavelaki, A. 2018. *Η Έννοια του Πνεύματος κατά την Αρχαία και τη Βυζαντινή Περίοδο. Μελέτη της Αρχαίας και της Βυζαντινής Φιλοσοφίας και Ιατρικής.* Athens: Ērodotos.

Kakoulidi, E. 1968. '*Ἡ Βιβλιοθήκη τῆς Μονῆς Προδρόμου–Πέτρας στὴν Κωνσταντινούπολη*', *Ἑλληνικά* 21: 3–39.

Kaldellis, A. 2007. *Hellenism in Byzantium: The Transformation of Greek Identity and the Reception of the Classical Tradition.* Cambridge: Cambridge University Press.

Kaldellis, A. 2013. *Ethnography After Antiquity: Foreign Lands and Peoples in Byzantine Literature.* Philadelphia: University of Pennsylvania Press.

Kaldellis, A. 2018. *Catalogue of Translations into Byzantine Greek From Texts in Any Other Language, 300–1453 AD* (Version III), available at https://www.academia.edu/36711128/Kaldellis_Catalogue_of_Translations_into_Byzantine_Greek_version_III_ (accessed 18 July 2019).

Kaliszuk, J. and S. Szyller. 2012. *Inwentarz rękopisów do połowy XVI wieku w zbiorach Biblioteki Narodowej.* Warsaw: Biblioteka Narodowa.

Kalopissi-Verti, S. 2004. 'Patronage and Artistic Production in Byzantium during the Palaiologan Period', in S. T. Brooks (ed.), *Byzantium: Faith and Power (1261–1557).* New York: Metropolitan Museum of Art, 76–97.

Kappes, C. (unpublished). 'The Dominican Presentation and Byzantine Reception of Thomas Aquinas in Byzantium', available at https://www.academia.edu/5503943/The_Dominican_Presentation_and_Byzantine_Reception_of_Thomas_Aquinas_in_Byzantium (accessed 27 March 2019).

Karayannopulos, J. 1958. *Das Finanzwesen des frühbyzantinischen Staates.* Munich: R. Oldenbourg.

Karlsson, G. H. and G. Fatouros. 1973. 'Aus der Briefsammlung des Anonymus Florentinus', *Jahrbuch der Österreichischen Byzantinistik* 22: 207–18.

Karpozilos, A. 1990. 'The Correspondence of Theodore Hyrtakenos', *Jahrbuch der Österreichischen Byzantinistik* 40: 275–84.

Karpozilos, A. 2008. 'Some Excerpts from Paulos Aiginetes in the *De Diagnosi* of Ioannes Aktouarios', in C. Stavrakos, A.-K. Wassiliou and M. Krikorian (eds.), *Hypermachos: Festschrift für Werner Seibt zum 65. Geburtstag*. Wiesbaden: Harrassowitz, 133–8.

Keil, G. 1969. *Der 'Kurze Harntraktat' des Breslauer 'Codex Salernitanus' und seine Sippe*. Rheinische Friedrich-Wilhelms-Universität Bonn: PhD thesis.

King, H. 1998. *Hippocrates' Woman: Reading the Female Body in Ancient Greece*. London: Routledge.

Kislinger, E. 1987. 'Der Pantokrator-Xenon, ein Trügerisches ideal?', *Jahrbuch der Österreichischen Byzantinistik* 37: 173–9.

Kissling, R. C. 1922. 'The Ὄχημα–Πνεῦμα of the Neo-Platonists and the De Insomniis of Synesius of Cyrene', *The American Journal of Philology* 43: 318–30.

Kleinman, A. 1988. *The Illness Narratives: Suffering, Healing and the Human Condition*. New York: Basic Books.

Koder, J. 1993. *Gemüse in Byzanz: die Versorgung Konstantinopels mit Frischgemüse im Lichte der Geoponika*. Vienna: Fassbaender.

Koetschet, P. 2016. 'Experiencing Madness: Mental Patients in Medieval Arabo-Islamic Medicine', in G. Petridou and C. Thumiger (eds), *Approaches to the Patient in the Ancient World*. Leiden: Brill, 224–44.

Kolovou, F. 2012. 'Ein Bischof *KAT'OIKONOMIAN* in spätbyzantinischen Urteilen: Synesios von Kyrene und Nikephoros Gregoras' Protheoria zu *De insomniis*', in L. M. Hoffmann and H. Seng (eds.), *Synesios von Kyrene: Politik – Literatur – Philosophie*. Turnhout: Brepols, 388–403.

König, J. 2005. *Athletics and Literature in the Roman Empire*. Cambridge: Cambridge University Press.

König, J. 2011. 'Self-Promotion and Self-Effacement in Plutarch's Table Talk', in F. Klotz and K. Oikonomopoulou (eds.), *The Philosopher's Banquet*. Oxford: Oxford University Press, 179–203.

Kontogiannopoulou, A. 2012. '*Η Προσηγορία Κυρ στη Βυζαντινή Κοινωνία*', *Βυζαντινά* 32: 209–26.

Kourousis, S. 1972. *Μανουὴλ Γαβαλᾶς εἶτα Ματθαῖος Μητροπολίτης Ἐφέσου (1271/2–1355/60)*. Athens: Myrtidēs.

Kourousis, S. 1978/9. '*Τὸ Ἐπιστολάριον Γεωργίου Λακαπηνοῦ καὶ Ἀνδρονίκου Ζαρίδου*,' *Ἀθηνᾶ* 77: 291–386.

Kourousis, S. 1980/2. '*Ὁ Ἀκτουάριος Ἰωάννης Ζαχαρίας Παραλήπτης τῆς Ἐπιστολῆς ι' τοῦ Γεωργίου Λακαπηνοῦ*,' *Ἀθηνᾶ* 78: 237–76.

Kourousis, S. 1984/8. *Τὸ Ἐπιστολάριον Γεωργίου Λακαπηνοῦ – Ἀνδρονίκου Ζαρίδου (1299 – 1315 ca.) καὶ ὁ Ἰατρὸς – Ἀκτουάριος Ἰωάννης Ζαχαρίας (1275 ca. – 1328/;). Μελέτη Φιλολογική*. Athens: Papadakēs.

Kourousis, S. 1985/9. '*Ὁ Ἀκτουάριος Ἰωάννης ὁ Ζαχαρίας* (1275 ca. – 1330 ca.) *Πρόδρομος Κακοδοξιῶν Βαρλαὰμ τοῦ Καλαβροῦ* (1290 ca. – 1348)', *Ἀθηνᾶ* 80: 385–406.

Kourousis, S. 1997/9. '*Ὁ Ἀκτουάριος Ἰωάννης Ζαχαρίας Συγγραφεὺς Ἀποδοθέντων Αὐτῷ μὴ Ἰατρικῶν Πονημάτων*', *Ἀθηνᾶ* 82: 27–84.

Kousis, A. P. 1933. '*Ἰωάννης ὁ Ἀκτουάριος*', in *Μεγάλη Ἑλληνικὴ Ἐγκυκλοπαίδεια*, vol. 13. Athens: Pyrsos, 361–7.

Kousis, A. P. 1946. 'Some New Informations on Antony Pyropoulos as Physician and on His Small Notice: '*Περὶ μέτρων καὶ σταθμῶν*' According the Codex 877 of the Iberian Monastery on Mount Athos and the Cod. med. gr. 27 of the National Library of Vienna', *Πρακτικὰ Ἀκαδημίας Ἀθηνῶν* 21: 9–18.

Krausmüller, D. 2006. 'The Rise of Hesychasm', in M. Angold (ed.), *The Cambridge History of Christianity,* vol. 5: *Eastern Christianity*. Cambridge: Cambridge University Press, 101–26.

Krischer, T. 1965. 'Herodots Prooimion', *Hermes* 93: 159–67.

Kroll, W. 1912. 'Hermippos', in *Real-Encyclopädie der classischen Alterthumswissenschaft*, vol. 7. Stuttgart: J. B. Metzler, 854–7.

Krueger, H. C. 1963. *Avicenna's Poem on Medicine*. Springfield: C. Thomas Publisher.

Krumbacher, K. 1897. *Geschichte der byzantinischen Litteratur: von Justinian bis zum Ende des oströmischen Reiches (527–1453).* Munich: Beck.

Kudlien, F. 1968a. *Die Sklaven in der griechischen Medizin in der klassischen und hellenistischen Zeit.* Wiesbaden: Steiner.

Kudlien, F. 1968b. 'Pneumatische Ärzte', in G. Wissowa (ed.), *Realencyclopädie der classischen Altertumswissenschaft*, vol. 11. Stuttgart: J. B. Metzler, Supplementband, 1097–108.

Kudlien, F. 1973. 'Empirie und Theorie in der Harnlehre des Johannes Aktuarios', *Clio Medica* 8: 19–30.

Kyritses, D. 1997. *The Byzantine Aristocracy in the Thirteenth and Early Fourtheenth Centuries.* Harvard University: PhD thesis.

Lacy, P. de. 1988. 'The Third Part of the Soul', in P. Manuli and M. Vegetti (eds.), *Le opere psicologiche di Galeno*. Naples: Bibliopolis, 43–63.

Laín Entralgo, P. 1950. *La historia clínica: Historia e teoria del relato patografico.* Madrid: Consejo superior de investigaciones cientificas.

Laiou, A. 1972. *Constantinople and the Latins. The Foreign Policy of Andronicus II 1282–1328.* Cambridge MA: Harvard University Press.

Laiou, A. 2000. 'The Byzantine Empire in the Fourteenth Century', in M. Jones (ed.), *The New Cambridge Medieval History,* vol. 6. *c.1300–c.1415.* Cambridge: Cambridge University Press, 795–824.

Laiou, A. 2003. 'Economic Concerns and Attitudes of the Intellectuals of Thessalonike', *Dumbarton Oaks Papers* 57: 205–23.

Lamagna, M. 2003a. 'La *Recensio amplior* inedita del *De urinis* di Avicenna', in A. Garzya and J. Jouanna (eds.), *Trasmissione e ecdotica dei testi medici greci.* Naples: D'Auria, 271–80.

Lamagna, M. 2003b. 'Il trattato *De urinis* di Stefano d'Atene e l'uroscopia Alessandrina', in I. Garofalo and A. Roselli (eds.), *Galenismo e medicina tardoantica fonti greche, latine e arabe.* Naples: Istituto Universitario Orientale, 52–73.

Lamagna, M. 2010. 'Gli *Scoli a Magno* di Stefano d'Atene', in V. Boudon-Millot, A. Garzya, J. Jouanna, and A. Roselli (eds.), *Storia della tradizione e edizione dei medici greci.* Naples: D'Auria, 241–57.

Lamagna, M. 2011. 'Per l'edizione del *De Urinis* attribuito ad Avicenna: studio complessivo della tradizione manoscritta', *Revue d'Histoire des Textes* 6: 27–59.

Lamagna, M. 2016. 'La revisione di una traduzione. Il lavoro di Giovanni Attuario sulla *Synopsis* di Cristodulo', in M. T. Santamaría Hernández (ed.), *Traducción y transmisión doctrinal de la Medicina grecolatina desde la Antigüedad hasta el Mundo Moderno: nuevas aportaciones sobre autores y textos*. Cuenca: Ediciones de la Universidad de Castilla-La Mancha, 51–63.

Lambeck, P. and A. F. Kollár. 1766–90. *Commentariorum de augustissima Bibliotheca caesarea Vindobonensi.* 9 vols. Vienna: Typis et sumptibus Joan. Thomae Nob. de Trattnern, Augustae Aulae typographi, et bibliopolae Vindobonensis.

Lambros, S. P. 1895–1900. *Catalogue of the Greek Manuscripts on Mount Athos*. 2 vols. Cambridge: Cambridge University Press.

Lampsides, O. 1938. 'Georges Chrysococcis, le médecin, et son oeuvre', *Byzantiniscshe Zeitischrift* 38: 310–22.

Langholf, V. 1990. *Medical Theories in Hippocrates: Early Texts and the 'Epidemics'*. Berlin: De Gruyter.

Langkavel, B. 1866. *Botanik der spaeteren Griechen*. Berlin: F. Berggold.

Lascaratos, J., Tsiamis, C. and A. Kostakis. 2003. 'Surgery for Iguinal Hernia in Byzantine Times (AD 324–1453): First Scientific Descriptions', *World Journal of Surgery* 27: 1165–9.

Lautner, P. 2013. '*Γνωστικῶς* and / or *ὑλικῶς*: Philoponus' Account of the Material Aspects of Sense-Perception', *Phronesis* 58: 378–400.

Lazaris, S. 2006. 'La production nouvelle en médecine vétérinaire sous les Paléologues et l'œuvre cynégétique de Dèmètrios Pépagôménos', in M. Cacouros and M.-H. Congourdeau (eds.), *Philosophie et Sciences à Byzance de 1204 à 1453*. Leuven: Peeters, 225–67.

Lazaris, S. 2010. *Art et science vétérinaire à Byzance*. Turnhout: Brepols.

Lebègue, H. 1924. *Catalogue des manuscrits alchimiques grecs*, vol. 1: *Les Parisini*. Brussels: Lamertin.

Lefort, J. 1998. 'La brève histoire du jeune Bragadin', in I. Ševčenko and I. Hutter (eds.), *ΑΕΤΟΣ. Studies in honour of Cyril Mango presented to him on April 14, 1998*. Stuttgart-Leipzig: Teubner, 210–19.

Letts, M. 2016. 'Questioning the Patient, Questioning Hippocrates: Rufus of Ephesus and the Pursuit of Knolwedge', in G. Petridou and C. Thumiger (eds), *Approaches to the Patient in the Ancient World*. Leiden: Brill, 81–103.

Lev, E. 2013. 'Mediators between Theoretical and Practial Medieval Knowledge: Medial Notebooks from the Cairo Genizah and their Significance', *Medical History* 57: 487–515.

Lev, E. and Z. Amar. 2008. *Practical Materia Medica of the Medieval Eastern Mediterranean According to the Cairo Genizah*. Leiden: Brill.

Leven, K.-H. 2004. "At Time These Ancient Facts Seem to Lie Before Me Like a Patient on a Hospital Bed'–Retrospective Diagnosis and Ancient Medical History', in H. F. J. Horstmanshoff and M. Stol (eds.), *Magic and Rationality in Ancient Near Eastern and Graeco-Roman Medicine*. Leiden: Brill, 369–86.

Leven, K.-H. (ed.). 2005a. *Antike Medizin: ein Lexikon*. Munich: Beck.

Leven, K.-H. (ed.). 2005b. 'Hypochonder', in K.-H. Leven (ed.), *Antike Medizin: ein Lexikon*. Munich: Beck, 448.

Levey, M. 1973. *Early Arabic Pharmacology*. Leiden: Brill.

Lewis, O. 2015. 'Marcellinus' De pulsibus: a Neglected Treatise on the Ancient "Art of Pulse"', *Scripta Classica Israelica* 34: 195–214.

Lewis, O. 2017. *Praxagoras of Cos on Arteries, Pulse and Pneuma. Fragments and Interpretation*. Leiden: Brill.

Lewis, O. and P. Gregoric. 2015. 'The Context of *De Spiritu*', *Early Science and Medicine* 20: 125–49.

Lewy, Y. 1978. *Chaldaean Oracles and Theurgy: Mysticism, Magic and Platonism in the Later Roman Empire*. Paris: Etudes Augustiniennes.

Lilla, S. R. C. 1985. *Codices Vaticani Graeci: codices 2162–2254*. Vatican City: in Bibliotheca Vaticana.

Lloyd, G. E. R. 1987. *The Revolutions of Wisdom*. Berkeley: University of California Press.

Lloyd, G. E. R. 2009. 'Galen's Un-Hippocratic Case-Histories', in C. Gill, T. Whitmarsh, and J. Wilkins (eds.), *Galen and the World of Knowledge*. Cambridge: Cambridge University Press, 115–31.

Louvaris, A. N. 2005. 'Fast and Abstinence in Byzantium', in W. Mayer and S. Trzcionka (eds.), *Feast, Fast or Famine: Food and Drink in Byzantium*. Brisbane: Australian Association for Byzantine Studies, 189–98.

Lucà, S. 1993. 'I Normanni e la 'Rinascita' del sec. XII', *Archivio Storico per la Calabria e la Lucanica* 60: 1–91.

Lucà, S. 2012. 'Testi medici e tecnico-scientifici del Mezzogiorno greco', in G. de Gregorio and M. Galante (eds.), *La produzione scritta tecnica scientifica nel Medioevo: libro e documento tra scuole e professioni*. Spoleto: Fondazione Centro italiano di studi sull'alto Medioevo, 551–605.

Luchner, K. 2004. *Philiatroi: Studien zum Thema der Krankheit in der griechischen Literatur der Kaiserzeit*. Göttingen: Vandenhoeck & Ruprecht.

Lucia, R. de. 1999. 'Doxographical Hints in Oribasius' Collectiones medicae', in P. J. van der Eijk (ed.), *Ancient Histories of Medicine. Essay in Medical Doxography and Historiography in Classical Antiquity*. Leiden: Brill, 473–89.

Lutz, A. 1963. 'Das Dynameron des sog. Nikolaos Myrepsos und das Antidotarium Nicolai', *Die Vorträge der Hauptversammlung der Internationalen Gesellschaft für Geschichte der Pharmazie, Neue Folge* 16: 97–133.

MacLachlan, R. 2006. *Epitomes in Ancient Literary Culture*. University of Cambridge: PhD thesis.

Macrides, R. J., Munitiz, J. A., and D. Angelov. 2013. *Pseudo-Kodinos and the Constantinopolitan Court: Offices and Ceremonies*. Farnham: Ashgate.

Magnus, H. 1901. *Die Augenheilkunde der Alten*. Breslau: Kern.

Majcherek, G. 2008. 'Academic Life of Late Antique Alexandria: A View from the Field', in M. El-Abbadi, O. Fathallah, and I. Serageldin (eds.), *What Happened to the Ancient Library of Alexandria*. Leiden, Brill: 191–206.

Makris, G. 2005. 'Alexios Apokaukos und sein Porträt im Codex Paris. gr. 2144', in S. Kolditz and R. C. Müller (eds.), *Geschehenes und Geschriebenes: Studien zu Ehren von Günther S. Henrich und Klaus-Peter Matschke*. Leipzig: Eudora-Verlag, 157–79.

Malakates, S. 1993. *Η Ουρολογία κατά τους Βυζαντινούς Χρόνους*. University of Athens: PhD thesis.

Maniatis, G. C. 2001. 'The Domain of Private Guild in the Byzantine Economy, Tenth to Fifteenth Centuries', *Dumbarton Oaks Papers* 55: 339–69.

Manolova, D. 2014. *Discourses of Science and Philosophy in the Letters of Nikephoros Gregoras*. Central European University, Budapest: PhD thesis, available at http://www.etd.ceu.hu/2015/manolova_divna.pdf (accessed 17 August 2018).

Manolova, D. 2017. 'Nikephoros Gregoras's *Philomathes* and *Phlorentios*', in A. Cameron and N. Gaul (eds.), *Dialogues and Debates from Late Antiquity to Late Byzantium*. Abingdon: Routledge, 203–19.

Mansfeld, J. 1992. *Heresiography in Context: Hippolytus' 'Elenchos' as a Source for Greek Philosophy*. Leiden: Brill.

Manzoni, T. 1998. 'The Cerebral Ventricles, the Animal Spirit and the Dawn of Brain Localization of Function', *Archives Italiennes de Biologie* 136: 103–52.

Manzoni, T. 2001. *Il cervello secondo Galeno*. Ancona: Il Lavoro Editoriale.

Marangon, P. 1984. 'Per una revisione dell'interpretazione di Pietro d'Abano', in P. Marangon (ed.), *Il pensiero ereticale nella Marca Trevigiana e a Venezia dal 1200 al 1350*. Padua: Francisci, 66–104.

Marciniak, P. 2007. 'Byzantine *Theatron* – A Place of Performance', in M. Grünbart (ed.), *Theatron. Rhetorische Kultur in Spätantike und Mittelalter*. Berlin: De Gruyter, 277–85.

Marganne, M.-H. 1994. *L'ophtalmologie dans l'Egypte gréco-romaine d'après les papyrus littéraires grecs*. Leiden: Brill.

Marganne, M.-H. 2006. 'Étiquettes de médicaments, listes de drogues, prescriptions et réceptaires dans l'Égypte gréco-romaine et byzantine', in F. Collard and E. Samama (eds.), *Pharmacopoles et Apothicaires: les «pharmaciens» de l'Antiquité au Grand Siècle*. Paris: L'Harmattan, 59–73.

Marketos, G. 1994. 'Hippocratic Medicine and Nephrology', *American Journal of Nephorology* 14: 264–9.

Martelli, M. 2017. 'Recipes Ascribed to the Scribe and Prophet Ezra in the Byzantine and Syriac Tradition', in L. Lehmhaus and M. Martelli (eds.), *Collecting Recipes: Byzantine and Jewish Pharmacology in Dialogue*. Berlin: De Gruyter, 195–219.

Martínez Manzano, T. 2015. 'Una interpolación bizantina de origen árabe en Dioscórides', *Estudios bizantinos* 3: 101–21.

Martini, E. and D. Bassi. 1906. *Catalogus codicum graecorum Bibliothecae Ambrosianae*. Milan: U. Hoepli.

Martini, U. de. 1964. 'Considerazioni sulla dottrina dello pneuma in Galeno', *Pagine di Storia della Medicina* 8: 41–7.

Mason, M. E. 1961. *Active Life and Contemplative Life: A Study of the Concepts from Plato to the Present*. Milwaukee: The Marquette University Press.

Massry, S. G. 2009. 'Isaac Judaeus Israeli: a Jewish founder of origins of nephrology', *Journal of Nephrology* 22 [Suppl. 14]: 8–11.

Massry, S. G., Smogorzewski, M., Hazani, E., and S. M. Shasha. 1997. 'Influence of Judaism and Jewish Physicians on Greek and Byzantine Medicine and Their Contribution to Nephrology', *American Journal of Nephrology* 17: 233–40.

Matschke, K.-P. 2002. 'Trade, Markets, and Money, Thirteenth–Fifteenth Centuries', in A. Laiou (ed.), *The Economic History of Byzantium*, vol. 1. Washington DC: Dumbarton Oaks, 771–806.

Matschke, K.-P. 2008. 'Beobachtungen zu den medizinischen Einrichtungen Konstantinopels in spätbyzantinischer Zeit und zur ärztlichen Versorgung des Kaiserhofes und der hauptstädtischen Bevölkerung', in *idem*, *Das spätbyzantinische Konstantinopel: alte und neue Beiträge zur Stadtgeschichte zwischen 1261 und 1453*. Hamburg: Kovac, 361–404.

Mattern, S. 1999. 'Physicians and the Roman Imperial Aristocracy: The Patronage of Therapeutics', *Bulletin of the History of Medicine* 73: 1–18.

Mattern, S. 2008. *Galen and the Rhetoric of Healing*. Baltimore: Johns Hopkins University Press.

Mattingly, C. 1991. 'The Narrative Nature of Clinical Reasoning', *Journal of American Ocupational Therapy* 45: 998–1005.

Mavroudi, M. 2002. *A Byzantine Book on Dream Intepretation: The Oneirocriticon of Achment and its Arabic Source*. Leiden: Brill.

Mavroudi, M. 2004. 'Exchanges with Arabic Writers during the Late Byzantine Period', in S. T. Brooks (ed.), *Byzantium: Faith and Power (1261–1557)*. New York: Metropolitan Museum of Art, 62–75.

Mavroudi, M. 2008. 'Arabic Words in Greek Letters: The Violet Fragment and More', in J. Lentin and J. Grand'Henry (eds.), *Moyen arabe et variétés mixtes de l'arabe à travers l'histoire*. Louvain-la-Neuve, 321–54.

Mavroudis, A. 1993. '*Ο Μιχαήλ Ιταλικός και ο Γαληνός*', *Ἑλληνικά* 43: 29–44.

Mavroudis, A. 2000. *Ἀρχιγένης Φιλίππου Ἀπαμεύς. Ὁ Βίος καὶ τὰ Ἔργα ἑνὸς Ἕλληνα Γιατροῦ στὴν Αὐτοκρατορικὴ Ῥώμη*. Athens: Akadēmia Athēnōn.

Maxwell-Stuart, P. G. 1981. *Studies in Greek Colour Terminology*. 2 vols. Leiden: Brill.

May, M. T. 1968. *Galen on the Usefulness of the Parts of the Body: Περὶ χρείας μορίων De usu partium*. 2 vols. Ithaca NY: Cornell University Press.

McCabe, A. 2007. *A Byzantine Encyclopaedia of Horse Medicine: The Sources, Compilation, and Transmission of the* Hippiatrica. Oxford: Oxford University Press.

McCabe, A. 2009. 'Imported materia medica, 4th–12th centuries, and Byzantine pharmacology', in M. Mango (ed.), *Byzantine Trade, 4th – 12th Centuries*. Farnham: Ashgate, 273–92.

McCormick, M. 2001. *The Origins of the European Economy: Communications and Commerce, A.D. 300–900*. Cambridge: Cambridge University Press.

McKendrick, S. 1999. *The British Library. A Summary Catalogue of Greek Manuscripts*, vol. 1. London: British Library.

McLaughlin, R. *The Roman Empire and the Indian Ocean*. Barnsley: Pen & Sword Military.

McVaugh, M. R. 1997. 'Bedside Manners in the Middle Ages', *Bulletin of the History of Medicine* 71: 201–23.

McVaugh, M. R. 2012. 'Losing Ground: The Disappearance of Attraction from the Kidney', in M. Horstmanshoff, H. King, and C. Zittel (eds.), *Blood, Sweat and Tears – The Changing Concepts of Physiology from Antiquity into Early Modern Europe*. Leiden: Brill, 103–37.

Medvedev, I. P. 1984. 'Tendances vers une renaissance dans la culture Byzantine tardive' *Βυζαντιακά* 4: 113–36.

Medvedev, I. P. 1993. 'The So-called *Θέατρα* as a Form of Communication of the Byzantine Intellectuals in the 14th and 15th centuries', in N. Moschonas (ed.), *Η Επικοινωνία στο Βυζάντιο*. Athens: Ethniko Idryma Ereunōn, 227–35.

Menchelli, M. 2013. 'Giorgio Oinaiotes lettore di Platone', in A. Rigo, A. Babuin, and M. Trizio (eds.), *Vie per Bisanzio*. Bari: Edizioni di Pagina, 833–55.

Mercati, G. 1926. *Scritti d'Isidoro, il cardinale ruteno, e codici a lui appartenuti che si conservano nella Biblioteca apostolica vaticana*. Rome: Biblioteca Apostolica Vaticana.

Mercati, G. and P. Franchi de' Cavalieri. 1923. *Codices Vaticani Graeci*, vol. 1, *Codices 1–329*. Vatican City: Bibliotheca Vaticana.

Mercier, R. 1984. 'The Greek "Persian Syntaxis" and the Zij-i Ilkhānī', *Archives internationales d'histoire des sciences* 34: 35–60.

Mergiali, S. 1996. *L'enseignement et les lettrés pendant l'époque des paléologues (1261–1453)*. Athens: Etaireia tōn Philōn tou Laou.

Meyendorff, J. 1971. 'Spiritual Trends in Byzantium in the Late Thirteenth and Early Fourteenth Centuries', in *Art et société à Byzance sous les Paléologues*. Venice: Institut hellénique d'études byzantines et post-byzantines, 53–71.

Meyendorff, J. 1974. 'Society and Culture in the Fourteenth Century. Religious Problems', in M. Berza and E. Stănescu (eds.), *Actes du XIVe Congrès international des études byzantines*, vol. 1: 69–92. Bucharest: Editura Academiei Republicii Socialiste România, 111–24.

Meyer, E. H. F. 1854–7. *Geschichte der Botanik*. 4 vols. Königsberg.

Meyier, K. A. de. 1955. *Codices Vossiani Graeci et Miscellanei*. Leiden: Bibliotheca Universitatis.

Miguet, T. 2017. 'Premiers jalons pour une étude complète de l'histoire du texte grec du *Viatique du Voyageur* (*Ἐφόδια τοῦ ἀποδημοῦντος*) d'Ibn al-Ǧazzār', *Revue d'Histoire des Textes* 12: 59–105.

Miller, J. I. 1969. *The Spice Trade of the Roman Empire, 29 B.C. to A.D. 641*. Oxford: Clarendon Press.

Miller, T. 1997. *The Birth of the Hospital in the Byzantine Empire*. [2nd edn.] Baltimore: Johns Hopkins University Press.

Miller, T. 2017. 'Medical Thought and Practice', in A. Kaldellis and N. Siniossoglou (eds.), *The Cambridge Intellectual History of Byzantium*. Cambridge: Cambridge University Press, 252–68.

Mioni, E. 1965. *Catalogo di manoscritti greci esistenti nelle bibliotheche italiane*, vol. 1. Rome: Istituto polografico e zecca dello Stato, Libreria dello Stato.

Mioni, E. 1972. *Bibliothecae divi Marci Venetiarum, Codices Graeci manuscripti. Codices in classes a prima usque ad quintam inclusi, Pars altera: Classis II, Codd. 121–198 – Classis III, IV, V*. Rome: Istituto polografico e zecca dello Stato, Libreria dello Stato.

Mioni, E. 1981. *Bibliothecae divi Marci Venetiarum, Codices Graeci manuscripti. Thesaurus antiquus*, vol. 1: *Codices 1–299*. Rome: Istituto polografico e zecca dello Stato, Libreria dello Stato.

Mioni, E. 1985. *Bibliothecae divi Marci Venetiarum, Codices Graeci manuscripti. Thesaurus antiquus*, vol. 2: *Codices 300–625*. Rome: Istituto polografico e zecca dello Stato, Libreria dello Stato.

Mitchell, P. D. 2011. 'Retrospective Diagnosis and the Use of Historical Text for Investigating Disease in the Past', *International Journal of Paleopathology* 1: 81–8.

Mitsakis, K. 1990. 'Byzantine and Modern Greek Parahymnography', in D. Conomos (ed.), *Studies in Eastern Chant*, vol. 5. Crestwood NY: St Vladimir's Seminary Press, 9–76.

Mondrain, B. 1999. 'Nicolas Myrepse et une collection de manuscrits médicaux dans la première moitié du XIVe siècle. A propos d'une miniature célèbre du Parisinus gr. 2243', in A. Garzya and J. Jouanna (eds.), *I testi medici greci: tradizione e ecdotica.* Naples: D'Auria, 403–18.

Mondrain, B. 2000a. 'Jean Argyropoulos professeur à Constantinople et ses auditeurs médecins, d'Andronic Eparque à Démétrios Angelos', in G. Makris and C. Scholz (eds.), *Πολύπλευρος νοῦς: Miscellanea für Peter Schreiner zu seinem 60. Geburtstag.* Munich: Saur, 223–50.

Mondrain, B. 2000b. 'Les Eparque, une famille de médecins collectionneurs de manuscrits aux Xve–XVIe siècles', S. Patoura (ed.), *Η Ελληνική Γραφή κατά τους 15ο και 16ο Αιώνες.* Athens: Ethniko Idryma Ereunōn, 145–63.

Mondrain, B. 2003. 'Comment était lu Galien à Byzance dans la première moitié du XVe siècle? Contribution à quelques aspects de l'histoire du texte', in A. Garzya and J. Jouanna (eds.), *Trasmissione e ecdotica dei testi medici greci.* Naples: D'Auria, 361–84.

Mondrain, B. 2010. 'Démétrios Angelos et la médecine: contribution nouvelle au dossier', in V. Boudon-Millot et al. (eds.), *Storia della tradizione e edizione dei medici greci, Atti del VI Colloquio Internazionale Paris 12–14 Aprile 2008.* Naples: D'Auria, 293–322.

Mondrain, B. 2014. 'La place de la *Collection hippocratique* à Byzance d'après les manuscrits', in J. Jouanna and M. Zink (eds.), *Hippocrate et les hippocratismes: Médecine, religion, société.* Paris, Académie des Inscriptions et Belles Lettres, 385–99.

Morgan, T. 1998. *Literate Education in the Hellenistic and Roman Worlds.* Cambridge: Cambridge University Press.

Morrisson, C. 2012. 'Weighing, Measuring, Paying Exchanges in the Market and the Marketplace', in C. Morrisson (ed.), *Trade and markets in Byzantium.* Washington DC: Dumbarton Oaks Research Library and Collection, 379–98.

Morrisson, C. and J.-C. Cheynet. 2002. 'Prices and Wages in the Byzantine World', in A. Laiou (ed.), *The Economic History of Byzantium*, vol. 1. Washington DC: Dumbarton Oaks, 815–78.

Moulinier-Brogi, L. 2004. 'La science des urines de Maurus de Salerne et les *Sinthomata magistri Mauri* inédits', in D. Jacquart and A. Paravicini-Bagliani (eds.), *La Scuola Medica Salernitana. Gli autori e i testi.* Florence: SISMEL, 261–81.

Moulinier-Brogi, L. 2010. 'La fortune du *De Urinis* de Maurus de Salerne et se *volgarizzamenti* inédits', *Mélanges de l'Ecole française de Rome* 122: 261–78.

Moulinier-Brogi, L. 2012. *L'uroscopie au Moyen Âge: "lire dans un verre la nature de l'homme".* Paris: Honoré Champion.

Munitiz, J. 1996. 'Dedicating a Volume: Apokaukos and Hippocrates', in C. Constantinidis, N. Panagiotakis, E. Jeffreys, and A. Angelou (eds.), *ΦΙΛΕΛΛΗΝ. Studies in Honour of Robert Browning.* Venice: Instituto Ellenico di Studi Zizantini e Postbizantini di Venezia, 267–80.

Musurillo, H. 1956. 'The Problem of Ascetical Fasting in the Greek Patristic Writers', *Traditio* 12: 1–64.

Muth, R. 1968. 'Urin', in G. Wissowa (ed.), *Realencyclopädie der classischen Altertumswissenschaft*, vol. 9. Stuttgart: J. B. Metzler, Supplementband, 1292–303.

Nagy, G. 1987. 'Herodotus the *Logios*', *Arethusa* 20: 175–84.

Neuburger, M. 1906–11. *Geschichte der Medizin*. 2 vols. Stuttgart: F. Enke.

Neuburger, M. 1937. 'The Early History of Urology', *Bulletin of the Medical Library Association* 25: 147–65.

Newton, F. 1994. 'Constantine the African and Monte Cassino: New Elements and the Text of the *Isagoge*', in C. Burnett and D. Jacquart (eds.), *Constantine the African and ʿAlī Ibn Al-ʿAbbās Al-Magūsī. The Pantegni and Related Texts*. Leiden: Brill, 16–47.

Nicol, D. 1993. *The Last Centuries of Byzantium, 1261–1453*. [2nd edn.] Cambridge: Cambridge University Press.

Nikitas, D. Z. 2001. 'Traduzioni greche di opera latine', in S. Settis (ed.), *I Greci: Storia, cultura, arte, società. 3. I Greci oltre la Grecia*. Turin: G. Einaudi, 1035–51.

Nutton, V. 1977. 'Archiatri and the Medical Profession in Antiquity', *Papers of the British School at Rome* 45: 191–226.

Nutton, V. 1984. 'From Galen to Alexander: Aspects of Medicine and Medical Practice in Late Antiquity', *Dumbarton Oaks Papers* 38: 1–14.

Nutton, V. 1985. 'Murders and Miracles: Lay Attitudes Toward Medicine in Classical Antiquity', in R. Porter (ed.), *Patients and Practitioners*. Cambridge University Press: Cambridge, 23–53.

Nutton, V. 1986. Review essay 'Miller, T. 1985. *The Birth of the Hospital in the Byzantine Empire*', *Medical History* 30: 218–21.

Nutton, V. 1993. 'Humoralism', in W. F. Bynum and R. Porter (eds.), *Companion Encyclopedia of the History of Medicine*. London: Routledge, 281–91.

Nutton, V. 1995. 'Medicine in Medieval Western Europe, 1000–1500', in L. Conrad et al. (eds.), *The Western Medical Tradition*. Cambridge: Cambridge University Press, 139–205.

Nutton, V. 2007. 'Galen in Byzantium', in M. Grünbart, E. Kislinger, A. Muthesius, and D. Stathakopoulos (eds.), *Material Culture and Well-being in Byzantium*. Vienna: Verlag der Österreichischen Akademie der Wissenschaften, 171–6.

Nutton, V. 2008. 'The Medical World of Rufus of Ephesus', in P. E. Pormann (ed.), *Rufus of Ephesus on Melancholy*. Tübingen: Mohr Siebeck, 139–58.

Nutton, V. 2013. *Ancient Medicine*. [2nd edn.] London: Routledge.

Oberhelman, S. 2015. 'Towards a Typology of Byzantine and Post-Byzantine Healing Texts', *Athens Journal of Health* 2.2: 133–46.

Odorico, P. 2017. 'Identité et craintes. Théodore Pédiasimos à Serrès au XIVe siècle', in A. Cuomo and E. Trapp (eds.), *Toward a Historical Sociolinguistic Poetics of Medieval Greek*. Turnhout: Brepols, 161–73.

Oikonomidès, N. 1979. *Hommes d'affaires grecs et latins à Constantinople: XIIIe–XVe siècles*. Montreal: Institut d'etudes medievales Albert-le-Grand.

Oldoni, M. 1994. 'Uroscopy in the Salerno School of Medicine', *American Journal of Nephrology* 14: 483–7.

Oldoni, M. 2004. 'Monastic Nephorology in the School of Salerno and in An Unpublished Treatise in Middlelatin and Italian Volgare of the Manuscript 2Qq C63 in the Public Library of Palermo', *Journal of Nephrology* 14: 334–6.

Omont, H. 1885. *Catalogue des manuscrits grecs de la Bibliothèque royale de Bruxelles*. Ghent: Imprimerie E. Vanderhaeghen.

Omont, H. 1886–8. *Inventaire sommaire des manuscrits grecs de la Bibliothèque nationale*. 3 vols. Paris: A. Picard.

Ouerfelli, M. 2008. *Le sucre: production, commercialisation et usages dans la Méditerranée médiévale*. Leiden: Brill.

Ousterhout, R. G. 1987. *The Architecture of the Kariye Camii in Istanbul*. Washington DC: Dumbarton Oaks Research Library and Collection.

Overwien, O. (2018). 'Der medizinische Unterricht der Iatrosophisten in der "Schule von Alexandria" (5.-7. Jh. n. Chr.): Überlegungen zu seiner Organisation, seinen Inhalten und seinen Ursprüngen', *Philologus* (erster Teil) 162(1): 2–14; (zweiter Teil) 162(2): 265–90.

Page, G. 2008. *Being Byzantine. Greek Identity Before the Ottomans*. Cambridge: Cambridge University Press.

Palmieri, N. 2001. 'Nouvelles remarques sur les commentaires à Galien de l'école médicale de Ravenne', in A. Debru and N. Palmieri (eds.), *Docente Natura. Mélanges de Médecine ancienne et médiévale offerts à Guy Sabbah*. Saint-Étienne: Publications de l'Université de Saint-Étienne, 209–46.

Papadakis, A. 1997. *Crisis in Byzantium. The Filioque Controversy in the Patriarchate of Gregory II of Cyprus (1283–1289)*. Crestwood NY: St Vladimir's Seminary Press.

Papazoglou, G. K. 1983. *Βιβλιοθῆκες στὴν Κωνσταντινούπολη τοῦ ΙΣΤʹ αἰῶνα*. Thessaloniki: [s.n.].

Paschetto, E. 1984. *Pietro d'Abano, medico e filosofo*. Florence: Nuovedizioni E. Vallecchi.

Paschos, E. A. and C. Simelidis. 2017. *Introduction to Astronomy by Theodore Metochites*. Hackensack NJ: World Scientific Publishing.

Pasquale Barbanti, M. di. 1998. *Ochema-pneuma e phantasia nel neoplatonismo: aspetti psicologici e prospettive religiose*. Catania: CUECM.

Pentogalos, G. 1970. *Οἱ Ἰατρικὲς Γνώσεις Ἰωσὴφ τοῦ Ῥακενδύτη καὶ ἡ Σχετικὴ Ἀνέκδοτη Ἐπιστολὴ τοῦ Μιχαὴλ Γαβρά*. Athens: *Ἀνακοίνωση στὴν Ἑλληνικὴ Ἑταιρεία Ἱστορίας τῆς Ἰατρικῆς*, 5–12.

Pentogalos, G. and J. G. Lascaratos. 1984. 'A Surgical Operation Performed on Siamese Twins During the Tenth Century in Byzantium', *Bulletin of the History of Medicine* 58: 99–102.

Perentidis, S. 1980. 'L'emploi du duel dans un texte grec du XIVe siècle', *Revue des Études Grecques* 93: 529–32.

Pérez Martin, I. 1989. 'Planudes y el Monasterio de Acatalepto: A propósito del 'Monacensis Gr.' 430 de Tucídides (ff. 4–5 y 83–5)', *Erytheia* 10: 303–7.

Peterson, D. W. 1974. *Galen's 'Therapeutics to Glaucon' and Its Early Commentaries*. Johns Hopkins University: PhD thesis.

Petridou, G. and C. Thumiger. (eds). 2016. *Approaches to the Patient in the Ancient World*. Leiden: Brill.

Phillips, W. D. Jr. 1986. 'Sugar Production and Trade in the Mediterranean at the Time of the Crusades', in V. P. Goss and C. V. Bronstein (eds.), *The Meetings of Two Worlds: Cultural Exchange Between East and West During the Period of the Crusades*. Kalamazoo MI: Medieval Institute Publications, Western Michigan University, 393–406.

Pietrobelli, A. 2010. 'Variation autour du *Thessalonicensis Vlatadon* 14: un manuscrit copié au xénon du Kral, peu avant la chute de Constantinople', *Revue des Études Byzantines* 68: 95–126.

Pingree, D. 1964. 'Gregory Chioniades and Palaeologan Astronomy', *Dumbarton Oaks Papers* 18: 133–60.

Pingree, D. 1971. 'The Astrological School of John Abramius', *Dumbarton Oaks Papers* 25: 189–215.

Plested, M. 2017. 'Aquinas in Byzantium', in A. Kaldellis and N. Siniossoglou (eds.), *The Cambridge Intellectual History of Byzantium*. Cambridge: Cambridge University Press, 542–56.

Polemis, I. 2007. '*Ἀρετὴ καὶ Λόγος: Παραδοσιακὰ Θέματα καὶ Νέοι Ἰδεολογικοὶ Προσανατολισμοὶ στὸν Ἐπιτάφιο Λόγο τοῦ Θεοδώρου Μετοχίτη γιὰ τὸν Ἰωσὴφ τὸν Φιλόσοφο*', in G. Andreiomenos (ed.), *Εὐκαρπίας Ἔπαινος*. Athens: Poreia, 923–44.

Pomata, G. 2005. '*Praxis Historialis*: The Uses of *Historia* in Early Modern Medicine', in G. Pomata and N. G. Siraisi (eds.), *Historia: Empiricism and Erudition in Early Modern Europe*. Cambridge MA: MIT Press, 105–46.

Pormann, P. 2003. 'The *Parisinus Graecus* 2293 as a Document of Scientific Activity in Swabian Sicily', *Arabic Sciences and Philosophy* 13: 137–61.

Pormann, P. 2005. 'The Physician and the Other: Images of the Charlatan in Medieval Islam', *Bulletin of the History of Medicine* 79: 189–227.

Pormann, P. 2010. 'Medical Education in Late Antiquity. From Alexandria to Montpellier', in M. Horstmanshoff (ed.), *Hippocrates and Medical Education*. Leiden: Brill, 419–41.

Pormann, P. 2011. 'The Formation of the Arabic Pharmacology Between Tradition and Innovation', *Annals of Science* 68: 493–515.

Pormann, P. 2013. 'Medical Epistemology and Melancholy: Rufus of Ephesus and Miskawayh', in W. V. Harris (ed.), *Mental Disorders in the Classical World*. Leiden: Brill, 223–44.

Pormann, P. and E. Savage-Smith. 2007. *Medieval Islamic Medicine*. Edinburgh: Edinburgh University Press.

Pournaropoulos, G. 1942. *Συμβολὴ εἰς τὴν Ἱστορίαν τῆς Βυζαντινῆς Ἰατρικῆς*. Athens: [s.n.].

Pradel, M. M. 2013. *Katalog der griechischen Handschriften der Bayerischen Staatsbibliothek München*, vol. 2. Wiesbaden: Harrassowitz.

Puntoni, V. 1896. 'Indice dei codici greci della Biblioteca Estense di Modena', *Studi italiani di filologia classica* 4: 379–536.

Putscher, M. 1973. *Pneuma, Spiritus, Geist: Vorstellungen vom Lebensantrieb in ihren geschichtlichen Wandlungen*. Wiesbaden: Steiner.

Ramsey, M. 2005. 'Uroscopy and Urinalysis: Tradition and Innovation in Diagnostic Practices', in P. Bourdelais and O. Faure (eds.), *Les nouvelles pratiques de santé: acteurs, objets, logiques sociales, XVIIIe–XXe siècles*. Paris: Belin, 27–49.

Rein, J. E. 1915. *Die Florentiner Briefsammlung: Codex Laurentianus S. Marco 356*. Helsinki: Suomalaisen Tiedeakatemian Kustantama.

Reiser, S. J. 1986. 'Creating Form out of Mass: The Development of the Medical Record', in E. Mendelsohn (ed.), *Transformation and Tradition in the Sciences: Essays in Honor of I. Benard Cohen*. Cambridge: Cambridge University Press, 303–16.

Reulos, M. and P. G. Bietenholz. 1985. 'Jean du Ruel', in P. G. Bietenholz (ed.), *Contemporaries of Erasmus. A Biographical Register of the Renaissance and Reformation*, vol. 1. Toronto: University of Toronto Press, 415.

Richler, B. 2015. 'Hebrew Translations of Isaac Israeli's Treatise on Urine', in K. Collins, S. Kottek, and H. Paavilainen (eds.), *Isaac Israeli: The Philosopher Physician*. Jerusalem: Muriel and Philip Berman Medical Library, 67–76.

Riddle, J. 1985. *Dioscorides on Pharmacy and Medicine*. Austin: University of Texas Press.

Riehle, A. 2011. 'Rhetorik, Ritual und Repräsentation. Zur Briefliteratur gebildeter Eliten im spätbyzantinischen Konstantinopel (1261–1328)', *Frühmittelalterliche Studien* 45: 259–76.

Rocca, J. 1997. 'Galen and the Ventricular System', *Journal of the History of the Neurosciences* 6: 227–39.

Rocca, J. 1998. 'Galen and Greek Pneuma Theory. The Limitations of Physiological Explanation', in K. Boudouris (ed.), *Philosophy and Medicine. II. Studies in Greek Philosophy, 29*. Athens: Ionia, 171–97.

Rocca, J. 2003. *Galen on the Brain: Anatomical Knowledge and Physiological Speculation in the Second Century AD*. Leiden: Brill.

Rocca, J. 2012. 'From Doubt to Certainty. Aspects of the Conceptualization and Interpretation of Galen's Natural Pneuma', in M. Horstmanshoff, H. King, and C. Zittel (eds.), *Blood, Sweat and Tears – The Changing Concepts of Physiology from Antiquity into Early Modern Europe*. Leiden: Brill, 629–59.

Romano, R. 1979/80. 'Sulla poesia di Nicola Callicle', *Annali di Facoltà di lettere e filosofia* 22: 61–75.

Roueché, M. 1999. 'Did Medical Students Study Philosophy in Alexandria?', *Bulletin of the Institute of Classical Studies* 43: 153–69.

Ruhland, W. (ed.). 1955. *Encyclopedia of Plant Physiology*, vol. 1. Berlin: Springer.

Runciman, S. 1970. *The Last Byzantine Renaissance*. Cambridge: Cambridge University Press.

Russell, N. 2004. *The Doctrine of Deification in the Greek Patristic Tradition*. Oxford: Oxford University Press.

Sanagustin, F. 2012. 'Māʾ al-Ward', in P. J. Bearman et al. (eds.), *Encyclopedia of Islam*. [2nd edn] Leiden: Brill, available at http://dx.doi.org/10.1163/1573-3912_islam_SIM_8797 (accessed 21 October 2018).

Sarton, G. 1927–48. *Introduction to the History of Science*. 3 vols. Baltimore: Published for the Carnegie Institution of Washington by the Williams & Wilkins Co.

Sato, T. 2015. *Sugar in the Social Life of Medieval Islam*. Leiden: Brill.

Savage-Smith, E. 1984. 'Hellenistic and Byzantine ophthalmology: Trachoma and Sequelae', *Dumbarton Oaks Papers* 38: 169–86.

Savage-Smith, E. 1995. 'Attitudes Toward Dissection in Medieval Islam', *Journal of the History of Medicine and Allied Sciences* 50: 67–110.

Scarborough, J. 1982. 'Roman Pharmacy and the Eastern Drug Trade: Some Problems as Illustrated by the Example of Aloe', *Pharmacy in History* 23: 135–43.

Scarborough, J. 1984. 'Early Byzantine Pharmacology', *Dumbarton Oaks Papers* 38: 213–32.

Scarborough, J. 2010. 'Teaching Surgery in Late Byzantine Alexandria', in M. Horstmanshoff (ed.), *Hippocrates and Medical Education*. Leiden: Brill, 230–60.

Schadelbauer, K. 1953. 'Alexandrinus(Alessandrini) von Neu(en)stein', *Neue deutsche Biographie*, vol. 1. Berlin: Duncker & Humblot, 196–7.

Schelenz, H. 1904. *Geschichte der Pharmazie*. Berlin: Springer.

Schipperges, H. 1955. 'Die frühen Übersetzer der arabischen Medizin in chronologischer Sicht', *Sudhoffs archiv für Geschichte der Medizin und der Naturwissenschaften* 39: 53–93.

Schmitt, W. O. 1968. 'Lateinische Literatur in Byzanz. Die Ubersetzungen des Maximos Planudes und die moderne Forschung', *Jahrbuch der Österreichischen Byzantinistik* 17: 127–47.

Schnorr von Carolsfeld, F. 1882. *Katalog der Handschriften der Königl. öffentlichen Bibliothek zu Dresden*, vol. 1. Leipzig: Teubner.

Schönauer, S. 1996. *Untersuchungen zum Steinkatalog des Sophrosyne: Gedichtes des Meliteniotes mit kritischer Edition des Verse 1107–1247*. Wiesbaden: Beerenverlag.

Schönberger, O. and E. Schönberger. 2010. *Lebenslehre in drei Dialogen: Hermodotos, Musokles, Hermippos*. Würzburg: Königshausen & Neumann.

Schöne, H. 1903. 'Zwei Listen chirurgischer Instrumente', *Hermes* 38: 280–4.

Serikoff, N. 2013. '"Syriac" Plant Names in a Fifteenth Century Greek Glossary (From the Wellcome Library Books and Manuscripts)', in B. Zipser (ed.), *Medical Books in the Byzantine World*. Bologna: Eikasmos, 97–115.

Ševčenko, I. 1962. *La vie intellectuelle et politique à Byzance sous les premiers Paléologues: Études sur la polémique entre Théodore Métochite et Nicéphore Choumnos*. Brussels: Byzantion.

Ševčenko, I. 1974. 'Society and Intellectual Life in the Fourteenth Century', in M. Berza and E. Stănescu (eds.), *Actes du XIVe Congrès international des études byzantines*, vol. 1: 69–92. Bucharest: Editura Academiei Republicii Socialiste România. [repr. Ševčenko, I. *Society and intellectual life in late Byzantium*. London: Variorum Reprints, 1981.]

Ševčenko, I. 1975. 'Theodore Metochites, the Chora, and the Intellectual Trends of his Time', in P. A. Underwood (ed.), *The Kariye Djami. Studies in the Art of the Kariye Djami and its Intellectual Background*. London: Routledge, vol. 4: 17–91.

Ševčenko, I. 1979. 'Vita: Theodore Metochites, Literary Statesman', *Harvard Magazine* 81: 1270–332.

Shaw, G. 1995. *Theurgy and the Soul: The Neoplatonism of Iamblichus*. University Park PA: Pennsylvania State University Press.

Shukurov, R. 2016. *The Byzantine Turks 1204–1461*. Leiden: Brill.

Sideras, A. 1974. 'Aetius und Oribasius', *Byzantinische Zeitschrift* 67: 110–30.

Sideras, A. 1994. *Die byzantinischen Grabreden: Prosopographie, Datierung, Überlieferung. 142 Epitaphien und Monodien aus dem byzantinischen Jahrtausend*. Vienna: Verlag der Österreichischen Akademie der Wissenschaften.

Siegel, R. E. 1968. *Galen's System on Physiology and Medicine*. Basel: Karger.

Siegel, R. E. 1970. *Galen on Sense Perception*. Basel: Karger.

Siegel, R. E. 1973. *Galen on Psychology, Psychopathology, and Function and Diseases of the Nervous System*. Basel: Karger.

Siegel, R. E. 1976. *Galen on the Affected Parts*. Basel: Karger.

Silbach, E. 1970. *Byzantinische Metrologie*. Düsseldorf: Brükken-Verlag.

Siraisi, N. 1981. *Taddeo Alderotti and His Pupils: Two Generations of Italian Medical Learning*. Princeton: Princeton University Press.

Siraisi, N. 1990. *Medieval & Early Renaissance Medicine*. Chicago: University of Chicago Press.

Slaveva-Griffin, S. 2018. 'Byzantine Medical Encyclopedias and Education', in P. T Keyser with J. Scarborough (eds.), *The Oxford Handbook of Science and Medicine in the Classical World*. Oxford: Oxford University Press, 965–86.

Smith, O. L. 1981/2. 'Tricliniana', *Classica et Mediaevalia* 33: 239–62.

Solomou, S. 2016. *Ο Πολιτικός Ρόλος των Μεγάλων Οικογενειών κατά την Παλαιολόγεια Περίοδο. Τα Πρόσωπα και τα Κείμενα. (1258–1453)*. University of Athens: PhD thesis, available at https://phdtheses.ekt.gr/eadd/handle/10442/39415 (accessed 28 March 2019).

Sonderkamp, J. A. M. 1984. 'Theophanes Nonnus: Medicine in the Circle of Constantine Porphyrogenitus', *Dumbarton Oaks Papers* 38: 29–41.

Sonderkamp, J. A. M. 1987. *Untersuchungen zur Überlieferung der Schriften des Theophanes Chrysobalantes (sog. Theophanes Nonnos)*. Bonn: R. Habelt.

Sournia, J.-C. et al. 1980–4. *Illustrierte Geschichte der Medizin*. 9 vols. Salzburg: Andreas.

Speranzi, D. 2010. 'Note codicologiche e paleografiche', in M. Bernabò (ed.), *La collezione di testi chirurgici di Niceta: Firenze, Biblioteca medicea laurenziana, Plut. 74.7*. Rome: Edizioni di storia e letteratura, 13–33.

Spruit, L. 2005. 'Ambrogio Leone', *Dizionario Biografico degli Italiani* 64: 560–2.

Staden, H. von. 1975. 'Experiment and Experience in Hellenistic Medicine', *Bulletin of the Institute of Classical Studies* 22: 178–99.

Staden, H. von. 1994. 'Author and Authority. Celsus and the Construction of a Scientific Self', in M. E. Vázquez Buján (ed.), *Tradición e innovación de la medicina latina de la antigüedad y de la Alta Edad Media*. Santiago de Compostela: Servicio de Publicacións e Intercambio Científico da Universidade de Santiago de Compostela, 103–17.

Staden, H. von. 1995. 'Anatomy as Rhetoric: Galen on Dissection and Persuasion', *Journal of the History of Medicine and Allied Sciences* 50: 47–66.

Staden, H. von. 2000. 'Body, Soul, and Nerves: Epicurus, Herophilus, Erasistratus, the Stoics, and Galen', in J. Wright and P. Potter (eds.), *Psyche and Soma: Physicians and Metaphysicians on the Mind-Body Problem from Antiquity to Enlightenment*. Oxford: Clarendon Press, 79–116.

Stannard, J. 1971. 'Byzantine Botanical Lexicography', *Episteme* 5: 168–87.

Stathakopoulos, D. 2004. 'Stiftungen von Spitälern in sptäbyzantinischer Zeit (1261–1453)', in M. Borgolte (ed.), *Stiftungen in Christentum, Judentum Islam vor der Moderne*. Berlin: Akademie Verlag.

Stathakopoulos, D. 2011. 'Review of B. Zipser, John the Physician's *Therapeutics*: A Medical Handbook in Vernacular Greek', *Medical History* 55: 120–1.

Stathakopoulos, D. 2012. 'The Location of Medical Practice in 13th-century Eastern Mediterranean', in G. Saint-Guillain and D. Stathakopoulos (eds.), *Liquid & Multiple: Individuals & Identities in the Thirteenth-Century Aegean*. Paris: Association des amis du Centre d'histoire et civilisation de Byzance, 135–54.

Stathakopoulos, D. 2013a. 'Disease and Where to Treat It: A Byzantine *vade mecum*', in B. Zipser (ed.), *Medical Books in the Byzantine World*. Bologna: Eikasmos, 19–34.

Stathakopoulos, D. 2013b. 'On Whose Authority? Regulating Medical Practice in the Twelfth and Early Thirteenth Century', in P. Armstrong (ed.), *Authority in Byzantium*. Farnham: Ashgate, 227–38.

Stathakopoulos, D. 2014. *A Short History of the Byzantine Empire*. London: I. B. Tauris.

Stathakopoulos, D. 2019. 'Galen in Non-Medical Byzantine Texts, 600–1453', in P. Bouras-Vallianatos and B. Zipser (eds.), *Brill's Companion to the Reception of Galen*. Leiden: Brill, 140–59.

Stathakopoulos, D. (forthcoming). 'Alexios Apokaukos: Apology for a Parvenu', in N. Gaul (ed.), *The Post-1204 Byzantine World: New Approaches and Novel Directions*. Abingdon: Routledge.

Stathakopoulos, D. (unpublished). 'Early Modern Translations of Late Byzantine Medical Texts: Contexts, Use and Dispersion'.

Stefec, R. 2012. 'Zur Geschichte der Handschriften des Francesco Patrizi und des Antonios Eparchos', *Νέα Ῥώμη: Rivista di Ricerche Byzantinistiche* 9: 245–60.

Stefec, R. 2014. 'Die Handschriften der Sophistenviten Philostrats', *Römische historische Mitteilungen* 56: 137–206.

Stettler, A. 1988. 'Fragen zur Harnschau in der Antike', *Antike Welt* 19: 60–2.

Stevenson, H. M. 1885. *Codices manuscripti palatini graeci Bibliothecae Vaticanae*. Rome: ex Typographeo Vaticano.

Stevenson, H. M. 1888. *Codices manuscripti graeci reginae suecorum et Pii PP. II Bibliothecae Vaticanae*. Rome: Typographeo Vaticano.

Stiernon, D. 1974. 'Joseph le Philosophe', in M. Viller (ed.), *Dictionnaire de spiritualité: ascétique et mystique, doctrine et histoire*, vol. 5. Paris: Beauchesne, 1388–92.

Stolberg, M. 2009. *Die Harnschau. Eine Kultur- und Alltagsgeschichte*. Köln: Böhlau. [English translation: 2015. *Uroscopy in Early Modern Europe*. Farnham: Ashgate.]

Strohmaier, G. 1998. 'Reception and Tradition: Medicine in the Byzantine and Arab World', in M. D. Grmek (ed.), *Western Medical Thought from Antiquity to the Middle Ages*. Cambridge MA: Harvard University Press, 139–69. [Originally published in German: 1996. 'Die Rezeption und die Vermittlung: die Medizin in der byzantinischen und in der arabischen Welt', in M. Grmek (ed.), *Die Geschichte des medizinischen Denkens*. Munich: Beck 151–81.]

Studemund, W. and Cohn, L. 1890. *Codices ex Bibliotheca Meermanniana Phillippici Graeci nunc Berolinenses* (*Verzeichniss der griechischen Handschriften der Königlichen Bibliothek zu Berlin 1*). Berlin: A. Asher.

Stur, J. 1930. 'Die Dermatologie des Johannes Aktuarios', *Archiv für Dermatologie und Syphilis* 159.3: 650–62.

Stur, J. 1931a. 'Die Gynäkologie des Johannes Aktuarios', *Archiv für Gynäkologie* 145.2: 551–65.

Stur, J. 1931b. 'Über Geschlechtskrankheiten bei Johannes Aktuarios', *Archiv für Dermatologie und Syphilis* 163.1: 181–4.

Tabanelli, M. 1964. *Studi sulla chirurgia bizantina. Paolo di Egina*. Firenze: Leo S. Olschki Editore.

Talamanca, M. 1977. Lo schema 'genus-species' nelle sistematiche dei giuristi romani', in *La filosofia greca e il diritto romano II* (*Atti Roma 1973*). Rome: Accademia Nazionale dei Lincei, 3–319.

Talbot, A.-M. 1975. *The Correspondence of Athanasius I, Patriarch of Constantinople: Letters to the Emperor Andronicus II, Members of the Imperial Family, and Officials.* Washington DC: Dumbarton Oaks Center for Byzantine Studies.

Talbot, A.-M. 1999. 'Epigrams in Context: Metrical Inscriptions on Art and Architecture of the Palaiologan Era', *Dumbarton Oaks Papers* 63: 75–109.

Talbot, A.-M. 2001. 'Building Activity in Constantinople under Andronikos II: The Role of Women Patrons in the Constructions and Restoration of Monasteries', in N. Necipoğlu (ed.), *Byzantine Constantinople: Monuments, Topography and Everyday Life.* Leiden: Brill, 329–43.

Talbot, A.-M. 2007. 'Mealtime in Monasteries: The Culture of the Byzantine Refectory', in L. Brubaker and K. Linardou (eds.), *Eat, Drink, and Be Merry (Luke 12:19) – Food and Wine in Byzantium.* Farnham: Ashgate, 109–25.

Taygetos, A. 2013. *Χαρίτωνος 'Περὶ Τροχίσκων'.* Thessaloniki: Kadmos.

Temkin, O. 1929. 'Krankengeschichte und Sinnsphäre der Medizin', *Kyklos* (Leipzig) 2: 42–66.

Temkin, O. 1951. 'On Galen's Pneumatology', *Gesnerus* 8: 180–9.

Temkin, O. 1962. 'Byzantine Medicine: Tradition and Empiricism', *Dumbarton Oaks Papers* 16: 97–115.

Temkin, O. 1973. *Galenism: Rise and Decline of a Medical Philosophy.* Ithaca NY: Cornell University Press.

Tétry, A. 1985. 'Jacques Goupyl', in *Dictionnaire de biographie française*, vol. 16. Paris: Librairie Letouzey.

Teza, E. 1903. 'Intorno ad un codice greco che contiene opere di Giovanni l'Attuario, medico bizantino', *Bollettino del Museo Civico di Padova* 6: 106–10.

Teza, E. 1903/4. 'I bagni: un capitolo, inedito in greco, dalle opera dell'Attuario, medico bizantino', *Atti del Reale Istituto Veneto di Scienze, Lettere ed Arti* 53: 299–317.

Thomas, J. P. 1987. *Private Religious Foundations in the Byzantine Empire.* Washington DC: Dumbarton Oaks Research Library and Collection.

Thomssen, H. and C. Probst. 1994. 'Die Medizin des Rufus von Ephesos', *Aufstieg und Niedergang der römischen Welt* II. 37.2: 1254–92.

Thorndike, L. 1923. 'Peter of Abano', in L. Thorndike (ed.), *A History of Magic and Experimental Science*, vol. 2. New York: The Macmillan Company, 874–947.

Thumiger, C. 2016. 'Patient Function and Physician Function in the Hippocratic Cases', in G. Petridou and C. Thumiger (eds.), *Approaches to the Patient in the Ancient World.* Leiden: Brill, 107–37.

Thumiger, C. 2018. 'The Professional Audiences of the Hippocratic *Epidemics*: Patient Cases in Hippocratic Scientific Communication', in P. Bouras-Vallianatos and S. Xenophontos (eds.), *Greek Medical Literature and Its Readers: From Hippocrates to Islam and Byzantium.* New York: Routledge, 48–64.

Tihon, A. 1987. 'Les tables astronomiques persanes à Constantinople dans la première moitié du XIVe siècle', *Byzantion* 57: 471–87.

Tihon, A. 1996. 'L'astronomie byzantine à l'aube de la Renaissance (de 1352 à la fin du XVe siècle)', *Byzantion* 66: 244–80.

Tihon, A. 2008. 'Chioniades, George (or Gregory)', in N. Koertge (ed.), *New Dictionary of Scientific Biography*, vol. 2. Detroit: Charles Scribner's Sons, 120–2.

Tihon, A. 2011. 'Barlaam de seminara traité sur la date de pâques', *Byzantion* 81: 362–411.

Tihon, A. 2017. 'Astronomy', in A. Kaldellis and N. Siniossoglou (eds.), *The Cambridge Intellectual History of Byzantium*. Cambridge: Cambridge University Press, 183–97.

Tinnefeld, F. 1995. 'Neue Formen der Antikenrezeption bei den Byzantinern der frühen Palaiologenzeit', *International Journal of the Classical Tradition* 1.3: 19–28.

Tinnefeld, F. 2003. 'Intellectuals in Late Byzantine Thessalonike', *Dumbarton Oaks Papers* 57: 153–72.

Todd, R. 1984. 'Philosophy and Medicine in John Philoponus' Commentary on Aristotle's *De Anima*', *Dumbarton Oaks Papers* 38: 103–10.

Totelin, L. M. V. 2009. *Hippocratic Recipes: Oral and Written Transmission of Pharmacological Knowledge in Fifth- and Fourth-Century Greece*. Leiden: Brill.

Totelin, L. M. V. 2012. 'And to End on a Poetic Note: Galen's Authorial Strategies in the Pharmacological Books', *Studies in History and Philosophy of Science Part A* 43.2: 307–15.

Totelin, L. M. V. 2015. 'When Foods Become Remedies in Ancient Greece: The Curious Case of Garlic and Other Substances', *Journal of Ethnopharmacology* 167: 30–7.

Totelin, L. M. V. 2018. 'Gone with the Wind: Laughter and the Audience of the Hippocratic Treatises', in P. Bouras-Vallianatos and S. Xenophontos (eds.), *Greek Medical Literature and Its Readers: From Hippocrates to Islam and Byzantium*. New York: Routledge, 30–47.

Toth, I. 2007. 'Rhetorical *Theatron* in Late Byzantium: The Example of Palaiologan Imperial Orations', in M. Grünbart (ed.), *Theatron. Rhetorische Kultur in Spätantike und Mittelalter*. Berlin: De Gruyter, 429–48.

Toulouse, S. 2016. 'Synésios de Cyrène', in R. Goulet (ed.), *Dictionnaire des philosophes antiques*, vol. 6. Paris: CNRS Éditions, 639–76.

Touwaide, A. 1999. 'Lexica medico-botanica byzantina. Prolégomènes à une etude', in L. Pérez Castro, F. Adrados, and L. de Cuenca (eds.), *Τῆς φιλίης τάδε δῶρα – Miscelánea léxica en memoria de Conchita Serrano*. Madrid: Consejo Superior de Investigaciones Científicas, 211–28.

Touwaide, A. 2000. 'On Uroscopy in Byzantium', in A. Diamandopoulos (ed.), *Ιστορία της Ελληνικής Νεφρολογίας*. Athens: Papazēsēs, 218–20.

Touwaide, A. 2002a. 'Arabic Medicine in Greek Translation: A Preliminary Report', *Journal of the International Society for the History of Islamic Medicine* 1: 45–53.

Touwaide, A. 2002b. 'Pseudo-Galen's *De urinis*: A Multifactorial Technique of Diagnosis and a Cultural Interpretation of Color', *American Journal of Nephrology* 22: 130–5.

Touwaide, A. 2003. 'Greek and Arabic Manuscripts of Dioscorides' *De materia medica*', in A. Touwaide, N. G. de Santo, G. Bellinghieri, and V. Savica (eds.), *Healing kidney diseases in antiquity*. Cosenza: Bios, 27–39.

Touwaide, A. 2004. 'Arabic Urology in Byzantium', *Journal of Nephrology* 17: 583–9.

Touwaide, A. 2007. 'Byzantine Hospital Manuals (*Iatrosophia*) as a Source for the Study of Therapeutics', in B. S. Bowers (ed.), *The Medieval Hospital and Medical Practice*. Farnham: Ashgate, 147–75.

Touwaide, A. 2008a. 'The Jujube Tree in the Eastern Mediterranean: A Case Study in the Methodology of Textual Archeobotany', in P. Dandle and A. Touwaide (eds.), *Health and Healing from the Medieval Garden*. Rochester NY: Boydell: 72–100.

Touwaide, A. 2008b. 'Medicina bizantina e araba alla corte di Palermo', in N. G. de Santo and G. Bellinghieri (eds.), *Medicina, scienza e politica al tempo di Federico II*. Naples: Istituto Italiano per gli Studi Filosofici, 39–55.

Touwaide, A. 2010. 'Transfer of Knowledge and Translation', in A. Classen (ed.), *Handbook of Medieval Studies: Terms, Methods, Trends*. Berlin: De Gruyter, 1368–99.

Touwaide, A. 2011. 'Arabic into Greek: The Rise of an International Lexicon of Medicine in the Medieval Eastern Mediterranean?', in J. Fumo, C. Fraenkel, F. Wallis, and R. Wisnovsky (eds.), *Vehicles of Transmission, Translation and Transformation in Medieval Textual Culture*. Turnhout: Brepols, 196–222.

Touwaide, A. 2013. 'Translation. A Case Study in Byzantine Science', *Medievalia* 165–70.

Touwaide, A. 2016a. 'Agents and Agencies? The Many Facets of Translation in Byzantine Medicine', in F. Wallis and R. Wisnovsky (eds.), *Medieval Textual Cultures: Agents of Transmission, Translation and Transformation*. Berlin: De Gruyter, 13–38.

Touwaide, A. 2016b. *A Census of Greek Medical Manuscripts: From Byzantium to the Renaissance*. Abingdon: Routledge.

Treadgold, W. T. (ed.). 1984. *Renaissances Before the Renaissance: Cultural Revivals of Late Antiquity and the Middle Ages*. Stanford CA: Stanford University Press.

Treu, M. 1899b. 'Der Philosoph Joseph', *Byzantinische Zeitschrift* 8: 1–64.

Tselikas, A. 1995. '*Τὰ Ἑλληνικὰ Γιατροσόφια: Μιὰ Περιφρονημένη Κατηγορία Χειρογράφων*', in T. Diamantopoulos (ed.), *Ἰατρικὰ Βυζαντινὰ Χειρόγραφα*. Athens: Ekdoseis Domos, 57–69.

Turyn, A. 1928. 'De Homeri et Ioannis Actuarii codicibus Varsoviensibus', *Studia Byzantina-EOS* 31: 505–11.

Turyn, A. 1972. *Dated Greek Manuscripts of the Thirteenth and Fourteenth Centuries in the Libraries of Italy*. 2 vols. Urbana: University of Illinois Press.

Ullmann, M. 1978. *Krankenjournale* (Rufus of Ephesus). Weisbaden: Harassowitz.

Valiakos, E. (with M. Marselos, N. Sakellaridis, Th. Constantinidis, and H. Skaltsa). 2015a. 'Ethnopharmacological Approach to the Herbal Medicine of the "Antidotes" in Nikolaos Myrepsos' Dynameron', *Journal of Ethnopharmacology* 163: 68–82.

Valiakos, E. 2015b. '*Το Δυναμερὸν του Νικολάου Μυρεψού*', *Βυζαντιακά* 32: 241–55.

Varella, E. 1995. 'Orientalische Elemente in der byzantinischen Heilkunde', *Medicina nei Secoli* 7: 29–40.

Vassis, I. 2005. *Initia Carminum Byzantinorum*. Berlin: De Gruyter.

Veen, M. van der and J. Morales. 2015. 'The Roman and Islamic Spice Trade: New Archaeological Evidence', *Journal of Ethnopharmacology* 167: 54–63.

Veit, R. 2015. 'Isaac Israeli: His Treatise on Urine (*De Urinis*) and Its Reception in the Latin World', in K. Collins, S. Kottek, and H. Paavilainen (eds.), *Isaac Israeli: The Philosopher Physician*. Jerusalem: Muriel and Philip Berman Medical Library, 77–114.

Verbeke, G. 1945. *L'évolution de la doctrine du Pneuma du stoicisme à S. Augustin*. Paris and Louvain: D. de Brouwer and Institut Supérieur de Philosophie.
Vieillard, C. 1903. *L'urologie et les médecins urologues dans la médecine ancienne: Gilles de Corbeil: sa vie, ses oeuvres, son poème des urines*. Paris: F. R. de Rudeval.
Visi, T. 2015. 'Tradition and Innovation: Isaac Israeli's Classification of the Colors of Urines', in K. Collins, S. Kottek, and H. Paavilainen (eds.), *Isaac Israeli: The Philosopher Physician*. Jerusalem: Muriel and Philip Berman Medical Library, 39–66.
Vogel, K. 1967. 'Byzantine Science', in J. M. Hussey (ed.), *The Cambridge Medieval History*, vol. 4: *The Byzantine Empire, Part II: Government, Church and Civilisation*. Cambridge: Cambridge University Press, 264–305.
Vogt, S. 2008. 'Drugs and Pharmacology', in R. J. Hankinson (ed.), *The Cambridge Companion to Galen*. Cambridge: Cambridge University Press, 304–22.
Volk, R. 1983. *Gesundheitswesen und Wohltätigkeit im Spiegel der byzantinischen Klostertypika*. Munich: Institut für Byzantinistik und Neugriechische Philologie der Universität.
Volk, R. 1990. *Der medizinische Inhalt der Schriften des Michael Psellos*. Munich: Institut für Byzantinistik und neugriechische Philologie der Universität.
Vries-van der Velden, E. de. 1987. *Théodore Métochite: une réévaluation*. Amsterdam: Gieben.
Wallis, F. 2000a. 'Inventing Diagnosis: Theophilus' *De urinis* in the Classroom', *Dynamis* 20: 31–73.
Wallis, F. 2000b. 'Signs and Senses: Diagnosis and Prognosis in Early Medieval Pulse and Urine Texts', *Social History of Medicine* 13: 265–78.
Wallis, F. 2005a. 'Gilles de Corbeil', in T. F. Glick, S. J. Livesey, and F. Wallis (eds.), *Medieval Science, Technology, and Medicine: An Encyclopedia*. London: Routledge, 198–9.
Wallis, F. 2005b. 'Maurus of Salerno', in in T. F. Glick, S. J. Livesey, and F. Wallis (eds.), *Medieval Science, Technology, and Medicine: An Encyclopedia*. London: Routledge, 334–5.
Ware, K. 1979. *The Orthodox Way*. London: Mowbray.
Warmington, E. H. 1974. *The Commerce Between the Roman Empire and India*. London: Curzon Press.
Watson, A. M. 1983. *Agricultural Innovation in the Early Islamic World*. Cambridge: Cambridge University Press.
Webster, C. 2016. 'Voice Pathologies and the 'Hippocratic Triangle'', in G. Petridou and C. Thumiger (eds), *Approaches to the Patient in the Ancient World*. Leiden: Brill, 166–99.
Wee, J. Z. 2016. 'Case History as Minority Report in the Hippocratic *Epidemics* 1', in G. Petridou and C. Thumiger (eds.), *Approaches to the Patient in the Ancient World*. Leiden: Brill, 138–65.
Wellmann, M. 1895. *Die pneumatische Schule bis auf Archigenes in ihrer Entwickelung*. Berlin: Weidmannsche Buchhandlung.
Wershub, P. 1970. *Urology: From Antiquity to the 20th Century*. St Louis: W. H. Green.
Whitmarsh, T. 2005. *The Second Sophistic*. Oxford: Oxford University Press.

Wilcox, J. 1985. *The Tranmission and Influence of Qusṭā ibn Lūqā's 'On the Difference between Spirit and Soul'*. The City University of New York: PhD thesis.
Wilcox, J. 1987. 'Our Continuing Discovery of the Greek Science of the Arabs: The Examples of Qusṭā ibn Lūqā', *Annals of Scholarship* 4: 57–74.
Wilkins, J. 2002. 'The Contribution of Galen, *De Subtiliante Diaeta* (*On the Thinning Diet*)', *Bulletin of the Institute of Classical Studies. Supplement* 77: 47–55.
Wilkins, J. 2003. 'Foreword', in O. Powell, *Galen: On the Properties of Foodstuffs*. Cambridge: Cambridge University Press, xi–xxi.
Wilkins, J. 2016. 'Treatment of the Man: Galen's Preventive Medicine in the *De Sanitate Tuenda*', in G. Petridou and C. Thumiger (eds), *Approaches to the Patient in the Ancient World*. Leiden: Brill, 413–31.
Willich [Wilichii], J. 1670. 'Urinarum probationes, illustratae scholis medicis, Hieronymi Reusneri Leorini', in *Actuarii Johannis Zachariae filii, Graeciae medici principis, De urinis libri VII. Accedunt huic editioni aliorum medicorum dissertationes de Urinis, Quorum nomina versa pagina indicat.* Utrecht: Ex Officina Gisberti à Zyll.
Wilson, L. 1959. 'Erasistratus, Galen, and the *Pneuma*', *Bulletin of the History of Medicine* 33: 293–314.
Wilson, N. 1996. *Scholars of Byzantium*. [rev. edn.] London: Duckworth.
Xenophontos, S. 2014. 'Psychotherapy and moralising rhetoric in Galen's newly discovered *Avoiding distress* (*Peri alypias*)', *Medical History* 58: 585–603.
Xenophontos, S. 2016. *Ethical Education in Plutarch: Moralising Agents and Contexts*. Berlin: De Gruyter.
Xenophontos, S. 2018. 'The Byzantine Plutarch: Self-identity and Model in Theodore Metochites' Essay 71 of the *Semeioseis Gnomikai*', in P. Mack and J. North (eds.), *The Afterlife of Plutarch. Bulletin of the Institute of Classical Studies Supplement* 137 London: Institute of Classical Studies, 23–39.
Zambon, M. 2005. 'Il significato filosofico della dottrina dell' ὄχημα dell'anima', in R. Chiaradonna (ed.), *Studi sull'anima in Plotino*. Naples: Bibliopolis, 307–35.
Zervan, V. (in collaboration with J. Kramer, C. Römer, M. Metzeltin, B. Pavlović, and A. M. Cuomo). 2019. *Die Lehnwörter im Wortschatz der spätbyzantinischen historiographischen Literatur*. Berlin: De Gruyter.
Zglinicki, F. 1982. *Die Uroskopie in der bildenden Kunst: eine kunst- und medizinhistorische Untersuchung über die Harnschau*. Darmstadt: Enrst Giebeler.
Zipser, B. 2003/4. 'Griechische Schrift, arabische Sprache und graeco-arabische Medizin: ein neues Fragment aus dem mittelalterlichen Sizilien', *Mediterranean Language Review* 15: 154–66.
Zipser, B. 2017. 'Revisions of Theophanes Chrysobalantes *De Curatione*', *Wellcome Open Research* 2:17, available at https://wellcomeopenresearch.org/articles/2-17/v2#article-reports (accessed 2 March 2018).
Zipser, B. 2018. 'Substitutes in John Archiatros's *Therapeutics*', in B. Pitarakis and G. Tanman (eds.), *Life Is Short, Art Long: The Art of Healing in Byzantium. New Perspectives*. Istanbul: Istanbul Research Institute, 187–98.
Zipser, B. 2019. 'Galen in Byzantine *iatrosophia*', in P. Bouras-Vallianatos and B. Zipser (eds.), *Brill's Companion to the Reception of Galen*. Leiden: Brill, 111–23.
Zytka, M. 2019. *A Cultural History of Bathing in Late Antiquity and Early Byzantium*. Abingdon: Routledge.

Index Rerum et Nominum

Index Locorum

Index Codicum Manu Scriptorum